T0329347

Antimicrobial Resistance in Agriculture

Antimicrobial Resistance in Agriculture

Perspective, Policy and Mitigation

Indranil Samanta
Department of Veterinary Microbiology
West Bengal University of Animal and Fishery Sciences
Kolkata, India

Samiran Bandyopadhyay
ICAR-Indian Veterinary Research Institute-Eastern Regional Station
Kolkata, India

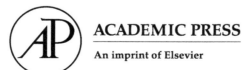

ACADEMIC PRESS

An imprint of Elsevier

Academic Press is an imprint of Elsevier
125 London Wall, London EC2Y 5AS, United Kingdom
525 B Street, Suite 1650, San Diego, CA 92101, United States
50 Hampshire Street, 5th Floor, Cambridge, MA 02139, United States
The Boulevard, Langford Lane, Kidlington, Oxford OX5 1GB, United Kingdom

Notices

Knowledge and best practice in this field are constantly changing. As new research and experience broaden our understanding, changes in research methods, professional practices, or medical treatment may become necessary.

Practitioners and researchers must always rely on their own experience and knowledge in evaluating and using any information, methods, compounds, or experiments described herein. In using such information or methods they should be mindful of their own safety and the safety of others, including parties for whom they have a professional responsibility.

To the fullest extent of the law, neither the Publisher nor the authors, contributors, or editors, assume any liability for any injury and/or damage to persons or property as a matter of products liability, negligence or otherwise, or from any use or operation of any methods, products, instructions, or ideas contained in the material herein.

Library of Congress Cataloging-in-Publication Data
A catalog record for this book is available from the Library of Congress

British Library Cataloguing-in-Publication Data
A catalogue record for this book is available from the British Library

ISBN: 978-0-12-815770-1

For information on all Academic Press publications visit
our website at https://www.elsevier.com/books-and-journals

Publisher: Charlotte Cockle
Acquisition Editor: Patricia Osborn
Editorial Project Manager: Susan Ikeda
Production Project Manager: Swapna Srinivasan
Cover Designer: Miles Hitchen

Typeset by TNQ Technologies

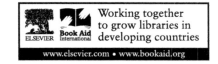

Contents

Foreword

The global community has been articulating serious concerns on the impact of antimicrobial resistance (AMR) on human development. AMR is considered as the most important challenge to human efforts in controlling communicable diseases. In an unprecedented way, the United Nations General Assembly has taken a serious note of burgeoning challenge of AMR and called upon all countries to initiate concerted actions to contain emergence and spread of AMR.

Recent report projects AMR causing 10 million deaths annually and wiping off a massive cumulative US$ 100 trillion from economy by 2050 as consequence of inaction to contain AMR. This report also estimates that mortality due to AMR shall exceed those due to cancers and road accidents put together. Moreover, most of these deaths will be in developing countries creating greater impact on health and economy. Data from the World Bank reveal that global exports will see a decrease of up to 3.5%, livestock production will diminish by 7.5% and additional health care—related costs will be staggering US$ 1 trillion by 2050.

Inextricable co-existence of human beings with animals, plants and environment since time immemorial has been both beneficial and malefic to human kind. Animals and plants sustain human life and are essential for food security for the growing human population. An ever-increasing and an unstoppable number of human infectious diseases arise from animals. A large part (60%) of all human infectious disease are transmitted from animals, 75% of all emerging infectious diseases originate from animals. Several pandemics in current millennium including severe acute respiratory syndrome, middle-east respiratory syndrome, influenza H5N1, influenza H1N1 and influenza H7N9 have animals as their sources. Around 1.67 million viruses are estimated to be enzootic with up to 50% of these having the potential to invade humans under conducive environment including deforestation and damage to local ecosystem.

The close and continuous contacts between humans and animals make the latter as a critical reservoir of infectious diseases to humans. One of the major drivers of AMR — perceived as the biggest challenge in global efforts to control communicable diseases — is the humongous irrational use of antimicrobial agents in the animal health sector, especially the use of antimicrobial agents for growth promotion of the animals.

The transmission of resistant pathogens and genes from animals to humans is a complex process influenced by several factors. The dynamics at human—animal interface require better understanding to facilitate institution of efficient control measures. It also requires close collaboration between human health, animal health and environment sectors in true spirit of One Health.

One Health is a validated, integrated and holistic approach that is being advocated by the World Health Organization (WHO), the Food and Agriculture Organization of the United Nations (FAO) and the World Organization for Animal Health (OIE) for combating health threats to humans and animals through human—animal—plant—environment interface. One Health concept warrants multisectoral, multidisciplinary, multiinstitutional and multilocation coordination, communication and collaboration to attain optimal health for people, domestic animals, wildlife, plants and environment. This makes it a complex philosophy with inherent barriers in successful implementation at the country level where silo and sector-specific approaches have been in vogue and well established.

It is heartening to note that this book aims to provide evidence-based information on various aspects of AMR in agriculture and their perceived impact on human health. The valuable information provided in this document may be utilized by policymakers and various groups of experts including academic and research personals engaged in zoonotic infection, veterinary microbiologists, veterinary medicine, medical microbiology and industrial microbiology, along with all veterinary and medical practitioners.

The book provides updated information encompassing all the genera of livestock and fish-originated pathogenic bacteria associated with AMR.

I am sure that the contents of this book shall be immensely helpful for not only academicians but also for progressive practitioners who wish to provide better care and management, and in the process, contributing to containment of AMR.

Dr Rajesh Bhatia
Former Director Communicable Diseases.
WHO Regional Office for South East Asia Region and
Former Regional Technical Adviser, AMR.
FAO Regional Office for Asia-Pacific.
New Delhi.

Preface

Antimicrobials have served as the most potent therapeutic agent for the last two to three decades saving the human and animal life. It is because of antibiotics we could have reduced the catastrophic effects of two World Wars that changed the human civilization in a significant way. Unfortunately, the infectious diseases are again returning back more intensely and threatening the human civilization as we failed to preserve the efficacy of antimicrobials. The United Nations has given the issue a parallel status to AIDS/tuberculosis to be discussed in the 71st UN General Assembly in New York in 2016. Antimicrobial resistance (AMR) is truly a 'One Health mega-concern' because it has three functional domains such as animals, human and environment. The resistance genes generated in the commensal or pathogens in animals or human can be transferred between them during the exchange of microbial pool. The resistant bugs become untreatable, as antimicrobials used in animals or human are mostly the same molecule and thus the resistance generated in one can affect the others. Tackling the resistance issue with One Health approach thus increases the therapeutic life span of the antibiotics. The World Health Organization (WHO) in collaboration with the Food and Agricultural Organization (FAO) and the World Organization for Animal Health (OIE) developed several joint strategies to combat the problem. Excess antibiotics are released in the environment through different excretory systems of the animals and human. Other than livestock and poultry manure, antibiotic residues from the pharmaceutical industry, human hospitals and agricultural fields are also the major sources of environmental contamination. The accumulated antibiotics contribute to the resistance gene pool present in the environmental bacteria. Thus the AMR is also considered as an ecological problem. The pollution with antibiotics is more pronounced in low- and middle-income countries because of lack of rigorous enforcement of the environmental protection laws. Furthermore, with the rising concern of AMR, global gross domestic product is anticipated to fall by 3.5%, causing around 28 million people to be slipped under poverty.

The authors felt a need for a comprehensive book to cover all the pertinent issues such as emergence of AMR in livestock, poultry, fishery, agriculture and the environment, as well as the approaches to tackle the issue. The book encompasses the biological properties, genome, antigenic characteristics, toxins and virulence factors, transmission, diagnosis and mechanism of AMR in all the bacterial genera associated with livestock, poultry and fishery. In the other part of the book, the authors narrated mechanism of cross-resistance with biocides, approaches, techniques and pitfalls of antimicrobial stewardship, alternative antiinfective therapy such as bacteriophage therapy, use of enzybiotics, phytobiotics, essential oils, nanomaterials, cellular immunotherapy, immunomodulators and vaccines. Moreover, how to tackle the problem with One Health approach and what are the challenges ahead to successfully combat AMR are incorporated.

We hope the book will cater the need by providing the basic and updated knowledge in AMR domain to the scientists/researchers, students, policymakers and all those common people who like to save our mother earth from the most devastating calamity. Any suggestions from any corner for the betterment of the book will be generously accepted.

Indranil Samanta
Samiran Bandyopadhyay
Kolkata
27 May 2019

Chapter 1

History of antimicrobial resistance

Definition

- **Antimicrobial:** Any substance of natural, semisynthetic or synthetic origin that kills or inhibits the growth of a microorganism but causes little or no damage to the host. It is a broader term and it can be classified into several groups according to the type of microbes on which it acts such as antibiotics (bacteria), antivirals (virus), antifungals (mould and yeast) and antiparasitic (malaria agent). On the basis of mode of action, antimicrobials are either microbicidal (lysis of microbes) or microbistatic (growth inhibition).
- **Antibiotic:** Low molecular weight substance produced by a microbe that at little concentrations inhibits or kills other bacteria.

History of chemotherapy

First evidence of chemotherapy was noticed in 1899 when Emmerich and Löw prepared extract from *Pseudomonas aeruginosa* (pyocyanase). The extract was found active against pathogenic bacteria although was toxic to the human cells. During the prechemotherapy (preantibiotic) era, case fatality rate of *Staphylococcus-* or *Streptococcus*-associated pneumonia, endocarditis and bacteraemia was 40%—97% (Newman et al., 1954). In First World War (1914—18), 70% of wound infections were treated with amputation as no antibiotic was available (Hirsch, 2008).

Paul Ehrlich (1854—1915, Germany) during his work with dyes noticed that specific aniline dyes can kill a specific group of microbes, not the others. Based on the idea of specificity, Ehrlich began his quest for "magic bullet" during 1904 to treat syphilis (sexually transmitted disease caused by *Treponema pallidum*). In Europe and United States, the syphilis was treated with mercury and arsenical compounds which had acute toxicity and poor efficacy. Paul Ehrlich and Alfred Bertheim identified the chemical structure of atoxyl, a less toxic arsenical drug used to treat African sleeping sickness. They started to synthesize numerous derivatives of atoxyl and the arsphenamine derivative (compound 606, Salvarsan) was found effective against syphilis in experimental rabbits, followed by limited human trials (Ehrlich and Halta, 1910). The era of chemotherapy thus began and Ehrlich was awarded with Nobel Prize in 1908 along with Metchnikoff. With the discovery of more antimicrobials (Table 1.1) and their introduction into the clinical practices such as sulphonamides (1935), penicillin (1941), streptomycin (1943), para-aminosalicylic acid (1944) and isoniazid (1952), the annual mortality rate due to infectious diseases decreased rapidly (Armstrong et al., 1999).

Discovery of antimicrobials/antibiotics and individual scientific contributions

William Roberts (1874) observed that *Penicillium glaucum* (a mould) can inhibit the growth of bacteria. John Tyndall also noted similar observations 2 years later (Roberts, 1874). Alexander Fleming (1881—1955, United Kingdom) discovered the first antibiotic "penicillin" in 1928. He observed that growth of *Staphylococcus aureus* was inhibited by a contaminant

TABLE 1.1 Discovery of major antimicrobials.

Antimicrobial	Scientist	Year
Streptomycin	Selman Abraham Waksman and Albert Schatz	1943
Tetracycline	Benjamin Minge Duggar, Yellapragada Subbarow (Lederle Laboratory Division of American Cyanamid Company)	1945
Chloramphenicol	David Gottlieb	1947
Erythromycin (Macrolide)	J. M. McGuire at Eli Lilly Company	1949
Pikromycin (Macrolide)	Brockmann and Henkel	1950
Colistin	Y. Koyama (Japan)	1950
Cycloserine	Kurosawa	1952
Vancomycin	Edmund Kornfeld at Eli Lilly Company	1953
Streptogramin	J. Charney	1953
Rifamycin	Piero Sensi, Maria Teresa Timbal, Pinhas Margalith (Milan, Italy)	1957
Quinolone	George Y. Lesher and team of Sterling–Winthrop Research Institute, New York	1962
Lincosamide	Upjohn	1963
Daptomycin	Researchers at Eli Lilly and Company	1980

blue mould (*Penicillium*) in culture dishes. The observation was converted to the concept that certain microbes produce diffusible substances that can inhibit the growth of other microorganisms. Fleming faced difficulties in purification of the "substance" extracted from the mould and the substance was unstable. After a decade, the Oxford team led by Howard Florey and Ernest Chain purified the substance (Chain et al., 1940). Penicillin was introduced into the clinical practice during 1940 and as a wonder drug it saved several lives during Second World War. Fleming, Chain and Florey were awarded with the Nobel Prize in 1945. Identification of core structure (6-aminopenicillanic acid) paved the way for development of numerous derivatives such as penicillinase-resistant penicillins (methicillin, oxacillin, nafcillin), aminopenicillins (ampicillin, amoxicillin, bacampicillin), carboxypenicillins (carbenicillin, ticarcillin) and ureidopenicillins (mezlocillin, azlocillin, piperacillin) (Wright, 1999).

Josef Klarer and Fritz Mietzsch (chemists of Bayer AG, Germany) first synthesized sulphonamide chrysoidine (KI-730, Prontosil), which was tested by Gerhard Domagk for antibacterial activity in animal models (Domagk, 1935). Prontosil was later confirmed as prodrug and its active component sulphanilamide was found to possess antibacterial activity, especially against streptococci. The sulphanilamide compounds were previously used in dye industry and the patent was already expired. Owing to off-patent nature and low production cost, numerous derivatives of sulphanilamide were developed by different companies. Introduction of sulpha drugs into the clinical practice reduced mortality by 2%–3% and increased life expectancy by 0.4–0.7 years (Jayachandran et al., 2010).

René Dubos (1939) first isolated tyrocidine (mixture of cyclic and linear polypeptide) having antibacterial activities (Lipmann et al., 1970). Gause and Brazhnikova (1944) extracted gramicidin S from *Brevibacillus brevis* and confirmed its antibacterial activities.

Discovery of other major antimicrobials and individual scientific contributions are described in Table 1.1.

Emergence of antibiotic-resistant bacteria historical perspective

Therapy with antibiotics fails when applied to resistant bacteria and it generates worse prognosis. The choice of antibiotic also becomes limited to treat multidrug-resistant organisms. As consequence, major medical advancements such as complex surgery, transplantation and chemotherapy are compromised (Hawkey, 2008). Annual mortality rate due to resistant bacteria is 50,000 each year across Europe and the United States alone, which will reach up to 10 million throughout the world by 2050 (O'Neill, 2014). The resistance is associated with increased resource utilization and cost because of prolonged hospital stay, use of mechanical ventilation, need for intensive care and invasive devices, excess surgery, additional isolation room and gloves, aprons, etc., need for postacute care and loss of man day (Friedman et al., 2016).

Few bacteria are intrinsically resistant to certain groups of antibiotics (e.g., *Pseudomonas*), whereas others develop resistance during therapy or contact with an antibiotic. The resistance gene can be transmitted through mobile genetic elements such as plasmids, integrons, etc., to other susceptible group of bacteria present in the gut or the environment. Transfer of resistant bacteria to human is a complex and multifactorial issue consisting of foods, water and probably all of the environmental components (Prescott, 2014). Details of resistance mechanism against different antibiotics generated in major bacterial species associated with livestock, poultry, fishery and environment are described in the following chapters. The resistance to antimicrobials is although an evolutionary conserved natural process and is not a "new" entity. Existence of natural product antibiotics was detected during 2 billion−40 million years ago, which indicates the similar "ancient" existence of the antibiotic resistance (Hall and Barlow, 2004). The metagenomic analysis of ancient DNA from Beringian permafrost sediments revealed the presence of antibiotic resistance genes against β-lactam, tetracycline and glycopeptides (D'Costa et al., 2011).

Emergence of penicillin-resistant *Staphylococcus* began in human patients during mid-1940s after the introduction of penicillin (Kirby, 1944). The penicillinase was detected although even before the clinical uses of penicillin (Bolhofer et al., 1960). Penicillin-resistant *Staphylococcus* became pandemic during 1950−60 with the spread of a specific *Staphylococcus* clone (phage-type 80/81) (Blair and Carr, 1960). It was followed by the generation of resistance to tetracycline and macrolides in 1950s. Introduction of methicillin (penicillinase-resistant) although cleared the phage type 80/81 from the

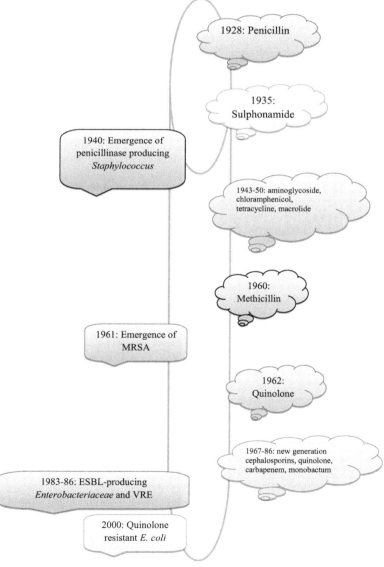

FIGURE 1.1 History of antibiotic discovery and associated development of antibiotic resistance.

population, methicillin-resistant *S. aureus* (MRSA) appeared in 1961 (Barber, 1961). The earliest MRSA strain (COL) was reported from three human patients in Colindale, United Kingdom (Jevons, 1961). Penicillin-resistant *Streptococcus pneumoniae* strains appeared in the community during late 1970s. Fig. 1.1 describes history of major antibiotic discovery and associated development of resistance.

One of the first reports of antibiotic resistance in livestock was detected in coliform bacteria in turkeys experimentally fed with streptomycin (Starr and Reynolds, 1951). Subsequent studies detected correlation between dietary intake of tetracycline and the generation of antibiotic-resistant streptococci in chicken (Barnes, 1958; Elliott and Barnes, 1959). First report of MRSA infection in animals was obtained from Belgium, which was associated with clinical mastitis in dairy cattle (Devriese et al., 1972).

The first recommendation to prohibit the subtherapeutic use of antibiotics in poultry was discussed in British Parliament during 1969, known as "Swann Report" (Britain and Swann, 1969). In the United States, the debate to ban the subtherapeutic usage of antibiotics in livestock and poultry began with the Council for Agricultural Science and Technology report (1981). World Health Organization (2000) recommended phase out prohibition of those antibiotics as growth promoters, which are also used in human therapy. Sweden (1986) and Denmark (avoparcin, 1995) are the first countries to ban the subtherapeutic use of antibiotics in livestock and poultry. In 1997, European Union (EU) banned the use of avoparcin as growth promoter in all the member countries. In 1999, EU banned certain antibiotics in livestock and poultry, which are commonly used in human such as tylosin, spiramycin, bacitracin and virginiamycin.

References

Armstrong, G.L., Conn, L.A., Pinner, R.W., 1999. Trends in infectious disease mortality in the United States during the 20th century. Journal of the American Medical Association 281 (1), 61−66.

Barber, M., 1961. Methicillin-resistant staphylococci. Journal of Clinical Pathology 14 (4), 385.

Barnes, E.M., 1958. The effect of antibiotic supplements on the faecal *Streptococci* (Lancefield group D) of poultry. British Veterinary Journal 114, 333−344.

Blair, J.E., Carr, M., 1960. Distribution of phage groups of *Staphylococcus aureus* in the years 1927 through 1947. Science 132 (3435), 1247−1248.

Bolhofer, W.A., Sheehan, J.C., Abrams, E.L., 1960. Totally synthetic penicillins. Journal of the American Chemical Society 82 (13), 3437−3441.

Britain, G., Swann, S.M.M., 1969. Report of the joint committee on the use of antibiotics in animal husbandry and veterinary medicine. HM Stationery Office.

Chain, E., Florey, H.W., Gardner, A.D., Heatley, N.G., Jennings, M.A., Orr-Ewing, J., Sanders, A.G., 1940. Penicillin as a chemotherapeutic agent. The Lancet 236 (6104), 226−228.

Council for Agricultural Science and Technology, 1981. Antibiotics in Animal Feeds. CAST, Ames, IA. Report 88.

D'Costa, V.M., King, C.E., Kalan, L., Morar, M., Sung, W.W., Schwarz, C., Froese, D., Zazula, G., Calmels, F., Debruyne, R., Golding, G.B., 2011. Antibiotic resistance is ancient. Nature 477 (7365), 457.

Devriese, L.A., Damme, L.V., Fameree, L., 1972. Methicillin (Cloxacillin)-resistant *Staphylococcus aureus* strains isolated from bovine mastitis cases. Zoonoses and Public Health 19 (7), 598−605.

Domagk, G., 1935. Ein beitrag zur chemotherapie der bakteriellen infektionen. DMW-Deutsche Medizinische Wochenschrift 61 (07), 250−253.

Ehrlich, P., Halta, S., 1910. Die Experimentelle Chemotherapie der Spirillosen, vol. 8. Julius Springer, Berlin.

Elliott, S.D., Barnes, E.M., 1959. Changes in serological type and antibiotic resistance of Lancefield group D *Streptococci* in chickens receiving dietary chlortetracycline. Microbiology 20 (2), 426−433.

Emmerich, R., Löw, O., 1899. Bakteriolytische Enzyme als Ursache der erworbenen Immunität und die Heilung von Infectionskrankheiten durch dieselben. Medical Microbiology and Immunology 31 (1), 1−65.

Friedman, N.D., Temkin, E., Carmeli, Y., 2016. The negative impact of antibiotic resistance. Clinical Microbiology and Infection 22 (5), 416−422.

Gause, G.F., Brazhnikova, M.G., 1944. Gramicidin S and its use in the treatment of infected wounds. Nature 154 (3918), 703.

Hall, B.G., Barlow, M., 2004. Evolution of the serine β-lactamases: past, present and future. Drug Resistance Updates 7 (2), 111−123.

Hawkey, P.M., 2008. The growing burden of antimicrobial resistance. Journal of Antimicrobial Chemotherapy 62 (Suppl. 1), i1−i9.

Hirsch, E.F., 2008. "The treatment of infected wounds," Alexis Carrel's contribution to the care of wounded soldiers during World War I. Journal of Trauma and Acute Care Surgery 64 (3), S209−S210.

Jayachandran, S., Lleras-Muney, A., Smith, K.V., 2010. Modern medicine and the twentieth century decline in mortality: evidence on the impact of sulfa drugs. American Economic Journal: Applied Economics 2 (2), 118−146.

Jevons, M.P., 1961. "Celbenin-resistant" staphylococci. The British Medical Journal 1, 124−125.

Kirby, W.M., 1944. Extraction of a highly potent penicillin inactivator from penicillin resistant staphylococci. Science 99 (2579), 452−453.

Lipmann, F., Roskoski, R., Gevers, W., Kleinkauf, H., 1970. Tyrocidine biosynthesis by three complementary fractions from *Bacillus brevis* (ATCC 8185). Biochemistry 9 (25), 4839−4845.

Newman, W., Torres, J.M., Guck, J.K., 1954. Bacterial endocarditis: an analysis of fifty-two cases. The American Journal of Medicine 16 (4), 535−542.

O'Neill, J., 2014. The Review on Antimicrobial Resistance. Available at: https://amr-review.org/sites/default/files/AMR%20Review%20Paper%20-%20Tackling%20a%20crisis%20for%20the%20health%20and%20wealth%20of%20nations_1.pdf.

Prescott, J.F., 2014. The resistance tsunami, antimicrobial stewardship, and the golden age of microbiology. Veterinary Microbiology 171 (3–4), 273–278.

Roberts, W., 1874. Studies on biogenesis. Philosophical Transactions of the Royal Society of London 164, 457–477.

Starr, M.P., Reynolds, D.M., 1951. Streptomycin resistance of coliform bacteria from turkeys fed streptomycin. American Journal of Public Health and the Nations Health 41 (11_Pt_1), 1375–1380.

World Health Organization, 2000. Available at: http://whqlibdoc.who.int/hq/2000/WHO_CDS_CSR_APH_2000.4.pdf.

Wright, A.J., 1999. The penicillins. In: Mayo Clinic Proceedings, vol. 74. Elsevier, pp. 290–307. No. 3.

Chapter 2

Use of antimicrobials and antibiotics in livestock, poultry, fishery and agriculture

Chapter outline

Use of antibiotics in animals and aquaculture — purpose and objective

There is no denying that livestock sector across the globe has witnessed a stupendous growth with a gradual but steady shift towards intensive farming practices, in recent years, only to meet the ever-increasing demand for animal protein for the growing world population. Increasing animal density, overcrowding, rapid urbanization, and deforestation, shrinkage of arable or grazing land — all are crucial to bringing a drastic and often irreversible change in the ecosystem, thereby rising infections and health problems in animals. As a consequence, the use of antibiotics has also been increased as the food animals in such environment demand aggressive health management that their production performance is maintained and preserved (Guardabassi, 2013; Magouras et al., 2017). Nevertheless, little information is available regarding the quality and quantity of antibiotic prescribed in animal sector, particularly in the developing and underdeveloped countries and that constitutes the major barrier for successful implementation of the antibiotic stewardship programme. In many countries, the surveillance system to monitor the antibiotic consumption, particularly in agriculture and animal sector, is not strong enough or nonfunctional. Even in many developed countries, such monitoring system started to function in full strength very recently. Thus, inadequacy of reliable data and the paucity of information are the major deterrent to provide an illustration of antimicrobials use (AMU) and in agriculture, animals and aquaculture sector.

Broadly, antibiotics are used in livestock or food animals for three purposes (Magouras et al., 2017; Van Boeckel et al., 2015; Landers et al., 2012):

(1) Therapeutic or curative treatment: This is conducted for the treatment of sick/diseased animals, to be particular, of animals exhibiting obvious clinical symptoms.

(2) Control treatment or metaphylaxis: Usually after the occurrence of disease/infection in a part of a group/herd or flock, this treatment protocol is followed with an objective to reduce the spread of infection to other animals at risk and also to reduce morbidity in animals already incubating the disease (Done et al., 2015; Checkley et al., 2010; Baptiste and Kyvsgaard, 2017).

(3) Prophylactic or preventive treatment: This is followed in an animal or a group of animals, before onset or indication of any clinical sign of infectious disease to prevent such occurrence (Checkley et al., 2010; Baptiste and Kyvsgaard, 2017).

(4) Nutritional treatment: In intensive livestock farming, it is not unusual to use antibiotic or antimicrobial agents as a growth promoter when antibiotics are used in subtherapeutic concentration. It is believed to improve feed conversion ratio by affecting the gut flora (Lee et al., 2012; Dibner and Richards, 2005).

Roughly, there are three avenues of antimicrobial uses in animals without any identifiable infectious illness. Landers et al., 2012, illustrated such nontherapeutic use of antibiotics using the data available for AMU in food animals in the United States (Landers et al., 2012). While 16% of the lactating dairy cattle in the United States were reported to receive antibiotics for clinical mastitis, the intramammary antimicrobial infusion was advocated for almost all dairy cattle as a prophylactic measure in the form of penicillin or other β-lactam drugs. In a similar way, about 10% of the beef feedlot cattle received antibiotic despite being healthy to prevent respiratory illness. About 42% of beef calves were reported to be treated with macrolide — tylosin to prevent liver abscess. Tylosin and tetracyclines were common antibiotics used as feed additives in 88% of the growing pigs in the United States for preventive or growth promotion purpose. Data suggested superfluous use of antibiotics in agriculture intended for nontherapeutic consumption. In the United States, about 74% of farm-animal received antibiotics in feed and 21% in drinking water (Anonymous, 2017). More importantly, the report stated that the sale of medically important antibiotics was three times higher in the animal sector than in human beings. In China, approximately 46% of 210,000 tons of antimicrobial produced was intended for consumption in animals (Li, 2017). Preventive use of antibiotics is not only intended for animals at risk but also during the impending stress of the animals because of weaning, prolonged transportation, confinement or over congestion (Anonymous, 2013a). There is no established recommendation for such prophylactic or metaphylactic use of antibiotic and concerned farm manager or veterinarians use their own dose or duration schedule based on his own experience. Many times, such nontherapeutic use is overseen by the concerned veterinarian. Thus, region-wise variation may be noted for this kind of nontherapeutic use of antibiotics.

For production purpose, the antibiotics are given in feed or water to promote faster growth. However, there is little scientific understanding of how antibiotics increase FCR (feed conversion ratio) and promote growth. It is thought that antibiotics in subtherapeutic dose modulate the gut microbiome, body metabolism, and adiposity resulting in higher body mass (Costa et al., 2017; Hughes and Heritage, 2004). Reduction of gastrointestinal infection is believed to mask the effect of catabolic hormone leading to increased body weight. Moreover, the effect of such growth promoter being more conspicuous in sick animals than in the healthy animals had led to the presumption that such growth promotion in animals was possibly mediated by reduction of infection burden (Hughes and Heritage, 2004). With burgeoning evidence of antimicrobial resistance in food animals, however, the use of antibiotics as growth promoter has no longer been permitted by the FDA since January 2017 (Siegner, 2019). They implemented a voluntary plan for the livestock industry to phase out such use for growth promotion. European countries also took such an initiative to curb the use of antibiotics in food animals, long before. Use of antibiotics as growth promoter was first prohibited by Sweden in 1986 followed by Denmark, the United Kingdom and other countries. All these countries have their own mechanism and monitoring system to review the trend of antimicrobial resistance and use in animals.

Recent trends of antibiotic usage — global scenario

In the human sector, few studies were conducted to reflect the global picture of antibiotic usage. Global Point Prevalence Survey (Global-PPS) of Antimicrobial Consumption and Resistance was conducted in 2015 to assess the international prevalence of antimicrobial use and resistance, with an emphasis on countries with low resources, support and expertise. The study based on data from 303 hospitals in 53 countries including 8 lower-middle-income and 17 upper-middle-income countries revealed that 34.4% of the inpatients of adult wards received at least one antimicrobial. The most frequently prescribed antimicrobials include penicillins with β-lactamase inhibitors, third-generation cephalosporins and fluoroquinolones in the most part of the globe. However, in Latin America, west and central Asia, carbapenems were most frequently prescribed. The study further pointed out the inherent weakness in the antimicrobial-consumption monitoring system in lower- and middle-income countries because of unavailability of proper tools to appraise antibiotic prescribing in hospitals, even in the human sector (Versporten et al., 2018). From such an observation, we can easily assume the status of such monitoring system in the animal sector in those countries. Very recently, the global trend in antimicrobial consumption in food animals was illustrated by Boeckel and co-workers (Van Boeckel et al., 2015). The workers estimated global average annual consumption of antimicrobials per kilogram of animal produced was 45 mg/kg, 148 mg/kg, and 172 mg/kg, for cattle, chicken, and pigs, respectively. Global consumption of antibiotic was projected to rise by 67% to reach 105,596 (±3605) tons in 2030 from 63,151 (±1560) tons in 2010. Although 66% of such drastic increase was attributed to the increased number of animals for food production, about 34% was only due to the shift towards intensive farming practices, particularly in middle-income countries. Asia alone is likely to see a 46% increase in antimicrobial consumption by 2030 to reach 51,851 tons, representing 82% of the current global antimicrobial consumption in food animals. This is possibly because of increased antibiotic consumption in the poultry and piggery sector where the same is expected to grow by 129% and 124%, respectively, by 2030. In a revised estimate, the authors predicted an approximate increase of 53% in global antimicrobial consumption in food-producing animals between 2013 (131,109 tons) and 2030 (200,235 tons) (Van Boeckel et al., 2017). Only in the BRICS countries, antibiotic consumption in food animals is expected to rise by 99% by 2030. The problem is likely to be more intense in low- and middle-income countries where the demand of animal-source protein is anticipated to be higher, about 725% increase in demand for poultry consumption being projected only in South Asia (Schar et al., 2018). In all, it is no less than a wake-up call for us to take initiatives to optimize the use of antibiotics in food animals so as to preserve their efficacy.

The exact data on AMU in food animals are not available from all countries. However, the sporadic figures are quite alarming. In 2012, in the United States, the AMU in food animals (32.2 million pounds/14.6 million kg) was more than four times higher than that in human (7.25 million pounds/3.29 million kg). Of all the antimicrobials sold for use in animals, majority belonged to tetracycline (12,439,729 pounds), penicillin (1,940,424 pounds), macrolides (1,284,931 pounds), sulphur drugs (817,958 pounds), aminoglycosides (473,761 pounds), lincosamides (419,100 pounds) and cephalosporins (58,667 pounds) and other compounds such as aminocoumarins, amphenicols, diaminopyrimidines, fluoroquinolones, glycolipids, pleuromutilins, polypeptides, quinoxalines and streptogramins (in total, 3,330,237 pounds). Most of these antibiotics (94%) sold for use in food animals were intended to be delivered through feed formulation or water; only 4% of the antibiotics were sold to be used in the injectable form. More importantly, many of these antimicrobials including those which are also considered to be highly or critically important in human medicine (macrolides, streptogramins and tetracyclines) were possibly sold over the counter without any prescription or veterinary oversight. Furthermore, the FDA report reads that nearly 70% of the 25 million pounds of medically important antibiotics sold for any purpose was consumed by food-producing animals (Basri, 2017). Of this, 43% was intended for use in cattle, 37% intended for use in swine, 9% intended for use in turkeys, 6% intended for use in chickens and 4% intended for use in other species/unknown. In the United States, medically important antibiotics approved for use in both food and nonfood-producing species include ceftiofur, lincomycin, ampicillin, penicillin, polymyxin B, sulfamethazine, chlortetracycline and oxytetracycline, which constituted about 60% of the domestic sales of all antimicrobials approved for use in food-producing animals (in 2016). The highest distribution and sell was recorded for tetracycline (70%), followed by penicillins (10%), macrolides (7%), sulfonamides (4%), aminoglycosides (4%), lincosamides (2%), fluoroquinolones ($\leq$1%) and cephalosporins (<1%). Among these antibiotics, while cephalosporin was mostly intended for use in cattle (80%), lincosamide (83%) and macrolide (61%) were intended for swine. About 72% of these antibiotics were designed for use as a feed additive, 23% to be in the water and only 5% was to be used by injection, intramammary, oral and topical route. The nonmedically important drugs, which accounted for 40% of the domestic sales of all antimicrobials approved for use in food-producing animals, were mostly comprised of ionophores. Of antimicrobials belonging this group, 55% were intended for use in cattle, 30% intended for use in chickens, 8% intended for use in swine and 7% intended for use in turkeys, as the FDA report stated. In total, 13,983,016 kg of the antimicrobial active ingredient was sold and distributed for use in food animals in the United States in 2016, of which medically important antibiotics shared 8,361,740 kg and nonmedically important class shared 5,621,276 kg. Timeline analysis during past 10 years (2009−16) showed a marginal increase (9%) in sales and distribution (domestic and export) of antimicrobials approved for use in food-producing animals; nevertheless, it decreased by 10% in 2016 when compared with that in 2015. A recent report given by the Natural Resources Defense Council in 2018 indicated that nearly 27.1% of all medically important antibiotics sold in the United States are used in piggery sector despite the initiative taken by the FDA to ban the use of antibiotics as a growth promoter in January 2017 (Wallinga, 2018). This is in stark contrast to data revealed from Denmark and the Netherlands where antibiotic use in pig production has fallen by 27% and 57%, respectively, since 2009.

During 2017, total quantity of active ingredient of antibiotic sold was about 282 tonnes, of which 72% was indicated for animal consumption in the United Kingdom. Thus, the consumption in animals has recorded a decrease of 35% from 2013 (436 tonnes) as per the report published by UK-VARSS 2017 (Peter Borriello, 2017). In animals, total sale of antibiotics was about 37 mg/kg when adjusted for animal population, which is a substantial drop from what sold in 2013 (40%). Species-wise, the majority of the antibiotics sold were indicated for use in pig and poultry (52%) followed by cattle (5.6%) and fish (1.2%). About 9.5% of the antibiotics were sold for use in nonfood animals. Among the various class of antibiotics sold during that period, tetracycline represented the major proportion ($\sim$37%) followed by β-lactams ($\sim$28%), trimethoprim/sulphonamides (11%), aminoglycosides (8.5%), macrolides (8.15%) and other antibiotics. In spite of the ban on antibiotic as a growth promoter, the premix route of administration remained the most common, accounting for 38% of all antibiotics sold in 2017. Nevertheless, the sale of critically important antibiotic (CIA) was reduced by 52%, since 2013. Antibiotic usage was about 131 mg/kg in pig production in 2017 and the total use was mostly represented by tetracycline (45%) followed by penicillins (17%), trimethoprim/sulphonamides (16%), macrolides (12%) and others. In comparison to 2015 (278 mg/kg), antibiotic use was dropped by more than 50% in 2017.

Since its inception in 1995, Danish Integrated Antimicrobial Resistance Monitoring and Research Programme (DANMAP) is instrumental to monitor trends in resistance among bacteria from animals, food and human, to monitor the consumption of antimicrobial agents, to determine the association between consumption and occurrence of resistance and to model transmission of resistance from animals to humans. Following discontinuation of antibiotics as growth promoter during 1994—99 in Denmark, the total antibiotic consumption in animals was decreased by 49% in 2016 than that in 1994, and as per the recent report of DANMAP-2016, the total antibiotic consumption in animals was estimated to about 104.4 tonnes active compound. Majority of the antibiotics was used in pigs (75%), followed by bovine (12%), fur animals (5%), poultry (2%), fish (2%), pet animals and horses (1% each) (Birgitte Borck and Korsgaard, 2016). For the piggery sector, the antibiotic consumption was decreased by 27% from 2009 to 2016 with a reduction in the use of tetracycline, pleuromutilin, and β-lactamase sensitive penicillin. Use of tetracycline alone dropped by 35% during this period, the report said. The use of CIA such as fluoroquinolone and cephalosporins was negligible in 2016 in Denmark. In contrast, use of colistin in pigs was increased by more than twofold during this span (864 Kg in 2016 from 409 Kg in 2009) — which may have potential public health implication as colistin is considered as last resort for treating human patients with carbapenem-resistant infection. Antibiotic consumption was considerably dropped also in cattle during this period. Interestingly, there was no record of the use of fluoroquinolone and approximately 11 kg of cephalosporins was used, of which higher generation cephalosporin constituted only negligible proportion. Use of cephalosporins was decreased by 83% in 2016 when compared with that in 2008. Importantly, use of intramammary antibiotic infusion was also restricted with initiatives from the Danish Agriculture and Food Council. In general, antibiotic consumption is low in the poultry sector in Denmark possibly because of the very high level of biosecurity in Danish poultry farms. Tetracycline and amoxicillin were the more frequently used antimicrobials in poultry in Denmark, as indicated in the report of DANMAP, 2016.

Swedish Antimicrobial Resistance Monitoring Programme (SVARM) has also been operational to monitor the use of antibiotics in animals, since long. The recent report from SVARM revealed that about 10,310 kg of antibiotics was sold for animals in 2017 against 16,364 kg in 2008 and this 37% drop in antibiotic sell could be attributed to the stringent antibiotic stewardship programme in Sweden, which restricted the use of CIA in the animal sector with increasing awareness among the prescribers. Sales of the CIAs such as cephalosporins, fluoroquinolones and colistin were dropped by 89%, 84% and 46%, respectively, since 2008 (OlssonAspevall, 2017).

There are sporadic reports on the use of antibiotics in animals from different countries. In 2013, Chinese Academy of Science reported that 162,000 tons of antibiotics are consumed in China each year, of which 52% was intended for food animals (Yu et al., 2019). The large-scale antibiotic consumption could be attributed to the pork industry in China. The situation is alarming as a recent report from China predicted that typical swine farms with the feedstock of 10,000 pigs could release about $4.0 \pm 1.3 \times 10^{17}$ gene copies of ARGs (antibiotic resistance genes) per day (Zhang et al., 2019). Again, Krishnaswamy et al., 2015 reported that about 38.5 million kg [84.9 million lbs] of antimicrobials were used in China's production of swine and poultry in 2012. While slightly more than 4.5 million kg [9.9 million lbs] of antimicrobials were used in poultry production, the figure is about 34 million kg [75 million lbs] in pigs. Group-wise, tetracycline and coccidiostats were frequently used in pigs and poultry, respectively (Krishnaswamy et al., 2015). In 2016, Chinese authority pushed for a reduction in antibiotic use in the animal sector and set a target to be achieved by 2020. Like in China, pig (392—423 mg/kg) industry was found to be the highest consumer of antibiotics in Japan, followed by beef cattle (45—67 mg/kg), broiler chickens (44—63 mg/kg) and dairy cattle (33—49 mg/kg). In 2013, 780.88 tons of active ingredients were sold for animal consumption of which tetracycline constituted the largest share (43.5%—46.2%). However, the medically important drugs such as third-generation cephalosporins and fluoroquinolones accounted for less than 1% of overall sales (Anonymous, 2017).

Details of the antimicrobials used in poultry

The use of antimicrobials in food-producing animals, especially in poultry, is a highly debated issue in current days. Other than its use in the treatment of the sick birds, antibiotics are also used in for a prophylactic or metaphylactic purpose and its use as a growth promoter is highly controversial. Birds have their unique physiological properties to impact drug absorption and distribution (Landoni and Albarellos, 2015). The crop of chicken influences the temporal pattern of drug absorption because of its acidic pH (4.5) and for being the storehouse of bacteria such as *Lactobacillus* spp. Tetracycline groups of drugs generally precipitated in crops of pigeons (pH 6.3) or turkeys (pH 6); however, in chickens, such precipitation is not common, thanks to the acidic pH. Conversely, the flora of chicken crop may interfere with the absorption of antibiotics belonging to macrolide—lincosamide—streptogramin (MLS) groups. In adult chicken, intestinal flora also contains a large number of *Lactobacillus* spp. In addition, efflux pumps (P-glycoprotein) and cytochrome P-450 enzyme (especially CYP3A), the enzymes responsible for the biotransformation of many drugs including antimicrobials in the enterocytes, reduce the bioavailability of many antimicrobials such as fluoroquinolones, oxytetracycline, doxycycline and MLS either because of rapid metabolism or interference in their absorption. Bioavailability of drugs in poultry is always compromised because of reduced glomerular filtration rate combined with low or absent tubular reabsorption.

In an effort to ensure rational use of antibiotic in the broiler industry, British Poultry Council's (BPC) antibiotic stewardship has been in place, since 2011 in the United Kingdom. About 82% of the total antibiotics used in poultry meat sector in the United Kingdom in 2016 were contributed by amoxicillin (44%) and tetracycline (38%). A number of measures taken up under this programme including a complete ban on colistin use (in 2016), stoppage of prophylactic use of antibiotics and use of fluoroquinolone and macrolides only as last resort — all resulted in 71% reduction in the total use of antibiotics from 2012 to 2016 (Anonymous, 2019). This pointed out the importance of stewardship programme in reducing the unnecessary use of antibiotics (Table 2.1).

TABLE 2.1 Details of the common antimicrobials used in broiler (Mehdi et al., 2018; Wongsuvan et al., 2018; Anonymous, 2012).

Sl No	Antimicrobials	Route	Indications	Dose	Withdrawal period
1	**β-Lactam** Penicillin-G Amoxicillin Ampicillin Ceftiofur	Oral SC (Ceftiofur) *In ovo* (in some countries)	*Escherichia coli, Pasteurella multocida, Salmonella* spp. and also for the control and treatment of necrotic enteritis (*Clostridium perfringens*)	Penicillin G: 300,000 −400,000 IU/L.	1 day
				Amoxicillin: 100 −200 ppm	5 days
				Ampicillin: 1.5 g/L	5 days
				Ceftiofur: 0.08−0.2 mg/chick	
2	**Polypeptides** (bacitracin)	Oral	necrotic enteritis	Prophylactic: 55−110 mg/kg feed Therapeutic: 200−400 mg/kg feed	No withdrawal period required.
3	**Aminoglycosides** Gentamicin Neomycin Streptomycin	SC, Oral	Infection with Gram-negative pathogens, colibacillosis	Gentamicin: 0.2−0.5 mg/chick SC 5.5 mg/kg IM (adults)	For meat, 7 days after the last administration. For kidneys and injection site, 45 days
				Neomycin: 70−140 g/ton (chicken) 22 mg/kg/day water medication (turkey)	7 days
				Streptomycin 20 mg/kg; 2.5−5.0 mg per chick (chicken) Spectinomycin 50−100 mg/kg BW	5 days
4	**Aminocyclitols** Hygromycin Spectinomycin Apramycin	Oral	Anthelmintic (hygromycin) Colibacillosis (spectinomycin) Colibacillosis, salmonellosis and other bacterial infections (apramycin)	Hygromycin (in feed) Spectinomycin (in drinking water) 2−5 mg/kg feed (apramycin)	0−14 days (apramycin)

Continued

TABLE 2.1 Details of the common antimicrobials used in broiler (Mehdi et al., 2018; Wongsuvan et al., 2018; Anonymous, 2012).—cont'd

Sl No	Antimicrobials	Route	Indications	Dose	Withdrawal period
5	**Macrolides, tiamulin and lincosamides** erythromycin, tylosin and tilmicosin		*Staphylococcus* infection (erythromycin) Mycoplasma infection, necrotic enteritis (tylosin) *Mycoplasma, Pasteurella multocida* and *Ornithobacterium rhinotracheale* infections (tilmicosin) Clostridium perfringens—induced necrotic enteritis and intestinal spirochaetosis (lincomycin)	Erythromycin 92.5—185 g/ton 115.6—250 mg/L	1 day
				Tylosin: 800—1000 g/ton, 500 mg/L	3—5
				Tilmicosin: 75 mg/L	12
				Tiamulin: 160—320 mg/kg, 250 mg/L	2
6	**Florfenicol**		Infections caused by *E. coli, Pasteurella* spp. and *Haemophilus* spp., *Chlamydia* spp. and *Mycoplasma* spp.	100 mg/L, over 2—4 days in drinking water	7 days
7	**Tetracycline** Chlortetracycline (CTC), tetracycline (T) and oxytetracycline (OTC)	Oral in feed or water	Effective against multiple pathogens including diseases such as chronic respiratory disease, fowl cholera and fowl coryza	CTC: 55—220 mg/kg or 110—280 mg/L	5—7 days
				T: 300 mg/kg or 45—100 mg/L	
				OTC: 100—400 mg/kg or 200 mg/L	
8	**Sulphonamide** (sulfachlorpyridazine, sulfadimethoxine, sulfamethazine, sulfaquinoxaline, sulfathiazole and the potentiated sulfonamides sulfachlorpyridazine/ trimethoprim, sulfadimethoxine/ ormetoprim and sulfaquinoxaline/ trimethoprim)		Coccidiosis and other bacterial infection	200 mg/kg, oral Trimethoprim sulfamethoxazole 360—400 mg/L drinking water/400 mg/kg feed/ 100 mg/kg PO q12h	Minimum 10 days
9	**Fluoroquinolones** Enrofloxacin Banned in many countries		Infections caused by *Mycoplasma, E. coli* and *Pasteurella* spp.	100 mg/L drinking water for 3—5 days 10 mg/kg for single pulse doses	3—7 days
10	**Ionophores** Salinomycin Monensin Maduramicin Lasalocid		Coccidiosis	Salinomycin: 50—70 mg/ kg feed	1 day
				Monensin: 80—125 mg/kg feed	
				Maduramicin: 5 mg/kg feed	5 days
				Lasalocid: 75—125 mg/kg feed	
11	Bacitracin methylene disalicylate[1]	4—50 g/ton as a growth promoter 100—200 g/ton for treatment of necrotic enteritis			

[1]*Banned in India since 2018*

Details of the antimicrobials used in pigs

For pigs, antibiotic consumption is relatively higher in pork-eating countries. In OECD countries, antimicrobial consumption per population correction unit (PCU) is much higher in pigs (172 mg/PCU) and poultry (148 mg/PCU) than in cattle (45 mg/PCU) (Gonzalez Ronquillo and Angeles Hernandez, 2017). In 2015, total AMU in the UK pig industry was about 200 tonnes, i.e., 260 mg per kg PCU — five times higher than in Denmark (46 mg/kg PCU) and the Netherlands (53 mg/kg PCU) and about 25 times higher than in Sweden (11 mg/kg PCU) (Rose and Nunan, 2016). In low- and middle-income countries, AMU was greatest in chickens (138 doses/1000 animal-days [interquartile range (IQR) 91.1—438.3]), followed by swine (40.2 [IQR 8.5—120.4]) and dairy cattle (10.0 [IQR 5.5—13.6]). However, for per kg of meat produced, AMU was the highest in swine, followed by chickens and cattle (Cuong et al., 2018). China is the largest producer and consumer of pig, and use of antibiotics in pig rearing in China has remained a much discussed and debated issue since the detection of plasmid-mediated colistin resistance gene (*mcr*-1) linked by many to the use of colistin as a feed additive in the porcine ration. Various studies indicated the use of antibiotics as feed additives in the majority of the pig rations, and prophylactically, antibiotics are often given to the herd rather than to the individual animal (Anonymous, 2013b). Apart from it, antibiotics are also used for the treatment of diseases such as enzootic pneumonia, *Streptococcus suis*, mycoplasma infections and swine dysentery (Table 2.2).

Details of the antimicrobials used in bovine

In dairy cattle, antibiotics are mostly used for the treatment of infections of which mastitis obviously comes first. In mastitis, antibiotics are often used prophylactically in the form of intramammary infusion, as dry cow therapy. Apart from it, antibiotics are often prescribed in metritis through the systemic or intrauterine application. Other bacterial diseases also warrant the need for antibiotics. In the face of outbreaks, farmers in consultation with veterinarians often prefer to keep their unaffected stocks under antibiotic therapy to prevent the spread of infection among healthy stocks. Some viral infection also requires antibiotic therapy to keep away the secondary infections. The most crucial factor which is frequently overlooked by the farmers or veterinary doctors is the actual body weight of the animal while prescribing or dispensing the antibiotics. Particularly at the field, body weight is often determined based on visual estimation, which is erroneous and eventually leads to overdosing/underdosing of the drugs. Such underdosed application runs the risk of being ineffective to cure the animals. On the other hand, overdosing may lead to toxicity. Besides, the resistant pathogens are likely to survive and propagate in more number in such cases. Therefore, antibiotics in bovines should always be given with adequate care such as to ensure proper dosing and duration. However, in feedlot cattle intended for beef production, antibiotics are given in premix feed often with an intention to increase FCR and body weight (Table 2.3).

Details of the antimicrobials used in aquaculture

As is the case in terrestrial animals, aquaculture has also been shifted towards intensification to meet the ever-increasing demand for human need. In parallel, the need for antibiotics is also increasing as a part of an aggressive disease management strategy. A survey conducted by the FAO in different countries revealed that 60 different veterinary medicine ingredients including 26 antibiotics are used in aquaculture. The antibiotics used in aquaculture belonged to a diverse group — β-lactam, nitrofurans, phenicols, macrolides, quinolones, sulphonamides, rifampicin and tetracycline. Studies conducted by the FAO revealed that oxytetracycline is the most frequently used antibiotic in aquaculture. The workers further emphasized that besides prophylactic uses, antibiotics are abused or overused because of improper diagnosis (Gonzalez Ronquillo and Angeles Hernandez, 2017). The use of antimicrobials is mainly intended for various fish diseases such as cold water diseases rainbow trout fry syndrome, bacterial kidney disease, enteric redmouth disease, furunculosis, piscirickettsiosis, bacterial gill disease, vibriosis, epitheliocystis, tenacibaculosis, rainbow trout gastroenteritis, red mark syndrome or cold water strawberry disease, etc. (Sekkin and Kum, 2011). Although data on the kind of antibiotics used in different countries are not available, most of the counties including many European countries use at least two CIAs in fish farming — tetracyclines and oxolinic acid, a third-generation quinolone. Studies pointed out wide variation in AMU ranging from 1 g per metric ton of production in Norway to 700 g per metric ton in Vietnam depending on the local or national regulation and government policies in this sector (Towers, 2014). An appreciable body of evidence suggested the metaphylactic use of antibiotics in aquaculture which is largely debated because it requires protracted antibiotic therapy in subtherapeutic concentration in the healthy fishes along with sick one, which is ineffective to completely clear out the infection, and the drug resistance is more likely to emerge (Towers, 2014) (Table 2.4).

TABLE 2.2 Details of the common antimicrobials used in pigs (Anonymous, 2012).

Sl No	Antimicrobials	Indications	Dose
1	**Penicillin and β-lactams**		
	Ampicillin	RTI, UTI, mastitis metritis agalactiae syndrome, synovitis	5—10 mg/kg BW QID
	Amoxicillin	UTI, wound infection, salmonellosis	10 mg/kg BW/BID
	Amoxicillin-cloxacillin	RTI, metritis, pyelonephritis, skin infection	
	Ampicillin-cloxacillin	RTI, metritis, pyelonephritis, skin infection	
	Benzathine penicillin	Swine erysipelas, tetanus, foot rot malignant oedema	12,000 IU/Kg BW
	Fortified procaine penicillin	Swine erysipelas, malignant oedema	4000—10,000, IU/Kg, BW
	Ceftiofur	RTI, UTI, mastitis metritis agalactiae syndrome, synovitis	3—5 mg/kg BW, IM
2	**Aminoglycosides**		
	Apramycin	Colibacillosis, salmonellosis and other bacterial infections	80—200 mg/kg feed
	Gentamicin	Piglet diarrhoea scours	4 mg/kg BW BID
	Neomycin	Bacterial enteritis	2.5—5 mg/kg BW BID IV/IM 10 mg/kg BW Oral
	Streptomycin	Pasteurellosis, enzootic pneumonia	10 mg/kg IM
3	Bambermycins		4 g/ton
4	Bacitracin methylene disalicylate[b]	10—30 grams/ton as a growth promoter 250 g/ton for treatment of swine dysentery and clostridial enteritis	
5	Carbadox*	Dysentery	20—50 ppm
6	**Fluoroquinolones**		
	Enrofloxacin	Swine Respiratory Disease	5 mg/kg BW oral or parental
7	**Lincosamides and macrolides**		
	Erythromycin	Swine erysipelas, pneumonia	2.2—6 mg/kg BW Oral
	Lincomycin	Infectious forms of arthritis and Mycoplasma pneumonia in swine	300 mg/27.2 Kg Or 20 g/ton of feed
	Tiamulin	Swine erysipelas, dysentery, mycoplasma arthritis	10—15 mg/kg BW
	Tylosin	Swine erysipelas, dysentery, pneumonia, arthritis	5—20 mg/kg BW oral
8	Florfenicol	RTI	10 mg of florfenicol per kg of body weight per day administered for 5 consecutive days (oral)/ 100 ppm
9	**Tetracycline**		
	Oxytetracycline	Swine erysipelas, scours, leptospirosis, joint ill, atrophic rhinitis	5—10 mg/kg BW/day
	Chlortetracycline		10—20 mg/kg BW oral
	Chlortetracycline bisulfate and sulfamethazine		
10	Sulphonamides		
	Sulfamethazine	45 mL of 25% solution for each 50 kg of body weight. Second and following days: one half of the above dosage.	
	Trimethoprim/ sulfadiazine	Mixed bacterial infection — alimentary/ genital/respiratory tract infection	15—30 mg/kg BW orally for 5 days

*Banned in the United States in 2016.
[b]Banned in India in 2018.

TABLE 2.3 Details of the common antimicrobials used in bovine (Anonymous, 2012).

Sl No	Antimicrobials	Indications	Dose	Sl No
1	**Penicillin and other β-lactams**			
	Fortified procaine penicillin	Anthrax, HS, BQ, mastitis, metritis, skin infection and other bacterial infection	4000–10,000, IU/Kg, BW	4–15 days with different penicillin products (meat) In milk, amoxicillin (60 h) and penicillin (72 h)
	Amoxicillin		10 mg/kg BW, IV/IM BID	
	Ampicillin		5–10 mg/kg BW, IV/IM	
	Ceftiofur	Mastitis, metritis, pneumonia, foot rot	1.1–2.2 mg/kg BW, IM/SC	3 days (meat) In some cases, no withdrawal period is mentioned
	Cefquinome	Mastitis, pneumonia	1 mg/Kg BW, IM for 5 days	5 days (meat) 12 h (milk)
2	**Fluoroquinolones**			
	Enrofloxacin	Acute and chronic mastitis, HS, BQ, pyometra, mastitis	2.5–5 mg/kg BW, oral/IM/IV	28 days for slaughter
3	**Lincosamide**			
	Lincomycin	RTI, mastitis, metritis and skin infection	10 mg/kg BW IM, IV, Oral BID	96 h for milk 7 days for meat (Food Animal Residue Avoidance Databank)
	Tylosin	Respiratory disease	10–16 mg/Kg BW IM up to 5 days	96 h (milk) 35 days (meat)
	Pirlimycin	Mastitis	50 mg Intramammary 2–8 treatment 24 h interval	36 h
4	Oxytetracycline	Pneumonia, CCBP, HS, BQ, pyometra, mastitis, wound, etc.	5–10 mg/kg IM/IV	15–22 days for short-acting and 28 days for long-acting
5	**Aminoglycosides**			
	Streptomycin[a]	Pasteurellosis, actinobacillosis, actinomycosis, etc.	10 mg/kg IM	Milk ~48 h
	Gentamicin[a]	Genitourinary tract infection	4 mg/kg BW IM/IV	18 months (meat) Food Animal Residue Avoidance Databank
6	**Sulphonamides**			
	Trimethoprim/ sulfadiazine	Alimentary tract and genital tract infection	15–60 mg/kg/day, PO, IV, or IM	3 days (but milk discard time is 7 days)

[a]Extra-label use of aminoglycosides is prohibited in many countries for its propensity to accumulate in the kidney for a lasting period.

TABLE 2.4 Details of the common antimicrobials used in aquaculture.

	Antimicrobials	Indication	Dose
1	Amoxicillin	Bacterial disease	0.2 ppm for 5 days
2	Oxytetracycline	Bacterial disease	4%–5% in fish feed for 5 days 2–10 mg/kg fish weight for 3–7 days
3	Chlortetracycline	Bacterial disease	7 g/100 kg for 5–7 days
4	Enrofloxacin	Bacterial disease	200 gm/80 Kg feed
5	Erythromycin	Water head mouth disease, gill rot disease, etc.	0.5 mg/100 kg fish weight for 6 days/1 ppm for 5 days
6	Florfenicol	Bacterial disease	10–15 mg/kg fish weight for 3–7 days
7	Sulfadiazine + trimethoprim	Ulcerative and systemic Aeromonas	5 g/100 kg for 7 days
8	Oxolinic acid	Redfin, red skin disease	10–20 mg/kg fish weight for 4–7 days

AMU in agriculture — current and future possible impacts

Although the use of an antimicrobial is regarded as the most important and crucial driver for the emergence of AMR, it is not very easy to understand and decipher how the use of antimicrobial in agriculture can impact human health. Moreover, we are yet to quantify the share of resistance burden of the public health that could be attributed to AMU in agriculture.

Landers et al., 2012, rightly, pointed out various complex interaction of elements in the physical environment (e.g., air, soil and water), social exchanges (e.g., between animals within a herd, farmers and animals, and domestic poultry and migratory birds), in processing steps (e.g., farming activities, transportation and storage) and in human use patterns (e.g., food preparation, meat consumption and susceptibility to infection) — which we all need to know to understand how antibiotic use in animals can affect human health, directly or indirectly (Landers et al., 2012). While the pathogens can be directly transferred to human beings by contact or consumption of contaminated feed of animal origin, indirect transfer entails various environmental components such as soil, water and air, which may carry the pathogens to human. At the same time, it is equally important to understand the consequential effect of phasing out of the use of antimicrobials, particularly CIA in animals on the farm economy. In their study, Landers et al., 2012, also deliberated various mathematical models proposed by different workers which estimated potential risk associated with the use of antimicrobials in animals by taking into account the prevalence of an infection caused by specific pathogens, its associated morbidity and proportion of that infection which might have been contributed by AMU in agriculture. However, by doing so, most of the workers undermined the potential benefits associated with AMU in sick animals by reducing the shredding of infective pathogens and thereby their spread in the environment. There are a number of studies which spoke volume of beneficial effects of the use of antibiotics in animals which included reduced morbidity and mortality, better feed conversion, growth, reproduction and production performance. However, scientists pointed out the potential risks associated with increased AMU in animals or agriculture — development and dissemination of formidable bugs causing increased human morbidity and mortality (Chattopadhyay et al., 2014). Taking a serious note of the potential impact of AMU in animals on human health, FDA made it mandatory for drug manufacturers perform risk analysis for any new drug to launch to ensure its safety and efficacy in animals and also to rule out any possible harmful effect on human health for its proposed use in animals. In the second OIE Global Conference on — "Antimicrobial Resistance and Prudent use of Antimicrobial Agents in Animals" held during 29—–31st October, 2018, Dr M. Ryan, Senior Policy Analyst, Trade and Agriculture Directorate, OECD, shared some interesting findings derived from a study conducted in European countries (Belgium, France, Germany, Sweden, Denmark, Netherland and Switzerland) to find out the associated economic benefit and costs of AMU in animals; lowering the use of antimicrobial had no adverse impact on animal production performance or farm economy. Even some farms increased profit margin albeit, at small scale, but this was against the generally conceived idea that complete or marginal withdrawal of antibiotics might have a disastrous impact on animal health and farm economy. The study reasserted the need for internal and external biosecurity of farms, enhanced natural immunity of the animals and better management practices to phase out the use of the CIA in animals (Ryan, 2018). A similar kind of study was conducted by Lhermie et al. (2018) to understand the farm impact of several potential policies aimed at decreasing AMU. The workers prepared a mathematical model in a dairy herd of 1000 cows with an average prevalence of nine most frequent bacterial dairy diseases found in western countries to extrapolate the increased net cost the farm had to bear on being prohibited from antimicrobial uses. The study showed a marginal increase in the net cost (ranging between $46 and $73 per cow per year) in case such prohibition was made (Lhermie et al., 2018). However, an inference drawn from both the studies cannot be generalized particularly for the developing world where the problem of AMR is looming large.

When there is an urgent call to reduce the AMU in animal/agriculture production, it must be borne into mind that AMR is a complex problem and the same cannot be surmounted with an easy and single window approach. Reduction in AMU in farm animals may not always lead to a direct and rapid reduction in AMR, as experienced in the case of VRE in a previous study (Guardabassi, 2013). The exceptional ability of the resistance pathogen and resistance gene(s) to disseminate and transmit made the control and containment of AMR herculean. Therefore, intervening in the dissemination and transmission pathways within animals and between animal and human may be another potential area for controlling AMR. Reservoirs and the transmission pathways of antimicrobial-resistant bacteria thus need to be explored so as to facilitate such intervention. The livestock farming and trade is a complex and heterogeneous structure, it is not easy to understand how it harbours and transmits the infectious pathogens including bugs in herd (Magouras et al., 2017). However, livestock trade has definite implication in the transmission of AMR pathogens in a similar way what previous workers observed in case of livestock-associated methicillin-resistant *Staphylococcus aureus* (LA-MRSA). On the other hand, colonization of LA-MRSA in nasal cavities of pig (Morcillo et al., 2011) or in bovine udder (Bhattacharyya et al., 2016) did not rule out the possibility of their shedding and transfer via indirect and direct route and now a colonization of LA-MRSA via the airborne route was established by another group of workers from Germany (Rosen et al., 2018). The similar genotypes and resistant phenotypes of the isolates of porcine and farmworker origin indicated how such pathogens can get an entry in human to establish colonization (Morcillo et al., 2011; Espinosa-Gongora et al., 2012). The pathogens like *E. coli* or *Enterococci*, which are periodically shed through faces, can spread to other in-contact animals or human and can contaminate the environment through the application of animal manure on the agricultural lands or during the grazing of the reservoir animals on the pasture. Manure application has long been known for being a major avenue for dissemination of AMR pathogens including ESBL producing or colistin-resistant mcr-1 harbouring *E. coli* (Blaak et al., 2014; Zheng et al., 2017), *Enterococcus faecalis* (Mangalappalli-Illathu et al., 2010) and even the methicillin-resistant *Staphylococcus scuiri* (Kumar et al., 2018). Such complexity lies in the transmission dynamics of AMR pathogen that even the common flies cannot be excluded out as a possible carrier of such resistant bugs (Blaak et al., 2014). In such a scenario, reducing AMU in animals can be important but not the only solution for rising AMR in public health. Nonetheless, optimization of the use of antimicrobials in animals is an essential step towards achieving that goal. Alternatives to antimicrobials, use of improved and reliable diagnostics, better infection, prevention and control measures may pave the way to reduce AMU in animals.

References

Anonymous, 2012. Current Indian Veterinary Index. Vet Ads Creation Pvt Ltd.

Anonymous, 2013. Management Approaches to Reduce Transportation Stress Risk for BRD, WSU Animal Science and Veterinary Medicine Extension. https://articles.extension.org/sites/default/files/Management Approaches to Reduce Transportation Stress Risk for BRD.pdf.

Anonymous, 2013. Responsible Use of Antimicrobials in Pig Production, Second. RUMA Alliance.

Anonymous, 2017. Farm Antibiotic Use in the United States. FDA. https://www.fda.gov/downloads/ForIndustry/UserFees/AnimalDrugUserFee ActADUFA/UCM.

Anonymous, 2019. Data | Nippon AMR One Health Report (NAOR) 2017. https://amr-onehealth.ncgm.go.jp/en/statistics/.

Anonymous, 2019. Antibiotic Stewardship. The British Poultry Council. https://www.britishpoultry.org.uk/category/issues/antibiotic-stewardship/.

Baptiste, K.E., Kyvsgaard, N.C., 2017. Do antimicrobial mass medications work? A systematic review and meta-analysis of randomised clinical trials investigating antimicrobial prophylaxis or metaphylaxis against naturally occurring bovine respiratory disease. Pathogens and Disease 75, 83. https://doi.org/10.1093/femspd/ftx083.

Basri, Z., 2017. Summary Report on Antimicrobials Sold or Distributed for Use in Food-Producing Animals. (FDA).

Bhattacharyya, D., Banerjee, J., Bandyopadhyay, S., Mondal, B., Nanda, P.K., Samanta, I., et al., 2016. First report on vancomycin-resistant *Staphylococcus aureus* in bovine and caprine milk. Microbial Drug Resistance 22, 675−681. https://doi.org/10.1089/mdr.2015.0330.

Birgitte Borck, H., Korsgaard, H., 2016. DANMAP - Use of Antimicrobial Agents and Occurrence of Antimicrobial Resistance in Bacteria from Food Animals, Food and Humans in Denmark.

Blaak, H., Hamidjaja, R.A., Van Hoek, A.H.A.M., De Heer, L., De Roda Husman, A.M., Schets, F.M., 2014. Detection of extended-spectrum beta-lactamase (ESBL)-producing *Escherichia coli* on flies at poultry farms. Applied and Environmental Microbiology 80, 239−246. https://doi.org/10.1128/AEM.02616-13.

Chattopadhyay, M.K., Zurek, L., Nosanchuk, J.D., 2014. Use of Antibiotics as Feed Additives: A Burning Question. https://doi.org/10.3389/fmicb.2014.00334.

Checkley, S.L., Campbell, J.R., Chirino-Trejo, M., Janzen, E.D., Waldner, C.L., 2010. Associations between antimicrobial use and the prevalence of antimicrobial resistance in faecal *Escherichia coli* from feedlot cattle in western Canada. Canadian Veterinary Journal 51, 853−861.

Costa, M.C., Bessegatto, J.A., Alfieri, A.A., Weese, J.S., Filho, J.A.B., Oba, A., 2017. Different antibiotic growth promoters induce specific changes in the cecal microbiota membership of broiler chicken. PLoS One 12, e0171642. https://doi.org/10.1371/journal.pone.0171642.

Cuong, N.V., Padungtod, P., Thwaites, G., Carrique-Mas, J.J., 2018. Antimicrobial usage in animal production: a review of the literature with a focus on low- and middle-income countries. Antibiotics (Basel) 7. https://doi.org/10.3390/antibiotics7030075.

Dibner, J.J., Richards, J.D., 2005. Antibiotic growth promoters in agriculture: history and mode of action. Poultry Science 84, 634−643. https://doi.org/10.1093/ps/84.4.634.

Done, H.Y., Venkatesan, A.K., Halden, R.U., 2015. Does the recent growth of aquaculture create antibiotic resistance threats different from those associated with land animal production in agriculture? The AAPS Journal 17, 513−524. https://doi.org/10.1208/s12248-015-9722-z.

Espinosa-Gongora, C., Broens, E.M., Moodley, A., Nielsen, J.P., Guardabassi, L., 2012. Transmission of MRSA CC398 strains between pig farms related by trade of animals. The Veterinary Record 170, 564. https://doi.org/10.1136/vr.100704.

Gonzalez Ronquillo, M., Angeles Hernandez, J.C., 2017. Antibiotic and synthetic growth promoters in animal diets: review of impact and analytical methods. Food Control 72, 255−267. https://doi.org/10.1016/j.foodcont.2016.03.001.

Guardabassi, L., 2013. Sixty years of antimicrobial use in animals: what is next? The Veterinary Record 173, 599−603. https://doi.org/10.1136/vr.f7276.

Hughes, P., Heritage, J., 2004. Antibiotic Growth-Promoters in Food Animals. In Assessing Quality and Safety of Animal Feeds. FAO, pp. 129−153.

Krishnaswamy, V., Otte, J., Silbergeld, E., 2015. Antimicrobial use in Chinese swine and broiler poultry production. Antimicrobial Resistance and Infection Control 4, 17. https://doi.org/10.1186/s13756-015-0050-y.

Kumar, D., Pornsukarom, S., Sivaraman, G.K., Thakur, S., 2018. Environmental dissemination of multidrug methicillin-resistant Staphylococcus sciuri after application of manure from commercial swine production systems. Foodbourne Pathogens and Disease 15, 210–217. https://doi.org/10.1089/fpd.2017.2354.

Landers, T.F., Cohen, B., Wittum, T.E., Larson, E.L., 2012. A review of antibiotic use in food animals: perspective, policy, and potential. Public Health Reports 127, 4–22. https://doi.org/10.1177/003335491212700103.

Landoni, M.F., Albarellos, G., 2015. The use of antimicrobial agents in broiler chickens. The Veterinary Journal 205, 21–27. https://doi.org/10.1016/j.tvjl.2015.04.016.

Lee, K.W., Ho Hong, Y., Lee, S.H., Jang, S.I., Park, M.S., Bautista, D.A., et al., 2012. Effects of anticoccidial and antibiotic growth promoter programs on broiler performance and immune status. Research in Veterinary Science 93, 721–728. https://doi.org/10.1016/j.rvsc.2012.01.001.

Lhermie, G., Tauer, L.W., Gröhn, Y.T., 2018. The farm cost of decreasing antimicrobial use in dairy production. PLoS One 13, e0194832. https://doi.org/10.1371/journal.pone.0194832.

Li, J., 2017. Current status and prospects for in-feed antibiotics in the different stages of pork production - a review. Asian-Australasian Journal of Animal Sciences 30, 1667–1673. https://doi.org/10.5713/ajas.17.0418.

Magouras, I., Carmo, L.P., Stärk, K.D.C., Schüpbach-Regula, G., 2017. Antimicrobial usage and -resistance in livestock: where should we focus? Frontiers in Veterinary Science 4, 148. https://doi.org/10.3389/fvets.2017.00148.

Mangalappalli-Illathu, A., Duriez, P., Masson, L., Diarra, M.S., Scott, A., Tien, Y.-C., et al., 2010. Dynamics of antimicrobial resistance and virulence genes in *Enterococcus faecalis* during swine manure storage. Canadian Journal of Microbiology 56, 683–691. https://doi.org/10.1139/W10-055.

Mehdi, Y., Létourneau-Montminy, M.-P., Gaucher, M.-L., Chorfi, Y., Suresh, G., Rouissi, T., et al., 2018. Use of antibiotics in broiler production: global impacts and alternatives. Anim Nutr 4, 170–178. https://doi.org/10.1016/j.aninu.2018.03.002.

Morcillo, A., Castro, B., González, J., Rodríguez-Alvarez, C., Novo, M., Sierra, A., et al., 2011. High prevalence of methicillin-resistant *Staphylococcus aureus* in pigs and slaughterhouse workers. Clinical Microbiology and Infections 17, S222.

Olsson, E., Aspevall, O., 2017. SWEDRES (SVRAM) – Consumption of Antibiotics and Occurrence of Antibiotic Resistance in Sweden.

Peter Borriello, S., 2017. UK-VARSS 2016 UK – Veterinary Antibiotic Resistance and Sales Surveillance Report.

Rose, E., Nunan, C., 2016. Antibiotic Use in the Pig Sector, pp. 1–5. www.saveourantibiotics.org.

Rosen, K., Roesler, U., Merle, R., Friese, A., 2018. Persistent and transient airborne MRSA colonization of piglets in a newly established animal model. Frontiers in Microbiology 9. https://doi.org/10.3389/fmicb.2018.01542.

Ryan, M., 2018. The economic benefits and costs of antimicrobial use in food animal production: what lessons can be drawn?. In: 2nd OIE Glob. Conf. Antimicrob. Resist. PRUDENT USE Antimicrob. AGENTS Anim., p. 5.

Schar, D., Sommanustweechai, A., Laxminarayan, R., Tangcharoensathien, V., 2018. Surveillance of antimicrobial consumption in animal production sectors of low- and middle-income countries: optimizing use and addressing antimicrobial resistance. PLoS Medicine 15, e1002521. https://doi.org/10.1371/journal.pmed.1002521.

Sekkin, S., Kum, C., 2011. Antibacterial Drugs in Fish Farms: Application and its Effects. Recent Adv. Fish Farms. InTech. https://doi.org/10.5772/26919.

Siegner, C., 2019. Use of Animal Antibiotics Dropped by a Third in 2017, FDA Says | Food Dive. https://www.fooddive.com/news/use-of-animal-antibiotics-dropped-by-a-third-in-2017-fda-says/544821/.

Towers, L., 2014. Antibiotics in Aquaculture Are They Needed? | the Fish Site. https://thefishsite.com/articles/antibiotics-in-aquaculture-are-they-needed.

Van Boeckel, T.P., Brower, C., Gilbert, M., Grenfell, B.T., Levin, S.A., Robinson, T.P., et al., 2015. Global trends in antimicrobial use in food animals. Proceedings of the National Academy of Sciences 112, 5649–5654. https://doi.org/10.1073/pnas.1503141112.

Van Boeckel, T.P., Glennon, E.E., Chen, D., Gilbert, M., Robinson, T.P., Grenfell, B.T., et al., 2017. Reducing antimicrobial use in food animals. Science (80-) 357, 1350–1352. https://doi.org/10.1126/science.aao1495.

Versporten, A., Zarb, P., Caniaux, I., Gros, M.F., Drapier, N., Miller, M., et al., 2018. Antimicrobial consumption and resistance in adult hospital in-patients in 53 countries: results of an internet-based global point prevalence survey. Lancet Global Health 6, e619–e629. https://doi.org/10.1016/S2214-109X(18)30186-4.

Wallinga, D., 2018. Better Bacon: Why It's High Time the U.S. Pork Industry Stopped Pigging Out on Antibiotics. NRDC. https://www.nrdc.org/resources/better-bacon-why-its-high-time-us-pork-industry-stopped-pigging-out-antibiotics.

Wongsuvan, G., Wuthiekanun, V., Hinjoy, S., Day, N.P.J., Limmathurotsakul, D., 2018. Antibiotic use in poultry: a survey of eight farms in Thailand. Bulletin of the World Health Organization 96, 94–100. https://doi.org/10.2471/BLT.17.195834.

Yu, A.Y., Rogers Van Katwyk, S., Hoffman, S.J., 2019. Probing popular and political discourse on antimicrobial resistance in China. Global Health Research and Policy 4, 6. https://doi.org/10.1186/s41256-019-0097-z.

Zhang, J., Lu, T., Chai, Y., Sui, Q., Shen, P., Wei, Y., 2019. Which animal type contributes the most to the emission of antibiotic resistance genes in large-scale swine farms in China? The Science of the Total Environment 658, 152–159. https://doi.org/10.1016/j.scitotenv.2018.12.175.

Zheng, B., Huang, C., Xu, H., Guo, L., Zhang, J., Wang, X., et al., 2017. Occurrence and genomic characterization of ESBL-producing, MCR-1-harboring *Escherichia coli* in farming soil. Frontiers in Microbiology 8. https://doi.org/10.3389/fmicb.2017.02510.

Chapter 3

The emergence of antimicrobial-resistant bacteria in livestock, poultry and agriculture

Chapter outline

Overview of antimicrobial use in animals

Owing to the rapid development of resistant bugs both in animal and human sector, the antimicrobial use (AMU) in animals especially as prophylactic or metaphylactic measure and as growth promoter has come under the scanner. Importantly, in many countries, a large proportion of antimicrobials used in animals belong to what was categorized as critically important antimicrobials by the World Health Organization (WHO). Intensive livestock farming marked an exuberant rise in AMU in animals because of high-density animal rearing and to meet the requirement of more products or growth. Thus modulation of the gut microbiome with prophylactic antimicrobial therapy with an intention to eliminate or minimize the pathogenic flora is a popular approach adopted by many farms — this remained a common practice even in the developed countries a few years back. All these practices helped the bugs flare and flourish in farms and their neighbouring environment.

Recently, Boeckel and coworkers gave an illustration of the global trend in antimicrobial consumption in food animals where they showed that global average annual consumption of antimicrobials per kilogram of animal produced was 45, 148 and 172 mg/kg for cattle, chicken and pigs, respectively (Van Boeckel et al., 2015). What is more worrisome is that the workers gave an estimated rise in global consumption of antibiotic by 67% in 2030 from 2010 — 67% of such rise was attributed to the increase in AMU in the animal sector. Only in the BRICS countries, antibiotic consumption in food animals is expected to rise by 99% by 2030. In total, this gave a bleak picture of AMU in animals and agriculture, and a detailed account of it is discussed in a separate chapter.

Resistant pathogens in livestock and poultry sector

β-Lactam resistance

Production of β-lactamase is known to cause resistance to *β-lactam* compounds, probably the most popular group of drugs among the clinicians because of their low toxicity. Food animals have been documented as potent reservoir of β-lactamase producers — extended-spectrum β-lactamase (ESBL) and AmpC type β-lactamase producing Gram-negative bacteria (GNB). Quite a good number of studies carried out in the People Republic of China reported the presence of such pathogens both in pigs and poultry. High prevalence of β-lactamase genes (AmpC, TEM, OXA-1 and GES) was detected in swine farms and pig wastewater treatment plants in northern China (Yang et al., 2019). Furthermore, multidrug resistance ESBL producers harbouring both the β-lactamase and PMQR genes were reported from the pig farms in Northwest China (Liu et al., 2018). ESBL producing *Escherichia coli* belonging to O13, O55, O133, O153, O157, O158, O166, rough and OUT serogroups were reported from pigs in India (Samanta et al., 2015). Recently, we showed how these pig farms could act as a potential source of β-lactamase or AmpC type β-lactamase producing *Enterobacteriaceae* (Samanta et al., 2018). Mandakini et al., 2015 reported ESBL-producing Shiga toxic *E. coli* and enteropathogenic *E. coli* in piglet diarrhoea from Northeast India (Mandakini et al., 2014). Poultry seems to be a potential reservoir of β-lactamase producers as reported from studies conducted in China (Qiao et al., 2018) and India (Kar et al., 2015; Mahanti et al., 2018; Brower et al., 2017). Likewise in bovine, mastitis was found a significant risk factor for having ESBL infection as reported from different parts of the world (Dahmen et al., 2013; Ali et al., 2016; Saishu et al., 2014), including India (Koovapra et al., 2016; Bandyopadhyay et al., 2015, 2018). Methicillin-resistant *Staphylococcus aureus* (MRSA) is one of the key pathogens which got immense attention because of recent emergence and spread of livestock-associated MRSA (LA-MRSA). MRSA, because of the presence of modified penicillin-binding protein, are resistant to β-lactam drugs and are often resistant to other antimicrobials, as well (Bandyopadhyay et al., 2015). In recent years, MRSA strains exhibiting resistance to vancomycin were reported from bovine and caprine mastitis in India (Bhattacharyya et al., 2016). Although carbapenem is not used in animals, the emergence of carbapenem resistance in food animals was recorded both from India (Ghatak et al., 2013) and abroad (Köck et al., 2018) — this is indeed alarming as carbapenems are regarded as last resort therapy for refractory and critical infections in human beings.

Fluoroquinolone resistance

Quinolone, a synthetic class of antibacterial, emerged as a unique compound against which resistance development was once considered a remote possibility. However, resistance has been noted against this compound since 1990, possibly because of their overuse in the treatment of genitourinary tract infection. Not only the problem is limited in the human sector but fluoroquinolone resistance has become an increasing concern in animal pathogens, as well. Simultaneous resistance to β-lactam and fluoroquinolone was noted among the ESBL-producing *Enterobacteriaceae* in animals both from India (Kar et al., 2015; Koovapra et al., 2016; Bandyopadhyay et al., 2018) and abroad (Dobiasova et al., 2013). In recent years, a study conducted in China revealed that most of the *Enterobacteriaceae* isolates were resistant to quinolones (nalidixic acid (81.5%) and norfloxacin (65.8%)), predominantly mediated by PMQR genes (Li et al., 2019). In India, we have conducted a series of study for exploring AMR (antimicrobial resistance) pattern of the GNB from various food animals including bovine, poultry and pigs — all the studies reflected that many of the *Enterobacteriaceae* isolates from food animals are concomitantly resistant to β-lactams and fluoroquinolones harbouring genes for ESBL and PMQR (Samanta et al., 2015; Mahanti et al., 2018; Koovapra et al., 2016; Bandyopadhyay et al., 2015, 2018).

Tetracycline resistance

Even after the introduction of various new generation antimicrobials, perhaps tetracycline remained the most prescribed and used drugs because of its wide availability, the spectrum of activity and cost-effectiveness, although its toxicity is still a critical concern. Bryan et al. (2004) investigated on the tetracycline resistance pattern of the *E. coli* isolate from diverse human and animal sources — the study indicated a higher distribution of tetracycline resistance determinants among porcine (78%) and chicken (47%) *E. coli* predominantly driven by *tet*A and *tet*B genes. Such predominance of *tet*A and *tet*B was also recorded among GNB isolated from bovine mastitis in eastern India (Das et al., 2017). High prevalence of tetracycline resistance (∼77%) was recorded among the *Campylobacter* isolates from diverse cattle samples as reported by Premarathne et al. (2017). This trend was also noticed in poultry (Abdi Hachesoo et al., 2014).

Macrolide resistance

Macrolides, such as tylosin, tilmicosin and spiramycin, constitute the mainstay of therapy for chronic respiratory diseases in poultry. Furthermore, macrolides at subtherapeutic concentration are used for improving feed conversion and growth promotion. Such use was often considered the primary attributing factor for the emergence of erythromycin-resistant campylobacteriosis — as erythromycin is one of the few alternatives used for treating campylobacteriosis in human beings. Berrang et al. (2007) reported that feeding of subtherapeutic tylosin phosphate lowered the number of *Campylobacter* in broiler carcass; however, such treatment increased the overall proportion of erythromycin-resistant *Campylobacter*. Prolonged exposure of the chicken to tylosin in feed at a growth-promoting dose (0.05 g/kg feed) facilitated the development of erythromycin-resistant *Campylobacter jejuni* or *Campylobacter coli*, possibly triggered by activation of CmeABC, a multidrug efflux pump (Lin et al., 2007). Gerchman et al. (2011) reported a strong correlation between macrolide resistance and point mutations in 23S rRNA genes among *Mycoplasma gallisepticum* of broiler origin. A similar observation was made with regard to macrolide—lincosamide—resistant *Mycoplasma synoviae*, a common nuisance for causing respiratory infections and synovitis in chicken and turkey (Lysnyansky et al., 2015). Macrolide resistance has also remained a burgeoning problem in other food animals such as pigs and cattle possibly because of the introduction of long-acting injectable macrolide with a long half-life and subtherapeutic use of macrolide in feed formulation. Macrolide resistance was predominantly noted in *Brachyspira* apart from staphylococci isolated from pigs and streptococci from cattle (Pyörälä et al., 2014). In a separate study conducted in Tibetan pigs, macrolide resistance was reported in *Mycoplasma hyopneumoniae*, a common pathogen to cause porcine enzootic pneumonia (Qiu et al., 2017). Use of tylosin as growth promoter was reported to significantly increase the recovery of erythromycin-resistant *enterococci* in the pig farms (Jackson et al., 2004). Holman and Chénier, 2013 reported increasing detection of *erm* genes in pigs fed with tylosin, which has been further reiterated by Birkegård et al. (2017) by establishing a positive correlation between the use of macrolide and increased detection of resistance genes such as ermB and ermF in pigs. However, another study did not provide any such clue for the increased detection of macrolide—lincosamide—streptogramin B resistance phenotypes among the pathogens in the manure samples from swine farms with no AMU (Zhou et al., 2009). A recent report from Iran showed that a large number of *S. aureus* isolates from bovine mastitis were tylosin-resistant (~55%) (Bahraminia et al., 2017).

Colistin resistance

It was probably the detection of plasmid-mediated colistin resistance gene *mcr-1* which made a hue and cry on the AMU in animals. It was way back in 2015 when plasmid-mediated colistin resistance was reported from China and exuberent use of colistin in fattening pig and poultry sector was incriminated for such resistance (Liu et al., 2016). Thereafter a series of reports came from different parts of the world, which were discussed in detail in the chapter on colistin resistance. Recently, Ghafur et al. (2019) reported *mcr-1*-positive GNB from Indian food samples. As colistin is the last therapy available against the carbapenem-resistant pathogens, scientists and clinicians all over the world looked at colistin resistance quite seriously.

Scientists across the globe are more concerned about AMU and AMR in food animals because of their direct impact over public health. However, AMR is also a serious issue when it comes to companion animals such as dogs — possibly because of the frequent use of antibiotics or transfer of resistant pathogens from the human. Of late, dogs were reported as a reservoir of such pathogens from the Scandinavian countries, Africa and China (Li et al., 2017; Schaufler et al., 2015; Damborg et al., 2015). Moreover, hospitalized pets were also documented as carbapenem-resistant pathogens (Gentilini et al., 2018). We have detected NDM (New Delhi metallo-β-lactamase) -producing *E. coli* in dogs from India (Genbank: LC427671.1; KJ624023.1).

Resistant pathogens in agriculture sector

Use of antimicrobials is limited in agriculture crops and plants. In the United States, application of antibiotics in plants accounts for only 0.5% of total antimicrobial usage. Most of the antibiotics are applied on plants by simple spraying; hence, the applied antibiotics are drained to the soils gradually. Moreover, the antibiotics are degraded or metabolically biotransformed through degradation of soil microbes. The draining out of antibiotics from crops or plants is more during rainy seasons. However, the accumulation of drained out antibiotics in the soil and aquatic reservoirs need to be taken into account for their possible implication on the environment. Besides, antibiotics may flow in the plants through the application of manure and contamination of the agricultural field or crops with faecal material and effluent from farm animals (Rashmi, 2017). In most of the European countries, use of antibiotics in the plant is limited to spraying of streptomycin to treat fire blight disease in apple and pear trees, caused by the phytopathogenic enterobacterium *Erwinia amylovora* (Thanner et al., 2016). This is important to introspect, as streptomycin-resistant strains of *E. amylovora*, *Pseudomonas* spp. and *Xanthomonas campestris* were documented in plants and many of them shared resistant genes harboured by the human, animal or soil bacteria (Sundin and Wang, 2018).

Dissemination

The spread of drug resistance determinants was studied vividly both in animal and human pathogens. While the animals treated with antibiotics can become a potent reservoir of resistant bugs because of incomplete or inappropriate dosing and duration schedule, the grazing land, vegetables and fresh fruits contaminated with animal manure may also turn out to be a source of such pathogens (Yazdankhah et al., 2018; Ortega-Paredes et al., 2018). Humans may get infection either by consuming such contaminated animal or plant products or via direct contact (Madec et al., 2017; Carattoli, 2008). On the other hand, humans may also carry such pathogens especially when they consume antibiotics without prescription or medical supervision and they can spread to others in contact human or animals. This problem is more intense for patients with chronic ailments in the healthcare premises where they usually receive antibiotics for a prolonged period and can spread it to inmates within a confined area. Once discharged, they may also transmit the same to their relative, friends and neighbours. Travellers may also become carrier when they contract such pathogens from their hospital admission or community interaction in the countries where such resistant pathogens are endemic (Lääveri et al., 2018). How AMU in animals can adversely affect antimicrobial efficacy in the long run and how the environment may act as an important reservoir for spreading of such resistant bugs were already discussed in detail in separate chapters.

Plasmid, transposon or mobile genetic elements and integrons are known to play an important role in the spread of such resistance genes. Ajiboye et al. (2009) screened several human and animal isolates for understanding the distribution of mobile elements — integrons and gene cassettes. In this study, they have detected class 1 integrons more frequently with gene cassettes such as aminoglycoside adenyltransferase A (aadA) and dihydrofolate reductase A (dfrA) (Ajiboye et al., 2009). We got quite similar findings when we screened the ESBL-producing *E. coli* and *Klebsiella pneumonia* from food animals (Kar et al., 2015; Koovapra et al., 2016). However, a putative transposable element, *ISEcp*-1, was responsible for mobilization and expression of CTX-M, the predominant ESBL gene, which was also previously observed by other workers from India (Arunagiri et al., 2013) or other countries (Tian et al., 2011). Conversely, it is not uncommon to see integron harbouring CTX-M genes as recorded by Dropa et al. (2015) in Brazil.

Human health impact

The use of antibiotics in food animals is often linked to the development of drug resistance in human and the exposure seems to be the highest at the places where intensive animal rearing is in practice. In many countries, the use of anti-microbials is four times higher than that in human being. Antibiotics used in animals may exert impact over human health in two possible ways.

Drug-resistant pathogens developed in animals may be transmitted to a human directly. LA-MRSA, which is equally pathogenic to hospital-associated MRSA emerged and adapted in animals, can infect human beings. LA-MRSA CC398 has been known to cause infection in livestock handlers; however, in recent days such infection was noticed among the rural people living in the vicinity of livestock farms possibly because of spillover from animals (Larsen et al., 2016). A recent study on LA-MRSA CC1 spa type t177 in nine Norwegian pig herds indicated that such MRSA strain had been possibly introduced in one farm by some infected farm worker and later the strain spread to other farms (Elstrøm et al., 2019). In addition to direct contact, foodborne transmission or transmission via environmental route or setting is also possible. Once established in the gut microbiome of the consumers/human beings, such resistant bugs may transfer their resistance determinants to other pathogenic strains. Many studies claimed foodborne transmission of drug-resistant *Salmonella* and *E. coli* from animals to human beings (Collignon, 2012).

Secondly, the antibiotic residue present in the consumable animal products — milk, meat, eggs — may expose the microbiome of the consumers to a low concentration of antibiotics for a prolonged period — which may be sufficient to exert selection pressure for development of resistant bugs. This is particularly important where critically important anti-microbials are used in animal farming, more importantly, when such antibiotics are used for the prophylactic purpose or for growth promotion and if the withdrawal period is not taken into account. Antimicrobial residue in poultry meat beyond the permissible limit has become a serious cause of concern (Muaz et al., 2018). Several studies from India indicated the presence of antibiotic residue in milk. Kumarswamy et al. (2018) reported the presence of β-lactam, tetracycline and enrofloxacin (Kumarswamy et al., 2018). Another study by Lundén (2015) reported that more than 88% of the samples were positive for neomycin or streptomycin and 23% for sulphonamides in addition to other antimicrobials such as β-lactam, macrolide and chloramphenicol in milk samples from Assam, India. A recent study conducted in Pakistan revealed the residue of antimicrobials such as tetracycline, ampicillin and streptomycin in poultry meat (Sajid et al., 2016). Another study from Korea showed that amoxicillin (15.5%), enrofloxacin (12.1%) and sulfamethoxazole (10.3%) were the most detectable antibiotics in poultry meat (Lee et al., 2018). Furthermore, Yamaguchi et al. (2015) detected antibiotics such as sulfonamides, fluoroquinolones and tilmicosin in pork, chicken and beef samples in Vietnam, of which sulfaclozine and fluoroquinolones were mainly detected in chicken samples and sulfamethazine in pork samples.

In general, infection with drug-resistant pathogens may lead to increased hospital stay/treatment duration, treatment expenses and ultimately increased mortality in human patients. Moreover, as suggested by a recent study, increased antibiotic exposure increases the risk of weight gain and obesity (Dutton et al., 2017).

Preventive strategy

AMR is probably the biggest threat faced by human civilization which has a far-reaching consequence beyond human or animal health. Apart from its catastrophic impact with extensive mortality and morbidity, the global economy will have a severe setback with around 28 million people slipped under poverty. Use of antimicrobials is thought the single most important driver for AMR; thus, O'Neil commission gave several recommendations to reduce the antimicrobial consumption (O'Neill et al., 2016).

1. Massive global campaigning on the menacing effect of AMR, so as to increase awareness and knowledge and also to stimulate appropriate governance.
2. Better infection, prevention and control measures with an objective to reduce the infection burden and its spread.
3. Reduce the AMU in agriculture to facilitate the reduction of antimicrobial selection pressure.
4. Improved surveillance and monitoring system to have reliable data on AMR in human, animal, agriculture and environment sectors.
5. Development of new and rapid diagnostics so that the antibiotics may be used or prescribed more wisely and selectively.
6. Development and use of vaccines to prevent the occurrence of infectious diseases in the livestock and companion animals.

Of late, the European Medicines Agency and the European Food Safety Authority gave certain outlines to reduce the AMU in animal husbandry (Murphy et al., 2017) — all were to categorically reduce the use of antimicrobials and development of AMR. The recommendations stressed on the development of appropriate strategies to monitor the burden of AMR development and antimicrobial consumption as well as target-oriented national strategies to reduce the AMU. Apart from an on-farm health plan, proper and improved husbandry and management procedures to reduce infection burden in animals and use of reliable diagnostics, the recommendations also emphasized on the need of responsible veterinarians for a judicious antibiotic prescription.

It is undeniable that we have only limited and effective alternatives against resistant bugs. Moreover, there are very few alternatives with proven clinical effectiveness when it comes to the treatment of diseases such as mastitis, metritis, diarrhoea and respiratory illness in animals where AMU in more. Nonetheless, some alternative approaches seem to have a promising impact in the near future. Details regarding these alternatives were discussed in a separate chapter.

CRISPR/Cas gene editing system

Because of their precision-guided ability to edit or eliminate the foreign or unwanted gene/genetic materials, CRISPR/Cas gene editing system may have a bright prospect in combating the rising concern of AMR. The target specificity of the system may help overcome the problem of destroying the commensals or healthy microbiome along with the pathogens, which is a usual outcome of conventional antimicrobial therapy. At the same time, the system may be exploited to transform resistant bacteria into sensitive one by eliminating the resistant genes; such approach was taken by a group, for resensitization of ESBL producers to β-lactams (Kim et al., 2015). Thus in the near future, its use as alternative antimicrobial cannot be undermined (Bikard and Barrangou, 2017).

Antibiotic conjugate

Antibiotics are fast acting with a short life span in their free form. Therefore, to increase the efficacy of antibiotics, conjugated form is often described. It can overcome the problem of limited bioavailability, shorter half-life, toxicity and repeated dosing and thus avert the adverse effect on patients (Cal et al., 2017).

Bacteriophage

Bacteriophages are long known for their potential antibacterial activities and thus tried for their efficacy against a wide range of bacterial pathogens. Genetically engineered phage-based delivery system was recently devised to combat the *S. aureus* infections (Park et al., 2017). Bovine mastitis, which is often thought for being refractory to antimicrobial therapy, was often investigated for phage therapy (Ganaie et al., 2018). Similarly, workers have also investigated the efficacy of phage therapy in bovine diarrhoea (Anand et al., 2015).

Antimicrobial peptides

The antimicrobial peptides are positively charged small amphipathic peptides which are active against a wide range of pathogens including bacteria. Despite intensive research on AMP (antimicrobial peptide) for a few decades, it is yet to gain a foothold for being effective clinically because of their instability in physiological condition and huge expenditure towards their production. Of late, Lam et al. (2016) developed structurally nanoengineered antimicrobial peptide polymers which are less toxic and more effective as antimicrobial agents (Lam et al., 2016).

Eubiotics, which include probiotics, prebiotics, organic acids, exogenous enzymes, essential oils and herbs, are now preferred as a growth promoter in animal feed in place of antibiotics (Dhama et al., 2014). In addition, enhancing host immunity and better infection control measures are the key aspects to reduce the infectious disease burden in animals, which can subsequently reduce AMR. Oral immunotherapy using chicken egg yolk immunoglobulin is known to reduce bacterial or viral infection. Use of herbs such as *Tinospora cordifolia* is also known to act as an effective immuno-modulator (More and Pai, 2017). Dietary supplementation of zinc was reported to reduce intestinal diseases in piglets as reported by many workers and thus dietary zinc may be a suitable alternative to conventional antimicrobial therapy in piglet diarrhoea (Mukhopadhya et al., 2019).

References

Abdi Hachesoo, B., Khoshbakht, R., Sharifi Yazdi, H., Tabatabaei, M., Hosseinzadeh, S., Asasi, K., 2014. Tetracycline resistance genes in *Campylobacter jejuni* and *C. Coli* isolated from poultry carcasses. Jundishapur Journal of Microbiology 7, e12129. https://doi.org/10.5812/jjm.12129.

Ajiboye, R.M., Solberg, O.D., Lee, B.M., Raphael, E., DebRoy, C., Riley, L.W., 2009. Global spread of mobile antimicrobial drug resistance determinants in human and animal *Escherichia coli* and Salmonella strains causing community-acquired infections. Clinical Infectious Diseases 49, 365–371. https://doi.org/10.1086/600301.

Ali, T., ur Rahman, S., Zhang, L., Shahid, M., Zhang, S., Liu, G., et al., 2016. ESBL-producing *Escherichia coli* from cows suffering mastitis in China contain clinical class 1 integrons with CTX-M linked to ISCR1. Frontiers in Microbiology 7. https://doi.org/10.3389/fmicb.2016.01931.

Anand, T., Vaid, R.K., Bera, B.C., Barua, S., Riyesh, T., Virmani, N., et al., 2015. Isolation and characterization of a bacteriophage with broad host range, displaying potential in preventing bovine diarrhoea. Virus Genes 51, 315–321. https://doi.org/10.1007/s11262-015-1222-9.

Arunagiri, K., Aparna, V., Menaka, K., Sekar, B., 2013. Characterization of ESBLs and ISEcp1 insertion sequences from *Klebsiella pneumoniae* and *Escherichia coli*. in a tertiary hospital in India. International Journal of Pharmacy and Pharmaceutical Sciences 5, 654–658.

Bahraminia, F., Emadi, S.R., Emaneini, M., Farzaneh, N., Rad, M., Khoramian, B., 2017. A high prevalence of tylosin resistance among *Staphylococcus aureus* strains isolated from bovine mastitis. Veterinary Research Forum an International Quarterly Journal 8, 121–125.

Bandyopadhyay, S., Samanta, I., Bhattacharyya, D., Nanda, P.K., Kar, D., Chowdhury, J., et al., 2015. Co-infection of methicillin-resistant *Staphylococcus epidermidis*, methicillin-resistant *Staphylococcus aureus* and extended spectrum β-lactamase producing *Escherichia coli* in bovine mastitis — three cases reported from India. Veterinary Quarterly 35, 56–61. https://doi.org/10.1080/01652176.2014.984365.

Bandyopadhyay, S., Banerjee, J., Bhattacharyya, D., Samanta, I., Mahanti, A., Dutta, T.K., et al., 2018. Genomic identity of fluoroquinolone-resistant bla CTX-M -15 -type ESBL and pMAmpC β-lactamase producing *Klebsiella pneumoniae* from buffalo milk, India. Microbial Drug Resistance 24. https://doi.org/10.1089/mdr.2017.0368 mdr.2017.0368.

Berrang, M.E., Ladely, S.R., Meinersmann, R.J., Fedorka-Cray, P.J., 2007. Subtherapeutic tylosin phosphate in broiler feed affects *Campylobacter* on carcasses during processing. Poultry Science 86, 1229–1233. https://doi.org/10.1093/ps/86.6.1229.

Bhattacharyya, D., Banerjee, J., Bandyopadhyay, S., Mondal, B., Nanda, P.K., Samanta, I., et al., 2016. First report on vancomycin-resistant *Staphylococcus aureus* in bovine and caprine milk. Microbial Drug Resistance 22, 675–681. https://doi.org/10.1089/mdr.2015.0330.

Bikard, D., Barrangou, R., 2017. Using CRISPR-Cas systems as antimicrobials. Current Opinion in Microbiology 37, 155–160. https://doi.org/10.1016/j.mib.2017.08.005.

Birkegård, A.C., Halasa, T., Græsbøll, K., Clasen, J., Folkesson, A., Toft, N., 2017. Association between selected antimicrobial resistance genes and antimicrobial exposure in Danish pig farms. Scientific Reports 7, 9683. https://doi.org/10.1038/s41598-017-10092-9.

Brower, C.H., Mandal, S., Hayer, S., Sran, M., Zehra, A., Patel, S.J., et al., 2017. The prevalence of extended-spectrum beta-lactamase-producing multidrug-resistant *Escherichia coli* in poultry chickens and variation according to farming practices in Punjab, India. Environmental Health Perspectives 125, 77015. https://doi.org/10.1289/EHP292.

Bryan, A., Shapir, N., Sadowsky, M.J., 2004. Frequency and distribution of tetracycline resistance genes in genetically diverse, nonselected, and nonclinical *Escherichia coli* strains isolated from diverse human and animal sources. Applied and Environmental Microbiology 70, 2503—2507. https://doi.org/10.1128/AEM.70.4.2503-2507.2004.

Cal, P.M.S.D., Matos, M.J., Bernardes, G.J.L., 2017. Trends in therapeutic drug conjugates for bacterial diseases: a patent review. Expert Opinion on Therapeutic Patents 27, 179—189. https://doi.org/10.1080/13543776.2017.1259411.

Carattoli, A., 2008. Animal reservoirs for extended spectrum β-lactamase producers. Clinical Microbiology and Infections 14, 117—123. https://doi.org/10.1111/j.1469-0691.2007.01851.x.

Collignon, P., 2012. Antibiotic resistance in human Salmonella isolates are related to animal strains. Proceedings of the Royal Society B: Biological Sciences 279, 2922—2923. https://doi.org/10.1098/rspb.2012.0349.

Dahmen, S., Métayer, V., Gay, E., Madec, J.-Y., Haenni, M., 2013. Characterization of extended-spectrum beta-lactamase (ESBL)-carrying plasmids and clones of *Enterobacteriaceae* causing cattle mastitis in France. Veterinary Microbiology 162, 793—799. https://doi.org/10.1016/j.vetmic.2012.10.015.

Damborg, P., Morsing, M.K., Petersen, T., Bortolaia, V., Guardabassi, L., 2015. CTX-M-1 and CTX-M-15-producing *Escherichia coli* in dog faeces from public gardens. Acta Veterinaria Scandinavica 57, 83. https://doi.org/10.1186/s13028-015-0174-3.

Das, A., Guha, C., Biswas, U., Jana, P.S., Chatterjee, A., Samanta, I., 2017. Detection of emerging antibiotic resistance in bacteria isolated from sub-clinical mastitis in cattle in West Bengal. Veterinary World 10, 517—520. https://doi.org/10.14202/vetworld.2017.517-520.

Dhama, K., Tiwari, R., Khan, R.U., Chakraborty, S., Gopi, M., Karthik, K., et al., 2014. Growth promoters and novel feed additives improving poultry production and health, bioactive principles and beneficial applications: the trends and advances-a review. International Journal of Pharmacology 10, 129—159. https://doi.org/10.3923/ijp.2014.129.159.

Dobiasova, H., Dolejska, M., Jamborova, I., Brhelova, E., Blazkova, L., Papousek, I., et al., 2013. Extended spectrum beta-lactamase and fluoroquinolone resistance genes and plasmids among *Escherichia coli* isolates from zoo animals, Czech Republic. FEMS Microbiology Ecology 85, 604—611. https://doi.org/10.1111/1574-6941.12149.

Dropa, M., Balsalobre, L.C., Lincopan, N., Matté, G.R., Matté, M.H., 2015. Complex class 1 integrons harboring CTX-M-2-encoding genes in clinical *Enterobacteriaceae* from a hospital in Brazil. Journal of Infection in Developing Countries 9, 890—897. https://doi.org/10.3855/jidc.6241.

Dutton, H., Doyle, M.-A., Buchan, C.A., Mohammad, S., Adamo, K.B., Shorr, R., et al., 2017. Antibiotic exposure and risk of weight gain and obesity: protocol for a systematic review. Systematic Reviews 6, 169. https://doi.org/10.1186/s13643-017-0565-9.

Elstrøm, P., Grøntvedt, C.A., Gabrielsen, C., Stegger, M., Angen, Ø., Åmdal, S., et al., 2019. Livestock-associated MRSA CC1 in Norway; introduction to pig farms, zoonotic transmission, and eradication. Frontiers in Microbiology 10. https://doi.org/10.3389/fmicb.2019.00139.

Ganaie, M.Y., Qureshi, S., Kashoo, Z., Wani, S.A., Hussain, M.I., Kumar, R., et al., 2018. Isolation and characterization of two lytic bacteriophages against *Staphylococcus aureus* from India: newer therapeutic agents against Bovine mastitis. Veterinary Research Communications 42, 289—295. https://doi.org/10.1007/s11259-018-9736-y.

Gentilini, F., Turba, M.E., Pasquali, F., Mion, D., Romagnoli, N., Zambon, E., et al., 2018. Hospitalized pets as a source of carbapenem-resistance. Frontiers in Microbiology 9. https://doi.org/10.3389/fmicb.2018.02872.

Gerchman, I., Levisohn, S., Mikula, I., Manso-Silván, L., Lysnyansky, I., 2011. Characterization of in vivo-acquired resistance to macrolides of *Mycoplasma gallisepticum* strains isolated from poultry. Veterinary Research 42. https://doi.org/10.1186/1297-9716-42-90.

Ghafur, A., Shankar, C., GnanaSoundari, P., Venkatesan, M., Mani, D., Thirunarayanan, M.A., et al., 2019. Detection of chromosomal and plasmid-mediated mechanisms of colistin resistance in *Escherichia coli* and *Klebsiella pneumoniae* from Indian food samples. Journal of Global Antimicrobial Resistance 16, 48—52. https://doi.org/10.1016/j.jgar.2018.09.005.

Ghatak, S., Singha, A., Sen, A., Guha, C., Ahuja, A., Bhattacharjee, U., et al., 2013. Detection of New Delhi metallo-beta-lactamase and extended-spectrum beta-lactamase genes in *Escherichia coli* isolated from mastitic milk samples. Transboundary and Emerging Diseases 60, 385—389. https://doi.org/10.1111/tbed.12119.

Holman, D.B., Chénier, M.R., 2013. Impact of subtherapeutic administration of tylosin and chlortetracycline on antimicrobial resistance in farrow-to-finish swine. FEMS Microbiology Ecology 85, 1—13. https://doi.org/10.1111/1574-6941.12093.

Jackson, C.R., Fedorka-Cray, P.J., Barrett, J.B., Ladely, S.R., 2004. Effects of tylosin use on erythromycin resistance in enterococci isolated from swine. Applied and Environmental Microbiology 70, 4205—4210. https://doi.org/10.1128/AEM.70.7.4205-4210.2004.

Kar, D., Bandyopadhyay, S., Bhattacharyya, D., Samanta, I., Mahanti, A., Nanda, P.K., et al., 2015. Molecular and phylogenetic characterization of multidrug resistant extended spectrum beta-lactamase producing *Escherichia coli* isolated from poultry and cattle in Odisha, India. Infection, Genetics and Evolution 29, 82—90. https://doi.org/10.1016/j.meegid.2014.11.003.

Kim, J.S., Cho, D.H., Park, M., Chung, W.J., Shin, D., Ko, K.S., et al., 2015. Crispr/cas9-mediated re-sensitization of antibiotic-resistant *Escherichia coli* harboring extended-spectrum β-lactamases. Journal of Microbiology and Biotechnology 26, 394—401. https://doi.org/10.4014/jmb.1508.08080.

Köck, R., Daniels-Haardt, I., Becker, K., Mellmann, A., Friedrich, A.W., Mevius, D., et al., 2018. Carbapenem-resistant *Enterobacteriaceae* in wildlife, food-producing, and companion animals: a systematic review. Clinical Microbiology and Infections. https://doi.org/10.1016/j.cmi.2018.04.004.

Koovapra, S., Bandyopadhyay, S., Das, G., Bhattacharyya, D., Banerjee, J., Mahanti, A., et al., 2016. Molecular signature of extended spectrum β-lactamase producing *Klebsiella pneumoniae* isolated from bovine milk in eastern and north-eastern India. Infection, Genetics and Evolution 44, 395—402. https://doi.org/10.1016/j.meegid.2016.07.032.

Kumarswamy, N., Latha, C., Menon, V., Sethukekshmi, C., Mercy, K., 2018. Detection of antibiotic residues in raw cow milk in Thrissur, India. Pharmaceutical Innovation Journal 7, 452—454.

Lääveri, T., Vlot, J.A., van Dam, A.P., Häkkinen, H.K., Sonder, G.J.B., Visser, L.G., et al., 2018. Extended-spectrum beta-lactamase-producing *Enterobacteriaceae* (ESBL-PE) among travellers to Africa: destination-specific data pooled from three European prospective studies. BMC Infectious Diseases 18, 341. https://doi.org/10.1186/s12879-018-3245-z.

Lam, S.J., O'Brien-Simpson, N.M., Pantarat, N., Sulistio, A., Wong, E.H.H., Chen, Y.-Y., et al., 2016. Combating multidrug-resistant gram-negative bacteria with structurally nanoengineered antimicrobial peptide polymers. Nature Microbiology 1, 16162. https://doi.org/10.1038/nmicrobiol.2016.162.

Larsen, J., Stegger, M., Andersen, P.S., Petersen, A., Larsen, A.R., Westh, H., et al., 2016. Evidence for human adaptation and foodborne transmission of livestock-associated methicillin-resistant *Staphylococcus aureus*. Clinical Infectious Diseases 63, 1349−1352. https://doi.org/10.1093/cid/ciw532.

Lee, H.-J., Cho, S.-H., Shin, D., Kang, H.-S., 2018. Prevalence of antibiotic residues and antibiotic resistance in isolates of chicken meat in Korea. Korean Journal for Food Science of Animal Resources 38, 1055−1063. https://doi.org/10.5851/kosfa.2018.e39.

Li, S., Liu, J., Zhou, Y., Miao, Z., 2017. Characterization of ESBL-producing *Escherichia coli* recovered from companion dogs in Tai'an, China. Journal of Infection in Developing Countries 11, 282. https://doi.org/10.3855/jidc.8138.

Li, P., Liu, D., Zhang, X., Tuo, H., Lei, C., Xie, X., et al., 2019. Characterization of plasmid-mediated quinolone resistance in gram-negative bacterial strains from animals and humans in China. Microbial Drug Resistance. https://doi.org/10.1089/mdr.2018.0405 mdr.2018.0405.

Lin, J., Yan, M., Sahin, O., Pereira, S., Chang, Y.-J., Zhang, Q., 2007. Effect of macrolide usage on emergence of erythromycin-resistant *Campylobacter* isolates in chickens. Antimicrobial Agents and Chemotherapy 51, 1678−1686. https://doi.org/10.1128/AAC.01411-06.

Liu, Y.-Y.Y., Wang, Y., Walsh, T.R., Yi, L.-X.X., Zhang, R., Spencer, J., et al., 2016. Emergence of plasmid-mediated colistin resistance mechanism MCR-1 in animals and human beings in China: a microbiological and molecular biological study. The Lancet Infectious Diseases 16, 161−168. https://doi.org/10.1016/S1473-3099(15)00424-7.

Liu, X., Liu, H., Wang, L., Peng, Q., Li, Y., Zhou, H., et al., 2018. Molecular characterization of extended-spectrum β-lactamase-producing multidrug resistant *Escherichia coli* from swine in Northwest China. Frontiers in Microbiology 9. https://doi.org/10.3389/fmicb.2018.01756.

Lundén, H., 2015. What's in the milk? Aflatoxin and antibiotic residues in cow's milk in Assam. Sweidish University of Agricultural Science, Uppasala. https://stud.epsilon.slu.se/8196/7/lunden_h_160112.pdf.

Lysnyansky, I., Gerchman, I., Flaminio, B., Catania, S., 2015. Decreased susceptibility to macrolide−lincosamide in *Mycoplasma synoviae* is associated with mutations in 23S ribosomal RNA. Microbial Drug Resistance 21, 581−589. https://doi.org/10.1089/mdr.2014.0290.

Madec, J.-Y., Haenni, M., Nordmann, P., Poirel, L., 2017. Extended-spectrum β-lactamase/AmpC- and carbapenemase-producing *Enterobacteriaceae* in animals: a threat for humans? Clinical Microbiology and Infections 23, 826−833. https://doi.org/10.1016/j.cmi.2017.01.013.

Mahanti, A., Ghosh, P., Samanta, I., Joardar, S.N., Bandyopadhyay, S., Bhattacharyya, D., et al., 2018. Prevalence of CTX-M-producing *Klebsiella* spp. in broiler, kuroiler, and indigenous poultry in West Bengal state, India. Microbial Drug Resistance 24, 299−306. https://doi.org/10.1089/mdr.2016.0096.

Mandakini, R., Dutta, T.K., Chingtham, S., Roychoudhury, P., Samanta, I., Joardar, S.N., et al., 2014. ESBL-producing Shiga-toxigenic *E. coli* (STEC) associated with piglet diarrhoea in India. Tropical Animal Health and Production 47, 377−381. https://doi.org/10.1007/s11250-014-0731-1.

Mandakini, R., Dutta, TK., Chingtham, S., Roychoudhury, P., Samanta, I., Joardar, SN., Pachauau, AR., Chandra, R., 2015 Feb. ESBL-producing Shiga-toxigenic E. coli (STEC) associated with piglet diarrhoea in India. Trop Anim Health Prod 47 (2), 377−381. https://doi.org/10.1007/s11250-014-0731-1.

More, P., Pai, K., 2017. Effect of *Tinospora cordifolia* (Guduchi) on the phagocytic and pinocytic activity of murine macrophages in vitro. Indian Journal of Experimental Biology 55, 21−26.

Muaz, K., Riaz, M., Akhtar, S., Park, S., Ismail, A., 2018. Antibiotic residues in chicken meat: global prevalence, threats, and decontamination strategies: a review. Journal of Food Protection 81, 619−627. https://doi.org/10.4315/0362-028X.JFP-17-086.

Mukhopadhya, A., O'Doherty, J.V., Sweeney, T., 2019. A combination of yeast beta-glucan and milk hydrolysate is a suitable alternative to zinc oxide in the race to alleviate post-weaning diarrhoea in piglets. Scientific Reports 9, 616. https://doi.org/10.1038/s41598-018-37004-9.

Murphy, D., Ricci, A., Auce, Z., Beechinor, J.G., Bergendahl, H., Breathnach, R., et al., 2017. EMA and EFSA joint scientific opinion on measures to reduce the need to use antimicrobial agents in animal husbandry in the European Union, and the resulting impacts on food safety (RONAFA). EFSA Journal 15. https://doi.org/10.2903/j.efsa.2017.4666.

Ortega-Paredes, D., Barba, P., Mena-López, S., Espinel, N., Zurita, J., 2018. *Escherichia coli* hyperepidemic clone ST410-A harboring bla CTX-M-15 isolated from fresh vegetables in a municipal market in Quito-Ecuador. International Journal of Food Microbiology 280, 41−45. https://doi.org/10.1016/j.ijfoodmicro.2018.04.037.

ONeill, J., et al., 2016. Tackling drug-resistant infections globally: final report and recommendations. Review of Antimicrobial Resistance 84.

Park, J.Y., Moon, B.Y., Park, J.W., Thornton, J.A., Park, Y.H., Seo, K.S., 2017. Genetic engineering of a temperate phage-based delivery system for CRISPR/Cas9 antimicrobials against *Staphylococcus aureus*. Scientific Reports 7, 44929. https://doi.org/10.1038/srep44929.

Premarathne, J.M.K.J.K., Anuar, A.S., Thung, T.Y., Satharasinghe, D.A., Jambari, N.N., Abdul-Mutalib, N.-A., et al., 2017. Prevalence and antibiotic resistance against tetracycline in *Campylobacter jejuni* and *C. Coli* in cattle and beef meat from Selangor, Malaysia. Frontiers in Microbiology 8. https://doi.org/10.3389/fmicb.2017.02254.

Pyörälä, S., Baptiste, K.E., Catry, B., van Duijkeren, E., Greko, C., Moreno, M.A., et al., 2014. Macrolides and lincosamides in cattle and pigs: use and development of antimicrobial resistance. The Veterinary Journal 200, 230−239. https://doi.org/10.1016/j.tvjl.2014.02.028.

Qiao, J., Alali, W.Q., Liu, J., Wang, Y., Chen, S., Cui, S., et al., 2018. Prevalence of virulence genes in extended-spectrum β-lactamases (ESBLs)-producing Salmonella in retail raw chicken in China. Journal of Food Science 83, 1048−1052. https://doi.org/10.1111/1750-3841.14111.

Qiu, G., Rui, Y., Zhang, J., Zhang, L., Huang, S., Wu, Q., et al., 2017. Macrolide-resistance selection in Tibetan pigs with a high load of *Mycoplasma hyopneumoniae*. Microbial Drug Resistance 24, 1043–1049. https://doi.org/10.1089/mdr.2017.0254.

Rashmi, H.B., 2017. Antibiotic resistance: role of fruits and vegetables in the food basket. International Journal of Pure and Applied Bioscience 5, 169–173. https://doi.org/10.18782/2320-7051.5327.

Saishu, N., Ozaki, H., Murase, T., 2014. CTX-M-type extended-spectrum β-lactamase-producing *Klebsiella pneumoniae* isolated from cases of bovine mastitis in Japan. Journal of Veterinary Medical Science 76, 1153–1156. https://doi.org/10.1292/jvms.13-0120.

Sajid, A., Kashif, N., Kifayat, N., Ahmad, S., 2016. Detection of antibiotic residues in poultry meat. Pakistan Journal of Pharmaceutical Sciences 29, 1691–1694.

Samanta, I., Joardar, S.N., Mahanti, A., Bandyopadhyay, S., Sar, T.K., Dutta, T.K., 2015. Approaches to characterize extended spectrum beta-lactamase/beta-lactamase producing *Escherichia coli* in healthy organized vis-a-vis backyard farmed pigs in India. Infection, Genetics and Evolution 36, 224–230. https://doi.org/10.1016/j.meegid.2015.09.021.

Samanta, A., Mahanti, A., Chatterjee, S., Joardar, S.N., Bandyopadhyay, S., Sar, T.K., et al., 2018. Pig farm environment as a source of beta-lactamase or AmpC-producing *Klebsiella pneumoniae* and *Escherichia coli*. Annals of Microbiology 68, 781–791. https://doi.org/10.1007/s13213-018-1387-2.

Schaufler, K., Bethe, A., Lübke-Becker, A., Ewers, C., Kohn, B., Wieler, L.H., et al., 2015. Putative connection between zoonotic multiresistant extended-spectrum beta-lactamase (ESBL)-producing *Escherichia coli* in dog feces from a veterinary campus and clinical isolates from dogs. African Journal of Disability 5. https://doi.org/10.3402/iee.v5.25334.

Sundin, G.W., Wang, N., 2018. Antibiotic resistance in plant-pathogenic bacteria. Annual Review of Phytopathology 56, 161–180. https://doi.org/10.1146/annurev-phyto-080417-045946.

Thanner, S., Drissner, D., Walsh, F., 2016. Antimicrobial resistance in agriculture. MBio 7. https://doi.org/10.1128/mBio.02227-15.

Tian, S.F., Chu, Y.Z., Chen, B.Y., Nian, H., Shang, H., 2011. ISEcp1 element in association with bla CTX-M genes of *E. coli* that produce extended-spectrum β-lactamase among the elderly in community settings. Enfermedades Infecciosas y Microbiologia Clinica 29, 731–734. https://doi.org/10.1016/j.eimc.2011.07.011.

Van Boeckel, T.P., Brower, C., Gilbert, M., Grenfell, B.T., Levin, S.A., Robinson, T.P., et al., 2015. Global trends in antimicrobial use in food animals. Proceedings of the National Academy of Sciences of the United States of America 112, 5649–5654. https://doi.org/10.1073/pnas.1503141112.

Yamaguchi, T., Okihashi, M., Harada, K., Konishi, Y., Uchida, K., Do, M.H.N., et al., 2015. Antibiotic residue monitoring results for pork, chicken, and beef samples in Vietnam in 2012–2013. Journal of Agricultural and Food Chemistry 63, 5141–5145. https://doi.org/10.1021/jf505254y.

Yang, F., Zhang, K., Zhi, S., Li, J., Tian, X., Gu, Y., et al., 2019. High prevalence and dissemination of β-lactamase genes in swine farms in northern China. The Science of the Total Environment 651, 2507–2513. https://doi.org/10.1016/j.scitotenv.2018.10.144.

Yazdankhah, S., Grahek-Ogden, D., Hjeltnes, B., Langsrud, S., Lassen, J., Norström, M., et al., 2018. Assessment of antimicrobial resistance in the food chains in Norway. European Journal of Nutrition and Food Safety 8, 237–239. https://doi.org/10.9734/EJNFS/2018/43854.

Zhou, Z., Raskin, L., Zilles, J.L., 2009. Macrolide resistance in microorganisms at antimicrobial-free swine farms. Applied and Environmental Microbiology 75, 5814–5820. https://doi.org/10.1128/AEM.00977-09.

Chapter 4

Emergence of antimicrobial resistant bacteria in aquaculture

Chapter outline

Background

There has been a sea change in the aquaculture industry in the last two decades with its dramatic growth and the way it catered the need for world food requirement. Because of quality dietary proteins, essential fatty acid, micronutrients and minerals, fish consumption has been increased manifold both in developed and in the developing countries. To meet the increasing demand of the growing consumers, aquaculture has grown more rapidly than any other agribusiness like terrestrial food animal production. With the increase in consumption of fishes, there has also been a significant increase in the production of high-value species of shrimp, salmon and bivalves and various other aquatic species (finfish, crustaceans, molluscs and others) across the globe with intensive aquaculture practise (Nakamura, 2006; Gopakumar, 2003). In 2014, about 70.5 million tonnes of foodfish and 26.1 million tons of aquatic algae were produced, indicating the rapid growth of aquaculture and within 40 years from 1962 to 2002, the contribution of aquaculture to fish consumption increased 10-fold. European aquaculture production is all set to reach 4 million tonnes by 2030 (Food and Agriculture Oraganization of the United Nations, 2016; Watts et al., 2017). On the other hand, the Asia-Pacific region contributed significantly in the global aquaculture production with region's capture fisheries totalled 44.7 million tonnes in 2002 (Nadarajah and Flaaten, 2017). In India, the total fish production during 2017—18 is estimated to be 12.60 million metric tonnes, which constitute about 6.3% of the global fish production (Anonymous, 2018a). World bank data suggested that total fish production in China in 2016 grew up to 81,500,000.00 metric tons from 3,085,600.00 metric tons in 1960 (Anonymous). This shows the peace at which the aquaculture is growing all over the world.

Like in other food-producing animals, the problem of antimicrobial resistance has also been cropped up in aquaculture despite the controls and regulation adopted by many countries (Smith, 2008; Cabello et al., 2016). This problem needs introspection in the developing countries where intensive aquaculture has gained massive momentum in the recent past, particularly in the Asia-Pacific region, and the regulation on antimicrobial usage in aquaculture is less stringent. Because of some inherent peculiarities, the problem of AMR (antimicrobial resistance) in aquaculture is quite unique and should be analysed from a different perspective — the antibiotics are dispersed in an aquatic system at relatively higher concentration when compared to livestock; fishes being physiologically compromised cannot metabolize most of the antibiotics and release active components in the environment; about 70%—80% of the drugs applied in aquaculture are dispersed in water system; all together it becomes the hotbed for the emergence and the persistence of AMR (Santos and Ramos, 2018).

Use of antimicrobials in aquaculture

Aquaculture is defined as the production of aquatic animals and plants within confined aquatic environment. In most circumstances, it is not possible to directly administer drugs individually. Therefore, the drugs including antibiotics are applied into the culture water in the form of mass medication — the practise escalates the chance of nontarget organisms being exposed to unnecessary antibiotics and thereby leads to the increased burden of antimicrobial resistance and toxicity (Korostynska et al., 2016). With growing demands for fish and fish products, it is necessary to enhance fish production and preserve their market value. However, there has been a shift towards semiintensive and intensive farming system from extensive aquaculture to ensure higher productivity and this ultimately leads to nutrient pollution and higher stocking density. Moreover, inadequate supply of clean water, use of animal manure and human waste as feed in many farms and contamination with waste products because of inadequate sewage treatment deteriorate the water quality substantially to provide a congenial environment for the fish pathogens (Strauss, Bardach, Santerre). Thus, in the countries where there is no stringent regulation, antimicrobials are used prophylactically to combat outbreaks of the infectious diseases that can severely impair the rate and quality of fish production. On the other hand in developed countries such as the United States, majority of fish farming enterprises are practised in closed infrastructures such as pond-like or tank structures. As the large commercial ponds are not regularly drained, the antibiotic residue may continue to sustain at a relatively high level affecting the growing fish and facilitating the resistant pathogens (Bryan et al., 2006). Besides, use of antimicrobials and their efficacy in aquaculture system depends on various factors such as disease burden of the particular farming system, diversity of the pathogens, their antibiotic sensitivity, water quality including salinity and other factors such as temperature and photoperiod.

Ecological factors are important with regard to the potency and stability of antibiotics in the aquatic environment. Presence of divalent cations such as Ca^{2+} and Mg^{2+} in marine water diminishes the biological activity of antimicrobials such as oxytetracycline, quinolones, flumequine, and oxolinic acid. Molecules such as oxytetracycline and quinolones are easily degraded photochemically and rapidly deactivated with the formation of complexes with divalent cations in seawater or binding to sediment and associated organic matter (Lunestad and Goksøyr, 1990; Leal et al., 2017).

Little information is available regarding the amounts of antimicrobials used in aquaculture as only a few countries used to monitor it in a regular manner. However, the usage of antimicrobials in aquaculture varies widely among countries. In Norway or Scotland, level of antibiotic use in aquaculture is about 0.02—0.39 g/tonne of harvested biomass in salmon aquaculture where the level goes up to about 660 g/tonne in Chile (Watts et al., 2017). Despite the fact that there is no direct evidence that antibiotics are being used as the growth promoter in aquaculture, prophylactic use of antibiotics is not uncommon in shrimp or salmon aquaculture. Moreover, because of the inherent problem of treating the affected fish individually, antibiotics are often used for the treatment of the entire population and this sometimes triggers the problem of AMR manifold (Cabello et al., 2016).

As water or other materials including untreated human and animal wastage manure are channelled in the aquatic environment, it becomes a perfect amalgamation of bacterial flora of diverse sources (Strauss; Zhu et al., 1990; Wohlfarth and Schroeder, 1979). Because of the genetic mobility and plasticity, the resistance gene(s) are often exchanged between and among the bacterial species irrespective of their source and host specificity (Khan et al., 2013). Therefore, aquatic farming is considered a hotspot for AMR. The prolonged and repeated use of antimicrobials even at a low concentration is able to sustain the selection pressure on the bacterial community to maintain their resistome. This also facilitates the transfer of resistome among fish and human pathogens (Rolain, 2013). As antimicrobials are stable and nonbiodegradable, they may persist for a prolonged period in the aquatic environment and facilitate the bacteria to acquire and maintain the resistance gene cassettes. A recent study conducted in Shanghai revealed that residue of antibiotics such as tetracyclines, fluoroquinolones, macrolides, β-lactams, sulfonamides and phenicols was detected in almost 52% of the finfish and shrimp samples (Wang et al., 2016). Similarly, other workers reported tetracycline, sulfonamide, quinolone, and macrolide antibiotics in the Haihe River Basin, China (Luo et al., 2011). Done and Halden, 2015 also reported the presence of antibiotics such as tetracycline (oxy- and 4-epoxytetracycline), macrolide (virginiamycin) and sulfonamide (sulfadimethoxine/ ormetoprim) in samples of farmed trout (*Oncorhynchus* spp.), tilapia (*Oreochromis* spp.) and salmon from 11 countries (Done and Halden, 2015). Besides antibiotics, various metal-based antifouling compounds (biocides) are also used in aquaculture to prevent or treat bacterial or parasitic diseases like copper oxide (Guardiola et al., 2012).

Antibacterial biocides and metals can co-select for antibiotic resistance when bacteria harbour resistance or tolerance genes towards both types of compounds. Moreover, studies indicated the presence of heavy metals such as cadmium, iron, lead, zinc and mercury in commercial fish-feed and the use of such premixed feed increases the chances of the soil and the water being contaminated with such heavy metals (Seiler and Berendonk, 2012). There are other ways of heavy metal contamination in aquaculture like from the waste products or agriculture runoff, as certain heavy metals are sourced from agriculture like cadmium in pesticides and fertilizers (Soler and Rovira, 1996). It is not uncommon to see that bacteria harbours both biocide/metal resistance genes (BMRGs) and antibiotic resistance genes (ARGs), and use of antibacterial biocides and metals can co-select for antibiotic resistance as well (Pal et al., 2015). The most common BMRGs which were detected to co-occur with ARGs were mercury resistance and quaternary ammonium compound resistance genes (*qacEΔ1*). Moreover, the association between cadmium/zinc and macrolide/aminoglycoside resistance genes was observed in recent past (Pal et al., 2015). Such co-resistance to antibiotics and heavy metals in *Enterobacteriaceae* spp. isolated from gills and intestines of *Acanthobrama marmid* was reported from Turkey (Toroglu et al., 2009). Furthermore, a study revealed a high degree of correlation between antibiotic resistance and heavy metal tolerance among the pathogens isolated from infected fish in Tuticorin, south-east coast of India (Kumar, Joseph, Fisheries JP-IJ of, 2011 U). Of late, different ARG(s) such as tetracycline resistance (*tet*B) (Furushita et al., 2003), carbapenem resistance (*bla*IMP) (Brouwer et al., 2018), quinolone resistance (*qnr*), aminoglycoside resistance (aac(6′)-Ib-cr) and ESBL gene(s) (Brahmi et al., 2018; Moremi et al., 2016) were reported in fish pathogens. These bacteria in the aquatic environment may contribute to spread the ARGs to other pathogens including those in human gut flora through the food chain.

AMR in open and closed system aquaculture

Open system culture is usually referred to the fish farming which is in natural waterbodies such as oceans, bays, estuaries, coastal lagoons, lakes or rivers. This kind of fish farming is conducted naturally and it lacks the scope of individualized or mass scale therapeutic intervention. Therefore, the prophylactic or therapeutic use of antimicrobials in such fish farming is expected to be low. However, the ocean, lakes or rivers are considered as the hotbed for accumulation and propagation of ARG(s). This is especially because of the various kinds of anthropogenic activities. Various reports pointed out the presence of ARG(s) in the samples collected from open water aquaculture (Yang et al., 2013). There are multiple avenues of antimicrobial contamination in the open water aquaculture. A major proportion of antibiotic contamination is usually caused by hospital wastewater and sewage from antibiotic treatment plants. Again most of the antibiotics used in human for medical treatment or used in livestock production are not metabolized and passed through to end up in the wastewater and cannot be removed by sewage treatment plants (Zhang et al., 2014; Huijbers et al., 2015; Anonymous, 2018b). These ultimately contaminate the open water system. Ultimately all these materials serve as a potent facilitator of diverse microbial pathogens and ARG(s) leading to a drastic shift of the microbiome which is being continuously transmuted with complex resistome (Seiler and Berendonk, 2012; Singer et al., 2016). Antimicrobial contamination at a higher concentration usually leads to the evolvement of bacterial pathogens with multiple resistance genes. This is particularly more important for the compounds that are chemically stable and may exist in the system without any chemical alteration for a relatively long period such as fluoroquinolones (for example, ciprofloxacin) and sulphonamides (such as sulfamethoxazole). Gradual accumulation and persistence of these compounds facilitate into the development of resistant bacterial community in the aquatic sediment. Thus, it is not surprising that a spectrum of gene(s) mediating resistance towards sulphonamide (*sul*1, *sul*2), tetracycline (*tet*B, *tet*C, *tet*M, *tet*W, *tet*O), quinolones (*qnr*A), aminoglycosides (*aadA*), β-lactams and carbapenem (TEM, SHV, CTX-M and NDM) were detected in aquatic sediment (Rolain, 2013; Luo et al., 2011; Done and Halden, 2015). It is noteworthy that although β-lactam compounds are biodegradable and readily destroyed, ARG(s) for β-lactams were also detected in aquatic sediment. The contribution of sewage or wastewater in the microbial resistance of open-water aquatic system was documented by Yang et al., (2013), who reported the presence of tetracycline-resistant pathogens harbouring transposons or plasmid identical to human pathogens in marine sediments. Again a recent study conducted in Pakistan showed how the wastewater from drug formulation factories can affect the drug residue and ARG(s) in the aquatic environment (Khan et al., 2013). High level of antibiotics such as oxytetracycline, trimethoprim, and sulfamethoxazole and ARG(s) such as *sul*1 and *dfrA1* were detected in the downstream river of the Lahore city as well as at the drug formulation facility of the city.

In contrast, closed system aquaculture is land-based farming of the aquatic species mainly in the raceways, tanks and ponds. This system segregates the farming process from the environment and the factors such as oxygenation, temperature and photoperiods are well-regulated in closed system aquaculture. It is often accompanied by the novel recirculation technology which helps to decontaminate the water using filtration processes and recycles it back into the aquaculture system. Thus, it is a near-zero discharge recirculating system which not only helps to maintain the water quality but also reduces the amount of waste discharge, antibiotics and chemicals to affect the environment or natural waterways. Because of the effective waste management and treatment, these recirculating aquaculture systems are often used for managing high-density stocks of fresh or marine fishes and become hot-bed for contagious or infectious diseases. Thus, it warrants the need for antibiotic medication either through premedicated feed or directly in the water. As there is a very little scope of fuelling water from an external source or the environment, it can be presumed that it is only the antibiotic applied in the system that continued to accumulate and facilitate the development of AMR. However, there is very little data on AMR in the closed aquaculture systems. Recent studies revealed that biofilter used for waste treatment in such cases may be a good reservoir for ARG(s) such as tetO, qnrA and tetE (Li et al., 2017).

AMR in integrated fish farming

Integrated aquaculture is a system of fish farming where other agricultural/livestock farming operations are simultaneously conducted in and around the fish pond. All the agricultural, aquatic and livestock farming practises are linked and cater to the need of each other. The by-products/wastes from one system are utilized as a valuable input to another system. This is considered profitable as such and widely practised in Asia and Africa (Vincke, 2003). In most of the cases, livestock such as poultry and pigs are reared with the aquatic system and the manure/biological waste from poultry or piggery units are used as manure and feed (fertilizer for phytoplankton) for fish and as manure for cropland.

Although such practice often maximizes the profit of the farmers, it may facilitate the transfer of AMR pathogens, zoonotic human pathogens and ARG(s) into the aquatic system. Similarly, the antimicrobial residues often become an issue causing selection pressure for sustenance and proliferation of AMR pathogens. Moreover, ARG(s) may get transferred from livestock pathogens to fish pathogens during such amalgamation (Wu et al., 2019; Chelossi et al., 2003; Labella et al., 2013; Neela et al., 2015). As such kind of integrated fish farming is often practised in pond where water content remains logged for a considerable duration, it thus becomes a breeding ground of AMR pathogens. Previous studies have indicated that integrated fish farming may serve as a potential reservoir for AMR pathogens and gene(s) (Neela et al., 2015; Hoa et al., 2011).

Spread of antimicrobial resistance in fish pathogens

Aeromonas salmonicida is one of the widely studied fish pathogens for AMR. This is a Gram-negative, facultative anaerobic, nonmotile bacterium responsible for causing furunculosis in freshwater fish. In 1971, Aoki and coworkers characterized R-plasmids from *A. salmonicida* conferring resistance to tetracycline, sulfonamides, phenicols and amino-glycosides (Aoki et al., 1971). Apart from these four, importantly, resistance to quinolone, the drug used in treatment of *Aeromonas* infection in human beings was also reported. Because of wide host adaptability, it is not impossible that MDR strains of *A. salmonicida* may also infect the in contact human beings or consumers. Recently, a multidrug-resistant, ESBL-producing *A. salmonicida* was detected in a 15-year-old boy who received medicinal leech therapy (Ruppé et al., 2018). While most of the *Aeromonas* sp. resistant to sulfonamides were found to carry sul1 and sul2 gene(s), many of them also carried dfrA/dfrB cassettes in the class 1 integrons (Kadlec et al., 2011). Apart from that, aad cassettes were also detected in many of the *Aeromonas* strains mediating aminoglycoside resistance. While the gene(s) tet(A) and tet(E) were more frequently found to trigger tetracycline resistance (Han et al., 2012; Agersø et al., 2007), point mutation in the gyrA (codon-83) was predominantly responsible for quinolone resistance among *Aeromonas* strains (Hu et al., 2016; Kim et al., 2011). No other mutation in the QRDR region (of gyrA and ParC) was reported for quinolone resistance. Recently, an unusual ColE1-type replicon plasmid bearing the gene chloramphenicol acetyltransferase (cat-pAsa7) was detected for phenicol resistance in *A. salmonicida* (Vincent et al., 2016). Patil et al., 2016, in a recent study, evaluated temporal trends in *Aeromonas* diversity and antibiotic resistance in two adjacent semiintensive aquaculture facilities to ascertain the effects of antibiotic treatment on antimicrobial resistance. Strains were more likely to be simultenously resistant to sulphadiazine, tetracycline and trimethoprim. Such MDR strains harbouring sul1, tetA and intI1 were detected particularly in pathogenic strains of *Aeromonas*. The study pointed out a strong linkage between prophylactic or systemic use of antibiotics and the development of AMR in aquaculture. Another study from Mexico showed that about 40% of the *Aeromonas* isolated from rainbow trout (19/48) were drug-resistant bearing the resistance genes such as blaCphA/IMIS, intI1 (6.2%) and blaSHV (Vega-Sánchez et al., 2014). Sequencing of the variable region of class 1 integrons revealed the presence of the gene cassette aadA1 (aminoglycoside transferase) that mediates streptomycin/spectinomycin resistance. Another study from Taiwan showed that many of the *Aeromonas hydrophila* isolates from tilapia were found to carry class 1, 2 and 3 integrons with aad2 and dfrA12 gene cassettes in class 1 integrons. Moreover, the quinolone resistance of these isolates was attributed to mutated gyrA and ParC gene(s) (Lukkana et al., 2012). Class 1 integrons were also detected in the *Aeromonas* isolates obtained from food fish, ornamental fish, shrimp, turtles and amphibians in China (Deng et al., 2016).

Edwardsiella tarda is a Gram-negative pathogen responsible for causing hemorrhagic septicemia in many commer-cially important fish species such as catfish, turbot, flounder and salmon. Naturally occurring R-plasmids, which confer resistance to five classes of antibiotics, namely sulfonamides, tetracyclines, streptogramins, phenicols and aminoglyco-sides, were identified in *E. tarda*. A multidrug-resistant *E. tarda* strain, CK41, isolated from Japanese flounder was found to carry a large plasmid which consists of potential virulence genes, transposases, plasmid maintenance genes, antibiotic-resistance genes (including kanamycin, tetracycline and streptomycin), conjugal transfer genes and unknown ORFs (open reading frames) (Yu et al., 2012). Recently, *E. tarda* isolated from farmed red hybrid tilapia was found resistant to novobiocin, ampicillin, spiramycin and chloramphenicol and heavy metals such as zinc, chromium, cooper and mercury (Lee and Wendy, 2017). *E. tarda* strain isolated from diseased fish at an epidemic-inflicted fish farm in China was reported to carry resistance determinants such as kn^R, catA3 and *tet*(A) to confer resistance to kanamycin, chloramphenicol and tetracycline, respectively (Sun et al., 2009). Again, the *E. tarda* isolates from diseased eels were found to carry two tetracycline resistance gene(s) including intact efflux pump encoded by tet(A) to mediate high level of tetracycline resistance (Lo et al., 2014). Besides, an *Edwardsiella ictaluri* isolate of catfish origin was found to carry an MDR IncA/C plasmid, pM07-1 conferring resistance to florfenicol, chloramphenicol, tetracycline, streptomycin, ampicillin, amoxicillin/clavulanic acid, ceftiofur and cefoxitin and reduced susceptibility to trimethoprim/sulfamethoxazole and ceftriaxone (Welch et al., 2009).

Yersinia ruckeri is a Gram-negative pathogen responsible for causing the enteric red mouth disease in several marine and freshwater fishes, characterized by subcutaneous haemorrhages in the throat, mouth, gill tips and fins and eventual erosion of the jaw and palate. Haemorrhages may be noticed in the internal organs also. This infection is more commonly detected in farms with poor water quality. The emergence of antibiotic resistance in this pathogen was linked to the application of antibiotics such as amoxicillin, oxolinic acid, oxytetracycline, sulphadiazine and trimethoprim (Kumar et al., 2015). Recently, *Y. ruckeri* strains isolated from trout fish farms were found resistant to florfenicol, erythromycin and oxytetracycline in Bulgaria (Orozova et al., 2015). Previous studies indicated at least 2% of the *Y. ruckeri* isolates resistant to florfenicol. Besides, the study also noted their resistance to oxolinic acid, oxytetracycline and potentiated sulphonamide (Rodgers, 2001). AmpC gene in *Y. ruckeri* isolates was observed to confer resistance to aminopenicillin and narrow spectrum cephalosporins (Mammeri et al., 2006). Other studies reported the tetracycline gene(s) such as tet(A) and tet(B) to cause OTC (oxytetracycline) resistance. Furthermore, Gibello et al., 2004 reported gyrA-83 mutation to mediate quinolone resistance (Gibello et al., 2004). However, no other tetracycline resistance gene(s) or mutation in the QRDR region could be detected. Other gene cassettes such as *sul2*, *strB* and *dfrA14* were reported to cause resistance to potentiated sulfonamides.

Photobacterium damselae subsp. *piscicida* (previously known as *Pasteurella piscicida*) is responsible for photo-bacteriosis (also known as pasteurellosis or pseudotuberculosis), a disease with chronic granulomatous lesions in the visceral organs of the fishes. Few studies on *Photobacterium*'s AMR pattern documented crucial role of plasmid and other mobile genetic elements for carriage of multiple drug-resistant genes. Kim and Aoki, 1993 reported the presence of Amp (for ampicillin) tet(A) (for tetracycline), floR, cat1 and cat2 (for phenicols, chloramphenicol) and aphA7 (for kanamycin) and sul1 (for sulfonamide) resistance gene(s) in the plasmid. Furthermore, transposon IS-26 was reported for mobilization of gene(s) such as tet(A) and aphA7 (Kim and Aoki, 1994). Further studies from Japan also revealed the involvement of multiple transposable elements in the mobilization of the resistant gene(s) such as *catA1*, *aphA7*, *tet(A)*, *tet(R)* and *sul2* in this fish pathogen (Kim et al., 2008). Apart from this, quinolone- and tetracycline- resistance were detected invariably among most of the fish pathogens such as *Flavobacterium psychrophilum*, which is responsible for bacterial cold water disease and rainbow trout fry syndrome in fishes. While quinolone resistance is mediated via mutation at gyrA-83 position, tetracycline resistance is caused by polymorphisms in the 16s rRNA (Izumi and Aranishi, 2004; Soule et al., 2005). Treatment of streptococcus, which is known to cause heavy economic loss in the fish industry, is also facing the problem of AMR after resistance noted to the mainstay of therapy — tetracycline and erythromycin. While *tet* determinants such as tet(M), tet(O) and tet(S) genes were found in most of the tetracycline-resistant isolates, ermB was reported in erythromycin-resistant isolates (Park et al., 2009).

Role of probiotics in AMR in the aquatic system

Probiotics can be defined as 'live microorganisms which, when administered in adequate amounts, confer a health benefit on the host' (Food and Agriculture (FAO) and World Health Organization (WHO) joint report (2001)). Way back in 1986, probiotics were first used in aquaculture when Kozasa used spores of *Bacillus toyoi* as feed additive to increase the growth rate of yellow tail, *Seriola quinqueradiata*. For many years, probiotic supplementation constitutes the Gram-positive bacteria such as lactic acid bacteria, particularly representative of the genera *Bifidobacterium*, *Lactobacillus* and *Streptococcus*. At present, many commercial probiotic formulations, prepared from various bacterial species such as *Bacillus* sp., *Lactobacillus* sp., *Enterococcus* sp., *Carnobacterium* sp., and the yeast *Saccharomyces cerevisiae* are available in the market. Apart from their presumed role in growth promotion and pathogen inhibition, probiotics are thought to play a crucial role to reduce stress response, improve nutritive digestibility and reproductive efficiency.

Thereby, it increases the overall production performance (Martínez Cruz et al., 2012). Probiotics are believed to exert their antibacterial effect due to multiple factors such as production of iron-scavenging siderophores, enzymes (e.g., proteases, amylases and lysozyme), hydrogen peroxide, organic acids and bacteriocins (Sharafi et al., 2013). Although bacteriocin-producing bacteria are often preferred as alternatives to classical antibiotics for their potential antibacterial effect, they often reported to carry AMR gene(s). Moreover, bacteria used as probiotics can also acquire the resistance gene(s) through mobile genetic element. Recently, several lactic acid bacteria of aquatic animal origin were reported to carry several AMR gene(s). Thus, the long-term implication of adding live bacterial population in aquaculture as probiotics need a serious introspection (Fukao and Yajim, 2012; Gueimonde et al., 2013).

Environment impact of AMR in aquaculture and its abatement

It is undeniable that the antimicrobials used or added to the aquaculture system will contaminate the environment in long term with the flow of water, wastage and other excreta into the ecosystem. The ultimate fate of antimicrobials and their persistence in the aquatic system depends on the route of administration and physiochemical properties of antimicrobials. The unabsorbed antimicrobials, which are used directly in the water or for topical or bath treatment, may contaminate the environment whenever there is an overflow of storage. Likewise, the leftover premedicated feed or unmetabolized drugs may also serve as a potential source of contamination. Distribution of the drugs between water and sediment phase also determines a lot for bioavailability of drugs to aquatic biota. Other physiochemical properties such as pH, temperature and presence of other materials in the aquatic environment determine the availability of functionally active antimicrobials. Because of the presence of divalent cations such as Ca^{2+} or Mg^{2+}, the bioavailability of tetracycline or OTC is substantially reduced because of chelation. In the marine aquatic system, the bioavailability of OTC reaches only upto 10%. Moreover, tetracyclines are highly sensitive to hydrolysis and often get degraded whenever there is a change in pH or increase in environmental temperature (Lunestad and Goksøyr, 1990). Likewise, macrolides are also hydrolyzed in acidic pH (Mitchell et al., 2015). In the presence of high-intensity light as occurred in the water surface, photodecomposition of tetracycline was recorded (Oka et al., 1989). Accumulation of antimicrobials is more common in the sediment because of direct deposition of the antibiotic-treated components and adsorption of drugs with the settling particles. The adsorption rate is substantially higher for the antimicrobials such as fluoroquinolones (Cardoza et al., 2005), followed by tetracycline, macrolides and sulphonamides. It is undeniable that there may be seepage of antimicrobials from the aquatic system to the environment and all that adds to the total burden of antimicrobials in the environment. There are multiple dimensions where the environment may be affected by such unwanted flow of antimicrobials from the aquatic system. The contamination of antimicrobials may have an adverse effect on soil microbes, earthworms, algae and other environmental organisms which may have a potential role in maintaining the natural ecosystem. Further impact on wildlife, terrestrial animals and others which may be potential recipient cannot be undermined. Majority of the antibiotics are not absorbed through the intestinal tract and are excreted via faeces and urine and thus add to the environmental burden of antimicrobials. The gradual accumulation of antibiotics and their biomagnification may lead to hazardous impact. Persistence of the antimicrobials is also an important factor and it has been estimated that the approximate half-life of the most of the antimicrobials is almost 2−3 weeks at 20°C and the degradation may increase at higher environmental temperature. Environmental or soil microorganisms may be adversely affected by the accumulation of antimicrobials. Tylosin was reported to reduce soil nitrogen mineralization at 37 ppm. The accumulation of antimicrobials in the aquatic system such as a river or marine sediment may enter into the human food chain also (Serrano, 2005). Studies conducted by Bakal and Stoskopf (2001) demonstrated that various factors such as salinity, pH and temperature may influence the adsorption of the drug molecules with sediments and once the condition favours, there may be release of such compounds in a free form which can be taken up by vertebrates and macroinvertebrates. Thus, the possibility of entering such compounds in the human food chain is substantially increased. Considering the prolonged half-life of the antimicrobial compounds, these may adversely affect the environmental microorganisms. The presence of antimicrobials may impair the microbial activity and lower their turnover capacity in the agricultural waste or other solid waste. Considering the prolonged half-life of the antimicrobial compounds, these may adversely affect the environmental microorganisms and affect the waste treatment and management process as the same largely depends on the microbial activity. Furthermore, agriculture waste and municipal solid waste are largely used for biogas production. However, the presence of antimicrobial residue may cut down anaerobic bacteria responsible for biogas production (Serrano, 2005). It is difficult to assume the total environmental impact as it has multidimensional areas where introspective research is warranted.

As it is clear that the impact of unscrupulous and uncontrolled use of antimicrobials in aquaculture may be long-lasting on the human and environmental health, strict control measure is necessary. Therefore, the following measures may be taken into account for abatement of AMR in aquaculture and thereby its impact over the ecosystem.

It is very important to detect and diagnose the food-borne and zoonotic bacteria in a pond environment. This can help the farmers and veterinarians take appropriate measures to reduce the burden of the pathogen and their dissemination to the environment.

Proper prophylactic control measures must be taken to attenuate the occurrence of infective fish pathogens so that usage of antimicrobials may be substantially reduced. Prevention and control of bacterial diseases in aquatic organisms are essential.

Continuous monitoring of antimicrobial resistance in human and food animals, which are particularly coming in close contact with the aquatic system, is important. This can give us an appraisal of emergence and amalgamation of AMR pathogens within aquatic and broader ecosystem.

Monitoring of the antimicrobial susceptibility is very important as it can do constant surveillance over changing dynamics of the resistance profile of the drug-resistant isolates prevalent in an aquatic system.

Effort must be made to reduce the use of antimicrobials in aquaculture with the adoption of better hygiene and proper prophylactic measures including vaccination so that the occurrence of infectious diseases can be reduced. Thereby, the requirement of antibiotics can be brought down substantially. The routine prophylactic use of antimicrobials can also be reduced with better hygienic management. Good aquaculture practise should promote the use of nonhuman antibiotics.

Application of manure in aquaculture is often incriminated as a major source of AMR bacteria and AMR gene(s). Therefore, it is necessary to avoid using manure in the aquatic system. That may further complicate the aquatic microflora with more resistant pathogens.

References

Agersø, Y., Bruun, M.S., Dalsgaard, I., Larsen, J.L., 2007. The tetracycline resistance gene tet(E) is frequently occurring and present on large horizontally transferable plasmids in *Aeromonas* spp. from fish farms. Aquaculture 266, 47−52. https://doi.org/10.1016/j.aquaculture.2007.01.012.

Anonymous, March 18, 2019. Total Fisheries Production (Metric Tons) | Data. World Bank. https://data.worldbank.org/indicator/ER.FSH.PROD.MT?view=chart.

Anonymous, 2018a. National Fisheries Development Board. Govt of India. NFDB. http://nfdb.gov.in/about-indian-fisheries.htm.

Anonymous, 2018b. Initiatives for Addressing Antimicrobial Resistance in the Environment: Current Situation and Challenges. https://wellcome.ac.uk/sites/default/files/antimicrobial-resistance-environment-report.pdf.

Aoki, T., Egusa, S., Kimura, T., Watanabe, T., 1971. Detection of R factors in naturally occurring *Aeromonas salmonicida* strains. Applied Microbiology 22, 716−717.

Bardach, J.E., Santerre, M.T., March 18, 2019. Use of Organic Residues in Aquaculture. http://archive.unu.edu/unupress/food/8F012e/8F012E02.htm.

Brahmi, S., Touati, A., Dunyach-Remy, C., Sotto, A., Pantel, A., Lavigne, J.-P., 2018. High prevalence of extended-spectrum β-lactamase-producing Enterobacteriaceae in wild fish from the mediterranean sea in Algeria. Microbial Drug Resistance 24, 290−298. https://doi.org/10.1089/mdr.2017.0149.

Brouwer, M.S.M., Rapallini, M., Geurts, Y., Harders, F., Bossers, A., Mevius, D.J., et al., 2018. *Enterobacter cloacae* complex isolated from shrimps from Vietnam encoding bla IMI-1, resistant to carbapenems but not cephalosporins. Antimicrobial Agents and Chemotherapy 00398−418. https://doi.org/10.1128/AAC.00398-18.

Bryan R, S., Sharpe, W.E., McCarty, T., 2006. Water Quality Concerns for Ponds, Penn State College of Agricultural Sciences Research, Extension, and Resident Education Programs. https://extension.psu.edu/water-quality-concerns-for-ponds.

Cabello, F.C., Godfrey, H.P., Buschmann, A.H., Dölz, H.J., 2016. Aquaculture as yet another environmental gateway to the development and globalisation of antimicrobial resistance. The Lancet Infectious Diseases 16, e127−e133. https://doi.org/10.1016/S1473-3099(16)00100-6.

Cardoza, L.A., Knapp, C.W., Larive, C.K., Belden, J.B., Lydy, M., Graham, D.W., 2005. Factors affecting the fate of ciprofloxacin in aquatic field systems. Water, Air, Soil Pollution 161, 383−398. https://doi.org/10.1007/s11270-005-5550-6.

Chelossi, E., Vezzulli, L., Milano, A., Branzoni, M., Fabiano, M., Riccardi, G., et al., 2003. Antibiotic resistance of benthic bacteria in fish-farm and control sediments of the Western Mediterranean. Aquaculture 219, 83−97. https://doi.org/10.1016/S0044-8486(03)00016-4.

Deng, Y., Wu, Y., Jiang, L., Tan, A., Zhang, R., Luo, L., 2016. Multi-drug resistance mediated by class 1 integrons in *Aeromonas* isolated from farmed freshwater animals. Frontiers in Microbiology 7. https://doi.org/10.3389/fmicb.2016.00935.

Done, H.Y., Halden, R.U., 2015. Reconnaissance of 47 antibiotics and associated microbial risks in seafood sold in the United States. Journal of Hazardous Materials 282, 10−17. https://doi.org/10.1016/j.jhazmat.2014.08.075.

Food and Agriculture Oraganization of the United Nations, 2016. FAO Yearbook: Fishery and Aquaculture Statistics. 2014. https://doi.org/10.5860/CHOICE.50-5350.

Fukao, M., Yajim, N., 2012. Assessment of Antibiotic Resistance in Probiotic Lactobacilli. Antibiot. Resist. Bact. - A Contin. Chall. New Millenn. InTech. https://doi.org/10.5772/30903.

Furushita, M., Shiba, T., Maeda, T., Yahata, M., Kaneoka, A., Takahashi, Y., et al., 2003. Similarity of tetracycline resistance genes isolated from fish farm bacteria to those from clinical isolates. Applied and Environmental Microbiology 69, 5336−5342. https://doi.org/10.1128/AEM.69.9.5336-5342.2003.

Gibello, A., Porrero, M.C., Blanco, M.M., Vela, A.I., Liebana, P., Moreno, M.A., et al., 2004. Analysis of the gyrA gene of clinical *Yersinia ruckeri* isolates with reduced susceptibility to quinolones. Applied and Environmental Microbiology 70, 599−602. https://doi.org/10.1128/AEM.70.1.599-602.2004.

Gopakumar, K., 2003. Indian aquaculture. Journal of Applied Aquaculture 13, 1−10. https://doi.org/10.1300/j028v13n01_01.

Guardiola, F.A., Cuesta, A., Meseguer, J., Esteban, M.A., 2012. Risks of using antifouling biocides in aquaculture. International Journal of Molecular Sciences 13, 1541−1560. https://doi.org/10.3390/ijms13021541.

Gueimonde, M., Sánchez, B., G. de los Reyes-Gavilán, C., Margolles, A., 2013. Antibiotic resistance in probiotic bacteria. Frontiers in Microbiology 4. https://doi.org/10.3389/fmicb.2013.00202.

Han, J.E., Kim, J.H., Choresca, C.H., Shin, S.P., Jun, J.W., Chai, J.Y., et al., 2012. Prevalence of tet gene and complete genome sequencing of tet gene-encoded plasmid (pAHH01) isolated from *Aeromonas* species in South Korea. Journal of Applied Microbiology 112, 631−638. https://doi.org/10.1111/j.1365-2672.2012.05237.x.

Hoa, P.T.P., Managaki, S., Nakada, N., Takada, H., Shimizu, A., Anh, D.H., et al., 2011. Antibiotic contamination and occurrence of antibiotic-resistant bacteria in aquatic environments of northern Vietnam. The Science of the Total Environment 409, 2894−2901. https://doi.org/10.1016/j.scitotenv.2011.04.030.

Hu, R., Du, N., Chen, N., Lin, L., Zhai, Y., Gu, Z., 2016. Molecular analysis of type II topoisomerases of *Aeromonas hydrophila* isolated from fish and levofloxacin-induced resistant isolates in vitro. Folia Microbiologica 61, 249−253. https://doi.org/10.1007/s12223-015-0432-9.

Huijbers, P.M.C., Blaak, H., De Jong, M.C.M., Graat, E.A.M., Vandenbroucke-Grauls, C.M.J.E., De Roda Husman, A.M., 2015. Role of the environment in the transmission of antimicrobial resistance to humans: a review. Environmental Science and Technology 49, 11993−12004. https://doi.org/10.1021/acs.est.5b02566.

Izumi, S., Aranishi, F., 2004. Relationship between gyrA mutations and quinolone resistance in *Flavobacterium psychrophilum* isolates. Applied and Environmental Microbiology 70, 3968−3972. https://doi.org/10.1128/AEM.70.7.3968-3972.2004.

Kadlec, K., von Czapiewski, E., Kaspar, H., Wallmann, J., Michael, G.B., Steinacker, U., et al., 2011. Molecular basis of sulfonamide and trimethoprim resistance in fish-pathogenic *Aeromonas* isolates. Applied and Environmental Microbiology 77, 7147−7150. https://doi.org/10.1128/AEM.00560-11.

Khan, G.A., Berglund, B., Khan, K.M., Lindgren, P.-E., Fick, J., 2013. Occurrence and abundance of antibiotics and resistance genes in rivers, canal and near drug formulation facilities–a study in Pakistan. PLoS One 8, e62712. https://doi.org/10.1371/journal.pone.0062712.

Kim, E.-H., Aoki, T., 1993. Drug resistance and broad geographical distribution of identical R plasmids of *Pasteurella piscicida* isolated from cultured yellowtail in Japan. Microbiology and Immunology 37, 103−109. https://doi.org/10.1111/j.1348-0421.1993.tb03186.x.

Kim, E.H., Aoki, T., 1994. The transposon-like structure of IS26-tetracycline, and kanamycin resistance determinant derived from transferable R plasmid of fish pathogen, *Pasteurella piscicida*. Microbiology and Immunology 38, 31−38. https://doi.org/10.1111/j.1348-0421.1994.tb01741.x.

Kim, M.J., Hirono, I., Kurokawa, K., Maki, T., Hawke, J., Kondo, H., et al., 2008. Complete DNA sequence and analysis of the transferable multiple-drug resistance plasmids (R Plasmids) from *Photobacterium damselae* subsp. piscicida isolates collected in Japan and the United States. Antimicrobial Agents and Chemotherapy 52, 606−611. https://doi.org/10.1128/AAC.01216-07.

Kim, J.H., Hwang, S.Y., Son, J.S., Han, J.E., Jun, J.W., Shin, S.P., et al., 2011. Molecular characterization of tetracycline- and quinolone-resistant *Aeromonas salmonicida* isolated in Korea. Journal of Veterinary Science 12, 41. https://doi.org/10.4142/jvs.2011.12.1.41.

Korostynska, O., Mason, A., Nakouti, I., Jansomboon, W., Al-Shamma', A., 2016. Monitoring use of antibiotics in aquaculture. Mar. Ocean Ecosyst. In: 16th Int. Multidiscip. Sci. GeoConference SGEM, pp. 1−8.

Kumar, G., Menanteau-Ledouble, S., Saleh, M., El-Matbouli, M., 2015. *Yersinia ruckeri*, the causative agent of enteric redmouth disease in fish. Veterinary Research 46, 103. https://doi.org/10.1186/s13567-015-0238-4.

Kumar, P., Joseph, B., 2011. Antibiotic and heavy metal resistance profile of pathogens isolated from infected fish in Tuticorin, South-East Coast of India. Indian Journal of Fisheries 58, 121−125. J Patterson.

Labella, A., Gennari, M., Ghidini, V., Trento, I., Manfrin, A., Borrego, J.J., et al., 2013. High incidence of antibiotic multi-resistant bacteria in coastal areas dedicated to fish farming. Marine Pollution Bulletin 70, 197−203. https://doi.org/10.1016/j.marpolbul.2013.02.037.

Leal, J.F., Henriques, I.S., Correia, A., Santos, E.B.H., Esteves, V.I., 2017. Antibacterial activity of oxytetracycline photoproducts in marine aquaculture's water. Environment and Pollution 220, 644−649. https://doi.org/10.1016/j.envpol.2016.10.021.

Lee, S.W., Wendy, W., 2017. Antibiotic and heavy metal resistance of *Aeromonas hydrophila* and *Edwardsiella tarda* isolated from red hybrid tilapia (*Oreochromis* spp.) coinfected with motile *Aeromonas* septicemia and *Edwardsiellosis*. Veterinary World 10, 803−807. https://doi.org/10.14202/vetworld.2017.803-807.

Li, S., Zhang, S., Ye, C., Lin, W., Zhang, M., Chen, L., et al., 2017. Biofilm processes in treating mariculture wastewater may be a reservoir of antibiotic resistance genes. Marine Pollution Bulletin 118, 289−296. https://doi.org/10.1016/j.marpolbul.2017.03.003.

Lo, D.Y., Lee, Y.J., Wang, J.H., Kuo, H.C., 2014. Antimicrobial susceptibility and genetic characterisation of oxytetracycline-resistant *Edwardsiella tarda* isolated from diseased eels. The Veterinary Record 175, 203. https://doi.org/10.1136/vr.101580.

Lukkana, M., Wongtavatchai, J., Chuanchuen, R., 2012. Class 1 integrons in *Aeromonas hydrophila* isolates from farmed nile *Tilapia* (*Oreochromis nilotica*). Journal of Veterinary Medical Science 74, 435−440. https://doi.org/10.1292/jvms.11-0441.

Lunestad, B., Goksøyr, J., 1990. Reduction in the antibacterial effect of oxy-tetracycline in sea water by complex formation with magnesium and calcium. Diseases of Aquatic Organisms 9, 67−72. https://doi.org/10.3354/dao009067.

Luo, Y., Xu, L., Rysz, M., Wang, Y., Zhang, H., Alvarez, P.J.J., 2011. Occurrence and transport of tetracycline, sulfonamide, quinolone, and macrolide antibiotics in the Haihe River basin, China. Environmental Science and Technology 45, 1827−1833. https://doi.org/10.1021/es104009s.

Mammeri, H., Poirel, L., Nazik, H., Nordmann, P., 2006. Cloning and functional characterization of the ambler Class C beta-lactamase of *Yersinia ruckeri*. FEMS Microbiology Letters 257, 57–62. https://doi.org/10.1111/j.1574-6968.2006.00148.x.

Martínez Cruz, P., Ibáñez, A.L., Monroy Hermosillo, O.A., Ramírez Saad, H.C., 2012. Use of probiotics in aquaculture. ISRN Microbiol 2012, 1–13. https://doi.org/10.5402/2012/916845.

Mitchell, S.M., Ullman, J.L., Teel, A.L., Watts, R.J., 2015. Hydrolysis of amphenicol and macrolide antibiotics: chloramphenicol, florfenicol, spiramycin, and tylosin. Chemosphere 134, 504–511. https://doi.org/10.1016/j.chemosphere.2014.08.050.

Moremi, N., Manda, E.V., Falgenhauer, L., Ghosh, H., Imirzalioglu, C., Matee, M., et al., 2016. Predominance of CTX-M-15 among ESBL producers from environment and fish gut from the shores of lake Victoria in Mwanza, Tanzania. Frontiers in Microbiology 7, 1862. https://doi.org/10.3389/fmicb.2016.01862.

Nadarajah, S., Flaaten, O., 2017. Global aquaculture growth and institutional quality. Marine Policy 84, 142–151. https://doi.org/10.1016/j.marpol.2017.07.018.

Nakamura, R., 2006. Aquaculture development in India: a model. BioScience 35, 96–100. https://doi.org/10.2307/1309846.

Neela, F.A., Banu, M.S.T.N.A., Rahman, M.A., Alam, M.F., Rahman, M.H., 2015. Occurrence of antibiotic resistant bacteria in pond water associated with integrated poultry-fish farming in Bangladesh. Sains Malaysiana 44, 371–377. https://doi.org/10.17576/jsm-2015-4403-08.

Oka, H., Ikai, Y., Kawamura, N., Yamada, M., Harada, K., Ito, S., et al., 1989. Photodecomposition products of tetracycline in aqueous solution. Journal of Agricultural and Food Chemistry 37, 226–231. https://doi.org/10.1021/jf00085a052.

Orozova, P., Chikova, V., Sirakov, I., 2015. Diagnostics and antibiotic resistance of *Yersinia ruckeri* strains isolated from trout fish farms in Bulgaria. International Journal of Development Research (IJDR) 5, 3013–3019.

Pal, C., Bengtsson-Palme, J., Kristiansson, E., Larsson, D.G.J., 2015. Co-occurrence of resistance genes to antibiotics, biocides and metals reveals novel insights into their co-selection potential. BMC Genomics 16, 964. https://doi.org/10.1186/s12864-015-2153-5.

Park, Y.-K., Nho, S.-W., Shin, G.-W., Park, S.-B., Jang, H.-B., Cha, I.-S., et al., 2009. Antibiotic susceptibility and resistance of *Streptococcus iniae* and *Streptococcus parauberis* isolated from olive flounder (*Paralichthys olivaceus*). Veterinary Microbiology 136, 76–81. https://doi.org/10.1016/j.vetmic.2008.10.002.

Patil, H.J., Benet-Perelberg, A., Naor, A., Smirnov, M., Ofek, T., Nasser, A., et al., 2016. Evidence of increased antibiotic resistance in phylogenetically-diverse *Aeromonas* isolates from semi-intensive fish ponds treated with antibiotics. Frontiers in Microbiology 7, 1875. https://doi.org/10.3389/fmicb.2016.01875.

Rodgers, C.J., 2001. Resistance of *Yersinia ruckeri* to antimicrobial agents in vitro. Aquaculture 196, 325–345. https://doi.org/10.1016/S0044-8486(01)00546-4.

Rolain, J.-M., 2013. Food and human gut as reservoirs of transferable antibiotic resistance encoding genes. Frontiers in Microbiology 4. https://doi.org/10.3389/fmicb.2013.00173.

Ruppé, E., Cherkaoui, A., Wagner, N., La Scala, G.C., Beaulieu, J.-Y., Girard, M., et al., 2018. In vivo selection of a multidrug-resistant *Aeromonas salmonicida* during medicinal leech therapy. New Microbes and New Infections 21, 23–27. https://doi.org/10.1016/j.nmni.2017.10.005.

Santos, L., Ramos, F., 2018. Antimicrobial resistance in aquaculture: current knowledge and alternatives to tackle the problem. International Journal of Antimicrobial Agents 52, 135–143. https://doi.org/10.1016/j.ijantimicag.2018.03.010.

Seiler, C., Berendonk, T.U., 2012. Heavy metal driven co-selection of antibiotic resistance in soil and water bodies impacted by agriculture and aquaculture. Frontiers in Microbiology 3, 399. https://doi.org/10.3389/fmicb.2012.00399.

Serrano, P.H., 2005. Responsible Use of Antibiotics in Aquaculture. Food and Agriculture Organization.

Sharafi, H., Alidost, L., Lababpour, A., Shahbani Zahiri, H., Abbasi, H., Vali, H., et al., 2013. Antibacterial activity of probiotic *Lactobacillus plantarum* HK01: effect of divalent metal cations and food additives on production efficiency of antibacterial compounds. Probiotics and Antimicrobial Proteins 5, 121–130. https://doi.org/10.1007/s12602-013-9130-6.

Singer, A.C., Shaw, H., Rhodes, V., Hart, A., 2016. Review of antimicrobial resistance in the environment and its relevance to environmental regulators. Frontiers in Microbiology 7, 1–22. https://doi.org/10.3389/fmicb.2016.01728.

Smith, P., 2008. Antimicrobial resistance in aquaculture. Revue Scientifique et Technique Office International des Epizooties 27, 243–264.

Soler, J.S., Rovira, J.S., 1996. Cadmium in Inorganic Fertilizers. Fertil. Environ. In: Springer Netherlands, Dordrecht, pp. 541–545. https://doi.org/10.1007/978-94-009-1586-2_95.

Soule, M., LaFrentz, S., Cain, K., LaPatra, S., Call, D., 2005. Polymorphisms in 16S rRNA genes of *Flavobacterium psychrophilum* correlate with elastin hydrolysis and tetracycline resistance. Diseases of Aquatic Organisms 65, 209–216. https://doi.org/10.3354/dao065209.

Strauss, M., n.d. Health (Pathogen) Considerations Regarding the Use of Human Waste in Aquaculture.

Sun, K., Wang, H., Zhang, M., Xiao, Z., Sun, L., 2009. Genetic mechanisms of multi-antimicrobial resistance in a pathogenic *Edwardsiella tarda* strain. Aquaculture 289, 134–139. https://doi.org/10.1016/j.aquaculture.2008.12.021.

Toroglu, S., Toroglu, E., Dincer, S., Kara, C., Kertmen, M., 2009. Resistances of antibiotics and heavy metals in *Enterobacteriaceae* spp. isolated from gills and intestines of *Achanthobrama marmid* (Heckel, 1843) from Sir Dam lake Turkey. Journal of Environmental Biology 30, 23–31.

Vega-Sánchez, V., Latif-Eugenín, F., Soriano-Vargas, E., Beaz-Hidalgo, R., Figueras, M.J., Aguilera-Arreola, M.G., et al., 2014. Re-identification of *Aeromonas* isolates from rainbow trout and incidence of class 1 integron and β-lactamase genes. Veterinary Microbiology 172, 528–533. https://doi.org/10.1016/j.vetmic.2014.06.012.

Vincent, A.T., Emond-Rheault, J.-G., Barbeau, X., Attéré, S.A., Frenette, M., Lagüe, P., et al., 2016. Antibiotic resistance due to an unusual ColE1-type replicon plasmid in *Aeromonas salmonicida*. Microbiology 162, 942–953. https://doi.org/10.1099/mic.0.000286.

Vincke, M.M.J., 2003. Integrated Livestock-Fish Production System. FAO. http://www.fao.org/3/ac155E/AC155E04.htm.

Wang, H., Wang, N., Wang, B., Zhao, Q., Fang, H., Fu, C., et al., 2016. Antibiotics in drinking water in Shanghai and their contribution to antibiotic exposure of school children. Environmental Science and Technology 50, 2692–2699. https://doi.org/10.1021/acs.est.5b05749.

Watts, J., Schreier, H., Lanska, L., Hale, M., 2017. The rising tide of antimicrobial resistance in aquaculture: sources, sinks and solutions. Marine Drugs 15, 158. https://doi.org/10.3390/md15060158.

Welch, T.J., Evenhuis, J., White, D.G., McDermott, P.F., Harbottle, H., Miller, R.A., et al., 2009. IncA/C plasmid-mediated florfenicol resistance in the catfish pathogen *Edwardsiella ictaluri*. Antimicrobial Agents and Chemotherapy 53, 845–846. https://doi.org/10.1128/AAC.01312-08.

Wohlfarth, G.W., Schroeder, G.L., 1979. Use of manure in fish farming-A review. Agricultural Wastes 1, 279–299. https://doi.org/10.1016/0141-4607(79)90012-X.

Wu, J., Su, Y., Deng, Y., Guo, Z., Mao, C., Liu, G., et al., 2019. Prevalence and distribution of antibiotic resistance in marine fish farming areas in Hainan, China. The Science of the Total Environment 653, 605–611. https://doi.org/10.1016/j.scitotenv.2018.10.251.

Yang, J., Wang, C., Shu, C., Liu, L., Geng, J., Hu, S., et al., 2013. Marine sediment bacteria harbor antibiotic resistance genes highly similar to those found in human pathogens. Microbial Ecology 65, 975–981. https://doi.org/10.1007/s00248-013-0187-2.

Yu, J.E., Cho, M.Y., Kim, J.W., Kang, H.Y., 2012. Large antibiotic-resistance plasmid of *Edwardsiella tarda* contributes to virulence in fish. Microbial Pathogenesis 52, 259–266. https://doi.org/10.1016/j.micpath.2012.01.006.

Zhang, X., Li, Y., Liu, B., Wang, J., Feng, C., Gao, M., et al., 2014. Prevalence of veterinary antibiotics and antibiotic-resistant *Escherichia coli* in the surface water of a livestock production region in Northern China. PLoS One 9, e111026. https://doi.org/10.1371/journal.pone.0111026.

Zhu, Y., Yang, Y., Wan, J., Hua, D., Mathias, J.A., 1990. The effect of manure application rate and frequency upon fish yield in integrated fish farm ponds. Aquaculture 91, 233–251. https://doi.org/10.1016/0044-8486(90)90191-O.

Chapter 5

Emergence of antimicrobial-resistant bacteria in environment

Chapter outline

Background

Environment can be defined as 'the complex of physical, chemical, and biotic factors (such as climate, soil, and living things) that act upon an organism or an ecological community and ultimately determine its form and survival'. Truly speaking, environment is the entire gamut of our surrounding and contains all the living and nonliving things, chemical, physical and climatic factors upon which we survive. The very air we breathe in, the water we take and the soil on which we live are all parts of the environment. In one word, everything on this mother planet is our environment. This gives an impression that how big and how complex our environment is and thus it cannot shy away of the fatal impact of antimicrobial resistance (AMR), probably the biggest and deadliest public health threat ever experienced by human civilization. Various scientific reports including the reports from UN agencies proclaimed the environment being the breeding and battle ground of AMR (FAO, 2018; Huijbers et al., 2015; Anonymous, 2018). A recent study conducted at the University of Exeter Medical School showed how resistant organism may evolve and propagate when exposed to antibiotic in subtherapeutic concentration. Metagenome and 16S rRNA analyses of sewage-derived bacteria exhibited increased propensity to acquire, mobilize and disseminate the *bla*CTX-M gene (Murray et al., 2018). This may just the tip of the iceberg of what is happening in the environment which houses millions of bacteria and is getting regularly contaminated with antibiotics from animal or human excreta, emission from hospital or pharmaceutical farms or other possible sources.

In nature, microorganisms produce antimicrobials as a part of their survival strategy to outcompete others in search of limited resources. Likewise, AMR is also a natural and unstoppable phenomenon used by the bacteria to shield themselves against antimicrobials. Since long, bacteria of this planet have evolved and gradually transmuted to respond to various stimuli from various stress factors, bioactive compounds and other anthropogenic activities. The more is the exposure, the more resistant they become. In the course of evolution, bacteria acquired gene(s) and modified gene(s)/genetic expression to ensure their nutrition and protection which include genes for transport or efflux pumps, genes for producing enzymes that can inactivate cytotoxic compounds including antibiotics. Many of such mechanisms, which bacteria acquired for some other purposes, eventually made them immune to antibiotics such as biofilm production, tolerance and persistence. Efflux pumps originally meant for physiological functions are not only instrumental for resistance to multiple drugs but also help bacteria acquire additional resistance determinants by lowering intracellular concentration of antimicrobials and facilitating mutation accumulation (Sun et al., 2014).

Antimicrobial Resistance in Agriculture. https://doi.org/10.1016/B978-0-12-815770-1.00005-5

Drivers and pathways

Understanding the drivers and transmission dynamics of the resistant pathogens is very important to know how the AMR is taking its strong foothold on various sectors. More than just overuse or abuse of antimicrobials, there are increasing evidences that other factors may contribute to AMR — quality of drugs, personal hygiene, water sanitation, sewage treatment and treatment of hospital, farm and pharmaceutical effusion, travel and migration quarantine. Apart from use of antimicrobials in human health and agricultural sector, which have been discussed in separate chapter, three major pathways were reported to contribute chemicals and antibiotics in the environment — municipal and industrial wastewater; land spreading of animal manure and sewage sludge and aquaculture (Singer et al., 2016).

Given the enormity of the bacteria present on our planet ($\sim 5 \times 10^{30}$) and their genetic variability, there lies immense scope and opportunity for genetic recombination, rearrangement and mutation, which can drive for emergence of novel antibiotic resistance genes (ARGs) anywhere, anytime (Bengtsson-Palme et al., 2018). Thus, nature has started to provide a platform for such emergence, long before we began to harness antimicrobials for our own benefit. Possibly, majority of such resistance gene(s)/mechanisms are still lurking in bacterial population and we are yet to know about them. However, this mere presence of resistance gene(s) in the nature is not sufficient for their entry and propagation in bacterial population unless pathogens are under selection pressure. Because of the associated fitness cost, usually such resistance gene(s)/factors are not selected during multiplication of bacteria, and even after acquiring, bacteria prefer to get rid of them in the absence of selection pressure. Moreover, the expression of the resistance gene(s) is usually not well-regulated and fine-tuned and the translated products of resistance gene(s) may interfere with the cellular function. This all eventually affect the fitness cost associated with resistance gene(s) (Bengtsson-Palme et al., 2018). In spite of negligible or absent fitness cost, bacteria are very unlikely to select resistance trait unless they are under strong selection pressure for it. Essentially, lower fitness cost and positive selection pressure are indispensable not only for acquisition and establishment of resistance gene onto bacterial genome and but also for their mobilization and spread (Melnyk et al., 2015; Harada & Asai, 2010). The mechanism of gene transfer that bacteria use is fundamentally different for those in eukaryotes. A recently mobilized resistance gene(s) is generally associated with increased fitness cost owing to maintain the burden of multiple copies of the gene(s) and their optimum expression level. However, once the gene is secured its holding in the mobile element, fitness cost is gradually reduced. If the fitness cost is not low or negligible, positive selection pressure is required for maintaining the resistance gene. Therefore, a conducive environment is important for both mobilization/transfer of resistance gene and maintenance of already mobilized one. If resistance determinants emerges naturally as the part of their survival strategy to have protected from the attack of the antimicrobials released by other microbes, environmental pool of such determinants often remains preserved, albeit mostly among the nonpathogenic natural flora (Bengtsson-Palme et al., 2018). Horizontal gene transfer or lateral gene transfer is commonly employed by bacteria to transfer resistance gene to ensure its (gene) reach to a larger bacterial community (Bengtsson-Palme et al., 2018). It is more frequent among the bacteria which are phylogenetically close and share same habitat, particularly in the presence of some stressor molecules — antibiotics, metals, biocides and numerous natural or synthetic biochemicals. Thus, such environmental stressors may facilitate transfer of resistance gene from environmental bacteria to opportunistic human pathogens in environmental setting. Most of the hitherto unknown resistance gene(s) are believed to be sequestered in exclusively environmental pathogens. In certain circumstances, environmental, plant or animal bacteria get entry in the human flora during accidental or voluntary consumption of raw food, contaminated drinking water or during interaction with domestic or wild animals, and then transfer of resistance gene(s) is not impossible (Martínez, 2012; Martínez, 2008). However, we are still at dark about the exact preconditions that make such carryover possible. Interestingly, human pathogens also use their environmental counterpart as a reservoir of resistance gene(s), so that the gene(s) can be recruited in future for re-emergence of resistant pathogens. Several soil bacteria such as *Burkholderia cepacia*, *Ochrobactrum intermedium* and *Stenotrophomonas maltophilia* were reported to not only serve as temporary reservoir of ARG but also to cause human infection in few favourable occasion (Johnning et al., 2013; Berg et al., 2013). Environment can thus acts as a constant source of resistance gene(s) in a vicious cycle which is not very easy to break.

In addition to antibiotics, a much wider breadth of chemicals that may also fall in the same line to select and maintain resistance gene(s) are biocides and metals. These are commonly used as microbicide or antiseptics or other purposes in domestic, industrial, health care and agriculture practice. According to the US Environmental Protection Agency, biocides are the group of substances in the form of 'preservatives, insecticides, disinfectants, and pesticides used for the control of organisms that are harmful to human or animal health or that cause damage to natural or manufactured products'. These substances are present in many commodities used in our daily life; toothpaste, household or utensil cleaners, sewage treatment materials, wipes and detergents, healthcare-related products, etc., are among the few. Common biocides include ethanol, formaldehyde, chlorhexidine, triclosan and quaternium ammonium compounds. Resistance to biocides is known for decades; however, biocides may also drive antibiotic resistance. This was recorded in a study by Akimitsu et al. (1999) who demonstrated that resistance to benzalkonium chloride was closely linked to oxacillin resistance in *Staphylococcus aureus*, as evidenced by higher oxacillin MIC (minimum inhibitory concentration) among benzalkonium chloride—resistant mutants of methicillin-resistant *S. aureus* (MRSA). As biocides are known to act on the microbes on multiple sites, biocide-resistance is often nonspecific and broad spectrum like resistance linked to increased expression of efflux pumps or change in the cell membrane permeability — all have the ability to reverse the antibiotic susceptibility as well. Plasmid-mediated resistance determinants to quaternary ammonium compounds (qacA, B, C, D and E), widely detected in *S. aureus*, *Pseudomonas* spp. and members of the *Enterobacteriaceae*, were reported to cause resistance to antibiotics belonging to trimethoprim, sulphonamides, oxacillin and aminoglycosides (Fraise, 2002). Similarly, presence of active drug efflux pumps may confer resistance to both antibiotics and biocides as seen in those strains constitutively expressing multiple antibiotic resistance proteins (Fraise, 2002). Apart from cross-resistance where the same gene/mechanism is involved for resistance to biocides and antibiotics, biocide resistance gene(s) may be present in the same plasmid with other ARG(s), a phenomenon known as co-resistance. This has been previously recorded in a gentamicin-resistant MRSA strain which carried resistance genes for aminoglycosides, ethidium bromide, benzalkonium chloride and chlorhexidine together in the same plasmid (Yamamoto et al., 1988). Moreover, altered physiological response, selective growth of rigid and resistant bacteria and increased alacrity of DNA repairing system are among the other important mechanisms by which bacteria resort to be antibiotic-resilient following biocide exposure (Anonymous (European Commission), 2009).

Environment gets a constant exposure of metal from household, industrial and automobile effluents, besides being contaminated from their (metal) uses in food, textiles, household, hospital products, agriculture and disinfectants. In general, bacteria use three different mechanisms to avert heavy metal toxicity — biosorption of toxic metals in cell membranes, cell walls and extracellular polymeric substance of biofilms; detoxification through reduction of intracellular ions, just as mediated by merA gene encoded reduction of Hg^{2+} to the less toxic Hg^0 to evade mercury toxicity; efflux pump mediated extrusion of toxic metals. Like biocides, metals are also regarded as important drivers for antibiotic resistance. Heavy metal may induce antibiotic resistance like arsenate linked with chloramphenicol resistance and copper/zinc linked tetracycline resistance were reported by a group of workers from China. Their study pointed out that relatively low heavy metal levels in polluted environments and in treated humans and animals might be sufficient to induce antibiotic resistance in bacteria (Chen et al., 2015). Metal-mediated antibiotic resistance may be observed in the form of cross-resistance or co-resistance (Pal et al., 2017; Seiler & Berendonk, 2012). Cross-resistance is usually mediated by the multidrug efflux pumps which use both the heavy metals and antibiotics as their substrate (Blanco et al., 2016). Co-resistance was reported in many instances when the gene(s) for both the metal and antibiotic resistance are carried in the form of gene cassette in mobile genetic element or plasmid (Pal et al., 2017; Seiler & Berendonk, 2012). Co-existence of resistant gene(s) for heavy metals such as cadmium, arsenic and copper and antibiotic resistance was reported in a novel composite staphylococcal cassette chromosome in a *Staphylococcus haemolyticus* isolate from bovine mastitis milk (Xue et al., 2015). This study emphasizes the possible link of metal use to the rise of antibiotic resistance in various settings.

Regulators

Waste water treatment plants (WWTP) receive sludge and effluents from various sources that are already contaminated with antibiotics, biocides, metals and ARGs, and the treatment is not always sufficient to eliminate these contaminants. On entering river, estuary or coastal water, WWTP discharge may have significant impact over the microbial community and its genetic makeup. Ultimately, it increases the risk of human exposure to resistant organism through contaminated recreational or coastal bathing water (Leonard et al., 2018; Leonard et al., 2015).

Use of manure slurry and sewage sludge on agricultural lands, a common practice with an aim to increase the soil fertility, has been viewed by many as an important driver for spreading antibiotic resistance in environment. Human and animal use of antibiotics, biocides and metals lead to contamination of both manure slurry and sewage sludge. Land spreading using these materials can thus serve as potential source for spread of such contaminants along with ARG(s) to farm workers, crops, agriculture run-off, aquatic bodies, groundwater, grazing domestic animals and wild animals, etc. Recent study demonstrated that such land spreading practice with treated or composted sludge may increase the spread of ARG(s) in environment — for example, use of pig slurry increases prevalence of *int1* gene (Tasho & Cho, 2016). Persistence of antibiotic residue depends on various factors — pH, soil condition, temperature, exposure to sunlight, etc. In general, antibiotics such as chloramphenicol and ceftiofur stay active for a short period — only for few days; however, antibiotics such as tetracyclines and fluoroquinolones may persist for as long as 300 days. The persistence may increase substantially in low temperature and absence of sunlight (Singer et al., 2016).

Another possible route of transmission and emergence of antibiotic-resistant pathogens is through aerosol route where pathogens resistant to antimicrobials, particularly to antifungal/fungicides, were recorded to spread through airborne transmission. Broadcast application of azole antifungal in crop cultivation has been presumed to play a role for emergence of azole-resistant *Aspergillus fumigatus*, a key pathogen involved in several life-threatening illnesses such as fungal pneumonia or invasive mycosis (Anders et al., 2012). Even studies found evidences to link human transmission of azole-resistant *A. fumigatus* with use of azole fungicides for plant and material protection. Thus, airborne transmission or bioaerosol is considered to be involved in such transmission of AMR (Alanio et al., 2011; Wirmann et al., 2018). All including air, water and waterbodies are known for being potent reservoir of antibiotic-resistant bacteria and ARG(s). Added to that, there is growing body of evidence to suggest that water treatment practices adopted to make drinking water safe for public consumption are accountable for preponderance of AMR — chlorination, a common water treatment practice, was reported to increase resistant bacterial count in drinking water (Armstrong et al., 1982; Shrivastava et al., 2004; Xi et al., 2009). Chlorinated sewage water had a higher proportion of bacteria resistant to ampicillin and cephalothin; what's more, potentially pathogenic species were also isolated from chlorinated and regrown sewage samples, including *Yersinia enterocolitica, Yersinia pestis, Pasteurella multocida* and *Hafnia alvei* (Murray et al., 1984). Livestock is often incriminated for contaminating water, as both antibiotic residues and ARG arising out of animals raised and reared under intensive system were detected to contaminate from surface water to nearby waterbodies (Zhang et al., 2014). The resistance problem may be more intense in the areas where use of poultry and cattle manure is rampant, as indicated in a study carried out in Southeastern China, particularly for the drugs such as tetracyclines, sulphonamides and macrolides, for which the corresponding resistance determinants (*tet, sul* and *erm*) have higher propensity to spread (Wang et al., 2016). In addition to livestock farming, antibiotics, such as streptomycin, tetracycline, oxolinic acid and gentamicin are also used in agriculture, primarily in tree fruits (apple, pear, peach and nectarine) for the treatment of bacterial spot of peach and nectarine (*Xanthomonas arboricola* pv. *pruni*) and fire blight of pear and apple (*Erwinia amylovora*), since long (Mayerhofer et al., 2009; Schnabel & Jones, 1999). Usually, antibiotics are sprayed to suppress pathogen growth on flowers and leaf surfaces before infection. Antibiotics applied through such route are considered short-lived without leaving any significant residue on harvested fruit. In 2009 in the United States, 16,465 kg (active ingredient) of antibiotics was applied on orchards, accounting for 0.12% of the total antibiotics used in animal agriculture (Stockwell & Duffy, 2012). Although there is little evidence that such use has any impact over the microbial community or abundance of mobile genetic elements in soil, its long-term impact on the microbial flora of plants, soils and waterbodies needs to be placed under scanner, especially when streptomycin-resistant gene(s) were reported in plant pathogens (*E. amylovora, Pseudomonas* spp. and *Xanthomonas campestris*) (Walsh et al., 2013; Duffy et al., 2014). Besides direct application of antibiotics, plant can also uptake antibiotics in their biomass from contaminated soil or groundwater. Such bioaccumulation may eventually lead to selection of the resistant bacterial population not only in the plant but also in the consumers — herbivores including insects, animals and human. Nevertheless, it depends on proportion of absorbed antibiotics being phytoextracted or transmitted in the consumable raw or processed food without any alteration in the physical or biological property, which still remains unclear. Certain antibiotics such as sulfathiazole, sulfadiazine, sulfamethazine, sulfadimethoxine, chlortetracycline and trimethoprim were demonstrated to be phytoextracted in plant biomass (Singer et al., 2016). Greenhouse studies conducted by scientists at the University of Minnesota revealed that all the three test crops — corn (*Zea mays* L.), green onion (*Allium cepa* L.) and cabbage (*Brassica oleracea* L. Capitata group) — used in their experiment were able to uptake antibiotic like tetracycline in a concentration-dependent manner when grown on manure-applied soils (Chander et al., 2005). Later on, the group extended their study involving three food crops, corn, lettuce and potato, grown on soil modified with liquid hog manure containing sulfamethazine, a common veterinary antibiotic, and was able to detect its presence in the leaves and potato tubers. It suggests that the root crops — potatoes, carrots and radishes, which are in direct contact with soil — are vulnerable for antibiotic contamination and bioaccumulation (Plants Uptake Antibiotics, n.d.). Again, use of antimicrobials in aquaculture also widens the scope for spreading and interchanging the resistant organism and resistant gene(s) with the surrounding aquatic environment. Furthermore, the spread of resistant bacteria and gene(s) from aquatic sources to human or animal microbial flora increases the burden of AMR in the environmental surrounding (Cabello et al., 2016). Little is known about the impact of antimicrobial residue present in groundwater, which is invariably contaminated with antibiotics because of irrigation, rainfall and other anthropogenic activities (Loos et al., 2010). Wastewater originated from healthcare units and livestock may also infiltrate to contaminate groundwater with considerable burden of residual antimicrobials (Bartelt-Hunt et al., 2011). However, effect of such contamination on emergence of AMR is still not known.

Prevention and control strategies

Multiple sources were identified to have definite role in contaminating the environment with antibiotic residue and ARG(s) — hospitals and healthcare units, livestock farms, agriculture and plant-based food production units, antibiotic manufacturing plants, all can have potential role. Although individual contribution of these factors to rising problem of AMR in environment is still unclear, each source needs to be managed and gridlocked with a view to reduce the burden of AMR in environment. Given the enormity of infective pathogens treated and diversity of antimicrobials used, hospital and healthcare units may serve as a potent source — a study conducted in 303 hospitals from 53 countries by Global-PPS of Antimicrobial Consumption and Resistance in 2015 documented that about 34.4% of the adult inpatients received at least one antimicrobial. Hence, it is important to reduce the burden of both bug and drug in hospital emission by hospital stewardship and IPC programmes to maintain optimum hygiene and sanitation in all hospital operation. Furthermore, it is important to ensure safe disposal of antimicrobial medicines and hazardous waste, which can be achieved by pretreatment of hospital waste before being discharged into the general sewage system. All hospital personnel should be educated and trained on hygiene, sanitation and safe disposal practices. Like hospitals, livestock farms, agriculture production units using antimicrobials as pesticides, and slaughterhouses are also considered as important sources to contaminate the environment with both commensal pathogens and antibiotic residues, which can only be diminished through improved biosecurity measures, better infection control strategy with proper vaccination and improved animal husbandry practices with a view to cut the antimicrobial usage in livestock and agriculture. Furthermore, pretreatment of waste from farms, slaughterhouse and agricultural lands before its discharge in general sewage can stop the bugs/antimicrobials/ARG(s) to enter into the environment. Another common source is the pharmaceutical industries which must wind down the release of antibiotic residue in the environment through waste disposal, for which a proper regulatory framework should be in place mentioning the prescribed limit of antibiotic in the discharge, and regular monitoring of the antibiotic residue in the waste to be discharged is essential. Although various protocols for wastewater treatment are there to reduce the burden of AMR in environment, most of the treatment protocols are not equally effective to reduce the antibiotic residues. It is therefore essential to optimize the treatment protocol depending on the type of antibiotic residue to be cut down. Moreover, limited facility with regard to waste management, lack of infrastructure and resources, poor regulation and absence of standard operating protocol are the major drawbacks which need to be addressed to put AMR stewardship into practice, particularly in developing and underdeveloped countries.

Innovative research is required for waste management or waste treatment such as composting and manure storage, biochar formation, anaerobic digestion, ozone and ultraviolet light treatment, etc. (Anonymous, n.d.). Moreover, it is important to know the role of wildlife as a reservoir of AMR pathogens as wild-animals may play a crucial role in spreading of such pathogens in environment in a covert and insidious manner (Dobiasova et al., 2013; Grobbel et al., 2018).

References

AKimitsu, N., Hamamoto, H., Inoue, R., Shoji, M., Akamine, A., Takemori, K., et al., 1999. Increase in resistance of methicillin-resistant *Staphylococcus aureus* to beta-lactams caused by mutations conferring resistance to benzalkonium chloride, a disinfectant widely used in hospitals. Antimicrobial Agents and Chemotherapy 43, 3042−3043.

Alanio, A., Cordonnier, C., Bretagne, S., 2011. Azole resistance in *Aspergillus fumigatus*—current epidemiology and future perspectives. Current Fungal Infection Reports 5, 168−178. https://doi.org/10.1007/s12281-011-0061-y.

Anders, A., Janzen, A.-L., Schlottmann, R., Wichert, M., Knop-Hammad, V., Gatermann, S., 2012. Fatal outcome of a bilateral community-acquired pneumonia due to *Aspergillus fumigatus*? International Journal of Medical Microbiology 302, 54.

Anonymous (European Commission), 2009. Effects of Biocides on Antibiotic Resistance Level 2 - Details on Effects of Biocides. DG Health and Consumers of the European Commission, pp. 1−25.

Anonymous, 2018. Initiatives for Addressing Antimicrobial Resistance in the Environment: Current Situation and Challenges. https://wellcome.ac.uk/sites/default/files/antimicrobial-resistance-environment-report.pdf.

Anonymous., n.d. MEDICINES drug-resistant microbes spread through trade, travel, and migration of people and animals. www.fao.org/antimicrobial-resistance.

Armstrong, J.L., Calomiris, J.J., Seidler, R.J., 1982. Selection of antibiotic-resistant standard plate count bacteria during water treatment. Applied and Environmental Microbiology 44, 308−316.

Bartelt-Hunt, S., Snow, D.D., Damon-Powell, T., Miesbach, D., 2011. Occurrence of steroid hormones and antibiotics in shallow groundwater impacted by livestock waste control facilities. Journal of Contaminant Hydrology 123, 94−103. https://doi.org/10.1016/j.jconhyd.2010.12.010.

Bengtsson-Palme, J., Kristiansson, E., Larsson, D.G.J., 2018. Environmental factors influencing the development and spread of antibiotic resistance. FEMS Microbiology Reviews 42, 68−80. https://doi.org/10.1093/femsre/fux053.

Berg, G., Alavi, M., Schmid, M., Hartmann, A., 2013. The rhizosphere as a reservoir for opportunistic human pathogenic bacteria. Mol. Microb. Ecol. Rhizosph. vol. 2, 1209−1216. https://doi.org/10.1002/9781118297674.ch116.

Blanco, P., Hernando-Amado, S., Reales-Calderon, J.A., Corona, F., Lira, F., Alcalde-Rico, M., et al., 2016. Bacterial multidrug efflux pumps: much more than antibiotic resistance determinants. Microorganisms 4. https://doi.org/10.3390/microorganisms4010014.

Cabello, F.C., Godfrey, H.P., Buschmann, A.H., Dölz, H.J., 2016. Aquaculture as yet another environmental gateway to the development and globalisation of antimicrobial resistance. The Lancet Infectious Diseases 16, e127−e133. https://doi.org/10.1016/S1473-3099(16)00100-6.

Chander, Y., Rosen, C.J., Kumar, K., Gupta, S.C., Baidoo, S.K., Chander, Y., et al., 2005. Antibiotic uptake by plants from soil fertilized with animal manure. Journal of Environmental Quality 34, 2082. https://doi.org/10.2134/jeq2005.0026.

Chen, S., Li, X., Sun, G., Zhang, Y., Su, J., Ye, J., 2015. Heavy metal induced antibiotic resistance in bacterium LSJC7. International Journal of Molecular Sciences 16, 23390−23404. https://doi.org/10.3390/ijms161023390.

Dobiasova, H., Dolejska, M., Jamborova, I., Brhelova, E., Blazkova, L., Papousek, I., et al., 2013. Extended spectrum beta-lactamase and fluoroquinolone resistance genes and plasmids among *Escherichia coli* isolates from zoo animals, Czech Republic. FEMS Microbiology Ecology 85, 604−611. https://doi.org/10.1111/1574-6941.12149.

Duffy, B., Holliger, E., Walsh, F., 2014. Streptomycin use in apple orchards did not increase abundance of mobile resistance genes. FEMS Microbiology Letters 350, 180−189. https://doi.org/10.1111/1574-6968.12313.

FAO, 2018. Summary Report of an FAO Meeting of Experts on Antimicrobial Resistance in the Environment. FAO Antimicrobial Resistance Working Group 1−3.

Fraise, A.P., 2002. Biocide abuse and antimicrobial resistance–a cause for concern? Journal of Antimicrobial Chemotherapy 49, 11−12. https://doi.org/10.1093/jac/49.1.11.

Grobbel, M., Schwarz, S., Feßler, A.T., Eichhorn, I., Brombach, J., Monecke, S., et al., 2018. Phenotypic and genotypic characteristics of *Staphylococcus aureus* isolates from zoo and wild animals. Veterinary Microbiology 218, 98−103. https://doi.org/10.1016/j.vetmic.2018.03.020.

Harada, K., Asai, T., 2010. Role of antimicrobial selective pressure and secondary factors on antimicrobial resistance prevalence in *Escherichia coli* from food-producing animals in Japan. Journal of Biomedicine and Biotechnology 2010, 1−12. https://doi.org/10.1155/2010/180682.

Huijbers, P.M.C., Blaak, H., De Jong, M.C.M., Graat, E.A.M., Vandenbroucke-Grauls, C.M.J.E., De Roda Husman, A.M., 2015. Role of the environment in the transmission of antimicrobial resistance to humans: a review. Environmental Science and Technology 49, 11993−12004. https://doi.org/10.1021/acs.est.5b02566.

Johnning, A., Moore, E.R.B., Svensson-Stadler, L., Shouche, Y.S., Joakim Larsson, D.G., Kristiansson, E., 2013. Acquired genetic mechanisms of a multiresistant bacterium isolated from a treatment plant receiving wastewater from antibiotic production. Applied and Environmental Microbiology 79, 7256−7263. https://doi.org/10.1128/AEM.02141-13.

Leonard, A.F.C., Zhang, L., Balfour, A.J., Garside, R., Gaze, W.H., 2015. Human recreational exposure to antibiotic resistant bacteria in coastal bathing waters. Environment International 82, 92−100. https://doi.org/10.1016/j.envint.2015.02.013.

Leonard, A.F.C., Yin, X.L., Zhang, T., Hui, M., Gaze, W.H., 2018. A coliform-targeted metagenomic method facilitating human exposure estimates to *Escherichia coli*-borne antibiotic resistance genes. FEMS Microbiology Ecology 94. https://doi.org/10.1093/femsec/fiy024.

Loos, R., Locoro, G., Comero, S., Contini, S., Schwesig, D., Werres, F., et al., 2010. Pan-European survey on the occurrence of selected polar organic persistent pollutants in ground water. Water Research 44, 4115−4126. https://doi.org/10.1016/j.watres.2010.05.032.

Martínez, J.L., 2008. Antibiotics and antibiotic resistance genes in natural environments. Science 321, 365−367. https://doi.org/10.1126/science.1159483 (80-).

Martínez, J.L., 2012. Bottlenecks in the transferability of antibiotic resistance from natural ecosystems to human bacterial pathogens. Frontiers in Microbiology 3, 265. https://doi.org/10.3389/fmicb.2011.00265.

Mayerhofer, G., Schwaiger-Nemirova, I., Kuhn, T., Girsch, L., Allerberger, F., 2009. Detecting streptomycin in apples from orchards treated for fire blight. Journal of Antimicrobial Chemotherapy 63, 1076−1077. https://doi.org/10.1093/jac/dkp055.

Melnyk, A.H., Wong, A., Kassen, R., 2015. The fitness costs of antibiotic resistance mutations. Evolutionary Applications 8, 273−283. https://doi.org/10.1111/eva.12196.

Murray, G.E., Tobin, R.S., Junkins, B., Kushner, D.J., 1984. Effect of chlorination on antibiotic resistance profiles of sewage-related bacteria. Applied and Environmental Microbiology 48, 73−77.

Murray, A.K., Zhang, L., Yin, X., Zhang, T., Buckling, A., Snape, J., et al., 2018. Novel insights into selection for antibiotic resistance in complex microbial communities. mBio 9. https://doi.org/10.1128/mBio.00969-18.

Pal, C., Asiani, K., Arya, S., Rensing, C., Stekel, D.J., Larsson, D.G.J., et al., 2017. Metal resistance and its association with antibiotic resistance. Advances in Microbial Physiology 70, 261−313. https://doi.org/10.1016/bs.ampbs.2017.02.001.

Plants Uptake Antibiotics. Plants Uptake Antibiotics | EurekAlert! Science News. Glob Source Sci News., n.d. https://www.eurekalert.org/pub_releases/2007-07/ssso-pua071107.php.

Schnabel, E.L., Jones, A.L., 1999. Distribution of tetracycline resistance genes and transposons among phylloplane bacteria in Michigan apple orchards. Applied and Environmental Microbiology 65, 4898−4907.

Seiler, C., Berendonk, T.U., 2012. Heavy metal driven co-selection of antibiotic resistance in soil and water bodies impacted by agriculture and aquaculture. Frontiers in Microbiology 3, 399. https://doi.org/10.3389/fmicb.2012.00399.

Shrivastava, R., Upreti, R.K., Jain, S.R., Prasad, K.N., Seth, P.K., Chaturvedi, U.C., 2004. Suboptimal chlorine treatment of drinking water leads to selection of multidrug-resistant *Pseudomonas aeruginosa*. Ecotoxicology and Environmental Safety 58, 277−283. https://doi.org/10.1016/S0147-6513(03)00107-6.

Singer, A.C., Shaw, H., Rhodes, V., Hart, A., 2016. Review of antimicrobial resistance in the environment and its relevance to environmental regulators. Frontiers in Microbiology 7, 1−22. https://doi.org/10.3389/fmicb.2016.01728.

Stockwell, V.O., Duffy, B., 2012. Use of antibiotics in plant agriculture. Revue Scientifique et Technique 31, 199−210.

Sun, J., Deng, Z., Yan, A., 2014. Bacterial multidrug efflux pumps: mechanisms, physiology and pharmacological exploitations. Biochemical and Biophysical Research Communications 453, 254−267. https://doi.org/10.1016/j.bbrc.2014.05.090.

Tasho, R.P., Cho, J.Y., 2016. Veterinary antibiotics in animal waste, its distribution in soil and uptake by plants: a review. The Science of the Total Environment 563−564, 366−376. https://doi.org/10.1016/j.scitotenv.2016.04.140.

Walsh, F., Smith, D.P., Owens, S.M., Duffy, B., Frey, J.E., 2013. Restricted streptomycin use in apple orchards did not adversely alter the soil bacteria communities. Frontiers in Microbiology 4, 383. https://doi.org/10.3389/fmicb.2013.00383.

Wang, N., Guo, X., Yan, Z., Wang, W., Chen, B., Ge, F., et al., 2016. A comprehensive analysis on spread and distribution characteristic of antibiotic resistance genes in livestock farms of Southeastern China. PLoS One 11, e0156889. https://doi.org/10.1371/journal.pone.0156889.

Wirmann, L., Ross, B., Reimann, O., Steinmann, J., Rath, P.-M., 2018. Airborne Aspergillus fumigatus spore concentration during demolition of a building on a hospital site, and patient risk determination for invasive aspergillosis including azole resistance. Journal of Hospital Infection 100, e91−e97. https://doi.org/10.1016/j.jhin.2018.07.030.

Xi, C., Zhang, Y., Marrs, C.F., Ye, W., Simon, C., Foxman, B., et al., 2009. Prevalence of antibiotic resistance in drinking water treatment and distribution systems. Applied and Environmental Microbiology 75, 5714−5718. https://doi.org/10.1128/AEM.00382-09.

Xue, H., Wu, Z., Li, L., Li, F., Wang, Y., Zhao, X., 2015. Coexistence of heavy metal and antibiotic resistance within a novel composite staphylococcal cassette chromosome in a Staphylococcus haemolyticus isolate from bovine mastitis milk. Antimicrobial Agents and Chemotherapy 59, 5788−5792. https://doi.org/10.1128/AAC.04831-14.

Yamamoto, T., Tamura, Y., Yokota, T., 1988. Antiseptic and antibiotic resistance plasmid in *Staphylococcus aureus* that possesses ability to confer chlorhexidine and acrinol resistance. Antimicrobial Agents and Chemotherapy 32, 932−935. https://doi.org/10.1128/AAC.32.6.932.

Zhang, X., Li, Y., Liu, B., Wang, J., Feng, C., Gao, M., et al., 2014. Prevalence of veterinary antibiotics and antibiotic-resistant *Escherichia coli* in the surface water of a livestock production region in northern China. PLoS One 9, e111026. https://doi.org/10.1371/journal.pone.0111026.

Chapter 6

β-Lactamase

Chapter outline

Overview, mechanism and diversity of β-Lactamase

Production of β-lactamase (BL) enzyme is the key contributing factor for the emergence of β-lactam resistance. The BL is a unique enzyme released by the bacteria to inactivate the antibiotics containing β-lactam rings such as penicillins, cephalosporins, cephamycins and carbapenems by hydrolysing 4-atom β-lactam ring and thereby rendering the compounds ineffective. Only carbapenems are relatively resistant to BL. Possibly, because of the extensive use of β-lactam drugs, BL started to spread to multiple pathogens, over the years. Penicillinase was the BL which was detected even before the discovery and introduction of penicillin in clinical practice. Later on, following the advent of penicillin, penicillinase enzyme started to spread rapidly and within a decade, penicillin-resistant *Staphylococcus* emerged as a significant problem with the production of staphylococcal penicillinase. More than 2000 naturally occurring BLs have been recorded, till date — they differ in the amino acid sequences and in their characteristic hydrolysis profile (Bonomo, 2017). Again, AmpC BL is first of this type of enzymes to be recorded in *Escherichia coli* in 1940. It was quite similar to penicillinase recorded in *Staphylococcus aureus*.

Based on the Bush Jacoby classification, the BLs may be broadly categorized into three groups — group 1, group 2 and group 3. Group 1 enzymes, the chromosomally encoded cephalosporinase, fall under molecular class C and usually are more active against cephalosporins, cephamycin and aztreonam than benzyl penicillin and cannot be inhibited by BL inhibitors such as clavulanic acid (CA) (Bush and Jacoby, 2010). While in many bacteria, such as *Citrobacter freundii*, *Enterobacter cloacae*, *Serratia marcescens* and *Pseudomonas aeruginosa*, production of these enzymes is low but inducible in the presence of β-lactams, in others such as *Acinetobacter baumannii* and *E. coli*, its production is constitutive because of missing induction components. Although *E. coli* inherently possess this group of cephalosporinase, its production is low under weak promoter. However, in the presence of β-lactam antibiotics, ACBL production may be induced and some organisms may overproduce the enzymes. Many bacteria were recently reported to promiscuously transmit chromosomal ACBL genes to plasmids, resulting in highly resistant *E. coli* and *Klebsiella pneumonia*. In contrast to ESBLs (extended spectrum β-lactamase), these strains are unaffected by BL inhibitors such as CA and capable of being cephamycin-resistant. ACBL-producing *E. coli* were reported from animal sources as well and few isolates were reported to be dual-type lactamases producers (DTL). Many of the ESBL strains (*E. coli* and *K. pneumonia*) recovered from food animals in our study were DTL types (Kar et al., 2015; Koovapra et al., 2016; Bandyopadhyay et al., 2018). The plasmid-mediated group 1 enzymes include CIT, EBC, DHA, CMY, FOX and MIR. A subgroup of group 1 enzyme (1e) is known for their extended spectrum activities against ceftazidime (CMY 10, CMY 19 and CMY 37). Occasionally, AmpC BLs are known to cause carbapenem resistance as reported in *E. coli* with upregulation in the expression of CMY-2 (van Boxtel et al., 2017), or extended-spectrum AmpC BLs were also reported to cause such carbapenem resistance (Mammeri et al., 2008).

Group 2 enzymes are the serine BLs that fall under the molecular classes A and D. Of them, the enzymes 2a constitute the penicillinase, abundant in Gram-positive cocci and are active against the benzyl penicillin or penicillin derivatives; however, their action is limited against cephalosporins and carbapenems. Enzymes of subgroup 2b, which include TEM-1, TEM-2 and SHV-1, are active against penicillin and early generation cephalosporins — cephaloridine and cephalothin — and they can be inhibited by BL inhibitors (Bush and Jacoby, 2010). TEM-1 was the first detected plasmid-mediated BL recorded in *E. coli* isolated from a patient of Greece in 1965. Subgroups 2e constitute the ESBL, probably the most discussed BL after MBL (metallo-β-lactamase) for its increasing threat to human health. Most of the early members of this group emerge with the amino acid substitution of the TEM-1, TEM-2 and SHV-1, broadening their spectrum of activity. ESBLs are the plasmid-mediated enzymes that can confer resistance to the newer group of cephalosporins — third- and fourth-generation cephalosporins (cefpodoxime, cefotaxime, ceftazidime and cefepime) and monobactam (aztreonam). In contrast, ESBL cannot affect carbapenems (imipenem, meropenem and itrapenem) and cephamycin (cefoxitin and cefotenan) and can be inhibited by BL inhibitors such as CA, sulbactum and tazobactum. It was way back in 1983 when ESBL was first reported and it was a point mutational variant of SHV-1. Soon, other BLs were reported to evolve from TEM-1 and 2 to show extended spectrum BL activities. These are classical ESBLs derived from mutation of the existing BL genes with wider hydrolytic potentiality. Another variant of ESBLs — CTX-M type — has been progressively replacing the TEM and SHV and becoming an emerging problem in human health and is considered as 'the CTX-M pandemic' (Cantón and Coque, 2006). CTX-M enzymes are classified into five main subgroups (group 1: CTX-M-1, group 2: CTX-M-2, group 8: CTXM-8, group 9: CTX-M-9 and group 25: CTX-M-25) (Bonnet, 2004). Although several other members of the *Enterobacteriaceae* family are ESBL producers, *K. pneumoniae* and *E. coli* have been most frequently reported. There are various reports suggesting the recent surge of CTX-M type of BLs all over the world. The CTX-M-type BL shows more than 90% sequence identity with BLs observed in *Kluyvera* spp., the possible progenitor of this ESBL variant (Poirel et al., 2002). The name, CTX-M, has originated from its hydrolytic efficiency against cefotaxime (Gazouli, 1998). In general, CTX-M-type ESBL producer exhibits appreciable sensitivity to ceftazidime. However, they are resistant to cefepime and mostly to aztreonam. Again, some variants of CTX-M-type ESBLs were recorded ceftazidime-resistant (Koovapra et al., 2016; Schneider et al., 2009). Several other plasmid-mediated or integron-associated ESBL types have been reported (PER (2be), VEB (2be), GES (2f), BES, TEL, SFO), albeit less frequently (Bonomo, 2017; Bush and Jacoby, 2010). Some of the enzymes under subgroup 2br — TEM 30, TEM-31 and SHV-10 are classified as inhibitor-resistant BL for their being refractory to the BL inhibitors such as CA (Bonomo and Rice, 1999).

The name OXA-type BLs has evolved from their oxacillin-hydrolysing capacity. The enzymes under subgroup 2d are known for the activity against cloxacillin and oxacillin, and they are inhibited by NaCl. Importantly, the enzymes from subgroups 2de and 2df have gained clinical significance because of their hydrolytic potentiality against extended spectrum cephalosporins and carbapenem, respectively. While OXA enzymes of 2de subgroup, derived from OXA 10, OXA 11, OXA 15 and OXA 35, were detected among *Pseudomonas aeruginosa* (Aubert, 2002; Evans and Amyes, 2014), those under 2df subgroup were reported in *A. baumannii* (chromosome-mediated) and *Enterobacteriaceae* (plasmid-mediated) (Bush and Jacoby, 2010; Evans and Amyes, 2014). In addition, cephalosporinase of subgroup 2e was reported exclusively in *Proteus* — these are exactly similar to ESBLs/ACBLs for their hydrolysis of ESCs (extended spectrum cephalosporin) (Bush and Jacoby, 2010).

ESBLs — origin and present status

New generation oxyimino-cephalosporins arrived as a new weapon in the hand of the clinicians to combat the increasing evidence of narrow spectrum BL causing resistance to penicillin, first- and second-generation cephalosporins. Undoubtedly third-generation cephalosporins were the first drug of this kind to overcome the increasing burden of ampicillin hydrolysing TEM-1 and SHV-1 BL, which became widespread among the *Enterobacteriaceae* family, especially in *E. coli* and *K. pneumoniae*, and it was preferred over aminoglycosides and polymyxins for lesser nephrotoxic effects (Extended Spectrum Beta La, 2012). However, the introduction and spread of plasmid-mediated ESBLs had become a major setback to what was regarded to initiate a new era of antibiotic therapy with the introduction of third-generation cephalosporins. Not that such the problem is limited in human patients and health-care premises only, but that acquisition of different virulence and such resistance factors may render the common commensal to pose a zoonotic threat with narrowed therapeutic armamentarium imposing a greater threat to public health (Xi et al., 2009; Leonard et al., 2018) and environmental safety (Bengtsson-Palme et al., 2018; Singer et al., 2016). Poultry, cattle and swine raised under the intensive farming system and with prolonged exposure of antibiotics as growth promoter are more likely to harbour significant populations of antibiotic-resistant bacteria, which may transfer to human through direct contact with the animals and through their meat, eggs and milk (Marshall and Levy, 2011). There is no gainsaying that continuous oral administration of low concentrations of antimicrobials — a decade old practice with an intention to increase feed conversion, weight gain and resistance to shipping stress-associated diseases in food animals — is indeed a key concern for facilitating resistance phenotype in animal biota (Reantaso et al., 2012).

Types and diversity

SHV-type BL is probably the most frequently encountered BL recorded at least a few years back. The first SHV-type ESBL was reported from Germany in 1983 and it derived from SHV-1 with a single amino acid substitution (serine-238-glycine) and the mutant enzyme exhibited hydrolytic potentiality against both cefotaxime and ceftazidime. Within a span of 10–15 years, SHV-type ESBLs producing *Enterobacteriaceae*, *P. aeruginosa* and *Acinetobacter* spp. were reported almost from every continent (Extended Spectrum Beta La, 2012). Presently, around 189 SHV variants have been recorded (Liakopoulos et al., 2016).

TEM-type ESBL has been derived from narrow-spectrum BL TEM variants — TEM-1 and TEM-2 (lysine for glutamate in 39th position of TEM-1 amino acid sequence). TEM-1, TEM-2 and TEM-13 are the BLs showing resistance mainly to penicillin group of drugs such as ampicillin and these variants do not have any hydrolytic capacity towards extended-spectrum cephalosporins (Paterson and Bonomo 2005). In 1982, the first TEM-type ESBL (TEM-12) was recorded in *Klebsiella oxytoca* isolate from a neonatal unit of a hospital from Liverpool, UK (Bois et al., 1995). Again in 1987, TEM-3-type ESBL was reported in a *K. pneumoniae* isolate from France. To date, more than 130 variants of TEM-type ESBL were recorded worldwide (Petit et al., 1990). A group of TEM-type ESBL was recorded, which exhibited not only wide spectrum of hydrolytic activities against new-generation cephalosporins but also they cannot be inhibited by BL inhibitors. These are called complex mutant TEM or inhibitor-resistant TEM BL (Chaibi et al., 1999). CTX-M-type ESBL has become pandemic and is being recorded all over the world including India (Cantón et al., 2012). Toho type BL (1 and 2) is similar to the CTX-M type recorded from Japan (Paterson et al., 2003). All these enzymes showed frank resistance to ceftazidime, cefotaxime and aztreonam. There were some striking differences in region-wise occurrence of the ESBL producers. While SHV- and TEM-type BLs were predominantly noted in the United States, other parts of the world experienced repeated outbreaks of CTX-M producing *K. pneumonia* and *E. coli* except in few instances where CTX-M-type ESBLs were reported in the United States (Wang et al., 2013). European Antibiotic Resistance Surveillance System reported a higher incidence of ESBL producers in European countries also. During 1980–90s, most of the ESBL producers belonged to SHV and TEM types and were exclusively associated with nosocomial outbreaks. Recent data suggested that with the implementation of stringent infection control strategies in Western Europe, the incidence of CTX-M type *K. pneumonia* outbreaks slightly decreased over the last few years; however, it was not true for Eastern Europe (Dhillon and Clark, 2012). In Latin American countries, the incidence of ESBL producers remained consistently high with the predominance of CTX-M types. The similar picture was noticed for Asian countries such as China, Japan (Hirakata et al., 2005), India (Odsbu et al., 2018), Pakistan (Habeeb et al., 2013), Saudi Arab (Mashwal et al., 2017) and Taiwan (Suwantarat and Carroll, 2016). Although ESBL producers are mostly predominated by *E. coli* and *K. pneumonia*, some other Gram-negative bacteria — *C. freundii*, *Enterobacter* spp., and *S. marcescens* — were also recorded for ESBL production (Kim and Lim, 2005).

Although several studies were carried out on ESBL producers in human from India, such reports have been truly limited in livestock. However, studies in other countries have indicated that food animals are an important reservoir of ESBL producers. In the recent past, bovine mastitis caused by ESBL-producing *Enterobacteriaceae* was reported from France (Dahmen et al., 2013). Again CTX-M-type ESBL producers were reported in bovine mastitis cases from Japan (Saishu et al., 2014) and China (Ali et al., 2016). Besides, ESBL-producing bacteria were isolated from raw milk, meat, meat products (Geser et al., 2012), broiler chicken (Brower et al., 2017), pigs (Dohmen et al., 2017), rabbit (Blanc et al., 2006), urinary tract infection of companion animals such as dogs and cats (Huber et al., 2013), wild animals (Guenther et al., 2011), domestic animal farm premises and other resources associated with animals (Nóbrega and Brocchi, 2014).

In India, multidrug-resistant ESBL and carbapenemase-producing *Enterobacteriaceae* were reported from a vaginal swab of the healthy swamp buffaloes in recent past (Singh, 2014). In our recent studies carried out at Eastern Regional Station, Kolkata ICAR-IVRI, we have detected both CTX-M-15 and SHV-12-type ESBL producing *K. pneumonia*, *K. oxytoca* and *E. coli* causing bovine mastitis. ESBL variants of CTX-M-15 and SHV-12 were invariably detected from the bovine milk samples collected from Jharkhand, Meghalaya, Odisha and West Bengal (Kar et al., 2015; Koovapra et al., 2016; Bandyopadhyay et al., 2015). Characterization of CTX-M type of ESBL producers revealed interesting findings in our study. Most of the strains of bovine and poultry origin carried CTX-M gene having 98%—100% similarity with CTX-M-15 (Koovapra et al., 2016). However, in another study conducted in pigs, most of the porcine isolates carried CTX-M-9 type of ESBL (Samanta et al., 2015). In our study, most of the ESBL producers recovered from animal isolates were multidrug-resistant. Recently ESBL producers from buffalo milk were found to harbour resistance genes to tetracycline, fluoroquinolone and aminoglycosides (Bandyopadhyay et al., 2018). In most of the strains, insertion sequence ISEcp1 was detected to facilitate the mobilization and expression of blaCTX-M-15. While our study in backyard poultry sector of West Bengal could hardly reveal any ESBL producer (Samanta et al., 2014), ESBL-producing *E. coli* were frequently detected from organized poultry sector in its neighbouring areas of Odisha (Kar et al., 2015). Furthermore, high prevalence of ESBLs was noted in commercial poultry farms from Western India (Brower et al., 2017). This indicates that frequent and exuberant use of antibiotic may confer substantial selection pressure for the emergence of such drug-resistant pathogens. Again, many of these ESBL producers from poultry or cattle were found resistant to BL inhibitors also. The class I integron of ESBL strains of bovine and avian origin in our study was found to carry several drug-resistant cassettes such as dfrA12/dfrA17 (dihydrofolate reductase-resistance to trimethoprim) and aadA2/aadA5 (aminoglycoside acetyltransferase-resistance to aminoglycosides). A recent study conducted by another group of workers from India also recorded a high prevalence of potential ESBL- and AmpC-producing *E. coli* in livestock and poultry from northeastern India (Tewari et al., 2019). A series of studies conducted from our laboratory in bovine and poultry showed that majority of the ESBLs were also AmpC-type BL producers (Kar et al., 2015; Koovapra et al., 2016; Bandyopadhyay et al., 2018; Mahanti et al., 2018). This was also further confirmed by Samanta et al., (2018) who reported that about 80% of the *K. pneumonia* isolates and all *E. coli* isolates from pigs or pig environment were AmpC-type BL producers. Rensing et al., 2019 also reported AmpC-type BL producers in the chicken carcass and mutton from Egypt — many of which also carried ESBL genes (Rensing et al., 2019). Both BLs can be transmitted to the surrounding environment to pose a considerable risk to public health as recorded in previous studies (Von Salviati et al., 2015; Laube et al., 2014).

Although several risk factors are established for health care or community-acquired ESBL infection in human, such evidence is poorly studied in animals. It is still unclear whether the extensive use of modern and newer antibiotic molecules such as third- or fourth-generation antibiotics led to the colonization of such ESBL producers in animals or not. Taking Indian perspective into context, it can be said that use of such expensive modern antibiotic molecules is still very limited in veterinary practices except for canines and high-yielding dairy cattle. However, our studies have revealed the presence of such ESC-resistant bugs in a range of animal hosts including yaks (Bandyopadhyay et al., 2009; Bandyopadhyay et al., 2012) and backyard piggery (Samanta et al., 2015) where the use of ESCs is negligible. Spreading of the bugs beyond hospital premises to the community and contamination of the environment may be an alternative source of infection for animals. Many of the bugs in animals also possess other resistance determinants for other antimicrobial agents such as quinolones, aminoglycosides and sulphonamides. Therefore, the use of other affordable antimicrobials may also put selection pressure for colonization and propagation of such bugs in livestock (Fig. 6.1).

Detection of β-lactamase production

Undoubtedly, diagnosis of ESBL infection is complex and requires appropriate laboratory setup and well-trained personnel for precise confirmation of ESBL production. As a part of the initial screening of ESBL production, following discs need to be used as per the recommendation of Clinical and Laboratory Standard Institute (CLSI) — cefpodoxime (10 μg), ceftazidime (30 μg), aztreonam (30 μg), cefotaxime (30 μ) and ceftriaxone (30 μg). Use of more than one disc usually increases the sensitivity of the test. The test should be performed using *K. pneumoniae* ATCC 700,603 (as positive control) and *E. coli* ATCC 25,922 (as negative control) as reference strains for quality control. The test isolates may be suspected as ESBL producer if it exhibits resistance to any of the five drugs screened. Details regarding the zone diameters of the drugs are given in Table 6.1.

Furthermore, in broth dilution method, isolates with MIC of ≥ 2 μg/mL for ceftazidime, aztreonam, cefotaxime or ceftriaxone is suspicious of ESBL production, and such isolates should be tested by suitable phenotypic confirmatory test. However, for cefpodoxime, organisms with MIC value of ≥ 8 μg/mL are considered for further investigation for ESBL production.

ESBL production is confirmed based on the fact that this group of enzymes can be inhibited by CA. Therefore, the synergy between the indicator cephalosporin and CA is used for confirmation of ESBL production. CLSI recommended the use of combination disk method which is described in brief.

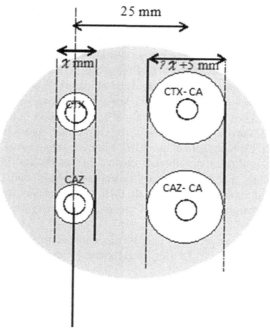

FIGURE 6.1 Combination disc method for detection of ESBL production. *CTX*, cefotaxime 30 μg; *CAZ*, ceftazidime 30 μg; *CTX-CA*, cefotaxime (30 μg) + clavulanic acid (10 μg); *CAZ-CA*, ceftazidime (30 μg) + clavulanic acid (10 μg).

TABLE 6.1 Zone diameter for initial screening of ESBL production.

	Drugs	Zones for isolates to be investigated	*Klebsiella pneumoniae* ATCC 700603	*Escherichia coli* ATCC® 25,922
1.	Cefpodoxime (10 μg)	≤17 mm	9−16 mm	23−28 mm
2.	Ceftazidime (30 μg)	≤22 mm	10−18 mm	25−32 mm
3.	Aztreonam (30 μg)	≤27 mm	9−17 mm	28−36 mm
4.	Cefotaxime (30 μg)	≤27 mm	17−25 mm	29−35 mm
5.	Ceftriaxone (30 μg)	≤25 mm	16−24 mm	29−35 mm

Combination disk method

In this method, following inoculation of the test isolate, two discs are placed — one is cephalosporin alone and another cephalosporin disc with CA. In our laboratory, this test is performed using cefotaxime (30 μg) or ceftazidime (30 μg) alone and with CA (10 μg). The discs should be placed with a distance of 25 mm, centre to centre. An increase of 5 mm (50%) or more in the zone of inhibition around the combined disc containing CA than the corresponding disc with cefotaxime or ceftazidime is considered positive for ESBL production. In general, laboratories should test all isolates of *E. coli* or *Klebsiella* spp. using both ceftazidime (the best indicator for TEM and SHV-derived ESBLs) and cefotaxime (the best indicator for CTX-M types).

Double-disc approximation test

This test is also known as double-disc synergy test (DDST). The plate is inoculated and processed as described in the combination disc method. A disc of amoxicillin-clavulanate (20 μg/10 μg) (Augmentin) is placed at the centre with the discs of extended-spectrum cephalosporins [cefpodoxime (30 μg), ceftazidime (30 μg) and cefotaxime (30 μg)] or aztreonam (30 μg) at the periphery with a centre to centre distance of 20 mm. This distance may vary from 16 to 30 mm and negative but suspected isolates may be retested with reduced distance. A clear extension of the edge of the inhibition zone of cephalosporin/aztreonam towards the augmentin disc is interpreted as positive for ESBL production.

Besides, many workers suggested disc replacement and three-dimensional methods, commercially available ESBL E-test and Vitek system for detection of phenotypic ESBL production. Although the current phenotypic tools such as combination disc method are popular and considered gold standard (Sittová et al., 2015), the process is time- and labour-consuming and lacks the desired sensitivity (Lupo et al., 2015). Detection of ESBL production in animal isolates is tricky, and false interpretation is often unavoidable because of the co-production of other BL or hyperproduction of ESBL or inhibitor-resistant BL (Kar et al., 2015; Koovapra et al., 2016; Bandyopadhyay et al., 2018). Workers rely on isoelectric focussing (Markovska et al., 2013), multiplex polymerase chain reaction (PCR) (Dallenne et al., 2010) or diagnostic microarray to determine ESBL variants. For rapid primary detection of SHV and CTX-M types of ESBLs, real-time PCR-based methods can be a better alternative (Sittová et al., 2015). But for determination of new or unknown variant, which is very common for frequent mutation of ESBL genes, sequencing of the entire coding region of the ESBL gene is to be conducted (D'Andrea et al., 2013).

Unlike ESBL, CLSI has not recommended any phenotypic confirmatory test for detection of AmpC-type BL. In general, *E. coli* isolates resistant to cefoxitin ($\leq$18 mm) or cefotetan ($\leq$16 mm) in disc diffusion test should be checked for Amp-type BL.

Cefoxitin-cloxacillin double-disk synergy test

Polsfuss et al., 2011 recommended the use of cefoxitin-cloxacillin double-disk synergy test (Polsfuss et al., 2011), which was found useful to detect AmpC BL production among *Enterobacteriaceae* isolates from food animals (Kar et al., 2015; Koovapra et al., 2016; Bandyopadhyay et al., 2018; Samanta et al., 2018). This test is based on the inhibitory effect of cloxacillin on AmpC BL where two disks containing 30 μg of cefoxitin and 30 μg of cefoxitin plus 200 μg of cloxacillin are placed on the surface of the MHA (Müller-Hinton agar) inoculated with test organism and was incubated at 35°C for 16−18 h. An increase of 4 mm or more in the cefoxitin-cloxacillin inhibition zones than the cefoxitin alone is considered indicative for AmpC BL production.

AmpC disk test

The test is based on the use of tris-EDTA to permeabilize a bacterial cell and release BL into the external environment. AmpC disks (filter paper disks containing tris-EDTA) are prepared in-house by applying 20 μL of a 1:1 mixture of normal saline and 100x tris-EDTA (1.0 M tris-HCl, pH ∼ 8.0, containing 0.1 M EDTA, filter sterilized) to sterile filter paper disks and the disks are dried before being stored at 2−8°C. The surface of a Mueller-Hinton agar plate is inoculated with a lawn of *E. coli* ATCC 25922 according to standard disk diffusion method. A rehydrated AmpC disks spotted with several colonies of each test organism along with a 30 μg cefoxitin disk are to be placed on the inoculated surface of the Mueller-Hinton agar. Following overnight incubation in an inverted position at 35°C in ambient air, the plates should be examined for either an indentation or a flattening of the zone of inhibition, indicating enzymatic inactivation of cefoxitin (positive result), or the absence of distortion, indicating no significant inactivation of cefoxitin (negative result).

Detection of β-lactamase production in *Staphylococcus* species by penicillin zone edge test

As we discussed Gram-positive bacteria especially *S. aureus* also produces penicillinase − a common phenomenon for resistance to penicillin and related antimicrobials in these bacteria. Penicillin zone edge test is performed to ascertain the production of BL/penicillinase based on the appearance of the inhibition zone edge in the disc diffusion test around a penicillin G disc (10 units). The test is considered positive when the edge is sharp (cliff) and negative when the appearance of the edge is fuzzy (beach). In addition, Papanicolas et al., 2014 also proposed the use of two chromogenic discs for detection of such penicillinase production (Papanicolas et al., 2014).

However, these phenotypic tests for detection of AmpC BL or penicillinase are also not without flaws and are time-consuming; therefore, molecular tests may be used as an alternative for conducting surveillance with a large number of samples and even in the screening of clinical samples to overcome the problem of the delayed report. Dallenne et al., 2010 described multiple sets of PCR to detect ESBL and AmpC BL gene; details of the oligonucleotides and amplicon size are described in Table 6.2. Similarly, different workers have reported that screening for blaZ gene can be a better alternative for rapid detection of BL in *S. aureus*.

TABLE 6.2 Primer details and amplicon size for detection of ESBL, AmpC-type b-lactamase.

Sl No	Details	Oligonucleotides	Sequence (5′-3′)	Amplicon size (bp)
1.	Multiplex I TEM, SHV and OXA-1-like	TEM variants including TEM-1 and TEM-2	CATTTCCGTGTCGCCCTTATTC	800
			CGTTCATCCATAGTTGCCTGAC	
		SHV variants including SHV-1	AGCCGCTTGAGCAAATTAAAC	713
			ATCCCGCAGATAAATCACCAC	
		OXA-1, OXA-4 and OXA-30	GGCACCAGATTCAACTTTCAAG	564
			GACCCCAAGTTTCCTGTAAGTG	
2.	Multiplex II CTX-M group 1, group 2 and group 9	MultiCTXMGp1_for	TTAGGAARTGTGCCGCTGYA	688
		MultiCTXMGp1-2_rev	CGATATCGTTGGTGGTRCCAT	
		MultiCTXMGp2_for	CGTTAACGGCACGATGAC	404
		MultiCTXMGp1-2_rev	CGATATCGTTGGTGGTRCCAT	
		MultiCTXMGp9_for	TCAAGCCTGCCGATCTGGT	561
		MultiCTXMGp9_rev	TGATTCTCGCCGCTGAAG	
3.	CTX-M group 8/25	CTX-Mg8/25_for	AACRCRCAGACGCTCTAC	326
		CTX-Mg8/25_rev	TCGAGCCGGAASGTGTYAT	
4.	Multiplex III ACC, FOX, MOX, DHA, CIT and EBC	MultiCaseACC_for	CACCTCCAGCGACTTGTTAC	346
		MultiCaseACC_rev	GTTAGCCAGCATCACGATCC	
		MultiCaseFOX_for	CTACAGTGCGGGTGGTTT	162
		MultiCaseFOX_rev	CTATTTGCGGCCAGGTGA	
		MultiCaseMOX_for	GCAACAACGACAATCCATCCT	895
		MultiCaseMOX_rev	GGGATAGGCGTAACTCTCCCAA	
		MultiCaseDHA_for	TGATGGCACAGCAGGATATTC	997
		MultiCaseDHA_rev	GCTTTGACTCTTTCGGTATTCG	
		MultiCaseCIT_for	CGAAGAGGCAATGACCAGAC	538
		MultiCaseCIT_rev	ACGGACAGGGTTAGGATAGY	
		MultiCaseEBC_for	CGGTAAAGCCGATGTTGCG	683
		MultiCaseEBC_rev	AGCCTAACCCCTGATACA	
5.	AmpC[a]	AmpCF	CCC CGC TTA TAG AGC AAC AA	634
		AmpCR	TCA ATG GTC GAC TTC ACA CC	
6.	*blaZ*[b]	blaZF1	TTC AAC ACC TGC TGC TTT CGG	326
		blaZR1	CCT TCA TTA CAC TCT TGG CGG TTT C	
		blaZF2[b]	CAA AGA TGA TAT AGT TGC TTA TTC TCC	421
		blaZR2	TGC TTG ACC ACT TTT ATC AGC	

[a](Samanta et al., 2018).
[b](Papanicolas et al., 2014; Ferreira et al., 2017).

Therapeutic strategies

There is a lack of literature regarding treatment of ESBL infection in animals. In human, carbapenem constitutes the mainstay of therapy. However, it is not recommended for animals. Furthermore, increasing evidence of carbapenemase producers in animals (Tewari et al., 2019; Zhang et al., 2013; Fischer et al., 2012, 2013; Bhardwaj et al., 2015; Webb et al., 2016) narrowed down such possibility, even if permission for carbapenem use can be sought for treating endangered species. The BL inhibitor potentiated cephalosporins/penicillin/carbenicillin like CA potentiated amoxycillin is another option which is advocated for ESBL infection and can be used in animals. Cephamycin, fluoroquinolones and amino-glycosides are also recommended for the treatment of ESBL infection (Dhillon and Clark, 2012). However, our observations with the ESBLs from food animals hardly indicate such possibility, as most of the ESBLs from bovine, poultry and pigs were resistant to amoxyclav because of co-production of AmpC BL/inhibitor-resistant TEM and many of them carried gene cassettes with multiple resistance determinants – sul1, tet, quinolone resistance determinants, etc. Thus the therapeutic armamentarium is limited in true sense. However, our *in vitro* studies reflected the efficacy of amikacin, ceftriaxone-tazobactam (Kar et al., 2015) and chloramphenicol (Koovapra et al., 2016) against ESBL producers from animals. Efficacy of chloramphenicol was also noted by Yadav et al., 2014. However, the use of chloramphenicol in food animals is not permitted. To counteract the cephalosporin resistant, Gram-negative organisms, broad-spectrum cephalosporin antibiotic should be used in a parental route instead of the oral route in food animals, as reported by some workers (Seiffert et al., 2013). Furthermore, the resistant feature of the isolates varies widely, as the ESBL-producing *E. coli* from bovine and poultry were found amikacin-sensitive while the same from pigs were amikacin-resistant (Kar et al., 2015; Bandyopadhyay et al., 2015; Samanta et al., 2015). Newer generation BL inhibitor such as avibactam was approved in human medicine – but it has a little scope in the veterinary sector. Thus the animal ESBL isolates need to be studied carefully and extensive clinical trial should be carried out to take a conclusive decision for recommendation to the veterinary clinicians.

References

Ali, T., ur Rahman, S., Zhang, L., Shahid, M., Zhang, S., Liu, G., et al., 2016. ESBL-producing *Escherichia coli* from cows suffering mastitis in China contain clinical class 1 integrons with CTX-M linked to ISCR1. Frontiers in Microbiology 7. https://doi.org/10.3389/fmicb. 2016.01931.

Aubert, D., 2002. OXA-35 is an OXA-10-related beta-lactamase from *Pseudomonas aeruginosa*. Journal of Antimicrobial Chemotherapy 48, 717–721. https://doi.org/10.1093/jac/48.5.717.

Bandyopadhyay, S, Biswas, T.K., Sasmal, D, Ghosh, M.K., Dutta, T.K., Das, S.C., et al., 2009. Virulence gene and antibiotic resistance profile of Shiga-toxin-producing Escherichia coli prevalent in captive yaks (Poephagus grunniens). Veterinary Microbiology 138, 403–404. https://doi.org/10.1016/j.vetmic.2009.04.016.

Bandyopadhyay, S., Lodh, C., Sarkar, M., Ghosh, M.K., Bera, A.K., Bhattacharyya, D., et al., 2012. Prevalence, molecular fingerprinting and drug resistance profile of enterovirulent Escherichia coli isolates from free-ranging yaks of Tawang district, Arunachal Pradesh, India. Tropical Animal Health and Production 44, 1063–1072. https://doi.org/10.1007/s11250-011-0041-9.

Bandyopadhyay, S., Samanta, I., Bhattacharyya, D., Nanda, P.K., Kar, D., Chowdhury, J., et al., 2015. Co-infection of methicillin-resistant *Staphylococcus epidermidis*, methicillin-resistant *Staphylococcus aureus* and extended spectrum β-lactamase producing *Escherichia coli* in bovine mastitis – three cases reported from India. Veterinary Quarterly 35, 56–61. https://doi.org/10.1080/01652176.2014.984365.

Bandyopadhyay, S., Banerjee, J., Bhattacharyya, D., Samanta, I., Mahanti, A., Dutta, T.K., et al., 2018. Genomic identity of fluoroquinolone-resistant bla CTX-M -15 -type ESBL and pMAmpC β-lactamase producing *Klebsiella pneumoniae* from buffalo milk, India. Microbial Drug Resistance 24, 0368. https://doi.org/10.1089/mdr.2017.0368 mdr.2017.

Bengtsson-Palme, J., Kristiansson, E., Larsson, D.G.J., 2018. Environmental factors influencing the development and spread of antibiotic resistance. FEMS Microbiology Reviews 42, 68–80. https://doi.org/10.1093/femsre/fux053.

Bhardwaj, M., Singh, B.R., Murugan, M.S., Prasannavadhana, Dubey, S., 2015. Emergence of carbapenemase producing pathogens in animals. Pharmaceutica Analytica Acta 6. https://doi.org/10.4172/2153-2435.1000379.

Blanc, V., Mesa, R., Saco, M., Lavilla, S., Prats, G., Miró, E., et al., 2006. ESBL- and plasmidic class C β-lactamase-producing *E. coli* strains isolated from poultry, pig and rabbit farms. Veterinary Microbiology 118, 299–304. https://doi.org/10.1016/j.vetmic.2006.08.002.

Bois, SK Du, Marriott, M.S., Amyes, S.G.B., 1995. TEM- and SHV-derived extended-spectrum β-lactamases: relationship between selection, structure and function. Journal of Antimicrobial Chemotherapy 35, 7–22. https://doi.org/10.1093/jac/35.1.7.

Bonnet, R., 2004. Growing group of extended-spectrum -lactamases: the CTX-M enzymes. Antimicrobial Agents and Chemotherapy 48, 1–14. https://doi.org/10.1128/AAC.48.1.1-14.2004.

Bonomo, R.A., 2017. β-Lactamases: a focus on current challenges. Cold Spring Harbor Perspectives in Medicine 7. https://doi.org/10.1101/cshperspect.a025239.

Bonomo, R.A., Rice, L.B., 1999. Inhibitor resistant class A β-lactamases. Frontiers in Bioscience 4, e34–41. https://doi.org/10.2741/Bonomo.

Brower, C.H., Mandal, S., Hayer, S., Sran, M., Zehra, A., Patel, S.J., et al., 2017. The prevalence of extended-spectrum beta-lactamase-producing multidrug-resistant Escherichia coli in poultry chickens and variation according to farming practices in Punjab, India. Environmental Health Perspectives 125, 77015. https://doi.org/10.1289/EHP292.

Bush, K., Jacoby, G.A., 2010. Updated functional classification of -lactamases. Antimicrobial Agents and Chemotherapy 54, 969–976. https://doi.org/10.1128/AAC.01009-09.

Cantón, R., Coque, T.M., 2006. The CTX-M beta-lactamase pandemic. Current Opinion in Microbiology 9, 466–475. https://doi.org/10.1016/j.mib.2006.08.011.

Cantón, R., González-Alba, J.M., Galán, J.C., 2012. CTX-M enzymes: origin and diffusion. Frontiers in Microbiology 3. https://doi.org/10.3389/fmicb.2012.00110.

Chaibi, E.B., Sirot, D., Paul, G., Labia, R., 1999. Inhibitor-resistant TEM -lactamases: phenotypic, genetic and biochemical characteristics. Journal of Antimicrobial Chemotherapy 43, 447–458. https://doi.org/10.1093/jac/43.4.447.

Dahmen, S., Métayer, V., Gay, E., Madec, J.-Y., Haenni, M., 2013. Characterization of extended-spectrum beta-lactamase (ESBL)-carrying plasmids and clones of Enterobacteriaceae causing cattle mastitis in France. Veterinary Microbiology 162, 793–799. https://doi.org/10.1016/j.vetmic.2012.10.015.

Dallenne, C., da Costa, A., Decré, D., Favier, C., Arlet, G., 2010. Development of a set of multiplex PCR assays for the detection of genes encoding important β-lactamases in Enterobacteriaceae. Journal of Antimicrobial Chemotherapy 65, 490–495. https://doi.org/10.1093/jac/dkp498.

Dhillon, R.H.P., Clark, J., 2012. ESBLs: a clear and present danger? Critical Care Research and Practice 2012, 1–11. https://doi.org/10.1155/2012/625170.

Dohmen, W., Dorado-García, A., Bonten, M.J.M., Wagenaar, J.A., Mevius, D., Heederik, D.J.J., 2017. Risk factors for ESBL-producing Escherichia coli on pig farms: a longitudinal study in the context of reduced use of antimicrobials. PLoS One 12, e0174094. https://doi.org/10.1371/journal.pone.0174094.

D'Andrea, M.M., Arena, F., Pallecchi, L., Rossolini, G.M., 2013. CTX-M-type β-lactamases: a successful story of antibiotic resistance. International Journal of Medical Microbiology 303, 305–317. https://doi.org/10.1016/j.ijmm.2013.02.008.

Evans, B., Amyes, S., 2014. OXA beta-lactamases. Clinical Microbiology Reviews 27, 241–263. https://doi.org/10.1128/CMR.00117-13.

Ferreira, A.M., Martins, K.B., Silva, V.R., Mondelli, A.L., Cunha, M.L., 2017. Correlation of phenotypic tests with the presence of the blaZ gene for detection of beta-lactamase. Brazilian Journal of Microbiology 48, 159–166. https://doi.org/10.1016/j.bjm.2016.10.011.

Fischer, J., Rodriguez, I., Schmoger, S., Friese, A., Roesler, U., Helmuth, R., et al., 2012. Escherichia coli producing VIM-1 carbapenemase isolated on a pig farm. Journal of Antimicrobial Chemotherapy 67, 1793–1795. https://doi.org/10.1093/jac/dks108.

Fischer, J., Rodríguez, I., Schmoger, S., Friese, A., Roesler, U., Helmuth, R., et al., 2013. Salmonella enterica subsp. enterica producing VIM-1 carbapenemase isolated from livestock farms. Journal of Antimicrobial Chemotherapy 68, 478–480. https://doi.org/10.1093/jac/dks393.

Gazouli, M., 1998. Two novel plasmid-mediated cefotaxime-hydrolyzing β-lactamases (CTX-M-5 and CTX-M-6) from Salmonella typhimurium. FEMS Microbiology Letters 165, 289–293. https://doi.org/10.1016/S0378-1097(98)00290-0.

Geser, N., Stephan, R., Hächler, H., 2012. Occurrence and characteristics of extended-spectrum β-lactamase (ESBL) producing Enterobacteriaceae in food producing animals, minced meat and raw milk. BMC Veterinary Research 8, 21. https://doi.org/10.1186/1746-6148-8-21.

Guenther, S., Ewers, C., Wieler, L.H., 2011. Extended-spectrum beta-lactamases producing E. coli in wildlife, yet another form of environmental pollution? Frontiers in Microbiology 2. https://doi.org/10.3389/fmicb.2011.00246.

Hirakata, Y., Matsuda, J., Miyazaki, Y., Kamihira, S., Kawakami, S., Miyazawa, Y., et al., 2005. Regional variation in the prevalence of extended-spectrum β-lactamase-producing clinical isolates in the Asia-Pacific region (SENTRY 1998-2002). Diagnostic Microbiology and Infectious Disease 52, 323–329.

Habeeb, M.A., Sarwar, Y., Ali, A., Salman, M., Haque, A., 2013. Rapid emergence of ESBL producers in E. coli causing urinary and wound infections in Pakistan. Pakistan Journal of Medical Sciences 29, 540–544.

Huber, H., Zweifel, C., Wittenbrink, M.M., Stephan, R., 2013. ESBL-producing uropathogenic Escherichia coli isolated from dogs and cats in Switzerland. Veterinary Microbiology 162, 992–996. https://doi.org/10.1016/j.vetmic.2012.10.029.

Kar, D., Bandyopadhyay, S., Bhattacharyya, D., Samanta, I., Mahanti, A., Nanda, P.K., et al., 2015. Molecular and phylogenetic characterization of multidrug resistant extended spectrum beta-lactamase producing Escherichia coli isolated from poultry and cattle in Odisha, India. Infection, Genetics and Evolution 29, 82–90. https://doi.org/10.1016/j.meegid.2014.11.003.

Kim, J., Lim, Y.M., 2005. Prevalence of derepressed AmpC mutants and extended-spectrum β-lactamase producers among clinical isolates of Citrobacter freundii, Enterobacter spp., and Serratia marcescens in Korea: dissemination of CTX-M-3, TEM-52, and SHV-12. Journal of Clinical Microbiology 43, 2452–2455. https://doi.org/10.1128/JCM.43.5.2452-2455.2005.

Koovapra, S., Bandyopadhyay, S., Das, G., Bhattacharyya, D., Banerjee, J., Mahanti, A., et al., 2016. Molecular signature of extended spectrum β-lactamase producing Klebsiella pneumoniae isolated from bovine milk in eastern and north-eastern India. Infection, Genetics and Evolution 44, 395–402. https://doi.org/10.1016/j.meegid.2016.07.032.

Laube, H., Friese, A., von Salviati, C., Guerra, B., Rösler, U., 2014. Transmission of ESBL/AmpC-producing Escherichia coli from broiler chicken farms to surrounding areas. Veterinary Microbiology 172, 519–527. https://doi.org/10.1016/j.vetmic.2014.06.008.

Leonard, A.F.C., Yin, X.L., Zhang, T., Hui, M., Gaze, W.H., 2018. A coliform-targeted metagenomic method facilitating human exposure estimates to Escherichia coli-borne antibiotic resistance genes. FEMS Microbiology Ecology 94. https://doi.org/10.1093/femsec/fiy024.

Liakopoulos, A., Mevius, D., Ceccarelli, D., 2016. A review of SHV extended-spectrum β-lactamases: neglected yet ubiquitous. Frontiers in Microbiology 7. https://doi.org/10.3389/fmicb.2016.01374.

Lupo, A., Papp-Wallace, K.M., Bonomo, R.A., Endimiani, A., 2015. Non-phenotypic tests to detect and characterize antibiotic resistance mechanisms in enterobacteriaceae. Antimicrobial Resistance in Food Safety 233−257. https://doi.org/10.1016/B978-0-12-801214-7.00012-0. Elsevier.

Mahanti, A., Ghosh, P., Samanta, I., Joardar, S.N., Bandyopadhyay, S., Bhattacharyya, D., et al., 2018. Prevalence of CTX-M-producing Klebsiella spp. in broiler, kuroiler, and indigenous poultry in West Bengal state, India. Microbial Drug Resistance 24, 299−306. https://doi.org/10.1089/mdr.2016.0096.

Mammeri, H., Nordmann, P., Berkani, A., Eb, F., 2008. Contribution of extended-spectrum AmpC (ESAC) β-lactamases to carbapenem resistance in *Escherichia coli*. FEMS Microbiology Letters 282, 238−240. https://doi.org/10.1111/j.1574-6968.2008.01126.x.

Markovska, R.D., Stoeva, T.J., Bojkova, K.D., Mitov, I.G., 2013. Epidemiology and molecular characterization of extended-spectrum beta-lactamase-producing *Enterobacter* spp., *Pantoea agglomerans*, and *Serratia marcescens* isolates from a Bulgarian hospital. Microbial Drug Resistance 20, 131−137. https://doi.org/10.1089/mdr.2013.0102.

Marshall, B.M., Levy, S.B., 2011. Food animals and antimicrobials: impacts on human health. Clinical Microbiology Reviews 24, 718−733. https://doi.org/10.1128/CMR.00002-11.

Mashwal, F.A., El Safi, S.H., George, S.K., Adam, A.A., Jebakumar, A.Z., 2017. Incidence and molecular characterization of the extended spectrum beta lactamase-producing *Escherichia coli* isolated from urinary tract infections in Eastern Saudi Arabia. Saudi Medical Journal 38, 811−815. https://doi.org/10.15537/smj.2017.8.18578.

Nóbrega, D.B., Brocchi, M., 2014. An overview of extended-spectrum beta-lactamases in veterinary medicine and their public health consequences. Journal of Infection in Developing Countries 8, 954−960. https://doi.org/10.3855/jidc.4704.

Odsbu, I., Khedkar, S., Lind, F., Khedkar, U., Nerkar, S., Orsini, N., et al., 2018. Trends in resistance to extended-spectrum cephalosporins and carbapenems among *Escherichia coli* and *Klebsiella* spp. isolates in a district in western India during 2004−2014. International Journal of Environmental Research and Public Health 15, 155. https://doi.org/10.3390/ijerph15010155.

Papanicolas, L.E., Bell, J.M., Bastian, I., 2014. Performance of phenotypic tests for detection of penicillinase in *Staphylococcus aureus* isolates from Australia. Journal of Clinical Microbiology 52, 1136−1138. https://doi.org/10.1128/JCM.03068-13.

Paterson, D.L., Bonomo, R.A., 2005. Extended-spectrum beta-lactamases: a clinical update. Clinical Microbiology Review 18, 657−686.

Paterson, D.L., Hujer, K.M., Hujer, A.M., Yeiser, B., Bonomo, M.D., Rice, L.B., et al., 2003. Extended-spectrum β-lactamases in *Klebsiella pneumoniae* bloodstream isolates from seven countries: dominance and widespread prevalence of SHV- and CTX-M-type β-lactamases. Antimicrobial Agents and Chemotherapy 47, 3554−3560. https://doi.org/10.1128/AAC.47.11.3554-3560.2003.

Petit, A., Gerbaud, G., Sirot, D., Courvalin, P., Sirot, J., 1990. Molecular epidemiology of TEM-3 (CTX-1) β-lactamase. Antimicrobial Agents and Chemotherapy 34, 219−224. https://doi.org/10.1128/AAC.34.2.219.

Poirel, L., Kampfer, P., Nordmann, P., 2002. Chromosome-encoded ambler class A -lactamase of *Kluyvera georgiana*, a probable progenitor of a subgroup of CTX-M extended-spectrum -lactamases. Antimicrobial Agents and Chemotherapy 46, 4038−4040. https://doi.org/10.1128/AAC.46.12.4038-4040.2002.

Polsfuss, S., Bloemberg, G.V., Giger, J., Meyer, V., Böttger, E.C., Hombach, M., 2011. Practical approach for reliable detection of AmpC beta-lactamase-producing Enterobacteriaceae. Journal of Clinical Microbiology 49, 2798−2803. https://doi.org/10.1128/JCM.00404-11.

Reantaso, M., Arthue, J.R., Subasinghe, R.P., 2012. Improving Biosecurity Through Prudent and Responsible Use of Veterinary Medicines in Aquatic Food Production doi:226.

Rensing, K.L., Abdallah, H.M., Koek, A., Elmowalid, G.A., Vandenbroucke-Grauls, C.M.J.E., al Naiemi, N., et al., 2019. Prevalence of plasmid-mediated AmpC in Enterobacteriaceae isolated from humans and from retail meat in Zagazig, Egypt. Antimicrobial Resistance and Infection Control 8, 45. https://doi.org/10.1186/s13756-019-0494-6.

Saishu, N., Ozaki, H., Murase, T., 2014. CTX-M-Type extended-spectrum β-lactamase-producing *Klebsiella pneumoniae* isolated from cases of bovine mastitis in Japan. Journal of Veterinary Medical Science 76, 1153−1156. https://doi.org/10.1292/jvms.13-0120.

Samanta, I., Joardar, S.N., Das, P.K., Das, P., Sar, T.K., Dutta, T.K., et al., 2014. Virulence repertoire, characterization, and antibiotic resistance pattern analysis of *Escherichia coli* isolated from backyard layers and their environment in India. Avian Diseases 58, 39−45. https://doi.org/10.1637/10586-052913-Reg.1.

Samanta, I., Joardar, S.N., Mahanti, A., Bandyopadhyay, S., Sar, T.K., Dutta, T.K., 2015. Approaches to characterize extended spectrum beta-lactamase/beta-lactamase producing *Escherichia coli* in healthy organized vis-a-vis backyard farmed pigs in India. Infection, Genetics and Evolution 36, 224−230. https://doi.org/10.1016/j.meegid.2015.09.021.

Samanta, A., Mahanti, A., Chatterjee, S., Joardar, S.N., Bandyopadhyay, S., Sar, T.K., et al., 2018. Pig farm environment as a source of beta-lactamase or AmpC-producing *Klebsiella pneumoniae* and *Escherichia coli*. Annals of Microbiology 68, 781−791. https://doi.org/10.1007/s13213-018-1387-2.

Schneider, I., Queenan, A.M., Markovska, R., Markova, B., Keuleyan, E., Bauernfeind, A., 2009. New variant of CTX-M-type extended-spectrum β-lactamases, CTX-M-71, with a Gly238Cys substitution in a klebsiella pneumoniae isolate from Bulgaria. Antimicrobial Agents and Chemotherapy 53, 4518−4521. https://doi.org/10.1128/AAC.00461-09.

Seiffert, S.N., Hilty, M., Perreten, V., Endimiani, A., 2013. Extended-spectrum cephalosporin-resistant gram-negative organisms in livestock: an emerging problem for human health? Drug Resistance Updates 16, 22−45. https://doi.org/10.1016/j.drup.2012.12.001.

Singer, A.C., Shaw, H., Rhodes, V., Hart, A., 2016. Review of antimicrobial resistance in the environment and its relevance to environmental regulators. Frontiers in Microbiology 7, 1−22. https://doi.org/10.3389/fmicb.2016.01728.

Singh, B.R., 2014. Carriage of multiple drug resistant bacteria in vagina of apparently healthy swamp buffaloes in Nagaland. Advances in Animal and Veterinary Sciences 2, 292−295. https://doi.org/10.14737/journal.aavs/2014/2.5.292.295.

Sittová, M., Röderová, M., Dendis, M., Hricová, K., Pudová, V., Horváth, R., et al., 2015. Application of molecular diagnostics in primary detection of ESBL directly from clinical specimens. Microbial Drug Resistance 21, 352–357. https://doi.org/10.1089/mdr.2014.0210.

Suwantarat, N., Carroll, K.C., 2016. Epidemiology and molecular characterization of multidrug-resistant gram-negative bacteria in Southeast Asia. Antimicrobial Resistance and Infection Control 5, 15. https://doi.org/10.1186/s13756-016-0115-6.

Tewari, R., Mitra, S., Ganaie, F., Das, S., Chakraborty, A., Venugopal, N., et al., 2019. Dissemination and characterisation of *Escherichia coli* producing extended-spectrum β-lactamases, AmpC β-lactamases and metallo-β-lactamases from livestock and poultry in Northeast India: a molecular surveillance approach. Journal of Global Antimicrobial Resistance 17, 209–215. https://doi.org/10.1016/j.jgar.2018.12.025.

van Boxtel, R., Wattel, A.A., Arenas, J., Goessens, W.H.F., Tommassen, J., 2017. Acquisition of carbapenem resistance by plasmid-encoded-AmpC-expressing *Escherichia coli*. Antimicrobial Agents and Chemotherapy 61. https://doi.org/10.1128/AAC.01413-16.

Von Salviati, C., Laube, H., Guerra, B., Roesler, U., Friese, A., 2015. Emission of ESBL/AmpC-producing *Escherichia coli* from pig fattening farms to surrounding areas. Veterinary Microbiology 175, 77–84. https://doi.org/10.1016/j.vetmic.2014.10.010.

Wang, G., Huang, T., Makam Surendraiah, P.K., Wang, K., Komal, R., Zhuge, J., et al., 2013. CTX-M β-lactamase-producing *Klebsiella pneumoniae* in suburban New York, New York, USA. Emerging Infectious Diseases 19, 1803–1810. https://doi.org/10.3201/eid1911.121470.

Webb, H.E., Bugarel, M., den Bakker, H.C., Nightingale, K.K., Granier, S.A., Scott, H.M., et al., 2016. Carbapenem-resistant bacteria recovered from faeces of dairy cattle in the high plains region of the USA. PLoS One 11. https://doi.org/10.1371/journal.pone.0147363 e0147363.

Xi, C., Zhang, Y., Marrs, C.F., Ye, W., Simon, C., Foxman, B., et al., 2009. Prevalence of antibiotic resistance in drinking water treatment and distribution systems. Applied and Environmental Microbiology 75, 5714–5718. https://doi.org/10.1128/AEM.00382-09.

Yadav, A., Sinha, D.K., Prasannavadhana, A., BR, S., 2014. Antibiogram with special reference to MDR and ESBL producing *E. coli* isolated from bovine calves. In: 8th Indian Assoc. Vet. Microbiol. Immunol. Spec. Infect. Dis., Bareilly: IVRI, p. 11.

Zhang, W.-J., Lu, Z., Schwarz, S., Zhang, R.-M., Wang, X.-M., Si, W., et al., 2013. Complete sequence of the bla(NDM-1)-carrying plasmid pNDM-AB from *Acinetobacter baumannii* of food animal origin. Journal of Antimicrobial Chemotherapy 68, 1681–1682. https://doi.org/10.1093/jac/dkt066.

Chapter 7

Carbapenem resistance

Chapter outline

Carbapenem is the group of drugs that is generally used to treat refractory infections caused by resistant Gram-negative bacteria including *Enterobacteriaceae* such as *Escherichia coli* and *Klebsiella pneumoniae*, particularly the extended-spectrum β-lactamase (ESBL) producers. However, extensive use of carbapenem in hospitals or health care setting has led to the development of carbapenem resistance in bacteria. The emergence and spread of carbapenem-resistant *Enterobacteriaceae* (CRE) or carbapenemase-producing *Enterobacteriaceae* (CPE) is the cause of serious clinical and public health concern as this group of drugs is considered as last resort of therapeutic option for the clinicians. Owing to extensive mortality associated with such infection by CRE, which may be as high as 40%–50% especially in blood stream infection, CRE/CPE are often referred as 'killer bacteria' (Mlynarcik et al., 2016). Former Director of Centers for Disease Control (CDC), Prof. Tom Friedman referred CRE as 'nightmare bacteria'. In general, CRE is consisted of a group of pathogens such as *E. coli, Enterobacter aerogenes, Enterobacter cloacae* complex, *K. pneumoniae* or *Klebsiella oxytoca*, which are not susceptible to carbapenem and other drugs such as extended-spectrum cephalosporins.

Infections caused by carbapenem-resistant pathogens are predominantly of nosocomial nature originated from healthcare setting. In most of the patients with CRE infection, the source was tracked down to long-term intensive medical care of the patients in hospitals. Apart from this, inadequate disinfection of the medical devices, cabinet and patients rooms, parenteral nutrition, mechanical ventilation, long term presence of indwelling catheter, previous exposure to carbapenem, glycopeptide or β-lactam drugs and immunosuppressive therapy were found to play important roles for such infection (Jeon et al., 2008; Jiao et al., 2015; Karaaslan et al., 2016; Kim et al., 2016; Kofteridis et al., 2014). Although it is believed that animals may play an important role for spread and dissemination of such pathogens, no such concrete evidence is available till date and there are only sporadic reports on occurrence of CRE in animals.

Carbapenem resistance – types and mechanism

It is noteworthy that carbapenem resistance is inherent in certain bacterial species such as *Stenotrophomonas maltophilia*, which possesses the intrinsic metallo-β-lactamase; therefore, carbapenem is not effective against them. On the other hand, many Gram-positive organisms often exhibit resistance to carbapenems because of mutated penicillin-binding protein.

The carbapenem resistance is mediated mostly by production of carbapenemase which causes the hydrolysis of the β-lactam ring leading to inactivation of the β-lactam or carbapenem group of drugs. The carbapenemase enzymes can be broadly categorized into two groups – one category of enzymes possess serine moiety at the active site, whereas the other, commonly known as metallo-β-lactamases, harbour divalent cations as cofactor for their enzymatic activity. Serine carbapenemases enzymes usually belong to class A or D group, whereas metallo-β-lactamases fall under class B.

Antimicrobial Resistance in Agriculture. https://doi.org/10.1016/B978-0-12-815770-1.00007-9

Class A carbapenemase may be chromosomal or plasmid-mediated and possess an active serine residue at position 70. This group includes β-lactamases or carbapenemases such as *K. pneumoniae* carbapenemase (KPC), SME, GES/IBC, IMI/ NMC-A and SFC-1, which were detected in bacteria such as *E. cloacae*, *Serratia marcescens* and *Klebsiella* spp. However, many of these enzymes are responsible for causing only reduced susceptibility to carbapenem with mildly elevated MIC (minimum inhibitory concentration). Thus in clinical setup, these gene(s) remained usually undetected. Majority of the enzymes of this group − NMC/IMI, SME and KPC − have the potentiality to hydrolyze the major β-lactams, such as carbapenems, cephalosporins, penicillins and aztreonam, and can be inhibited by clavulanate (CA) and tazobactam (TZB). Although the fourth member GES enzyme was originally introduced as an ESBL variant, over time it was found that GES has a low-grade hydrolytic activity against imipenem and therefore was lately included as carbapenemase (Queenan and Bush, 2007). Of all these class A carbapenemases, SME, NMC and IMI are chromosomally mediated and are not linked to any mobile genetic element. Therefore, the occurrence of such enzymes is relatively less. While SME (*S. marcescens* enzyme) was sporadically reported in *S. marcescens* isolates in the United States, IMI (imipenem-hydrolyzing β-lactamase) and NMC-A (not metalloenzyme carbapenemase) − were detected in *E. cloacae* isolates from the United States, France and Argentina. Other two enzymes of class A carbapenemases − KPC and GES − are usually plasmid-mediated. The KPC was first detected in a *K. pneumoniae* clinical isolate from North Carolina in 1996. Thereafter, various variants of KPC − KPC-1, KPC-2, KPC-3 and KPC-4 − have been detected from other parts of the United States, Israel, Scotland and China. KPC enzymes were recorded to hydrolyze most of the β-lactam compounds including cefotaxime, aztreonam, imipenem and meropenem. However, KPC is weakly active against cefoxitin and ceftazidime. The GES variant was first described in 2000 as IBC class of β-lactamase (integron-borne β-lactamase) in an *E. cloacae* isolate in Greece and GES-1 (Guiana extended-spectrum) in a *K. pneumoniae* isolate from French Guiana. GES family of enzymes were reported to be carried by integron from many parts of the world − Greece, France, Portugal, South Africa, French Guiana, Brazil, Argentina, Korea and Japan.

Enzymes such as OXA β-lactamase fall under the group of class D carbapenemase, although most of the enzymes under OXA β-lactamase do not possess the carbapenemase activity. These were originally plasmid-mediated β-lactamase among *Enterobacteriaceae* and *Pseudomonas aeruginosa*, which have the property of hydrolyzing penicillin, oxacillin and cloxacillin. First extended-spectrum OXA β-lactamase, OXA-11, was reported in 1993 followed by other extended variants such as OXA-15, OXA-18 and OXA-45. The first OXA enzyme having carbapenemase activity was detected also in 1993 in an *Acinetobacter baumannii* strain from a patient in Scotland in 1985. OXA-23 subfamily was also reported from other countries such as Brazil, United Kingdom, Korea and other parts of the world. Other OXA β-lactamases with carbapenemase activity include OXA-24, OXA-48, OXA-50, OXA-51, OXA-55, OXA-58, OXA-60 and OXA-62. Most of these were reported in *A. baumannii* and *P. aeruginosa*. Although these OXA variants show considerable carbapenemase activity, their hydrolyzing potency against cephalosporins may be weak.

Enzymes under class B carbapenemase, more commonly known as metallo-β-lactamases, contain zinc at their active site for hydrolysis. Several enzymes fall in this group such as IMP (Zhao and Hu, 2011a), VIM (Zhao and Hu, 2011b), NDM (Zhang et al., 2013), SPM (Carvalhaes et al., 2013), GIM (Hamprecht et al., 2013), SIM (Carvalhaes et al., 2013), AIM (Leski et al., 2013), DIM (Leski et al., 2013), FIM (Leski et al., 2013) and POM (Thaller et al., 2011). Most of them are active against all classes of β-lactam agents including all penicillins and cephalosporins except for aztreonam. Unlike, class A carbapenemase, which can be inhibited by clavulanic acid and TZB, class B enzymes cannot be inhibited by β-lactamase inhibitors. However, as the active site of class B enzymes contains zinc ion, they can be inhibited by metal ion chelators like EDTA. Although the metallo-β-lactamases were first detected and characterized in chromosomal gene(s) of the environmental opportunistic bacteria such as *Bacillus cereus*, *Aeromonas* spp. and *S. maltophilia*, epidemiologically predominant class B enzymes were detected within a variety of integron structures associated with plasmid and transposon facilitating their transfer and dissemination across the bacterial species. Thus the spread of these kinds of carbapenemases − VIM, IMP, GIM and SIM − has been established across the globe. Transferable imipenem resistance mediated by the enzyme IMP-1 was first detected in a *P. aeruginosa* isolate in Japan and then in *Bacillus fragilis*. Later on a variant of IMP-1, i.e., IMP-2 was detected in *A. baumannii* isolate from Italy. Subsequently, this enzyme has been reported from various parts of the world. Another metallo-β-lactamase − VIM (Verona integron−encoded metallo-β-lactamase) − was first detected in Italy and France. There are about 14 variants of VIM of which VIM-2 is probably the most frequently detected metallo-β-lactamase in the world. The enzyme SPM-1 (Sao Paulo metallo-β-lactamase) was detected first in Sao Paulo, Brazil. Details of different carbapenemase are illustrated in Table 7.1.

Although class 3 β-lactamases are not considered as true carbapenemase, their overexpression or overproduction may lead to carbapenem resistance. A major proportion of *Enterobacteriaceae* exhibit resistance to carbapenem due to change

TABLE 7.1 Characteristics of the bacterial carbapenemases.

Sl No	Class	Types	Organisms	Specificity	Substrates	Carriage	Inhibitors
1	A	SME, IMI, KPC, GES/IBC and SFC-1	*Serratia marcescens, Pseudomonas aeruginosa, Klebsiella pneumoniae* and *Escherichia coli, Enterobacter cloacae, Citrobacter freundii*	Active serine in the position 70	Majority of the carbapenems, cephalosporins, penicillins and monobactams	Plasmid or chromosomally mediated (SME, NMC and IMI are chromosomally mediated)	Clavulanate (CA) and tazobactam (TZB)
2	B	B1, B2 and B3 (IMP, VIM, NDM, SPM, GIM, SIM, AIM, DIM, FIM, POM)	Gram-negative bacteria	Contains divalent cations such as Zn^{2+}	All penicillins, cephalosporins and carbapenem but monobactams are not affected	Plasmid, Insertion sequence Few are chromosomal	Metal chelators like EDTA
3	D	OXA-24, OXA-48, OXA-50, OXA-51, OXA-55, OXA-58, OXA-60 and OXA-62	*Acinetobacter* spp. and *Pseudomonas* spp.		Hydrolyze penicillin oxacillin, cloxacillin and carbapenems Potency against other cephalosporins may be weak	Plasmid	CA/TZB (variable)

in the outer membrane protein — porin. Any change in the structure or function of porin channels may lead to the failure in diffusion of carbapenems in the periplasm and thereby carbapenem resistance may ensue. Such phenomenon has been observed in carbapenem-resistant *K. pneumoniae* with loss of outer membrane porin proteins, OmpK35 and OmpK36. Such resistance has been noted in *P. aeruginosa* also. Carbapenem molecules enter the bacterial cell via the outer membrane protein OprD and bacteria with diminished expression of OprD may show carbapenem resistance. Similarly active drug efflux pump may cause expulsion of carbapenem from bacterial cells lowering the intracellular availability of the drugs and its antibacterial effect. Overexpression of such drug efflux pumps may cause multiple drug resistance such as resistance to quinolone, penicillins, cephalosporins and aminoglycosides.

Detection of carbapenem resistance

As carbapenem resistance is one of the major health hazards faced by the world community, it is very important to notice and identify such resistance in bacteria at the earliest. As such pathogens can transfer or propagate their resistance characteristics rapidly either by clonal propagation of the resistant isolates or by transfer of resistance genes to native bacteria, it is important to detect such pathogens to facilitate the outbreak investigation and evaluation of potential colonization.

Routine disk diffusion assay and broth microdilution assays are indicative of carbapenem resistance. Four drugs — namely imipenem, doripenem, ertapenem and meropenem — may be used for such purpose. The break points as per the recommendations of Clinical and Laboratory Standards Institute are tabulated (Tables 7.2 and 7.3) below (CLSI, 2017).

Isolates not susceptible to carbapenem may be screened by standard phenotypic tests to confirm carbapenemase or metallo-β-lactamase production. Such tests include modified Hodge test (MHT), CarbaNP test and imipenem inactivation test. Lately the matrix-assisted laser desorption ionization—time-of-flight mass spectrometry (MALDI-TOF MS) has

TABLE 7.2 Breakpoints for carbapenems in disc diffusion tests.

		Current disk diffusion zone diameters (mm)		
		Zone size interpretation		
Sl No	Carbapenems	Susceptible	Intermediate	Resistant
1.	Doripenem (10 μg)	≥23	20−22	≤19
2.	Ertapenem (10 μg)	≥22	20−21	≤18
3.	Imipenem (10 μg)	≥23	20−21	≤18
4.	Meropenem (10 μg)	≥23	20−21	≤18

TABLE 7.3 Breakpoints for carbapenems in MIC tests.

		Current MIC breakpoints (μg/mL)		
		MIC interpretation		
Sl No	Carbapenems	Susceptible	Intermediate	Resistant
1.	Doripenem	≤1	2	≥4
2.	Ertapenem	≤0.5	1	≥2
3.	Imipenem	≤1	2	≥4
4.	Meropenem	≤1	2	≥4

become popular to detect such carbapenemase production. However, none of these tests can guide the clinicians about the types of carbapenemase production. A diagnostic flow diagram proposed by Lee et al. (2003) may be an useful guide for clinical microbiologists to detect the type of metallo-β-lactamase in Gram-negative bacteria (Lee et al., 2003). The process includes testing the imipenem nonsusceptible isolates with MHT using Zn^{2+} added imipenem disc and further testing of the MHT positive isolates using a disc containing 10 μg of imipenem and a disc with 750 μg of EDTA and 2 mg of sodium mercaptoacetic acid (SMA). The isolates positive in the second screening should be again evaluated by polymerase chain reaction (PCR)—based screening for *bla*IMP and *bla*VIM gene(s).

The following phenotypic tests may be performed for detection of metallo-β-lactamase or carbapenemase production by different Gram-negative pathogens.

EDTA-disk synergy test

This test is performed using two different discs - one of 10 μg of imipenem (IPM) and a second disc containing 10 μL of 0.5 M EDTA which are placed at 15 mm distance (edge-to-edge). After incubating overnight at 37°C, the presence of an expanded growth inhibition zone between the two disks will be interpreted as positive for synergy. To increase the sensitivity, a modified form of the test, known as extended EDTA-disk synergy test, is also used where discs containing ceftazidime (30 μg) and meropenem (10 μg) and a reduced concentration of EDTA (10 μL of 0.1 M) are placed at 10 mm distance (edge-to-edge) (Fig. 7.1).

Imipenem-EDTA disc synergy test

This method was developed to detect metallo-β-lactamase production using metal chelating and metallo-β-lactamase inhibitory properties of EDTA (Yong et al., 2002). This test is conducted using two discs: one containing imipenem (10 μg) only and another with imipenem (10 μg) and EDTA (750 μg). Another disk containing only 750 μg EDTA is also placed as a control. After overnight incubation, the established zone diameter difference of ≥7 mm between imipenem disk and imipenem plus EDTA is interpreted as EDTA synergy positive (Fig. 7.2).

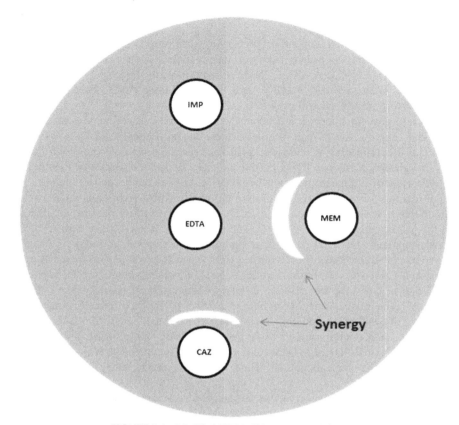

FIGURE 7.1 Modified EDTA-disk synergy (EDS) test.

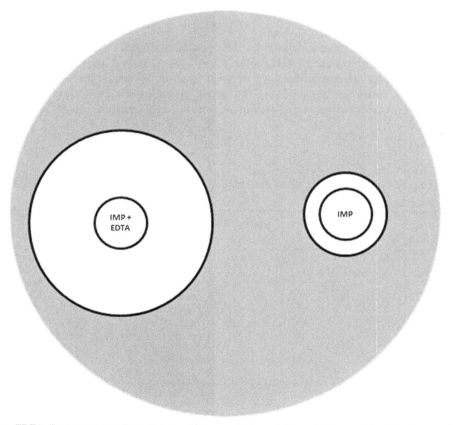

FIGURE 7.2 Imipenem–EDTA disc synergy test: Zone diameter difference of ≥7 mm between imipenem disk and imipenem plus EDTA is interpreted as EDTA synergy positive.

Modified Hodge test

MHT is useful for testing isolate for epidemiological or infection control purposes. This test is based on the principle that carbapenemase-producing strains or the test isolate can cause inactivation of a carbapenem and this ultimately enable the pan-susceptible indicator strain, usually *E. coli* ATCC 25922 to grow towards the imipenem or meropenem disc resulting in a cloverleaf-like indentation. With each test, MHT-positive *K. pneumoniae* ATCC BAA-1705 and MHT-negative *K. pneumoniae* ATCC BAA-1706 should be used for control study.

Carba NP test is relatively easy to interpret biochemical test for rapid detection of carbapenemase production by Gram-negative bacteria. This employs the change of colour of the medium because of hydrolysis of carbapenem (especially imipenem) by bacterial lysate leading to change in pH of the medium supplemented with indicator such as phenol red. Although the test fairly detects KPC and NDM producers, class D carbapenemase or the enzymes that lead to low grade or suboptimum hydrolysis of imipenem may not be properly detected with this technique.

Similarly carbapenem inactivation method (CIM) is a simple and low cost technique which can detect the carbapenemase production within 8–10 h. It was first described in 2015. In this test, a 10 μg meropenem disk is incubated with the aqueous suspension of the test organism for 2 h at 35^0 C. The disk will be inactivated or degraded, provided that the test organism produces carbapenemase. To check such degradation or inactivation, the disk is usually incubated with a carbapenem susceptible indicator strain. Recently, a modified CIM test was developed by Pierce et al. (2017) and the same was found 99% sensitive and 100% specific. In this modified test, the workers recommended to incubate the meropenem disk in tryptic soy broth suspension of the test bacteria instead of aqueous suspension for an extended period.

Double-disk synergy test is the most convenient technique used for detection of metallo-β-lactamase production. This test is based on the inhibition of enzyme by chelating agents such as EDTA or SMA. In this test, an imipenem (10 μg) or ceftazidime (30 μg) disk with a disk containing either 750 μg of EDTA or 750 μg of EDTA and 2 mg of SMA is placed on MH agar plate streaked with test isolate at a distance of 10 mm and incubated overnight. Synergistic inhibition zone produced by the test isolate in the presence of chelating agent is considered as positive for metallo-β-lactamase production.

Nucleic acid detection or molecular detection of the carbapenem resistance is getting popularity because of multiple advantages of nucleic acid–based molecular tests like rapid results than the conventional tests, definite identification of the carbapenemase resistance gene and direct detection from clinical specimen without the need for culture. However, it may be possible to detect such resistance gene in some isolates which are phenotypically susceptible to carbapenems. Such kind of weak phenotypic expression was recorded in some isolates with *bla*KPC gene possibly because of low level of KPC expression (Kitchel et al., 2010).

PCR is relatively established molecular technique for detection of *bla*NDM-1 gene. In our laboratory, two different PCR protocols were found effective to detect NDM-producing isolates of animal origin (data unpublished). The details regarding the PCR condition and oligonucleotides are detailed in table. Besides, other sets of PCR primers are also available, which may also be used for this purpose. The details regarding the PCR conditions, oligonucleotides for detection of important carbapenemase or metallo-β-lactamase gene(s) are described in the following table (Table 7.4).

TABLE 7.4 Oligonucleotides and details of polymerase chain reaction (PCR) conditions for detection of carbapenem resistance gene(s).

Gene(s)	Oligonucleotides	Amplicon size (bp)	PCR condition	PCR reaction	Reference
NDM-1 1st set	F:GGGCAGTCGCTTCCAACGGT R:GTAGTGCTCAGTGTCGGCAT	475 bp	Initial denaturation 10 min at 94°C; 36 cycles of amplification consisting of 30 s at 94°C, 40 s at 52°C, and 50 s at 72°C; and 5 min at 72°C for the final extension.	1× PCR buffer [10 mM Tris-HCl (pH 8.3), 50 mM KCl], 1.5 mM MgCl2, 0.15 mM of each deoxynucleotide triphosphate, 0.1 μM of each primer, and 1 U of DNA polymerase.	(Manchanda et al., 2011; Shanthi et al., 2014)

Continued

TABLE 7.4 Oligonucleotides and details of polymerase chain reaction (PCR) conditions for detection of carbapenem resistance gene(s).—cont'd

Gene(s)	Oligonucleotides	Amplicon size (bp)	PCR condition	PCR reaction	Reference
NDM 2nd set	NDMF2: GGTTTGGCGATCTGGTTTTC NDMR2:CGGAATGGCTCATCACGATC	621	Initial denaturation 10 min at 94°C; 36 cycles of amplification consisting of 30 s at 94°C, 40 s at 52°C, and 50 s at 72°C; and 5 min at 72°C for the final extension	1× PCR buffer (10 mM Tris-HCl [pH 8.3], 50 mM KCl), 1.5 mM MgCl2, 0.125 mM each deoxynucleotide triphosphate, 0.1 μM each primer, and 2 U of Taq polymerase	Nordmann et al. (2011)
Multiplex for IMP, VIM and KPC	IMPF: TTGACACTCCATTTACDG IMPR: GATYGAGAATTAAGCCAC YCT	139 bp	Initial denaturation 10 min at 94°C; 30 cycles of amplification consisting of 40 s at 94°C, 40 s at 55°C, and 1 min at 72°C; and 7 min at 72°C for the final extension.	Multiplex PCR to be carried out in a 50 μL reaction mixture containing 1× PCR buffer (10 mM Tris −HCl, pH 8.3/50 mM KCl/ 1.5 mM MgCl), 200 μM of each dNTP, 0.5 pmol/μL of IMP and VIM primers and 0.2 pmol/μL of KPC primers and 1 U of Taq polymerase	Dallenne et al. (2010)
	VIMF: GATGGTGTTTGGTCGCATA VIMR: CGAATGCGCAGCACCAG	390			
	KPCF: CATTCAAGGGCTTTCTTGC TGC KPCR: ACGACGGCATAGTCATTTGC	538			
Subclass of IMP	IMP1F: TGAGCAAGTTATCTGTATTC IMP1R: TTAGTTGCTTGGTTTTGATG	740	Initial denaturation 3 min at 94°C; 35 cycles of 1 min at 94°C, 1 min at 55°C, and 2 min at 72°C; and finally, 7 min at 72°C.	1× PCR buffer (10 mM Tris-HCl [pH 8.3], 50 mM KCl), 1.5 mM MgCl2, 200 μM each deoxynucleotide triphosphate, 0.1 μM each primer, and 2 U of Taq polymerase	Yan et al. (2001)
	IMP2F: GGCAGTCGCCCTAAAACAAA IMP2R: AGTTACTTGGCTGTGATGG	737			
Subclass of VIM	VIM1F: TTATGGAGCAGCAACGATGT VIM1R: CAAAAGTCCCGCTCCAACGA	920			
	VIM2F: AAAGTTATGCCGCACTCACC VIM2R: TGCAACTTCATGTTATGCCG	865			
OXA-48 like	OXA48F: AACGGGCGAACCAAG-CATTTT OXA48R: TGAGCACTTCTTTTGTGATGGCT	585/597	Initial denaturation 5 min at 94°C; 35 cycles of 1 min at 95°C, 1 min at 52°C, and 1 min at 72°C, and finally, 5 min at 72°C.	The PCR reaction mixture consists of 0.5 μL DNA (50 ng) in 24.5 μL complete reaction buffer with MgCl2 (containing 100 mmol/L Tris-HCl [pH 8.8], 500 mmol/L KCl, 1% Triton X-100, 15 mmol/L MgCl2), dNTP (10 mM, 0.5 μL), 15 pmol of each primer (0.5 μL) and IU Taq DNA polymerase	Mlynarcik et al. (2016)
OXA-23 like	OXA-23F:GTGGTTGCTTCTCTTTTTCT OXA23R: ATTTCTGACCGCATTTCCAT	736	Initial denaturation 5 min at 94°C; 35 cycles of 1 min at 95°C, 1 min at 56°C, and 1 min at 72°C, and finally, 5 min at 72°C.		
SME(1−5)	SMEF:TATGGAACGATTTCTTGGCG SMER:CTCCCAGTTTTGTCACCTAC	300	Initial denaturation 5 min at 94°C; 35 cycles of 1 min at 95°C, 1 min at 56°C, and 1 min at 72°C, and finally, 5 min at 72°C.		
GIM	GIMF:TCGACACACCTTGGTCTGAA GIMR:AACTTCCAACTTTGCCATGC	477			

MALDI-TOF MS is used by many workers for detection of carbapenem resistance as it requires less time. The principal is based on the degradation or hydrolysis of carbapenem by carbapenemase enzymes released by the test organism. The test organism is incubated with carbapenem compounds for about 2–4 h, and measurable mass increase in degraded carbapenem products indicates the presence of carbapenemase or MBL producers. However, overincubation may lead to further degraded products of lower molecular mass leading to false positive interpretation. In contrast, it may take relatively extended period of incubation like 24 h to detect the carbapenemases like OXA-48, which shows low degrading or hydrolytic activity.

Spread in animals

There are only few reports on occurrence of carbapenem-resistant pathogens in animals. This may be due to the fact that carbapenems are not registered for use in animals. A recently published systemic review revealed that the occurrence of CRE, predominantly *Escherichia* and *Klebsiella*, has been reported among a range of animals including pigs, poultry, cattle, seafood, dogs, cats, horses, pet birds, swallows, wild boars, wild stork, gulls and black kites from five continents — Africa, America, Asia, Australia and Europe. The carbapenemases that were detected in animals or farm environment belonged to VIM, KPC, NDM, OXA and IMP types (Köck et al., 2018). Recently, a group of workers from the United States reported the occurrence of carbapenem-resistant multiple bacterial species including *E. coli* and *Proteus mirabilis* in environmental samples of a swine farm. The isolates were positive for the metallo-β-lactamase gene *bla*IMP-27 carried on IncQ1 plasmids. No such carbapenem-resistant isolate could be recovered from rectal swab or fecal samples collected from pigs. Although the isolates were resistant to meropenem, cephalosporins, sulfonamides and tetracyclines, they were susceptible to aminoglycosides and fluoroquinolones and possessed additional antimicrobial resistance genes located on the IncQ1 plasmid, including sul-2, sat-1 and aph(3′)-Ia. The investigator hypothesized that use of ceftiofur might have been responsible for acquisition of blaIMP-27 gene and subsequent development of carbapenem resistance (Köck et al., 2018). Previously also, Zhang et al., 2013 reported blaNDM-1-mediated carbapenem resistance in *E. coli*, *A. baumannii* and *Acinetobacter calcoaeticus* isolates recovered from lung samples of the diseased pigs (Zhang et al., 2013). Again in Germany, Fischer and co-workers reported VIM-1-type carbapenemase producing *E. coli* and *Salmonella enterica* subsp. *enterica* from two fattening pig farms and one broiler farm, respectively (Fischer et al., 2012, 2013). Carbapenem-resistant *P. aeruginosa* with *bla*VIM-2 and *A. baumannii* with *bla*OXA-23 and bla*OXA*-58 gene(s) were reported in cattle, swine and poultry from Lebanon (Zhang et al., 2013). From India, carbapenem-resistant *E. coli* and *K. pneumoniae* were reported from bovine milk and poultry, although the isolates were not positive for carbapenemase (Kar et al., 2015; Koovapra et al., 2016). This kind of carbapenem resistance was possibly mediated by overproduction of blaCTX-M ESBL and loss of porin (Shanthi et al., 2014; Nordmann et al., 2011). Similarly, Singh et al. (2012) also reported such kind of carbapenem (meropenem) resistance among nontyphoidal *Salmonella* isolated from human, animals and meat samples from India (Singh et al., 2012).

Previously, Poirel et al. (2012) reported occurrence of carbapenem-resistant *Acinetobacter* genomospecies in bovine rectal swab from France. All the isolates harboured a blaOXA-23 gene, which is known to be widely prevalent in *A. baumannii*. In one isolate, transposon Tn2008 was identified, whereas in rest of the isolates the IS*Aba1* element of Tn2008 had been truncated by a novel insertion sequence termed IS*Acsp2* (Poirel et al., 2012). Carbapenem-resistant bacteria were also reported in the bovine fecal samples from high plain region of the United States (Webb et al., 2016). On the basis of phenotypic tests, a total of 28 isolates including *E. coli*, *Aeromonas*, *A. baumannii* and *Pseudomonas* were studied using whole-genome assembly. All the three *E. coli* isolates harboured AmpC β-lactamase gene blaCMY-2 along with truncated ompF gene. The *A. baumannii* isolate was detected with Ambler class D carbapenemase blaOXA-497. Of the 18 *Aeromonas* isolates including 17 *Aeromonas veronii* and 1 *Aeromonas allosaccharophila*, all the *A. veronii* isolates harboured a blacphA-like gene. The six *Pseudomonas* isolates were detected with conserved domain of various carbapenemase-producing genes — viz., Ambler class B (blaIMP), class C (blaAmpC) and class D (blaOXA) β-lactamases. Despite sporadic reports on carbapenem-resistant pathogens in animals or their surroundings, there is hardly any convincing evidence to support that animals can contribute to human infection with such pathogens. Poirel et al., 2014 proposed two main factors for dissemination of carbapenem resistance in human pathogen. One is the increased use of carbapenem to treat the increasing burden of infections caused by pathogens resistant to extended-spectrum cephalosporins. Another factor which causes the spread of such pathogens is increased human movement worldwide by migration and tourism (Poirel et al., 2014).

Therapeutic strategies

Carbapenems are often considered as the last resort of therapy for infection with other bugs such as ESBL-producing *Enterobacteriaceae*. However, little is available as therapeutic option for treating the infections of carbapenem-resistant pathogens. In most of the cases, the plasmid with carbapenem resistance gene also harbours resistance determinants for other antimicrobials such as tetracycline, aminoglycosides and quinolones and thereby transforms the isolates virtually untreatable. Limited therapeutic options and high mortality make infections caused by carbapenem-resistant pathogens challenging for the clinicians. Till date, the clinicians have to rely on the older antimicrobials only for this purpose, including polymyxins, tigecycline and fosfomycin, particularly to treat the cases of invasive infections (Bowers and Huang, 2016). Of them, colistin and tigecycline were reported effective when monotherapy is advocated (Garnacho-Montero et al., 2015). Recently, Rogers et al., 2013 reported successful treatment of two separate cases of urinary tract infections caused by *Enterobacteriaceae* harbouring blaNDM-1 enzyme (one with *E. coli* and another with *E. cloacae*). While oral therapy with nitrofurantoin was successful in one case, combination of colistin and rifampicin was required in the second patient (Rogers et al., 2013). In a recent paper, Trecarichi and Tumbarello, 2017 summarized the therapeutic outcome of infections caused by carbapenem-resistant pathogens mainly caused by KPC producers and less frequently by VIM either alone or in association with KPC barring a single case where carbapenem resistance was caused by blaCTXM-15 enzyme combined with porin loss (Trecarichi and Tumbarello, 2017). The observation was made in perspective of three regions — reports from European countries, United States and Brazil. The study did not include CRE infections caused by NDM or OXA-48 production. Resistance was noted against the mainstay of therapy against CRE such as colistin, gentamicin and tigecycline. Resistance was found to be as high as 50% and 80% for colistin and gentamicin, respectively. Finally, it has been noted that combination therapy with two or more *in vitro* active agents was more effective than monotherapy in reducing mortality. Although the use of carbapenems in treatment of CRE infections is not widely recommended, the authors pointed out its usefulness in association with other active drugs for treating the infections with CRE isolates with carbapenem MICs ≤8 mg/L, particularly in combination with colistin or high-dose tigecycline or aminoglycosides. However, for isolates with MIC ≥8 mg/L, a combination of two or even three antibiotics — colistin, high-dose tigecycline, aminoglycoside and fosfomycin — was found effective (Rafailidis and Falagas, 2014).

It is true that an alternative and effective therapeutic strategy is required for treating the infections caused by carbapenemase producers. However, till date, we have only limited therapeutic option. Ceftazidime—avibactam combination has been reported to show *in vitro* antibacterial efficacy to KPC producers (Falcone and Paterson, 2016). However, the combination was poorly effective against OXA enzymes or metallo-β-lactamase producers. Sufficient clinical trial is lacking with avibactam combination; however, the reports that came out of the two trials are not very promising (Shields et al., 2016; Temkin et al., 2016). Furthermore, several novel antimicrobial compounds were recorded to showcase *in vitro* antibacterial efficacy against the carbapenem-resistant pathogens. Such compounds include avibactam with other extended-spectrum cephalosporins or monobactams such as ceftaroline fosamil—avibactam and aztreonam—avibactam, carbapenem with novel β-lactamase inhibitors such as meropenem—vaborbactam and imipenem/cilastatin—relebactam, new generation aminoglycosides (plazomicin) and tetracycline (eravacycline). However, none of them were found universally effective against all kinds of carbapenemases. But, indeed, these compounds may provide suitable alternative for the mainstay therapy (Bassetti et al., 2016). Nevertheless, sufficient clinical trials are necessary to provide a conclusive evidence in this regard.

References

Bassetti, M., Peghin, M., Pecori, D., 2016. The management of multidrug-resistant *Enterobacteriaceae*. Current Opinion in Infectious Diseases 29, 583—594. https://doi.org/10.1097/QCO.0000000000000314.

Bowers, D.R., Huang, V., 2016. Emerging issues and treatment strategies in carbapenem-resistant *Enterobacteriaceae* (CRE). Current Infectious Disease Reports 18, 48. https://doi.org/10.1007/s11908-016-0548-3.

Carvalhaes, C.G., Cayô, R., Assis, D.M., Martins, E.R., Juliano, L., Juliano, M.A., et al., 2013. Detection of SPM-1-producing *Pseudomonas aeruginosa* and class D β-lactamase-producing *Acinetobacter baumannii* isolates by use of liquid chromatography-mass spectrometry and matrix-assisted laser desorption ionization—time of flight mass spectrometry. Journal of Clinical Microbiology 51, 287—290. https://doi.org/10.1128/JCM.02365-12.

CLSI, 2017. Performance Standards for Antimicrobial Susceptibility Testing.

Dallenne, C., da Costa, A., Decré, D., Favier, C., Arlet, G., 2010. Development of a set of multiplex PCR assays for the detection of genes encoding important B-lactamases in *Enterobacteriaceae*. Journal of Antimicrobial Chemotherapy 65, 490—495. https://doi.org/10.1093/jac/dkp498.

Falcone, M., Paterson, D., 2016. Spotlight on ceftazidime/avibactam: a new option for MDR Gram-negative infections. Journal of Antimicrobial Chemotherapy 71, 2713—2722. https://doi.org/10.1093/jac/dkw239.

Fischer, J., Rodriguez, I., Schmoger, S., Friese, A., Roesler, U., Helmuth, R., et al., 2012. *Escherichia coli* producing VIM-1 carbapenemase isolated on a pig farm. Journal of Antimicrobial Chemotherapy 67, 1793—1795. https://doi.org/10.1093/jac/dks108.

Fischer, J., Rodríguez, I., Schmoger, S., Friese, A., Roesler, U., Helmuth, R., et al., 2013. *Salmonella enterica* subsp. enterica producing VIM-1 carbapenemase isolated from livestock farms. Journal of Antimicrobial Chemotherapy 68, 478—480. https://doi.org/10.1093/jac/dks393.

Garnacho-Montero, J., Amaya-Villar, R., Ferrándiz-Millón, C., Díaz-Martín, A., López-Sánchez, J.M., Gutiérrez-Pizarraya, A., 2015. Optimum treatment strategies for carbapenem-resistant *Acinetobacter baumannii* bacteremia. Expert Rev Anti Infect Ther 13, 769—777. https://doi.org/10.1586/14787210.2015.1032254.

Hamprecht, A., Poirel, L., Gottig, S., Seifert, H., Kaase, M., Nordmann, P., 2013. Detection of the carbapenemase GIM-1 in *Enterobacter cloacae* in Germany. Journal of Antimicrobial Chemotherapy 68, 558—561. https://doi.org/10.1093/jac/dks447.

Jeon, M.-H., Choi, S.-H., Kwak, Y.G., Chung, J.-W., Lee, S.-O., Jeong, J.-Y., et al., 2008. Risk factors for the acquisition of carbapenem-resistant *Escherichia coli* among hospitalized patients. Diagnostic Microbiology and Infectious Disease 62, 402—406. https://doi.org/10.1016/j.diagmicrobio.2008.08.014.

Jiao, Y., Qin, Y., Liu, J., Li, Q., Dong, Y., Shang, Y., et al., 2015. Risk factors for carbapenem-resistant *Klebsiella pneumoniae* infection/colonization and predictors of mortality: a retrospective study. Pathogens and Global Health 109, 68—74. https://doi.org/10.1179/2047773215Y.0000000004.

Kar, D., Bandyopadhyay, S., Bhattacharyya, D., Samanta, I., Mahanti, A., Nanda, P.K., et al., 2015. Molecular and phylogenetic characterization of multidrug resistant extended spectrum beta-lactamase producing *Escherichia coli* isolated from poultry and cattle in Odisha, India. Infection, Genetics and Evolution 29, 82—90. https://doi.org/10.1016/j.meegid.2014.11.003.

Karaaslan, A., Soysal, A., Altinkanat Gelmez, G., Kepenekli Kadayifci, E., Söyletir, G., Bakir, M., 2016. Molecular characterization and risk factors for carbapenem-resistant Gram-negative bacilli colonization in children: emergence of NDM-producing *Acinetobacter baumannii* in a newborn intensive care unit in Turkey. Journal of Hospital Infection 92, 67—72. https://doi.org/10.1016/j.jhin.2015.09.011.

Kim, S., Russell, D., Mohamadnejad, M., Makker, J., Sedarat, A., Watson, R.R., et al., 2016. Risk factors associated with the transmission of carbapenem-resistant *Enterobacteriaceae* via contaminated duodenoscopes. Gastrointestinal Endoscopy 83, 1121—1129. https://doi.org/10.1016/j.gie.2016.03.790.

Kitchel, B., Rasheed, J.K., Endimiani, A., Hujer, A.M., Anderson, K.F., Bonomo, R.A., et al., 2010. Genetic factors associated with elevated carbapenem resistance in KPC-producing *Klebsiella pneumoniae*. Antimicrobial Agents and Chemotherapy 54, 4201—4207. https://doi.org/10.1128/AAC.00008-10.

Köck, R., Daniels-Haardt, I., Becker, K., Mellmann, A., Friedrich, A.W., Mevius, D., et al., 2018. Carbapenem-resistant *Enterobacteriaceae* in wildlife, food-producing, and companion animals: a systematic review. Clinical Microbiology and Infections. https://doi.org/10.1016/j.cmi.2018.04.004.

Kofteridis, D.P., Valachis, A., Dimopoulou, D., Maraki, S., Christidou, A., Mantadakis, E., et al., 2014. Risk factors for carbapenem-resistant *Klebsiella pneumoniae* infection/colonization: a case-case-control study. Journal of Infection and Chemotherapy 20, 293—297. https://doi.org/10.1016/j.jiac.2013.11.007.

Koovapra, S., Bandyopadhyay, S., Das, G., Bhattacharyya, D., Banerjee, J., Mahanti, A., et al., 2016. Molecular signature of extended spectrum β-lactamase producing *Klebsiella pneumoniae* isolated from bovine milk in eastern and north-eastern India. Infection, Genetics and Evolution 44, 395—402. https://doi.org/10.1016/j.meegid.2016.07.032.

Lee, K., Lim, Y.S., Yong, D., Yum, J.H., Chong, Y., 2003. Evaluation of the hodge test and the imipenem-EDTA double-disk synergy test for differentiating metallo—Lactamase-producing isolates of *Pseudomonas* spp. and *Acinetobacter* spp. Journal of Clinical Microbiology 41, 4623—4629. https://doi.org/10.1128/JCM.41.10.4623-4629.2003.

Leski, T.A., Bangura, U., Jimmy, D.H., Ansumana, R., Lizewski, S.E., Li, R.W., et al., 2013. Identification of blaOXA-51-like, blaOXA-58, blaDIM-1, and blaVIM carbapenemase genes in hospital *Enterobacteriaceae* isolates from Sierra Leone. Journal of Clinical Microbiology 51, 2435—2438. https://doi.org/10.1128/JCM.00832-13.

Manchanda, V., Gupta, S., Chopra, R., Verma, N., Kaur, I., Rai, S., et al., 2011. Development of TaqMan real-time polymerase chain reaction for the detection of the newly emerging form of carbapenem resistance gene in clinical isolates of *Escherichia coli*, *Klebsiella pneumoniae*, and *Acinetobacter baumannii*. Indian Journal of Medical Microbiology 29, 249. https://doi.org/10.4103/0255-0857.83907.

Mlynarcik, P., Roderova, M., Kolar, M., 2016. Primer evaluation for PCR and its application for detection of carbapenemases in *Enterobacteriaceae*. Jundishapur Journal of Microbiology 9, e29314. https://doi.org/10.5812/jjm.29314.

Nordmann, P., Poirel, L., Carrer, A., Toleman, M.A., Walsh, T.R., 2011. How to detect NDM-1 producers. Journal of Clinical Microbiology 49, 718—721. https://doi.org/10.1128/JCM.01773-10.

Pierce, V.M., Simner, P.J., Lonsway, D.R., Roe-Carpenter, D.E., Johnson, J.K., Brasso, W.B., et al., 2017. Modified carbapenem inactivation method for phenotypic detection of carbapenemase production among *Enterobacteriaceae*. Journal of Clinical Microbiology 55, 2321—2333. https://doi.org/10.1128/JCM.00193-17.

Poirel, L., Berçot, B., Millemann, Y., Bonnin, R.A., Pannaux, G., Nordmann, P., 2012. Carbapenemase-producing *Acinetobacter* spp. in Cattle, France. Emerging Infectious Diseases 18, 523—525. https://doi.org/10.3201/eid1803.111330.

Poirel, L., Stephan, R., Perreten, V., Nordmann, P., 2014. The carbapenemase threat in the animal world: the wrong culprit. Journal of Antimicrobial Chemotherapy 69, 2007—2008. https://doi.org/10.1093/jac/dku054.

Queenan, A.M., Bush, K., 2007. Carbapenemases: the versatile -lactamases. Clinical Microbiology Reviews 20, 440—458. https://doi.org/10.1128/CMR.00001-07.

Rafailidis, P.I., Falagas, M.E., 2014. Options for treating carbapenem-resistant *Enterobacteriaceae*. Current Opinion in Infectious Diseases 27, 479–483. https://doi.org/10.1097/QCO.0000000000000109.

Rogers, B.A., Sidjabat, H.E., Silvey, A., Anderson, T.L., Perera, S., Li, J., et al., 2013. Treatment options for New Delhi metallo-beta-lactamase-harboring *Enterobacteriaceae*. Microbial Drug Resistance 19, 100–103. https://doi.org/10.1089/mdr.2012.0063.

Shanthi, M., Sekar, U., Kamalanathan, A., Sekar, B., 2014 Oct. Detection of New Delhi metallobeta lactamase-1 (NDM-1) carbapenemase in Pseudomonas aeruginosa in a singlecentre in southern India. Indian J Med Res 140 (4), 546–550.

Shields, R.K., Potoski, B.A., Haidar, G., Hao, B., Doi, Y., Chen, L., et al., 2016. Clinical outcomes, drug toxicity, and emergence of ceftazidime-avibactam resistance among patients treated for carbapenem-resistant *Enterobacteriaceae* infections: Table 1. Clinical Infectious Diseases 63, 1615–1618. https://doi.org/10.1093/cid/ciw636.

Singh, S., Agarwal, R.K., Tiwari, S.C., Singh, H., 2012. Antibiotic resistance pattern among the Salmonella isolated from human, animal and meat in India. Tropical Animal Health and Production 44, 665–674. https://doi.org/10.1007/s11250-011-9953-7.

Temkin, E., Torre-Cisneros, J., Beovic, B., Benito, N., Giannella, M., Gilarranz, R., et al., 2016. Ceftazidime-avibactam as salvage therapy for infections caused by carbapenem-resistant organisms: a case series from the compassionate-use program. Antimicrobial Agents and Chemotherapy 61. https://doi.org/10.1128/AAC.01964-16. AAC.01964-16.

Thaller, M.C., Borgianni, L., Di Lallo, G., Chong, Y., Lee, K., Dajcs, J., et al., 2011. Metallo-β-Lactamase production by *Pseudomonas otitidis* : a species-related trait. Antimicrobial Agents and Chemotherapy 55, 118–123. https://doi.org/10.1128/AAC.01062-10.

Trecarichi, E.M., Tumbarello, M., 2017. Therapeutic options for carbapenem-resistant *Enterobacteriaceae* infections. Virulence 8, 470–484. https://doi.org/10.1080/21505594.2017.1292196.

Webb, H.E., Bugarel, M., den Bakker, H.C., Nightingale, K.K., Granier, S.A., Scott, H.M., et al., 2016. Carbapenem-resistant bacteria recovered from faeces of dairy cattle in the high plains region of the USA. PLoS One 11, e0147363. https://doi.org/10.1371/journal.pone.0147363.

Yan, J.J., Hsueh, P.R., Ko, W.C., Luh, K.T., Tsai, S.H., Wu, H.M., et al., 2001. Metallo–lactamases in clinical *Pseudomonas* isolates in taiwan and identification of VIM-3, a novel variant of the VIM-2 enzyme. Antimicrobial Agents and Chemotherapy 45, 2224–2228. https://doi.org/10.1128/AAC.45.8.2224-2228.2001.

Yong, D., Lee, K., Yum, J.H., Shin, H.B., Rossolini, G.M., Chong, Y., 2002. Imipenem-edta disk method for differentiation of metallo–lactamase-producing clinical isolates of *Pseudomonas* spp. and *Acinetobacter* spp. Journal of Clinical Microbiology 40, 3798–3801. https://doi.org/10.1128/JCM.40.10.3798-3801.2002.

Zhang, W.-J., Lu, Z., Schwarz, S., Zhang, R.-M., Wang, X.-M., Si, W., et al., 2013. Complete sequence of the bla(NDM-1)-carrying plasmid pNDM-AB from *Acinetobacter baumannii* of food animal origin. Journal of Antimicrobial Chemotherapy 68, 1681–1682. https://doi.org/10.1093/jac/dkt066.

Zhao, W.-H., Hu, Z.-Q., 2011. IMP-type metallo-β-lactamases in Gram-negative bacilli: distribution, phylogeny, and association with integrons. Critical Reviews in Microbiology 37, 214–226. https://doi.org/10.3109/1040841X.2011.559944.

Zhao, W.-H., Hu, Z.-Q., 2011. Epidemiology and genetics of VIM-type metallo-β-lactamases in Gram-negative bacilli. Future Microbiology 6, 317–333. https://doi.org/10.2217/fmb.11.13.

Chapter 8

Resistance to fluoroquinolones

Chapter outline

Overview

Quinolones and fluoroquinolones (FQs) are widely used in human and veterinary medicine for treatment of bacterial infections. Nalidixic acid, the first quinolone compound derived from an antimalarial drug chloroquine, was discovered in 1962. Basically quinolones are synthetically derived by modification of 1-alkyl-1,8-naphthyridin-4-one-3-carboxylic acid. In 1965, it was introduced in clinical practice. However, use of nalidixic acid was rather limited owing to poor absorption through gastrointestinal tract and narrow spectrum activity particularly in the urinary tract infection (UTI). To broaden the spectrum and increase its absorption and bioavailability, quinolone was structurally modified with addition of fluorine atom to develop FQ in 1980s. Among various FQs, ciprofloxacin and norfloxacin were first approved for clinical use in 1980. Later enrofloxacin was the first FQ introduced for use in dogs and cats in 1989. Later other FQ compounds such as orbifloxacin, difloxacin and marbofloxacin were introduced for use in pet animals.

FQs received wide acceptability to the clinicians because of their enhanced bactericidal property against both replicating and dormant bacteria and for being able to achieve bactericidal concentration in bone and cerebrospinal fluid. Thus overprescription from medical fraternity leads to emergence of FQ-resistance through plasmid-mediated mechanism and chromosomal mutation. Although FQs are regarded as broad spectrum antibacterial agent, they are not effective against anaerobic pathogens, streptococci and enterococci. However, their excellent efficacy was found against *Staphylococcus* and *Enterobacteriaceae* involved in UTI. Based on their spectrum of activity, FQs are categorized into four groups — first to fourth generations (Table 8.1).

Use of FQs such as enrofloxacin, marbofloxacin, danofloxacin, difloxacin, ibafloxacin, sarafloxacin and orbifloxacin were approved in the treatment of animals.

Resistance mechanism

FQs impart bactericidal action by impairing the enzymes DNA gyrase (topoisomerase II) and topoisomerase IV involved in bacterial DNA replication. Bacterial DNA usually remains in supercoiled state and for replication, DNA needs to be uncoiled with its strands separated. DNA gyrase is instrumental for cut, separation and sealing of the DNA strands. The exact mechanism by which FQs inhibit gyrase is not known. However, it is thought that FQs inhibit ligase domain keeping nuclease domains free to cause DNA fragmentation. By inhibiting topoisomerase IV, the enzyme responsible for relaxation of DNA after replication, FQs cause trapping of intercoiled DNA and cell death. First- and second-generation FQs selectively inhibit DNA gyrase, whereas third- and fourth-generation FQs inhibit topoisomerase IV and thus are more effective against Gram-positive pathogens.

Antimicrobial Resistance in Agriculture. https://doi.org/10.1016/B978-0-12-815770-1.00008-0

TABLE 8.1 Different generations of quinolone and fluoroquinolones.

Sl no	Generations	Drugs
1.	First generation	Flumequine Oxolinic acid Rosoxacin
2.	Second generation	Ciprofloxacin Lomefloxacin Norfloxacin Ofloxacin Pefloxacin Fleroxacin Nadifloxacin Rufloxacin
3.	Third generation	Sparfloxacin Levofloxacin Balofloxacin Grepafloxacin Pazufloxacin Temafloxacin
4.	Fourth generation	Gatifloxacin Moxifloxacin Clinafloxacin Sitafloxacin Prulifloxacin

Although there are ample guidelines on reserved use of FQs only in refractory cases, resistance to FQ is on the rise. Within a period of 5 years, FQ resistance has grown up to 20% in 2006 from 6% in 2001 in United States. Likewise, FQ-resistant (FQ^R) *Klebsiella pneumonia* were reported to increase up to 50% in 2012 from 11% in 2005. Interestingly, it was reported that FQ^R *Campylobacter* were persistently detected in the poultry even after on-farm FQ use had been withdrawn and the workers commented that ban on FQs in poultry might not be sufficient to mitigate the problems of quinolone resistant *Campylobacter* in poultry products (Price et al., 2007).

Mutations in the chromosomal target enzymes

As we discussed previously, quinolones target bacterial type II topoisomerase enzymes — DNA gyrase and DNA topoisomerase IV — and the most common mechanism responsible for FQ-resistance is mediated via mutations of the gene(s) encoding these target enzymes. The mutations are usually recorded in a short region of DNA sequences, known as quinolone resistance-determining region (QRDR). Single amino acid alteration in QRDR region of gyrase and topoisomerase IV may lead to such resistance. QRDR region is located to amino terminal domains of GyrA (residues 67–106 for *Escherichia coli* numbering) or ParC (residues 63–102). Usually combined mutations in QRDR of GyrA and ParC were observed among highly resistant Gram-negative bacteria (GNB) (Bagel et al., 1999; Chen et al., 1996). In various scientific reports, it has been documented that the most common sites of mutation in GyrA are at Ser83 followed by Asp87 in *E. coli*. While the amino acid substitutions such as Ser83Trp and Ser83Leu were found to cause reduced affinity of quinolone compounds towards gyrase-DNA complexes, mutations in the Asp87 position substantially reduce catalytic efficiency of DNA gyrase. In ParC gene, the common sites of mutations leading to a quinolone resistance among *E. coli* are Ser-80–Arg (Ile can also be found) and Glu-84–Val (Gly can also be found) (Nakamura et al., 1989; Kumagai et al., 1996; Yang et al., 2018; Vila et al., 1996).

Price et al. (2007) reported FQ^R *Campylobacter jejuni* and *Campylobacter coli* obtained from feedlot cattle farms in multiple states in the United States. All the FQ^R *C. coli* and most of the *C. jejuni* isolates carried a single Thr-86-Ile mutation in GyrA. However, mutations in other positions of GyrA (such as Arg-285-Lys, Asn-203-Ser and Ser-22-Gly) were also noticed in case of FQ^R *C. jejuni*. In addition, the workers observed another mutation — Arg-285-Lys among ciprofloxacin-sensitive isolates — indicated that this mutation might not be directly linked to quinolone resistance. FQs usually target either DNA gyrase or topoisomerase IV depending on their relative sensitivity towards these enzymes.

Most of the quinolone drugs which are in clinical use have more affinity to gyrase in GNB and topoisomerase IV in Gram-positive bacteria with few exceptions. Thus the magnitude of FQ resistance depends on mutation in the respective genes of enzymes and sensitivity of the enzyme to the given FQ compound (Redgrave et al., 2014; Hooper and Jacoby, 2015; Aldred et al., 2014). Once FQ resistance develops because of mutation at the primary target, they start to exert antibacterial action using the secondary target. However, it is not uncommon to notice mutation in both the targets. There are several reports on high level of quinolone resistance associated with mutations in both gyrase and topoisomerase IV. Many bacterial species such as *Mycobacterium* spp., *Campylobacter* spp., *Corynebacterium* spp., *Treponema pallidum* and *Helicobacter pylori* do not possess topoisomerase IV (Chen et al., 1996). In these bacteria DNA gyrase remains the only target for quinolone compounds.

Mutations at other domains such as GyrB and ParE are also known to contribute towards quinolone resistance, although the frequency of such resistance is much less in clinical isolates. Two such kinds of mutations were noted in GyrB of *E. coli* (Redgrave et al., 2014; Aldred et al., 2014). While the first one Asp-426—Asn is reported to be associated with higher resistance towards both quinolone and FQ, the second mutation at Asp-426-Asn causes nalidixic acid resistance with hypersusceptibility to FQs. Sorlozano et al. (2007) described the mutation at position 458 (Ser → Ala) within the QRDR of ParE of ESBL-producing *E. coli* responsible for high level of FQ resistance (Sorlozano et al., 2007). In other GNB also, mutations in ParE region was reported to cause FQ resistance (Kim et al., 2010).

Efflux pump—mediated resistance

Owing to small size and intrinsic surface charges, FQs can easily enter the bacterial cells. The FQ molecules pass through outer cell membrane and cytoplasmic membrane via porin channels by simple diffusion. Thus porin channels play an important role for the entry of FQ molecules in the cell. With reduction of the porin channels, intracellular accumulation of drug molecules tends to reduce substantially and makes the bacteria resistant. However, reduction of porin channel alone is not sufficient for FQ resistance. Endogenous drug efflux pumps are important to mediate such resistance, as recent studies reported. Other than plasmid-borne efflux pumps, there are chromosomal drug efflux pumps such as major facilitator superfamily (MFS) pumps such as *NorA* in *Staphylococcus aureus* and resistance nodulation division (RND) family pumps in Gram-negative pathogens. In GNB such drug efflux pumps consisted of three components — an outer membrane protein, efflux pump domain in the cytoplasmic membrane and a fusion protein which joins the two components. Very recently, presence of such RND efflux pumps were recorded in multidrug-resistant *Helicobacter pullorum* isolates from broiler and free-range chickens in Hyderabad, India (Qumar et al., 2016). Chromosomal mutation of the gene(s) regulating the efflux pumps may cause overexpression of such pumps leading to higher minimum inhibitory concentration (MIC) to quinolones/FQs. Exposure of the bacteria to FQs for a longer period, possibly a fallout of inadvertent use of antimicrobials or for therapeutic purpose, may result into selective selection of the bacteria with mutants with overexpressed drug efflux pumps such as *patAB* in *Streptococcus pneumoniae* and *acrAB-TolC* in *Salmonella typhimurium* and *E. coli* (Hooper, 2001). In many circumstances, such overexpressed efflux pumps may be instrumental along with other resistance mechanisms such as mutation in GyrA/ParC or presence of Plasmid-mediated quinolone resistance (PMQR). Such instance was observed in highly FQ[R] isolates of *S. pneumoniae* with overexpressed patAB and mutated ParC (Garvey et al., 2011).

Plasmid-mediated quinolone resistance

It was way back in 1998 when transferrable quinolone resistance gene was first described in a large multidrug-resistant plasmid of a porin-deficient *K. pneumoniae* strain from the United States. Unlike the chromosomal mutation—driven quinolone resistance, which can be transmitted only vertically from generation to generation, plasmid-mediated resistance may be transferred both vertically and horizontally. PMQR gene(s) usually confer low to moderate degree of FQ resistance ($\leq$10-fold). However, higher degree of resistance ($\approx$250-fold) was also reported. Such degree of resistance usually depends on plasmid copy number and level of resistance gene expression. To date, three classes of PMQR gene(s) were described with three distinct mechanisms of resistance — qnr proteins, the aminoglycoside acetyltransferase AAC(6′)-Ib-cr and the efflux pumps qepA and OqxAB (Hooper and Jacoby, 2015; Aldred et al., 2014; Strahilevitz et al., 2009; Poirel et al., 2012).

The qnr proteins were extensively studied and these proteins usually consist of about 200 amino acids and belong to the pentapeptide repeat family. Till date, six different qnr genes were described. The first reported qnr was qnrA made up of 218 amino acids followed by discovery of other qnr such as qnrS, qnrB, qnrC, qnrD and qnrVC, which was lately detected in *Vibrio cholera*. These genes differ in sequence by 35% from each other. Further several allelic variants were also reported for these qnr gene(s). Currently seven alleles were reported for qnrA (qnrA1-7) and qnrVC. Furthermore, 1 allele for qnrC, 2 for qnrD, 9 for qnrS and 78 for qnrB were described. These qnr proteins share structural homology with McbG and MfpA, which are also members of pentapeptide repeat family and instrumental in resistance towards gyrase inhibitors (Poirel et al., 2012). Recent structural analysis of qnr proteins revealed that these proteins bind with gyrase and topoisomerase IV to prevent access of the quinolone molecules to cleavage complexes of the target enzymes and intercalation of quinolone with the enzymes is no longer possible (Redgrave et al., 2014; Aldred et al., 2014). Furthermore, similar to McbG and MfpA, qnr proteins appear to reduce the binding of gyrase and topoisomerase with DNA and thus reduce the available enzyme targets on chromosome (Aldred et al., 2014). The qnr genes are thought to have originated from chromosomal gene(s) of aquatic bacteria such as *Vibrio splendidus* and *Shewanella algae* (Poirel et al., 2012). Furthermore, the progenitor of qnrB was traced from aquatic *Citrobacter* (Jacoby et al., 2011). All the qnr genes were detected in the plasmid of varying sizes ranging from 7 to more than 300 kb. The plasmid usually contains other resistance determinants against β-lactams, aminoglycosides, chloramphenicol, tetracycline, sulfonamides, trimethoprim and rifampin. Insertion sequences such as IS*CR1* or ISEcp1 or *ISEcl2* elements or Tn3 transposon structures were found in association for qnr determinants facilitating their acquisition and transfer.

The other PMQR determinant AAC(6′)-Ib-cr is a variant of the enzyme aminoglycoside acetyltransferase with two mutations at codons 102 (Trp → Arg) and 179 (Asp → Tyr). While the wild-type AAC(6′)-Ib can acetylate and inactivate the aminoglycosides such as kanamycin, tobramycin and amikacin, the mutant is capable to acetylate more efficiently the amino nitrogen on the piperazinyl substituent of the FQs (Aldred et al., 2014; Jacoby et al., 2014). Thus the FQs having such unsubstituted nitrogen of the C7 piperazine ring such as ciprofloxacin or norfloxacin are usually affected by AAC(6′)-Ib-cr. This PMQR gene is more frequently detected among *K. pneumoniae* and *E. coli*. In humans, the overall detection rate varies from 0.4 to as high as 34%. However, recently it has been detected in *Salmonella* (Lu et al., 2015) and *E. coli* isolates from chicken (Ferreira et al., 2018), *E. coli* of porcine origin (Poirel et al., 2012) and *K. pneumoniae* isolates from buffalo milk (Bandyopadhyay et al., 2018). Mostly this gene is found in the drug-resistant cassette of the integron in the MDR plasmid where other genes encoding resistance to sulphonamides (*sul1*) or higher generation cephalosporins (*bla*CTX-M-15) also coexist. Mobile genetic element — IS*26* — was found to be associated in higher frequency with AAC(6′)-Ib-cr (Hooper and Jacoby, 2015).

The third group of PMQR determinants falls under the group of efflux pumps where three genes have been recognized till date — qepA1, qepA2 and OqxAB (Jacoby et al., 2014). The qepA, quinolone efflux pump, is a 53 kDa protein consisting of 511 amino acids which belongs to the MFS group. The progenitor of qepA is not known but it is thought *Actinomycetales* species may be the natural reservoir, as qepA has a significant similarity with membrane transporter of *Actinomycetales*. Although qepA was initially detected in human clinical isolates of *E. coli* from Japan and Belgium, its occurrence in human clinical isolates is low. In contrast, qepA was frequently detected in animal isolates. In general, qepA confers resistance to hydrophilic FQs such as enrofloxacin, ciprofloxacin and norfloxacin with 8- to 32-fold increase in MIC. However, qepA did not alter the susceptibility pattern of the isolate towards moderately hydrophilic (pefloxacin, sparfloxacin, levofloxacin and moxifloxacin) or hydrophobic (nalidixic acid) quinolone or FQs. In most of the animal isolates, qepA was found to coexist with 16S rRNA or ribosomal methylase rmtB mediating resistance to aminoglycosides in the same plasmid. Insertion elements such as IS*26* elements and IS*CR3C* were found to drive mobilization and expression of qepA gene (Redgrave et al., 2014; Hooper and Jacoby, 2015; Aldred et al., 2014; Strahilevitz et al., 2009; Jacoby et al., 2014). Two variants of qepA — qepA1 and qepA2 — were described with difference in two amino acids. The oqxAB is the MDR pumps belonging to the resistance−nodulation−cell division efflux systems (Redgrave et al., 2014; Hooper and Jacoby, 2015; Aldred et al., 2014; Strahilevitz et al., 2009; Kim et al., 2009a). This was first detected in *E. coli* isolates from swine manure. Originally the oqxAB was recorded to drive resistance to olaquindox which is generally used as growth promoter in pigs. However, the oqxAB is active against many other drug molecules such as chloramphenicol, trimethoprim and quinolones like ciprofloxacin, flumequine, norfloxacin and nalidixic acid. Like qepA, oqxAB was also found to be linked with mobilizing element IS*26* element and ESBL gene(s) such as *bla*CTX-M alleles (Kim et al., 2009a).

Present status

It is important to note that despite multifaceted mechanism operational for FQ resistance, several FQ^R clones have successfully established their foothold globally. One of such examples is EMRSA-15 belonging to the MLST type ST22. Recent studies reported how the introduction of FQ in the United Kingdom in 1980 facilitated the spread of a subclone ST22A2 of EMRSA-15 with acquired FQ resistance throughout the globe by 2014 (Redgrave et al., 2014; Das et al., 2013; Holden et al., 2013). It has been postulated that as the FQs are excreted through skin, introduction and subsequent use of FQs in clinical medicine could have expedited the sustenance and proliferation of the FQ^R subclone ST22A2.

With regard to animal pathogens, few studies were conducted to assess the FQ resistance especially in dairy and poultry. Recently, Balakrishnan et al. (2016) characterized 30 *E. coli* isolates from 92 milk samples collected from cases of bovine mastitis for FQ resistance. The phenotypic resistance varies from 23.33% to 63.33% and mutation scan screening of the QRDR of GyrA and parC revealed mutation at 83rd and 87th amino acid position of GyrA gene and at 80th and 108th amino acid position of parC gene. Similarly, a study conducted on FQ^R *E. coli* from milk samples from cases of bovine mastitis in Taiwan revealed similar kind of mutation in GyrA and parC (Su et al., 2016). Another study from Mangalore revealed that both mutation in the QRDR of GyrA gene (87th position) and plasmid-borne quinolone resistance determinants (qnrS, qnrA and qnrB) are responsible for quinolone resistance in nontyphoidal *Salmonella* from chicken in Mangalore, India (Olukemi Adesiji et al., 2017). However, Samanta et al. (2014) did not find any *qnr* gene(s) among *E. coli* isolates in the backyard poultry and their environment in West Bengal, India. The finding suggested that emergence of plasmid-mediated FQ resistance might have a direct linkage with their usage. In other parts of the world, FQ^R *Enterobacteriaceae* were recovered from poultry. One study in Brazil documented predominance of PMQR determinants such as *qnrB* among FQ^R *Enterobacteriaceae* in healthy poultry population with qnrS and AAX(6′)-Ib-cr in very low frequency (Ferreira et al., 2018). The gene qnrB was located in small-sized plasmid pPAB19-3 favouring its easy dissemination. Lu et al. (2015) characterized quinolone-resistant *Salmonella enterica serovar Indiana* isolates from chicken farm and slaughterhouse samples. All the isolates carried mutation in GyrA gene. Although the other PMQR determinants — qnrA, qnrB, qnrS and qepA — were not detected in any of the isolates, AAC(6′)-Ib-cr was found in higher frequency (>90%). Likewise, quinolone-resistant *Salmonella enterica* isolated from chickens, ducks and pigs at animal clinics in Guangdong, People's Republic of China, were found to carry mutation in GyrA gene in addition to the PMQR determinates such as AAC(6′)-Ib-cr, oqxAB (9.1%) and qnrS (Cao et al., 2017). Mutation in the QRDR region along with PMQR determinants was reported to cause frequent quinolone resistance among *E. coli* isolates from diverse animals in Taiwan. Proportions of nalidixic acid resistance were found as high as 72.0% in swine, 81.9% in chickens, 81.0% in turkeys, 64.0% in ducks and 73.2% in geese (Yeh et al., 2017). Another report from China revealed the presence of *Salmonella enterica serovar Indiana* and *California* isolates of chicken origin with concurrent resistance to cefotaxime, amikacin and ciprofloxacin (Wang et al., 2017). PMQR determinants — AAC(6′)-Ib-cr, oqxAB, qnrB, qepA and qnrD — were detected in many of the isolates. A study conducted in the Moravian regions of the Czech Republic also revealed that PMQR genes are involved for quinolone resistance of the *E. coli* isolates from environment of the poultry houses and cloacal swab of turkeys (Hricová et al., 2017). However, such PMQR genes could be detected among a small number of poultry-associated nalidixic acid (NAL)-resistant *E. coli* in the Annaba city, Algeria (Laarem et al., 2017). An extensive study was conducted to assess the FQ^R *E. coli* in individual fecal samples from preweaned dairy calves, postpartum cows and in environmental samples from 23 Swedish dairy farms (Duse et al., 2016). The authors reported such pathogens in higher frequency in the dairy farm environment and in postpartum cows. Animal feed and water troughs along with farm environments were found as potential source for pathogens to young calves. Although the isolates were genotypically diverse, few genotypes such as MLVA type-1 and 2 were more predominantly detected in several farms indicating possibility of transfer of such pathogens across the farms through newly introduced/purchased animals. Recently, Yang et al., 2018 reported that almost 23% of the *E. coli* isolates from bovine mastitis were quinolone resistant and 65% of the quinolone-resistant strains harbour PMQR gene(s), of which AAC(6′)-Ib-cr was predominant followed by oqxA/B, qepA4, qnrS and qnrB2 (Yang et al., 2018). The study also indicated high rate of co-existence of both ESBL and FQ^R gene(s) in same isolate. This has been also previously observed by workers from India who detected various quinolone resistance gene(s) among ESBL producers from bovine and buffalo milk (Koovapra et al., 2016; Kar et al., 2015; Bandyopadhyay et al., 2018).

Detection

Phenotypic detection of quinolone resistance depends on disk diffusion test or determination of MIC for agents such as nalidixic acid and ciprofloxacin. The FDA had given the guidelines for determining nonsusceptibility towards nalidixic acid and ciprofloxacin. In general, for *E. coli* and *Salmonella* spp, isolates with MIC_{CIP} with less than 0.06 μg/mL are categorized as susceptible while the isolates with $MIC_{CIP} \geq 0.12$ μg/mL are categorized as intermediate and resistant. As per new guidelines, $MIC_{CIP} \geq 0.12$ μg/mL is used as a marker of lower susceptibility towards ciprofloxacin — an indicator of emerging quinolone/FQ resistance. Similarly, MIC for nalidixic acid (MIC_{NAL}) is also used to categorize the quinolone resistance pattern. Isolates with $MIC_{NAL} \leq 16$ μg/mL are considered as susceptible, while $MIC_{NAL} \geq 32$ μg/mL are categorized as resistant.

TABLE 8.2 Breakpoints for determination of quinolone resistance.

SI No	Quinolones/fluoroquinolones	Disk diffusion test			MIC		
		S	I	R	S	I	R
1.	Ciprofloxacin 5 µg	≥21	16–20	≤15	≤1	2	≥4
	Campylobacter *jejuni* and Campylobacter *coli*				≤0.5		≥1
	Salmonella sp.	≥31	21–30	≤20	≤0.06	0.12–0.5	≥1.0
2.	Levofloxacin 5 µg	≥17	14–16	≤13	≤2	4	≥8
	Salmonella sp.				0.12	0.25–1	2
3.	Gatifloxacin 5 µg	≥18	15–17	≤14	≤2	4	≥8
4.	Gemifloxacin 5 µg	≥20	16–19	≤15	≤0.25	0.5	≥1
5.	Grepafloxacin 5 µg	≥18	15–17	≤14	≤1	2	≥4
6.	Ofloxacin 5 µg	≥16	13–15	≤12	≤2	4	≥8
	Salmonella sp.				0.12	0.25–1	2
7.	Lomefloxacin 10 µg	≥22	19–21	≤18	≤2	4	≥8
8.	Norfloxacin 10 µg	≥17	13–16	≤12	≤4	8	≥16
9.	Nalidixic acid 30 µg	≥19	14–18	≤13	≤16		≥32
	C. jejuni and *C. coli*				≤16		≥32
	Salmonella sp.	≥19	14–18	≤13	≤16		≥32
10.	Pefloxacin 5 µg (surrogate test for ciprofloxacin in *Salmonella* sp.)	≥24		≤23			

For *Enterobacteriaceae* isolates, CSLI had given standard breakpoints for most of the quinolones and FQs for disk diffusion test and determination of MIC. Monitoring FQ resistance in *Campylobacter* is important, particularly the isolates of avian origin. The FDA has provided guidelines to summarize the respective breakpoints for *C. jejuni* and *C. coli* (Table 8.2). The conventional phenotypic detection methods were found insufficient to detect FQ resistance among *Salmonella enterica* possibly because of the fact that traditional phenotypic methods cannot detect several emerging FQ resistance and the recent changes that were documented in pharmacokinetics and pharmacodynamics of FQ drugs. Moreover, the failures of FQ therapy to recover the patients infected with isolates with low level of FQ resistance had prompted CLSI to provide separate guidelines with revised MIC breakpoints for ciprofloxacin, levofloxacin and ofloxacin for detection of FQ resistance in *Salmonella*. Such guidelines were also given by the FDA and EUCAST with regard to MIC$_{CIP}$. However, to overcome the difficulties faced by several laboratories to interpret ciprofloxacin disk diffusion results or where MIC$_{CIP}$ or MIC for other FQs cannot be determined, CLSI and EUCAST both recommended to use pefloxacin 5 µg as surrogate marker for detection of FQ resistance in *Salmonella* (Deak et al., 2015). Therefore, the revised guideline for *Salmonella* is separately mentioned in the table.

Although the phenotypic detection methods give a clear picture on the susceptibility of individual isolates to various antimicrobial agents of quinolone and FQ groups, they can hardly give an idea about the resistant mechanism operational in an isolate. As it has been discussed previously that FQ resistance can be driven by various chromosomal and plasmid-mediated determinants, it is important to appraise what kind of resistance mechanisms are responsible for emergence of FQ resistance in various sectors from epidemiological point. Plasmid-mediated mutation may spread rapidly across the species because of horizontal transmission and may require immediate attention. Various PMQR determinants as detailed in earlier are responsible for only low level of FQ resistance and thus phenotypic detection methods may fail to identify such isolates. Therefore, molecular tools may be of great help in such circumstances. In general, such resistance mechanism can be explored by polymerase chain reaction (PCR)-based detection of such genes and sequencing whenever required. Various PCR methods with multiple primer sets are available. For the help of the readers, a list of oligonucleotides with respective PCR conditions for some well-studied gene(s) is given herewith. Readers can go through the details with help of references for respective PCR conditions (Table 8.3).

TABLE 8.3 Oligonucleotides and details of polymerase chain reaction (PCR) conditions for detection of quinolone resistance gene(s).

Sl No	Genes	Oligonucleotides	Amplicon size	PCR condition	References
1.	GyrA	F:AAA TCT GCC CGT GTC GTT GGT R: GCC ATA CCT ACG GCG ATA CC	344 bp	Initial denaturation: 5 m at 95°C; 15 cycles of amplification consisting of 95°C for 30 s, 53°C for 1 m, 72°C for 1 m followed by 20 cycles of 95°C for 1 m, 55°C for 1 m, 72°C for 1 m and 10 m at 72°C for the final extension.	Vila et al. (1995)
2.	GyrB	F: GCACGTGAAGCTGCGCGTAA R: CTGTGGTAGCGCAGCTTATC	316 bp	Initial denaturation: 5 m at 94°C; 30 cycles of amplification consisting of 94°C for 30 s, 50°C for 30 s, 72°C for 1 m and 10 m at 72°C for the final extension.	Kim et al. (2010)
3.	ParC	AAACC TGTTCAGCGCCGCATT GTGGTGCCGTTAAG CAAA	395 bp	Initial denaturation: 5 m at 95°C; 15 cycles of amplification consisting of 95°C for 30 s, 53°C for 1 m, 72°C for 1 m followed by 20 cycles of 95°C for 1 m, 55°C for 1 m, 72°C for 1 m and 10 m at 72°C for the final extension.	Vila et al. (1996)
4.	ParC (alternate)	F: CTG AAT GCC AGC GCC AAA TT R: GCG AAC GAT TTC GGA TCG TC	168 bp	Initial denaturation: 5 m at 94°C; 35 cycles of amplification consisting of 94°C for 1 m, 55°C for 1 m, 72°C for 1 m and 10 m at 72°C for the final extension.	Kim et al. (2009b)
5.	ParE	F: CAGGAAGTGATCGATAACAG R: GACAGGGCGTTGACTACCGA	241 bp	Initial denaturation: 5 m at 94°C; 30 cycles of amplification consisting of 94°C for 30 s, 50°C for 30 s, 72°C for 1 m and 10 m at 72°C for the final extension.	Kim et al. (2010)
6.	qnrA	F: ATT TCT CAC GCC AGG ATT TG F: GAT CGG CAA AGG TTA GGT CA	516 bp	Initial denaturation: 5 m at 95°C; 35 cycles of amplification consisting of 95°C for 1 m, 56°C for 1 m, 72°C for 1 m and 10 m at 72°C for the final extension.	Kar et al. (2015)
7.	qnrB	F: GAT CGT GAA AGC CAG AAA GG R:ATG AGC AAC GAT GCC TGG TA	476 bp		Kar et al. (2015)
8.	qnrS	F: GCA AGT TCA TTG AAC AGG GT R: TCT AAA CCG TCG AGT TCG GCG	428 bp		Kar et al. (2015)
9.	qnrC	F: GGG TTG TAC ATT TAT TGA ATC G R: CAC CTA CCC ATT TAT TTT CA	307 bp	Initial denaturation: 5 m at 94°C; 35 cycles of amplification consisting of 94°C for 1 m, 50°C for 1 m, 72°C for 1 m and 10 m at 72°C for the final extension.	Kim et al. (2009b)
10.	qnrD	F: CGA GAT CAA TTT ACG GGC AAT A R: AAC AAG CTG AAG CGC CTG	533 bp		Cavaco et al. (2009)
11.	qepA	F: GCA GGT CCA GCA GCG GGT AG 3' R: CTT CCT GCC CGA GTA TCG TG 3'	218 bp	Initial denaturation: 5 m at 94°C; 35 cycles of amplification consisting of 94°C for 30 s, 50°C for 30 s, 72°C for 1 m and 10 m at 72°C for the final extension.	Ferjani et al. (2015)
12.	AAC(6')-lb-cr	F:TTG CGA TGC TCT ATG AGT GGCTA R:CTCGAA TGC CTG GCG TGT TT	482bp	Initial denaturation: 5 m at 95°C; 20 cycles of amplification consisting of 95°C for 1 m, 50°C for 1 m, 72°C for 1 m; followed by 20 cycles with 95°C for 1 m, 53°C for 1 m, 72°C for 1 and 10 m at 72°C for the final extension.	Kim et al. (2009b)

Continued

TABLE 8.3 Oligonucleotides and details of polymerase chain reaction (PCR) conditions for detection of quinolone resistance gene(s).—cont'd

Sl No	Genes	Oligonucleotides	Amplicon size	PCR condition	References
13.	oqxA	F: CTC GGC GCG ATG ATG CT R: CCA CTC TTC ACG GGA GAC GA	392 bp	Initial denaturation: 5 m at 94°C; 35 cycles of amplification consisting of 94°C for 45 s, 57°C for 45 s, 68°C for 1 m and 10 m at 72°C for the final extension.	Kim et al. (2009a)
14.	oqxB	F: CGA AGA AAG ACC TCC CTA CCC R: CGC CGC CAA TGA GAT ACA	512 bp	Initial denaturation: 5 m at 94°C; 35 cycles of amplification consisting of 94°C for 45 s, 64°C for 45 s, 72°C for 1 m and 10 m at 72°C for the final extension.	

Therapeutic strategies

The new-generation quinolones along with β-lactam constitute the mainstay of therapy for community-acquired infection in most of the countries. Therefore, preserving the utility of quinolones, particularly the higher groups of FQs, is essential while deciding on the therapeutic regimen planning against different infections. Two aspects are important in the development of new FQ — broadening the antibacterial efficacy of the compounds and improvement in the pharmacokinetic properties of the drugs with increased bioavailability. Although the first-generation quinolones are effective against GNB, their usage is restricted only in UTI because of poor tissue distribution. The second-generation FQs — ciprofloxacin, ofloxacin and norfloxacin — are more active against GNB with sufficient tissue distribution. The third-generation FQ — levofloxacin — is usually more effective against Gram-positive bacteria such as *S. pneumonia*; however, its efficacy is poor than ciprofloxacin against *Pseudomonas aeruginosa*. The fourth-generation FQs such as moxifloxacin and gatifloxacin are more effective against refractory pathogens such as Gram-positive anaerobes.

Thus depending on the kind, site and nature of infection drug regimen should be decided. Bacteria with mutation in the gyrase and DNA topoisomerase usually exhibit resistance to FQs.

The mutant prevention concentration (MPC) is very important for deciding on the therapeutic regimen for quinolone-resistant strains. MPC represents the threshold value above which the selective proliferation of resistant mutants is expected to occur rarely. Thus if the concentration of the desired FQ is maintained at sufficiently high level, only the isolates with multiple resistance conferring mutations will be able to survive and the chance of emergence of new resistant strains will be substantially reduced. Such case is possible with FQ with improved antibacterial efficacy and pharmacodynamics property such as increased bioavailability. This was further substantiated by the study of Strahilevitz and Hooper, (2005), which revealed that the use of two different FQs — one acting on DNA gyrase and another on DNA topoisomerase IV — reduced the frequency of resistant *S. aureus* strains. Likewise, such low-resistance frequency was observed for the compounds where multiple mutations are required for development of resistance. While mutation of either of DNA gyrase or topoisomerase gene may cause resistance to second- and third-generation FQ, resistance to C-8 methoxy FQs (fourth generation) such as gatifloxacin and moxifloxacin requires simultaneous mutations in both the gene(s) (Sanders et al., 2011; Mah et al., 2007). Thus in infection caused by *S pneumoniae*, use of C-8 methoxy FQ compounds is more effective. In case of *P. aeruginosa*, FQ should be used in combination with a β-lactam compound to increase treatment efficacy and to reduce the chance of emergence of resistant strains (Sivagurunathan et al., 2008). Efflux pumps are also operational in *P. aeruginosa* to increase MICs to FQ and thus use of appropriate EPI may reduce the resistance frequency (Sivagurunathan et al., 2008).

Despite all the best efforts, preservation of FQ efficacy may not be an easy task to achieve. Even with selection of the best drug with optimum antibacterial potency and improved pharmacokinetic and pharmacodynamics properties, this may become herculean task to attain. There are three factors that can be attributed for preservation of the efficacy of higher generation quinolones. Continued use of quinolones in agriculture, animal husbandry and aquaculture, suboptimal treatment or dosing regimen and the natural variation in the susceptibility of individual bacterial strains to different quinolones can come in a big way of such endeavour. Suboptimum drug regimen is an important factor as exposure of the bacterial strains to a concentration ranging between MIC and MPC may favour the emergence of mutant strains. Such concentration range is known as mutation selection window, which favours the selection of the bacterial strains with single mutation. Ultimately, such strains may emerge as highly resistant with multiple mutations over the time defeating the outcome of more refined treatment regimen. Thus restriction over nonjustifiable use of FQ and adoption of proper therapeutic regimen is also required along with the proper understanding of the pharmacological properties of newer compounds and improvement of their antibacterial efficacy.

References

Aldred, K.J., Kerns, R.J., Osheroff, N., 2014. Mechanism of quinolone action and resistance. Biochemistry 53, 1565–1574. https://doi.org/10.1021/bi5000564.

Bagel, S., Hüllen, V., Wiedemann, B., Heisig, P., 1999. Impact of gyrA and parC mutations on quinolone resistance, doubling time, and supercoiling degree of *Escherichia coli*. Antimicrobial Agents and Chemotherapy 43, 868–875.

Balakrishnan, S., Antony, P.X., Mukhopadhyay, H.K., Pillai, R.M., Thanislass, J., Padmanaban, V., et al., 2016. Genetic characterization of fluoroquinolone-resistant *Escherichia coli* associated with bovine mastitis in India. Veterinary World 9, 705–709. https://doi.org/10.14202/vetworld.2016.705-709.

Bandyopadhyay, S., Banerjee, J., Bhattacharyya, D., Samanta, I., Mahanti, A., Dutta, T.K., et al., 2018. Genomic identity of fluoroquinolone-resistant bla CTX-M -15 -type ESBL and pMAmpC β-lactamase producing *Klebsiella pneumoniae* from buffalo milk, India. Microbial Drug Resistance 0368. https://doi.org/10.1089/mdr.2017.0368 mdr.2017.

Cao, T.-T., Deng, G.-H., Fang, L.-X., Yang, R.-S., Sun, J., Liu, Y.-H., et al., 2017. Characterization of quinolone resistance in *Salmonella enterica* from farm animals in China. Journal of Food Protection 80, 1742–1748. https://doi.org/10.4315/0362-028X.JFP-17-068.

Cavaco, L.M., Hasman, H., Xia, S., Aarestrup, F.M., 2009. qnrD, a novel gene conferring transferable quinolone resistance in *Salmonella enterica* serovar Kentucky and Bovismorbificans strains of human origin. Antimicrobial Agents and Chemotherapy 53, 603–608. https://doi.org/10.1128/AAC.00997-08.

Chen, C.-R., Malik, M., Snyder, M., Drlica, K., 1996. DNA gyrase and topoisomerase IV on the bacterial chromosome: quinolone-induced DNA cleavage. Journal of Molecular Biology 258, 627–637. https://doi.org/10.1006/jmbi.1996.0274.

Das, S., Anderson, C.J., Grayes, A., Mendoza, K., Harazin, M., Schora, D.M., et al., 2013. Nasal carriage of epidemic methicillin-resistant *Staphylococcus aureus* 15 (EMRSA-15) clone observed in three Chicago-area long-term care facilities. Antimicrobial Agents and Chemotherapy 57, 4551–4553. https://doi.org/10.1128/AAC.00528-13.

Deak, E., Skov, R., Hindler, J.A., Humphries, R.M., 2015. Evaluation of surrogate disk tests for detection of ciprofloxacin and levofloxacin resistance in clinical isolates of *Salmonella enterica*. Journal of Clinical Microbiology 53, 3405–3410. https://doi.org/10.1128/JCM.01393-15.

Duse, A., Persson Waller, K., Emanuelson, U., Ericsson Unnerstad, H., Persson, Y., Bengtsson, B., 2016. Occurrence and spread of quinolone-resistant *Escherichia coli* on dairy farms. Applied and Environmental Microbiology 82, 3765–3773. https://doi.org/10.1128/AEM.03061-15.

Ferjani, S., Saidani, M., Amine, F.S., Boutiba-Ben Boubaker, I., 2015. Prevalence and characterization of plasmid-mediated quinolone resistance genes in extended-spectrum β-lactamase-producing enterobacteriaceae in a Tunisian hospital. Microbial Drug Resistance 21, 158–166. https://doi.org/10.1089/mdr.2014.0053.

Ferreira, J.C., Penha Filho, R.A.C., Kuaye, A.P.Y., Andrade, L.N., Berchieri Junior, A., Darini, A.L.D.C., 2018. Identification and characterization of plasmid-mediated quinolone resistance determinants in Enterobacteriaceae isolated from healthy poultry in Brazil. Infection, Genetics and Evolution 60, 66–70. https://doi.org/10.1016/j.meegid.2018.02.003.

Garvey, M.I., Baylay, A.J., Wong, R.L., Piddock, L.J.V., 2011. Overexpression of patA and patB, which encode ABC transporters, is associated with fluoroquinolone resistance in clinical isolates of *Streptococcus pneumoniae*. Antimicrobial Agents and Chemotherapy 55, 190–196. https://doi.org/10.1128/AAC.00672-10.

Holden, M.T.G., Hsu, L.-Y., Kurt, K., Weinert, L.A., Mather, A.E., Harris, S.R., et al., 2013. A genomic portrait of the emergence, evolution, and global spread of a methicillin-resistant *Staphylococcus aureus* pandemic. Genome Research 23, 653–664. https://doi.org/10.1101/gr.147710.112.

Hooper, D.C., 2001. Emerging mechanisms of fluoroquinolone resistance. Emerging Infectious Diseases 7, 337–341. https://doi.org/10.3201/eid0702.700337.

Hooper, D.C., Jacoby, G.A., 2015. Mechanisms of drug resistance: quinolone resistance. Annals of the New York Academy of Sciences 1354, 12–31. https://doi.org/10.1111/nyas.12830.

Hricová, K., Röderová, M., Pudová, V., Hanulík, V., Halová, D., Julínková, P., et al., 2017. Quinolone-resistant *Escherichia coli* in poultry farming. Central European Journal of Public Health 25, 163–167. https://doi.org/10.21101/cejph.a4328.

Jacoby, G.A., Strahilevitz, J., Hooper, D.C., 2014. Plasmid-mediated quinolone resistance. In: Plasmids Biol. Impact Biotechnol. Discov., vol. 2. American Society of Microbiology, pp. 475–503. https://doi.org/10.1128/microbiolspec.PLAS-0006-2013.

Kar, D., Bandyopadhyay, S., Bhattacharyya, D., Samanta, I., Mahanti, A., Nanda, P.K., et al., 2015. Molecular and phylogenetic characterization of multidrug resistant extended spectrum beta-lactamase producing *Escherichia coli* isolated from poultry and cattle in Odisha, India. Infection, Genetics and Evolution 29, 82–90. https://doi.org/10.1016/j.meegid.2014.11.003.

Kim, H.B., Wang, M., Park, C.H., Kim, E.-C., Jacoby, G.A., Hooper, D.C., 2009. oqxAB encoding a multidrug efflux pump in human clinical isolates of Enterobacteriaceae. Antimicrobial Agents and Chemotherapy 53, 3582–3584. https://doi.org/10.1128/AAC.01574-08.

Kim, H.B., Park, C.H., Kim, C.J., Kim, E.-C., Jacoby, G.A., Hooper, D.C., 2009. Prevalence of plasmid-mediated quinolone resistance determinants over a 9-year period. Antimicrobial Agents and Chemotherapy 53, 639–645. https://doi.org/10.1128/AAC.01051-08.

Kim, M.S., Jun, L.J., Shin, S.B., Park, M.A., Jung, S.H., Kim, K., et al., 2010. Mutations in the gyrB, parC, and parE genes of quinolone-resistant isolates and mutants of *Edwardsiella tarda*. Journal of Microbiology and Biotechnology 20, 1735–1743.

Koovapra, S., Bandyopadhyay, S., Das, G., Bhattacharyya, D., Banerjee, J., Mahanti, A., et al., 2016. Molecular signature of extended spectrum β-lactamase producing *Klebsiella pneumoniae* isolated from bovine milk in eastern and north-eastern India. Infection, Genetics and Evolution 44, 395–402. https://doi.org/10.1016/j.meegid.2016.07.032.

Kumagai, Y., Kato, J.-I., Hoshino, K., Akasaka, T., Sato, K., Ikeda, H., 1996. Quinolone-resistant mutants of *Escherichia coli* DNA topoisomerase IV parC gene. Antimicrobial Agents and Chemotherapy 40, 710–714.

Laarem, M., Barguigua, A., Nayme, K., Akila, A., Zerouali, K., El Mdaghri, N., et al., 2017. Occurrence of plasmid-mediated quinolone resistance and virulence genes in avian *Escherichia coli* isolates from Algeria. Journal of Infection in Developing Countries 11, 143. https://doi.org/10.3855/jidc.8643.

Lu, Y., Zhao, H., Liu, Y., Zhou, X., Wang, J., Liu, T., et al., 2015. Characterization of quinolone resistance in *Salmonella enterica* serovar Indiana from chickens in China. Poultry Science 94, 454–460. https://doi.org/10.3382/ps/peu133.

Mah, F.S., Romanowski, E.G., Kowalski, R.P., Yates, K.A., Gordon, Y.J., 2007. Zymar (gatifloxacin 0.3%) shows excellent gram-negative activity against *Serratia marcescens* and *Pseudomonas aeruginosa* in a New Zealand white rabbit keratitis model. Cornea 26, 585–588. https://doi.org/10.1097/ICO.0b013e318033a6f2.

Nakamura, S., Nakamura, M., Kojima, T., Yoshida, H., 1989. gyrA and gyrB mutations in quinolone-resistant strains of *Escherichia coli*. Antimicrobial Agents and Chemotherapy 33, 254–255.

Olukemi Adesiji, Y., Kogaluru Shivakumaraswamy, S., Kumar Deekshit, V., Shivani Kallappa, G., Karunasagar, I., 2017. Molecular characterization of antimicrobial multi-drug resistance in non-typhoidal Salmonellae from chicken and clam in Mangalore, India. The Journal of Biomedical Research. https://doi.org/10.7555/JBR.31.20160094.

Poirel, L., Cattoir, V., Nordmann, P., 2012. Plasmid-mediated quinolone resistance; interactions between human, animal, and environmental ecologies. Frontiers in Microbiology 3, 1–7. https://doi.org/10.3389/fmicb.2012.00024.

Price, L.B., Lackey, L.G., Vailes, R., Silbergeld, E., 2007. The persistence of fluoroquinolone-resistant Campylobacter in poultry production. Environmental Health Perspectives 115, 1035–1039. https://doi.org/10.1289/ehp.10050.

Qumar, S., Majid, M., Kumar, N., Tiwari, S.K., Semmler, T., Devi, S., et al., 2016. Genome dynamics and molecular infection epidemiology of multi-drug resistant Helicobacter pullorum isolates obtained from broiler and country chickens in India. Applied and Environmental Microbiology 83, 02305–02316. https://doi.org/10.1128/AEM.02305-16. AEM.

Redgrave, L.S., Sutton, S.B., Webber, M.A., Piddock, L.J.V., 2014. Fluoroquinolone resistance: mechanisms, impact on bacteria, and role in evolutionary success. Trends in Microbiology 22, 438–445. https://doi.org/10.1016/j.tim.2014.04.007.

Samanta, I., Joardar, S.N., Das, P.K., Das, P., Sar, T.K., Dutta, T.K., et al., 2014. Virulence repertoire, characterization, and antibiotic resistance pattern analysis of *Escherichia coli* isolated from backyard layers and their environment in India. Avian Diseases 58, 39–45. https://doi.org/10.1637/10586-052913-Reg.1.

Sanders, M.E., Moore, Q.C., Norcross, E.W., Sanfilippo, C.M., Hesje, C.K., Shafiee, A., et al., 2011. Comparison of Besifloxacin, gatifloxacin, and moxifloxacin against strains of *Pseudomonas aeruginosa* with different quinolone susceptibility patterns in a rabbit model of keratitis. Cornea 30, 83–90. https://doi.org/10.1097/ICO.0b013e3181e2f0f3.

Sivagurunathan, N., Krishnan, S., Rao, J.V., Nagappa, A.N., Subrahmanyam, V.M., Vanathi, B.M., 2008. Synergy of gatifloxacin with cefoperazone and cefoperazone-sulbactam against resistant strains of *Pseudomonas aeruginosa*. Journal of Medical Microbiology 57, 1514–1517. https://doi.org/10.1099/jmm.0.2008/001636-0.

Strahilevitz, J., Hooper, D.C., 2005. Dual targeting of topoisomerase IV and gyrase to reduce mutant selection: direct testing of the paradigm by using WCK-1734, a new fluoroquinolone, and ciprofloxacin. Antimicrobial Agents and Chemotherapy 49, 1949–1956. https://doi.org/10.1128/AAC.49.5.1949-1956.2005.

Strahilevitz, J., Jacoby, G.A., Hooper, D.C., Robicsek, A., 2009. Plasmid-mediated quinolone resistance: a multifaceted threat. Clinical Microbiology Reviews 22, 664–689. https://doi.org/10.1128/CMR.00016-09.

Sorlozano, A., Gutierrez, J., Jiménez, A., De Dios Luna, J., Martínez, J.L., 2007. Contribution of a new mutation in parE to quinolone resistance in extended-spectrum-β-lactamase-producing *Escherichia coli* isolates. *Journal of Clinical Microbiology* 45, 2740–2742.

Su, Y., Yu, C.-Y., Tsai, Y., Wang, S.-H., Lee, C., Chu, C., 2016. Fluoroquinolone-resistant and extended-spectrum β-lactamase-producing *Escherichia coli* from the milk of cows with clinical mastitis in Southern Taiwan. Journal of Microbiology, Immunology, and Infection 49, 892–901. https://doi.org/10.1016/j.jmii.2014.10.003.

Vila, J., Ruiz, J., Goñi, P., Marcos, A., Jimenez de Anta, T., 1995. Mutation in the gyrA gene of quinolone-resistant clinical isolates of Acinetobacter baumannii. Antimicrobial Agents and Chemotherapy 39, 1201–1203. https://doi.org/10.1128/AAC.39.5.1201.

Vila, J., Ruiz, J., Goñi, P., De Anta, M.T., 1996. Detection of mutations in parC in quinolone-resistant clinical isolates of *Escherichia coli*. Antimicrobial Agents and Chemotherapy 40, 491–493.

Wang, Y., Zhang, A., Yang, Y., Lei, C., Jiang, W., Liu, B., et al., 2017. Emergence of *Salmonella enterica* serovar Indiana and California isolates with concurrent resistance to cefotaxime, amikacin and ciprofloxacin from chickens in China. International Journal of Food Microbiology 262, 23–30. https://doi.org/10.1016/j.ijfoodmicro.2017.09.012.

Yang, F., Zhang, S., Shang, X., Wang, L., Li, H., Wang, X., 2018. Characteristics of quinolone-resistant *Escherichia coli* isolated from bovine mastitis in China. Journal of Dairy Science. https://doi.org/10.3168/jds.2017-14156.

Yeh, J.-C., Lo, D.-Y., Chang, S.-K., Chou, C.-C., Kuo, H.-C., 2017. Prevalence of plasmid-mediated quinolone resistance in *Escherichia coli* isolated from diseased animals in Taiwan. Journal of Veterinary Medical Science 79, 730–735. https://doi.org/10.1292/jvms.16-0463.

Chapter 9

Resistance to aminoglycoside, tetracycline and macrolides

Chapter outline

Aminoglycoside resistance

Aminoglycoside (AG) is an important group of natural or semisynthetic antibiotics used in veterinary and medical science, especially for the treatment of Gram-negative bacteria (GNB). Drugs such as streptomycin, kanamycin, neomycin, gentamicin, amikacin, netilmicin and tobramycin fall under this group. AGs exhibit the bactericidal action by binding the highly conserved region of 16S rRNA and 30S ribosomal subunit. Such interaction leads to translational errors in amino acid synthesis and disruption in bacterial protein synthesis (Krause et al., 2016). Even after the introduction of newer generation β-lactam compounds and fluoroquinolones, which have more potent antibacterial potential, AGs are still preferred choice to treat complicated infection with GNB like *Pseudomonas aeruginosa* particularly in combination with β-lactam drugs because of their broad-spectrum bactericidal properties and synergistic antibacterial effect with other antimicrobials (β-lactam) (Tschudin-Sutter et al., 2018).

Resistance mechanism

Resistance to AG involves three major pathways or mechanisms:

1. The most important pathway is via enzymatic modification of the AGs, particularly by AG-modifying enzymes.
2. Modification of the drug target like a mutation of the ribosomal target subunit or 16S rRNA.
3. Reduced permeability or increased drug efflux to reduce effective drug concentration within the bacterial cell.

Antimicrobial Resistance in Agriculture. https://doi.org/10.1016/B978-0-12-815770-1.00009-2

Enzymatic modification of aminoglycoside

Enzymatic modification mediated by AG-modifying enzyme is the most important and well-studied mechanism for AG resistance. These enzymes are usually responsible for covalent modification of the drugs to weaken their interaction with 16sRNA (Smith and Baker, 2005; Serpersu et al., 2008). In general, three categories of enzymes were reported:

I. Aminoglycoside N-acetyltransferases (AAC) — they cause N acetylation
II. Aminoglycoside phosphoryl transferases (AHP) to cause O phosphorylation
III. Aminoglycoside nucleotidyltransferase (ANT) to cause O adenylation

Based on the site of modification, these enzymes are divided into various groups. Similarly, AAC can be divided into AAC(1), AAC(2′), AAC(3) and AAC(6′) depending on the acetylation they cause to 1, 2′, 3 and 6′ amino groups. Again, AAC(3) is subdivided into three categories AAC(3)-I, AAC(3)-II and AAC(3)-III. Most importantly, these enzymes are carried on R factors or mobile genetic elements (MGE) such as integron and transposon and thus can be transferred to other bacteria via horizontal gene transfer. Furthermore, these enzymes may coexist with resistance determinants to other antimicrobial compounds such as chloramphenicol, sulfonamides, β-lactam and other antiseptics in the MGE, making the pathogen multidrug resistant (MDR). Such MDR strains were reported in food (YuanTing et al., 2017) and companion animals (Jackson et al., 2015).

Reduced drug uptake or increased efflux

The reduced intracellular concentration of AG is another important mechanism responsible for AG resistance. AGs are cationic molecules which enter the bacterial cell via self-mediated uptake through lipopolysaccharide (LPS) and outer membrane using energy-dependent transport across the cytoplasmic membrane. Thus, modification of LPS and low-energy bacterial population may be responsible for AG resistance. Aminoarabinose substitution of the lipid A moiety controlled by PhoP/PhoQ regulatory system is thought responsible for such impermeability of bacterial cell as observed in *P. aeruginosa* (Poole, 2005). This kind of modification by the PhoP/PhoQ system was previously documented in colistin resistance also. The energy-deficient small colony variants are another recalcitrant population where drug influx is substantially affected because of a reduction in energy-dependent uptake process across the cell membrane (Biswas et al., 2009). In case of *P. aeruginosa*, another resistance phenomenon called adaptive resistance was documented. Such phenomenon is characterized by the development of a refractory bacterial population over a period of time once the initial killing of the bacterial population with rapid accumulation of the drug is over (Barclay et al., 1996; Gilleland et al., 1989). Overexpression of anaerobic respiratory gene(s) and lower metabolic pH are thought responsible for such adaptive response (Pang et al., 2019). Other than this, OMPs (outer membrane proteins) such as OpmG and OpmI were also reported for intrinsic AG resistance in *P. aeruginosa* (Jo et al., 2003). In *Escherichia coli*, an oligonucleotide transporter protein called OppA is reported to mediate drug transport. Thus, *E. coli* isolates which are lacking OppA may become AG-resistant (Rodriguez and Costa, 1999).

Several efflux pumps were also documented to mediate AG resistance. Although most of the resistance nodulation division (RND) efflux pumps are involved for spilling out the lipophilic compounds, recent evidence has shown that several RND pumps are also known to confer AG resistance (Anes et al., 2015). Such RND pumps mediating resistance towards cationic AG compounds include AcrD of *E. coli* (Rosenberg et al., 2000), AmrAB-OprA and BpeAB-OprB of *Burkholderia pseudomallei* (Mima and Schweizer, 2010; Moore et al., 1999) and MexXY—OprM of *P. aeruginosa* (Morita et al., 2012; Guénard et al., 2014). Like for other RND efflux systems, these pumps are also thought to be functional for extruding the toxic compounds especially those interfere with protein synthesis and thus these systems are modulated by exposure to AG compounds.

Ribosomal protection and alteration of drug target

Although enzymatic modification of drug molecules, cell membrane impermeability and drug efflux system were mostly studied for AG resistance, recent studies showed that posttranscriptional modification or methylation of ribosomal RNA (rRNA) might play a critical role in AG resistance (Doi and Arakawa, 2007; Lioy et al., 2014). Such methylation of rRNA is thought to be an intrinsic and integrated characteristic of the bacteria synthesizing the antibiotics as a part of their self-defense strategy. It seems that nosocomial pathogens or other infective pathogens acquire such resistance characteristics in the process of evolution. Nevertheless, the evolutionary pathway is yet to be clearly understood. First such kind of modification enzyme — aminoglycoside resistance methyltransferase (*armA*) — was detected in a plasmid pCTX-M-3 of *Citrobacter freundii* from Poland (Galimand et al., 2005; Zacharczuk et al., 2011). The gene *armA* was recorded to co-exist with another resistance factor such as CTX-M type extended-spectrum β-lactamase (ESBL) and gene(s) responsible for resistance to streptomycin—spectinomycin, sulfonamides and trimethoprim as a part of MDR cassettes of an MGE (Wei et al., 2014). Later, the gene *armA* was detected among other GNB such as *E. coli, Klebsiella pneumoniae, Enterobacter cloacae, Salmonella enterica, Shigella flexneri* and *Acinetobacter baumannii*. Additional methylases such as *rmtA* and *rmtB* were also detected in pathogens such as *P. aeruginosa* (Yamane et al., 2007). Ribosomal modification is known to confer broad-spectrum resistance towards AG including the newer generation and clinically relevant AG molecules such as tobramycin.

Status in animals

AGs have been extensively used in both food and companion animals for serious infections affecting digestive, respiratory and genitourinary tract, diarrhoea and septicaemia because of their efficacy against Gram-negative pathogens including *P. aeruginosa*. Different drugs under AGs such as apramycin, gentamicin, kanamycin, paromomycin, neomycin, framycetin, streptomycin and amikacin are used in animals in oral, injectable and intramammary routes (Wagner et al., 2014). Therefore, the problem of AG resistance emerged in animals and even GNB isolated from human patients were traced back to veterinary use of AGs for their gentamicin resistance previously (Johnson et al., 1994). Furthermore, a systematic analysis reflecting the abundance of AG resistance genes among various animal pathogens including coliform bacteria, bacteria with zoonotic potential such as *Salmonella* spp., *Campylobacter* spp. and livestock-associated methicillin-resistant *Staphylococcus aureus* (MRSA) underlined the high probability of transmission of AG resistance from animals to humans through the transfer of zoonotic or commensal foodborne bacteria and/or their MGE (van Duijkeren et al., 2019). Bovine mastitis was reported to harbour AG-resistant pathogens such as *P. aeruginosa* (Chuanchuen et al., 2008), *Nocardia farcinica* (Kogure et al., 2010) in addition to *Enterobacteriaceae* (Bandyopadhyay et al., 2018) and *S. aureus*. Turutoglu et al. (2009) reported MRSA or methicillin-sensitive *S. aureus* (MSSA) isolates from bovine mastitis resistant to gentamicin, neomycin and kanamycin bearing AG-modifying enzyme. A recent study by Belaynehe et al. (2017) reported occurrence of AG-modifying enzymes among isolates of *E. coli* exhibiting high levels of AG resistance in Korean cattle farms. Besides, *E. coli* isolated from diarrhoeic neonatal calves harboured AG adenyltransferase types: aadA1, aadA2, aadA5, aadA7 and aadA23, conferring resistance to streptomycin and spectinomycin; and AG acetyltransferase gene, aac(3)-Id, which confers resistance to gentamicin and sisomicin (Ahmed et al., 2009).

Poultry isolates — *E. coli* (Zhang et al., 2012) and *Salmonella* (Doosti et al., 2016) — were also recorded to harbour AG-resistant determinants in high frequency, possibly because of extensive use of AG in poultry farming. Waste from the cattle or dairy farms can be a major source of AG-resistant bacteria (particularly to kanamycin, gentamicin and streptomycin) in the surrounding environment as revealed in a study from Bangladesh (Ahmed et al., 2013). Pigs were found as a potent reservoir for AG-resistant pathogens as documented in various studies — AG-resistant *Enterococci* were isolated from pigs in Thailand (Lan et al., 2016); such kinds of resistant *Trueperella pyogenes* of swine origin were reported from China (Dong et al., 2017) and Urumova et al., 2015 also reported AG resistance among *E. coli* isolates from pig in Belgium.

Detection

Currently, most of the veterinary diagnostic laboratories follow disk diffusion assay or determination of MIC (minimum inhibitory concentration) to evaluate the AG susceptibility profile of bacterial isolates. However, it is very important to know the molecular basis of such resistance, at least to understand cycling or transfer of such AMR gene(s) in the animal—human—environment interface. Existence of multifaceted resistance mechanism and multiple genes (s) mediating to AG resistance make this an uphill task. However, some important and predominant genes may be screened to understand the molecular epidemiology of AG resistance in food animals. The polymerase chain reaction (PCR) with oligonucleotides of such gene(s) is described in Table 9.1.

Therapeutic strategies

The major hurdles for successful and uninterrupted use of AGs in clinical settings are their toxicity and emergence of resistance. New resistant strains with a plasmid bearing various forms of AG-modifying enzymes are difficult to tackle. Despite this fact, scientists have developed new compounds such as amikacin, tobramycin, isepamicin and dibekacin,

TABLE 9.1 Oligonucleotides for amplification of aminoglycoside resistance genes.

Sl No	Aminoglycosides	Genes	Oligonucleotides (3′-5′)	Tm	References
1	Gentamicin	aac(3)-IV	AGTTGACCCAGGGCTGTCGC	63	Maynard et al. (2004)
			GTGTGCTGCTGGTCCACAGC		
2		ant(2″)-I	GGG CGC GTC ATG GAG GAG	67	Cameron et al. (1986)
			TATCGCGACCTGAAAGCGGC		
3		aac(3)-II	TGA AAC GCT GAC GGA GCC TC	54	Vliegenthart et al. (1989)
			GTC GAA CAG GTA GCA CTG AG		
4	Neomycin	aph(3′)-III	AACGTCTTGCTCGAGGCCGCG	52	Oka et al. (1981)
			GGCAAGATCCTGGTATCGGTCTGCG		
5		aph(3′)-II	GCTATTCGGCTATGACTGGGC	63	Aarestrup (2003)
			CCACCATGATAT TCGGCAAGC		
6		aph(3′)-I	GCCGATGTGGATTGCGAAAA	68	Melano (2003)
			GCTTGATCCCCAGTAAGTCA		
7	Streptomycin	strA	CCA ATC GCA GAT AGA AGG C	55	Scholz et al. (1989)
			CTT GGT GAT AAC GGC AAT TC		
8		strB	GGA TCG TAG AAC ATA TTG GC	56	
			ATC GTC AAG GGA TTG AAA CC		
9		aadA2	ATT TGC TGG TTA CGG TGA CC	56	Rahmani et al. (2013)
			CTT CAA GTA TGA CGG GCT GA		
10		aadE	TCA AAA CCC CTA TTA AAG CC	60	Ouoba et al. (2008)
			ATCCTTCGGCGCGATTTTG		

which are poorly affected by modifying enzymes (Kondo and Hotta, 1999; Vakulenko and Mobashery, 2003). With the use of crystallography, the structures of AG-modifying enzymes were studied and this was useful to understand the drug (AG) binding domains of the enzymes. Thus, significant efforts were made to develop specific inhibitors of such binding domains, although with limited success. Various derivatives and dimers of neamine and kanamycin were tried and such compounds showed promising results as inhibitors of modifying enzymes (Ramirez and Tolmasky, 2017). Likewise, dimers of neamine exhibited antibiotic efficacy with little or no effect by the modifying enzymes (Labby and Garneau-Tsodikova, 2013). Crystallographic image of APH (3′)-IIIa revealed its high degree of resemblance with eukaryotic protein kinase. Thus, the development of compounds with selective inhibitory efficacy towards APH(3′)-IIIa with little effect over host kinase is a new challenge. Target modification at the ribosomal site is also responsible for complicating the resistance problem with regard to the AG group of drugs. Thus, our weapons are limited in the real sense, and till date, no significant development was made to overcome or for reversal of AG resistance.

Tetracycline resistance

Tetracyclines are broad-spectrum antibiotics, effective against a wide range of Gram-positive bacteria (GPB) and GNB, chlamydia, mycoplasmas, rickettsia and protozoan parasites (Chopra and Roberts, 2001). Since its discovery in 1945, chlortetracycline and oxytetracycline, the first members of this group, have been extensively used in human and veterinary medicine. Later on, the semisynthetic tetracyclines such as doxycycline and minocycline and glycylcyclines derivative such as tigecyclines came into practice. Tetracyclines exhibit bacteriostatic activity by inhibition of ribosomal protein synthesis. Interaction of the drug molecules with ribosome prevents the attachment of amino-acyl tRNA to the 'A' site of ribosome, which leads to reversible inhibition of protein synthesis.

Mechanism of tetracycline resistance:

Till date, four possible ways have been explored to cause acquired tetracycline resistance (Grossman, 2016; Nguyen et al., 2014):

1. Efflux pumps
2. Ribosomal protection
3. Enzymatic degradation of the drug molecules
4. Mutations in rRNA with resulting in reduced drug binding affinity

Apart from these, some bacteria may be naturally resistant to tetracycline.

Efflux pumps

In total, 28 different classes of well-characterized energy-dependent efflux pumps have been reported in GPB and GNB, till date. They exchange a proton for a monocationic magnesium—tetracycline complex and act as antiporter to reduce intracellular concentration of drugs. Although this class of efflux pump is predominantly detected among the tetracycline-resistant GNB such as *E. coli*, they are poorly effective against the second-generation tetracycline — doxycycline and minocycline and totally ineffective against the glycylcyclines such as tigecycline (Blanco et al., 2016). The largest group constitutes the drug-proton antiporters efflux pumps which have a structural similarity with the pumps under major facilitator superfamily (MFS) class. The regulation of *tet* gene is differently controlled for GPB and GNB. In case of GNB, two gene(s) control the expression of *tet* gene; in the absence of tetracycline, the repressor protein *tetR* binds with the operator of the structural efflux gene(s) and blocks its expression and in the presence of magnesium—tetracycline complex, repressors are usually released from the operator to allow the expression of *tet* genes (Kamionka et al., 2004). In case of GPB, *tet* genes such as *tet*(K) and *tet*(X) are controlled by translational attenuation (Alekshun and Levy, 2007; Roberts, 1996).

Ribosomal protection

Till date, about 12 classes of such ribosomal protection proteins (RPPs) were documented as to protect bacterial ribosome from binding the antibiotic tetracycline (Biswas et al., 2009; Barclay et al., 1996). They have sequence homology among them and are thought to be derived from *otrA*, a tetracycline resistance gene of *Streptomyces rimosus*, natural producer of oxytetracycline. RPPs are about 72.5 kDA cytoplasmic proteins which share structural similarity to ribosomal elongation factors. Basically, their interaction with ribosome is thought to cause allosteric disruption of tetracycline binding sites. This leads to release of tetracycline from ribosome with bacterial protein synthesis machineries started functioning normally. Among these RPPs, *tetO* and *tet*M were studied in depth. Although *tetO* can be present both in plasmid (as in case of *Campylobacter*) or chromosome (such as in *Streptococcus* and *Staphylococcus*), *tet*M is usually transmitted by conjugative transposons (Tn916 and Tn1545) among *Streptococcus* and a large population of GPB and GNB (Connell et al., 2003; Li et al., 2013; Taylor et al., 2009).

Enzymatic inactivation

Two different genes were reported to cause enzymatic inactivation of tetracycline — *tet*(X) and tet*(37)*. These are basically FAD-dependent monooxygenase which causes hydroxylation of C11a carbon of the tetracycline in presence of NADPH and O_2. The hydroxylated tetracyclines have reduced binding affinity towards ribosomes and soon undergo nonenzymatic degradation. The gene *tet*(X) was reported among large number of MDR GNB — *E. cloacae, Comamonas testosteroni, E. coli, K. pneumonia, Delftia acidovorans* and among other members of *Enterobacteriaceae* and *Pseudomonadaceae* (Markley and Wencewicz, 2018).

Mutations in rRNA

Mutation in 16s RNA is another process for tetracycline resistance because of decreased affinity to the drugs. This was first detected in a GPB, *Propionibacterium acnes*, where a G1058C mutation was detected in a conserved region — helix 34, the major factor for accurate peptide chain termination and translation. Such mutation was reported to cause increased MIC to tetracycline, doxycycline and minocycline. Again, in *Helicobacter pylori* triple mutations in the stem loop of helix 31 of the 16s rRNA, A965U/G966U/A967C was reported to cause high level of tetracycline resistance (Gerrits et al., 2003).

In addition, several multidrug transporters were also found to play an important role for tetracycline resistance. In *E. coli*, two such multidrug efflux pumps were recorded — EmrE multidrug transporter and AcrAB-Tolc efflux systems (Blanco et al., 2016; Aghazadeh et al., 2014). EmrE efflux system belongs to the small multidrug resistance family and overproduction of emrE protein was recorded to induce low level of tetracycline resistance. Similarly upregulation of AcrAB efflux system may also lead to tetracycline resistance. Two different efflux systems of RND superfamily — MexCD-OprJ and MexAB-OprM — along with reduced permeability were shown to confer tetracycline resistance in *P. aeruginosa*. Further deficiency or mutation leading to the structural alteration of outer membrane protein like OmpF which allows the entry of magnesium-bound tetracycline in the cell may lead to tetracycline resistance.

Diagnosis

Phenotypic detection of tetracycline resistance relies on the conventional disc diffusion test and determination of MIC using agar dilution and broth dilution method. A more convenient alternative may be E-test to determine MIC for tetracycline. The microorganisms other than streptococci such as *Enterobacteriaceae, P. aeruginosa, Acinetobacter, Staphylococci and Enterococci* are considered resistant to tetracycline if the diameter of the zone of growth inhibition is 14 mm, as intermediate if zone diameter is between 15 and 18 mm and as susceptible if the zone diameter is ≥ 19 mm using a disc with 30 µg of tetracycline. Likewise, with regard to MIC values, the pathogens are considered resistant to tetracycline if MIC ≥ 16 µg/mL, intermediate in case of MIC is 8 µg/mL and susceptible if MIC ≤ 4 µg/mL.

Although most of the laboratories rely on phenotypic detection methods, molecular detection tools may be used additionally for exploring the resistance mechanism. For amplification of *tet*(A), *tet*(B), *tet*(C), *tet*(D), *tet*(E) and *tet*(Y), Maynard et al. (2003) described the PCR carried out in 50 µL mixture containing 29.6 µL of H2O, 5.0 µL of 10X PCR buffer, 5.0 µL of 2 mM deoxynucleoside triphosphates, 1 U of Taq polymerase and 25 pmol of each primer; the following conditions were followed for running the PCR: 5 min at 94°C, followed by 30 cycles of 94°C for 30 s, 50°C for 30 s and 72°C for 1.5 min and a final extension at 72°C for 5 min. Hedayatianfard et al. (2014) reported slightly different PCR condition — initial denaturation at 94°C for 5 min followed by 30 cycles of denaturation at 94°C for 45 s, annealing at 55°C for 1 min, extension at 72°C for 1 min and a final extension at 72°C for 5 min — what they followed for multiplication of *tet*(M) and *tet*(O) in 50 µL reaction mixture containing 50 mM KCl, 10 mM Tris-HCl (pH 9.0), 1.5 mM MgCl2, 200 µM dNTPs, 20 pmol of each primer, 2 U Taq DNA polymerase and 4 µL of DNA (Table 9.2).

TABLE 9.2 Oligonucleotides for amplification of tetracycline resistance genes.

SI no.	Genes	Oligonucleotides	Amplicon size	
1	tet (M)-F	GTG GAC AAA GGT ACA ACG AG	406	Ng et al. (2001)
2	tet (M)-R	CGG TAA AGT TCG TCA CAC AC		
3	tet (O)-F	AAC TTA GGC ATT CTG GCT CAC	515	
4	tet (O)-R	TCC CAC TGT TCC ATA TCG TCA		
5	tet(S)-F	CAT AGA CAA GCC GTT GAC C	667	
6	tet(S)-R	ATG TTT TTG GAA CGC CAG AG		
7	tet(A)-F	GTGAAACCCAACATACCCC	888	Maynard et al. (2003)
8	tet(A)-R	GAAGGCAAGCAGGATGTAG		
9	tet(B)-F	CCTTATCATGCCAGTCTTGC	774	
10	tet(B)-R	ACTGCCGTTTTTTCGCC		
11	tet(C)-F	ACTTGGAGCCACTATCGAC	881	
12	tet(C)-R	CTACAATCCATGCCAACCC		
13	tet(D)-F	TGGGCAGATGGTCAGATAAG	827	
14	tet(D)-R	CAGCACACCCTGTAGTTTTC		
15	tet(E)-F	TTAATGGCAACAGCCAGC	853	
16	tet(E)-R	TCCATACCCATCCATTCCAC		
17	tet(Y)-F	ACCGCACTCATTGTTGTC	823	
18	tet(Y)-R	TTCCAAGCAGCAACACAC		

Present status

Tetracycline resistance has been exhaustively studied among human and animal bacterial isolates for its extensive use in both human and veterinary medicine. A study on tetracycline resistance pattern of 1263 unique *E. coli* isolates from humans, cats, cows, deer, turkeys, ducks, sheep, geese, dogs, pigs, horses, chickens and goats in Minnesota and western Wisconsin region revealed that more than 78%, 47% and 41% of the *E. coli* isolates from pigs, chickens and turkeys, respectively, were tetracycline-resistant with MIC_{TET} reaching about ≥ 233 µg/mL for many of the isolates (Bryan et al., 2004). Molecular typing revealed predominance of *tet* gene(s) such as *tet*(A) and *tet*(B), which were detected among 35% and 63% of the *E. coli* isolates, respectively. Among others, *tet*(C), *tet*(D) and *tet*(M) were detected, as well. In South Korea, more than 90% of the 155 *E. coli* from beef cattle were found tetracycline-resistant and majority of them carried tetracycline resistance gene *tet*(A) (46.5%) followed by *tet*(B) (45.1%) and *tet*(C) (5.8%). The isolates with *tet*(B) exhibited higher MIC values to tetracycline, chlortetracycline, oxytetracycline, doxycycline and minocycline. Only two of them carried multiple tetracycline resistance gene(s). Conjugation experiments showed that the *tet* gene(s) might be transferred to recipients by IncFIB replicon in most of the isolates (Shin et al., 2015). Schwarz et al. (1998) investigated tetracycline resistantance feature of 838 staphylococcal isolates from cattle, cats, dogs, ducks, guinea pigs, horses, mink, pigeons, pigs, rabbits and turkeys and about 27.2% of the isolates were tetracycline-resistant harbouring several tetracycline resistance (*tet*) genes — *tet*(K), *tet*(L), *tet*(M) or *tet*(O). While the *tet*(M) gene was found predominantly in the resistant *Staphylococcus intermedius* isolates, *tet*(K) was found in other staphylococcal species. Investigation carried out by Kyselková et al., 2015 on the spread of tetracycline resistance at a conventional dairy farm where chlortetracycline is prophylactically used as intrauterine suppository after each calving revealed that the calves in that farms got colonized with tetracycline-resistant bacteria in their early ages and *tet*(O), *tet*(Q) and *tet*(W) were predominantly detected in the fresh excrements of heifers and adult cows, the soils from farm proximity and also in soils of the field which were previously treated with farm manures. This study pointed out how small dairy farms can play a role in contaminating the surrounding environment with antibiotic resistance genes (Kyselková et al., 2015). Furthermore, Al-Bahry et al. (2016) investigated on the diversity of tetracycline-resistant genes of 118 *E. coli* isolates of 201 samples collected from chicken intestine, human feces and treated sewage effluent. On using single and multiplex PCR only seven tetracycline-resistant genes (A, B, C, M, Q, W, 32) were found. Of them *tet*(A) was the predominant followed by *tet*(B) and *tet*32. Most of the tetracycline-resistant strains exhibited a high variation of resistance genes with only few strains harboured a combination of four resistance genes tet (A/B/C/32) and tet (A/B/M/32) (Al-Bahry et al., 2016). Tetracycline-resistant bacteria were reported in food animals from Indian subcontinent. Recently, Khan et al. (2018) reported that about 60% of the *Campylobacter jejuni* isolates from poultry meat, and related samples at retail shops in Northern India were resistant to tetracycline (Khan et al., 2018). Again 24.4% of the *S aureus* isolates from four cattle slaughterhouses of Kerala, South India, were found tetracycline-resistant (Gowda et al., 2017). Almost similar trend was noticed by another group of workers for *S. aureus* isolated from cattle and pigs in Punjab, a western province of India (Zehra et al., 2017). Tetracycline resistance was also noted among the MRSA (Bandyopadhyay et al., 2015) and ESBL producers (Bandyopadhyay et al., 2018) isolated from bovine mastitis in Eastern India.

Macrolide resistance

Macrolides (MLs) are natural compounds consisting of large macrocyclic lactone ring attached to amino or neutral sugars and some of the MLs with the bacteriostatic property are used as antibiotics. The most common MLs which are used as antibiotics include erythromycin, roxithromycin, azithromycin and clarithromycin. Other ML antibiotics are fidaxomicin, telithromycin, oleandomycin, spiramycin, troleandomycin (used in Italy and Turkey) and tylosin (in animals). Besides, some macrocyclic lactone derivatives have antifungal (amphotericin B, nystatin), antiparasitic (ivermectin) and immunomodulatory properties (tacrolimus, pimecrolimus and sirolimus). Reversibly binding to P site on the 50S subunit of the bacterial ribosome, MLs inhibit the peptidyl transferase from adding the nascent peptide attached to tRNA to the next amino acid. Thus, the protein biosynthesis is impeded (Dinos, 2017). Lincosamides are chemically distinct from MLs as they do not have lactone ring. However, they are similar in mode of action.

MLs are effective against most of the GPB (except enterococci) and some GNB. Because of their activity against atypical pathogens such as *Mycoplasma pneumoniae, Treponema pallidum, Bordetella pertussis, Chlamydia trachomatis, Chlamydophila pneumoniae, Legionella* spp., *Campylobacter* spp. *and Borrelia* spp, MLs are often advocated in lower respiratory tract infection, community-acquired pneumonia and acute nonspecific urethritis in human being. Besides, clarithromycin and azithromycin were found effective against *Haemophilus influenzae* and *Mycobacterium avium* complex. Again, fidaxomicin is active against *Clostridium difficile* causing colitis and diarrhoea. In animals, MLs are used against a wide spectrum of pathogens — pathogens involved in bovine respiratory disease (BRD) or shipping fever (*Mannheimia haemolytica, Pasteurella multocida, Histophilus somni* or *Mycoplasma bovis*), foot rot or interdigital necrobacillosis (*Fusobacterium necrophorum* and *Porphyromonas levii*), pink eye (*Moraxella bovis*), swine enzootic pneumonia (*Mycoplasma hyopneumoniae, Actinobacillus pleuropneumoniae, P. multocida* and *Haemophilus parasuis*) (Pyörälä et al., 2014), canine giardiasis, pyoderma, papillomatosis and lyme disease (Yağci et al., 2008; Hansmann, 2009; Silva et al., 2014; Zygner et al., 2008), chronic respiratory disease (*Mycoplasma gallisepticum*) and necrotic enteritis in poultry (Stipkovits and Kempf, 1996; Cooper and Songer, 2016). MLs are absorbed poorly when given orally. But once absorbed, they can diffuse appreciably in all body fluid except for cerebrospinal fluid (CSF). Because of limited diffusion in CSF, MLs are not effective in bacterial meningitis. However, MLs are concentrated well in leucocytes and can easily be transported to the site of infection in adequate concentration.

Resistance mechanism

Bacteria can acquire resistance to ML and lincosamide in three ways (Weisblum, 1998; Gaynor and Mankin, 2010). Modification of the target (23S ribosomal RNA) is the most primitive one to be detected for ML resistance in staphylococci shortly after the clinical debut of erythromycin in 1953. The modification of 23S rRNA is caused by methylation of adenine nucleotide (A2058 *E. coli* numbering) under the control of the *erm* gene (erythromycin ribosomal methyltransferase) disrupting the bondage with desoamine sugar. Subsequently, *erm* gene was detected in a number of organisms including Gram-positive species, spirochetes and anaerobes conferring resistance to MLs, lincosamides and streptogramin B, collectively known as MLS$_B$ phenotype (Cetin et al., 2008). Nearly 40 *erm* genes have been reported so far and broadly they are classified in four categories — *erm*(A), *erm*(B), *erm*(C) and *erm*(F). While *erm*(A) and *erm*(C) are predominantly detected among *Staphylococcus* sp., *erm*(B) is found in *Streptococcus* and *Enterococcus* sp. The *erm*(F) class is reported in Bacteroides and other anaerobic bacteria. The *erm* gene(s) are carried by plasmid or transposons and hence can be transferred independently. As in case of MRSA, *erm*(A) gene is predominantly carried by transposon *Tn554* (Abbas, 2015), and in methicillin-sensitive isolates (MSSA) plasmid-borne *erm*(C) gene is most frequently detected (Cuny et al., 2013).

Intrinsic resistance to MLs can be mediated by chromosomally encoded active efflux pumps present in GNB (RND) and GPB (ABC — ATP-binding-cassette transporter superfamily and MFS) (Zechini and Versace, 2009; Handzlik et al., 2013). The acquired ML resistance was first reported in *Staphylococcus epidermidis* mediated by plasmid-borne *msr*(A) gene encoding for the efflux pump of the ABC transporter family (Poole, 2012). Later on, *msr*(A) gene has been reported in several staphylococci. Likewise, *mef*(A) gene was reported in *S. pneumoniae, Streptococcus pyogenes* and in other species of streptococci to ensue efflux pump-mediated ML resistance (Del Grosso et al., 2002).

Enzymatic modification of MLs was reported in *Enterobacteriaceae* mediated by enzymes such as esterase and phosphotransferase, although its clinical significance is negligible as MLs are not used against *Enterobacteriaceae*. Nonetheless, such enzymatic inactivation of MLs was reported in few clinical isolates of *S. aureus,* mediated by the gene *mph*(C) (Matsuoka et al., 2003). Likewise, lincosamide nucleotidyltransferases encoded by the genes *lnu*(A) and *lnu*(B) conferring frank resistance to lincomycin were reported in *S. aureus,* coagulase-negative *staphylococci* and *Enterococcus faecium.*

Status in animals

ML resistance is not a new phenomenon in animal or veterinary pathogens. Way back in 1990, ML resistance was reported in *S. aureus* and several CoNS isolates of bovine mastitis from Assam, India (Buragohain and Dutta, 1990). Furthermore, the workers reiterated their observation among *Staphylococcus, Streptococcus* and *Micrococcus* isolates from bovine mastitis (Buragohain and Dutta, 1998). While some European countries recorded ML-resistant *Streptococcus uberis* and *Streptococcus agalactiae* from bovine mastitis (France, Finland and the Netherlands), in countries such as Sweden and Norway, no such resistance towards erythromycin and clindamycin has been reported (Pyörälä et al., 2014). Again erythromycin (and/or pirlimycin) resistance was reported among the CoNS isolates carrying resistance gene(s) such as *erm*(B), *erm*(C), *msr*(A), *mph*(C) and *lnu*(A) from bovine subclinical mastitis in Germany (Lüthje and Schwarz, 2006). Isolates carrying *erm* methylase genes or the exporter gene *msr*(A) showed higher MICs than those harbouring only *mph*(C) or *lnu*(A) genes coding inactivating enzymes indicating target modification or efflux pumps as more potent resistance mediator than inactivating enzymes. Recently, Wipf et al. (2017) reported a novel MLS$_B$ gene *erm*(48) in a plasmid of *Staphylococcus xylosus* isolate from bovine mastitis milk. In addition, the plasmid also carried *mph*(C) and *mrs*(A) genes.

MLs are often advocated for treatment of BRD or bronchopneumonia in small ruminants. Recent studies have indicated ML resistance among *P. multocida* and *M. haemolytica* associated with BRD syndrome (Michael et al., 2012; Desmolaize et al., 2011). ML resistance gene(s) such as rRNA methylase *erm*(42), ML transporter gene *msr*(E) and the ML phosphotransferase *mph*(E) were detected in *P. multocida* isolates (Kadlec et al., 2011). Olsen et al. (2015) also reported the importance of mutation at rRNA methylase causing ML resistance among the BRD pathogens such as *M. haemolytica* and *P. multocida*. Recently Anholt et al. (2017) reported ML resistance among the pathogens associated with BRD such as *M. haemolytica*, *M. bovis*, *P. multocida*, *H. somni* and *T. pyogenes* at an alarming proportion (90.2% of the isolates). ML resistance was also noted among the *P. multocida* isolates associated with swine pneumonia in Taiwan (Yeh et al., 2017). In general, although ML resistance is considered rare among the *P. multocida* and *M. haemolytica* strains from BRD in EU, isolated studies indicated that ML resistance may be as high as 25% in *P. multocida* and 35% in *M. haemolytica*. Likewise, about 17% − 18% of the *H. somni* isolates exhibited nonsusceptibility towards tilmicosin and tulathromycin (Pyörälä et al., 2014). ML resistance mediated by a mutation in the 23S rRNA genes by *erm*(B) and efflux pumps (*mef*(A) and *msr*(D)) was observed among the *Streptococcus suis* isolates from clinically infected human and pigs (Huang et al., 2014). ML resistance was also noted among the *S. epidermidis* and *S. intermedius*, associated with canine pyoderma (Schwarz and Blobel, 1990; Boerlin et al., 2001). The gene(s) *erm*(B) and *vat*(E) genes encoding resistance to streptogramins were detected in one *E. faecium* isolate from dog (Leener et al., 2005).

Detection of macrolide and lincosamide resistance

Detection of inducible clindamycin resistance is an important criterion for determining the therapeutic regimen for *Staphylococcus* especially with regard to macrolide−lincosamide−streptogramin B (MLS$_B$) resistance characteristics. Clindamycin resistance may be inducible or constitutive. Inducible clindamycin-resistant test (or more commonly known as D-test) is conducted to determine the clindamycin sensitivity profile of the erythromycin-resistant *Staphylococcus*, as routine drug sensitivity assay frequently fails to detect inducible clindamycin resistance. This test is done for an erythromycin-resistant *S. aureus* isolate using a clindamycin (2-μg) and an erythromycin (15-μg) disks placed approximately 15 mm apart and flattening of the zone of inhibition around the clindamycin disk proximal to the erythromycin is considered a positive result for inducible clindamycin resistance (positive for 'D-zone test') (Rich et al., 2005). In case of group B *Streptococcus* (*S. agalactiae*), such inducible test can also be employed to determine inducible clindamycin resistance by conducting the assay on Mueller Hinton agar supplemented with 5% defibrinated horse blood using erythromycin and clindamycin disks. As discussed previously, blunting of the clindamycin inhibition zone proximal to the erythromycin disk indicated an inducible type of MLS$_B$ resistance. Susceptibility to clindamycin with no blunting is defined as M phenotype where resistance is possibly mediated by efflux mechanism (De Mouy et al., 2001).

In the case of *Mycoplasma*, such as *M. bovis*, determination of ML or lincosamide susceptibility is difficult to interpret, as there are no CLSI-approved MIC cutoff values for veterinary *Mycoplasma* species. Kong et al. (2016) recommended to use CLSI-approved interpretative criteria for other respiratory bovine pathogens to understand the implication of *M. bovis* sensitivity testing (clindamycin (susceptible, ≤0.5 μg/mL; resistant, ≥4 μg/mL), tulathromycin (susceptible, ≤16 μg/mL; resistant, ≥64 μg/mL), florfenicol (susceptible, ≤2 μg/mL; resistant, ≥8 μg/mL) and MLs (susceptible, ≤16 μg/mL; resistant, ≥64 μg/mL)) (Kong et al., 2016).

As discussed earlier, MLS$_B$ phenotype is a crucial concern for the bacterial pathogens involved in BRD, particularly *M. haemolytica* and *P. multocida*. Rose et al. (2012) reported a multiplex PCR to determine the three types of MLS$_B$ phenotypes for this class of pathogens: (1) Type I phenotype with high resistance to lincosamides and low to moderate resistance to ML and streptogramin B antibiotics is seen in pathogens harbouring *erm* gene. (2) Pathogens with type II phenotype are usually ML-resistant without concomitant lincosamide resistance and they do not possess *erm* gene but *msr*(E) and *mph*(E) encoding a ML efflux pump and a ML-inactivating phosphotransferase, respectively. (3) Type III phenotypes are exhibited by the pathogens which carry all the three gene(s) and are resistant to a comprehensive set of MLs. Details of oligonucleotides and PCR are given in Table 9.3. In addition, other workers made a thorough investigation to establish a correlation between mutation in the domains II and V of the two 23S rRNA alleles and ribosomal proteins L4 and L22 and acquired resistance to MLs such as tylosin and tilmicosin in *M. bovis* (Kong et al., 2016; Lerner et al., 2014). Details are given in Table 9.3. Likewise, Gerchman et al. (2011) also detailed a nested PCR protocol to determine the molecular basis for ML resistance in *M. gallisepticum*.

TABLE 9.3 Oligonucleotides and polymerase chain reaction details for determining resistance to macrolides.

Target	Oligonucleotides	Annealing temperature	Amplicon size	Reference
erm(42)		68°C	173 bp	Rose et al. (2012)
mph(E)	F: ATGCCCAGCATATAAATCGC R: ATATGGACAAAGATAGCCCG		271 bp	
msr(E)	F: TATAGCGACTTTAGCGCCAA R: GCCGTAGAATATGAGCTGAT		395 bp	
rrnA	F: GGATATCTAACGCCGTGTCT R: GTACTGGTCAGCTCAACAC	50°C	5041	(Kong et al., 2016; Lerner et al., 2014)
rrnB	F:GCATGCAAGGTTAAGCAG R: CTAATTCCAAGTGCCACTAGCG	50°C	2848	
L4	F: TTTAGAAAAAAGAAATGAAGACAA R: CTACTCATATTGGCGATCTAGTT	49°C	603	
L22	F:ATGAGTACTCAACAAGCTAAAGCA R: AATGCTATTGATAAATTAGATGTT	49°C	329	

Strategies

MLs are widely used for the treatment of food animals for long. In general, MLs are indicated for the treatment of respiratory and genital infections, foot lesions and mastitis in large ruminants, pneumonia, enteritis and arthritis in pigs and CRD and necrotic enteritis in poultry. The first ML introduced in veterinary use was spiramycin followed by erythromycin and tylosin. MLs are considered as critically important for veterinary medicine (Kirst, 2005). However, there are many issues with regard to ML use in veterinary medicine which needs introspection. Following many of the old recommendation, in-feed MLs are used for a long duration (~5 weeks) just like growth promoter which always increases the possibility of developing resistance. MLs in the form of one-shot therapy such as tilmicosin are also under scanner for such implication. There are also concerns regarding MLs used in combination with other antibiotics (Zaheer et al., 2013). Reports have suggested a strong correlation between the use of ML such as tylosin as a growth promoter in pigs and the development of ML-resistant *Campylobacter* spp. Thus, the practise of using MLs for growth promotion may have a strong bearing over the emergence of ML-resistant bacteria in animals in the long run (Pyörälä et al., 2014). Nevertheless, the use of antibiotics as a growth promoter has been restricted or absolutely banned in different countries. MLs or lincosamides are not absolutely necessary in most of the diseases where alternatives are available except few occasions such as swine dysentery, enzootic pneumonia, mycoplasmal arthritis (in pig) and CRD (in poultry). However, in BRD, MLs are used because of their better tissue penetration and intracellular concentration. However, use of MLs is always preferred than drugs belonging to groups such as fluoroquinolones and extended-spectrum cephalosporins, which are critically important for human despite their efficacy against BRD pathogens.

References

Aarestrup, F.M., 2003. Antimicrobial susceptibility and occurrence of resistance genes among *Salmonella enterica* serovar Weltevreden from different countries. Journal of Antimicrobial Chemotherapy 52, 715−718. https://doi.org/10.1093/jac/dkg426.

Abbas, A., 2015. Prevalence of M LSB resistance and observation of erm A & erm C genes at a tertiary care hospital. Journal of Clinical and Diagnostic Research 9, DC08−DC10. https://doi.org/10.7860/JCDR/2015/13584.6112.

Aghazadeh, M., Hojabri, Z., Mahdian, R., Nahaei, M.R., Rahmati, M., Hojabri, T., et al., 2014. Role of efflux pumps: MexAB-OprM and MexXY(-OprA), AmpC cephalosporinase and OprD porin in non-metallo-β-lactamase producing *Pseudomonas aeruginosa* isolated from cystic fibrosis and burn patients. Infection, Genetics and Evolution 24, 187−192. https://doi.org/10.1016/j.meegid.2014.03.018.

Ahmed, A.M., Younis, E.E.A., Osman, S.A., Ishida, Y., El-khodery, S.A., Shimamoto, T., 2009. Genetic analysis of antimicrobial resistance in *Escherichia coli* isolated from diarrheic neonatal calves. Veterinary Microbiology 136, 397−402. https://doi.org/10.1016/j.vetmic.2008.11.021.

Ahmed, S., Hossain, M.I., Hossan, T., Islam, K.M.R., Uddin, B., Rahman, M.B., et al., 2013. The central cattle Breeding and Dairy Farm, Bangladesh waste contributes in emergence and spread of aminoglycoside-resistant bacteria. Advances in Bioscience and Biotechnology 4, 278−282. https://doi.org/10.4236/abb.2013.42A038.

Al-Bahry, S., Al-Sharji, N., Yaish, M., Al-Musharafi, S., Mahmoud, I., 2016. Diversity of tetracycline resistant genes in *Escherichia coli* from human and environmental sources. The Open Biotechnology Journal 10, 289–300. https://doi.org/10.2174/1874070701610010289.

Alekshun, M.N., Levy, S.B., 2007. Molecular mechanisms of antibacterial multidrug resistance. Cell 128, 1037–1050. https://doi.org/10.1016/j.cell.2007.03.004.

Anes, J., McCusker, M.P., Fanning, S., Martins, M., 2015. The ins and outs of RND efflux pumps in *Escherichia coli*. Frontiers in Microbiology 6. https://doi.org/10.3389/fmicb.2015.00587.

Anholt, R.M., Klima, C., Allan, N., Matheson-Bird, H., Schatz, C., Ajitkumar, P., et al., 2017. Antimicrobial susceptibility of bacteria that cause bovine respiratory disease complex in Alberta, Canada. Frontiers in Veterinary Science 4. https://doi.org/10.3389/fvets.2017.00207.

Bandyopadhyay, S., Samanta, I., Bhattacharyya, D., Nanda, P.K., Kar, D., Chowdhury, J., et al., 2015. Co-infection of methicillin-resistant *Staphylococcus epidermidis*, methicillin-resistant *Staphylococcus aureus* and extended spectrum β -lactamase producing *Escherichia coli* in bovine mastitis — three cases reported from India. Veterinary Quarterly 35, 56–61. https://doi.org/10.1080/01652176.2014.984365.

Bandyopadhyay, S., Banerjee, J., Bhattacharyya, D., Samanta, I., Mahanti, A., Dutta, T.K., et al., 2018. Genomic identity of fluoroquinolone-resistant bla CTX-M -15 -type ESBL and pMAmpC β-lactamase producing *Klebsiella pneumoniae* from Buffalo Milk, India. Microbial Drug Resistance 24, 1345–1353. https://doi.org/10.1089/mdr.2017.0368.

Barclay, M.L., Begg, E.J., Chambers, S.T., Thornley, P.E., Pattemore, P.K., Grimwood, K., 1996. Adaptive resistance to tobramycin in *Pseudomonas aeruginosa* lung infection in cystic fibrosis. Journal of Antimicrobial Chemotherapy 37, 1155–1164. https://doi.org/10.1093/jac/37.6.1155.

Belaynehe, K.M., Shin, S.W., Hong-Tae, P., Yoo, H.S., 2017. Occurrence of aminoglycoside-modifying enzymes among isolates of *Escherichia coli* exhibiting high levels of aminoglycoside resistance isolated from Korean cattle farms. FEMS Microbiology Letters 364. https://doi.org/10.1093/femsle/fnx129.

Biswas, L., Biswas, R., Schlag, M., Bertram, R., Gotz, F., 2009. Small-colony variant selection as a survival strategy for *Staphylococcus aureus* in the presence of *Pseudomonas aeruginosa*. Applied and Environmental Microbiology 75, 6910–6912. https://doi.org/10.1128/AEM.01211-09.

Blanco, P., Hernando-Amado, S., Reales-Calderon, J.A., Corona, F., Lira, F., Alcalde-Rico, M., et al., 2016. Bacterial multidrug efflux pumps: much more than antibiotic resistance determinants. Microorganisms 4. https://doi.org/10.3390/microorganisms4010014.

Boerlin, P., Burnens, A.P., Frey, J., Kuhnert, P., Nicolet, J., 2001. Molecular epidemiology and genetic linkage of macrolide and aminoglycoside resistance in *Staphylococcus intermedius* of canine origin. Veterinary Microbiology 79, 155–169. https://doi.org/10.1016/S0378-1135(00)00347-3.

Bryan, A., Shapir, N., Sadowsky, M.J., 2004. Frequency and distribution of tetracycline resistance genes in genetically diverse, nonselected, and nonclinical *Escherichia coli* strains isolated from diverse human and animal sources. Applied and Environmental Microbiology 70, 2503–2507. https://doi.org/10.1128/AEM.70.4.2503-2507.2004.

Buragohain, J., Dutta, G.N., 1990. A new type of macrolide resistance in staphylococci from bovine subclinical mastitis. Research in Veterinary Science 49, 248–249.

Buragohain, J., Dutta, G.N., 1998. Antibiotic resistance patterns among isolates from bovine mammary origin. Indian Journal of Comparative Microbiology, Immunology and Infectious Diseases 19, 110–113.

Cameron, F.H., Groot Obbink, D.J., Ackerman, V.P., Hall, R.M., 1986. Nucleotide sequence of the AAD(2′) aminoglycoside adenylyltransferase determinant aadB. Evolutionary relationship of this region with those surrounding aadA in R538-1 and dhfrII in R388. Nucleic Acids Research 14, 8625–8635. https://doi.org/10.1093/nar/14.21.8625.

Cetin, E.S., Gunes, H., Kaya, S., Aridogan, B.C., Demirci, M., 2008. Macrolide—lincosamide—streptogramin B resistance phenotypes in clinical staphylococcal isolates. International Journal of Antimicrobial Agents 31, 364–368. https://doi.org/10.1016/j.ijantimicag.2007.11.014.

Chopra, I., Roberts, M., 2001. Tetracycline antibiotics: mode of action, applications, molecular Biology, and epidemiology of bacterial resistance. Microbiology and Molecular Biology Reviews 65, 232–260. https://doi.org/10.1128/MMBR.65.2.232-260.2001.

Chuanchuen, R., Wannaprasat, W., Ajariyakhajorn, K., Schweizer, H.P., 2008. Role of the MexXY multidrug efflux pump in moderate aminoglycoside resistance in *Pseudomonas aeruginosa* isolates from *Pseudomonas mastitis*. Microbiology and Immunology 52, 392–398. https://doi.org/10.1111/j.1348-0421.2008.00051.x.

Connell, S.R., Tracz, D.M., Nierhaus, K.H., Taylor, D.E., 2003. Ribosomal protection proteins and their mechanism of tetracycline resistance. Antimicrobial Agents and Chemotherapy 47, 3675–3681.

Cooper, K.K., Songer, J.G., 2016. Necrotic enteritis of poultry. Clostridial Diseases of Animals 123–137. https://doi.org/10.1002/9781118728291.ch10.

Cuny, C., Layer, F., Köck, R., Werner, G., Witte, W., 2013. Methicillin susceptible *Staphylococcus aureus* (MSSA) of clonal complex CC398, t571 from infections in humans are still rare in Germany. PLoS One 8, e83165. https://doi.org/10.1371/journal.pone.0083165.

De Mouy, D., Cavallo, J.D., Leclercq, R., Fabre, R., 2001. Antibiotic susceptibility and mechanisms of erythromycin resistance in clinical isolates of *Streptococcus agalactiae*: French multicenter study. Antimicrobial Agents and Chemotherapy 45, 2400–2402. https://doi.org/10.1128/AAC.45.8.2400-2402.2001.

Del Grosso, M., Iannelli, F., Messina, C., Santagati, M., Petrosillo, N., Stefani, S., et al., 2002. Macrolide efflux genes mef(A) and mef(E) are carried by different genetic elements in *Streptococcus pneumoniae*. Journal of Clinical Microbiology 40, 774–778. https://doi.org/10.1128/JCM.40.3.774-778.2002.

Desmolaize, B., Rose, S., Wilhelm, C., Warrass, R., Douthwaite, S., 2011. Combinations of macrolide resistance determinants in field isolates of *Mannheimia haemolytica* and *Pasteurella multocida*. Antimicrobial Agents and Chemotherapy 55, 4128–4133. https://doi.org/10.1128/AAC.00450-11.

Dinos, G.P., 2017. The macrolide antibiotic renaissance. British Journal of Pharmacology 174, 2967–2983. https://doi.org/10.1111/bph.13936.

Doi, Y., Arakawa, Y., 2007. 16S ribosomal RNA methylation: emerging resistance mechanism against aminoglycosides. Clinical Infectious Diseases 45, 88−94. https://doi.org/10.1086/518605.

Dong, W.-L., Kong, L.-C., Wang, Y., Gou, C.-L., Xu, B., Ma, H.-X., et al., 2017. Aminoglycoside resistance of *Trueperella pyogenes* isolated from pigs in China. Journal of Veterinary Medical Science 79, 1836−1839. https://doi.org/10.1292/jvms.16-0597.

Doosti, A., Mahmoudi, E., Jami, M.S., Mokhtari-Farsani, A., 2016. Prevalence of aadA1, aadA2, aadB, strA and strB genes and their associations with multidrug resistance phenotype in *Salmonella typhimurium* isolated from poultry carcasses. The Thai Journal of Veterinary Medicine 46, 691−697.

Galimand, M., Sabtcheva, S., Courvalin, P., Lambert, T., 2005. Worldwide disseminated armA aminoglycoside resistance methylase gene is borne by composite transposon Tn1548. Antimicrobial Agents and Chemotherapy 49, 2949−2953. https://doi.org/10.1128/AAC.49.7.2949-2953.2005.

Gaynor, M., Mankin, A.S., 2010. Macrolide antibiotics: binding site, mechanism of action, resistance. Frontiers in Medicinal Chemistry 2, 21−35. https://doi.org/10.2174/978160805205910502010021.

Gerchman, I., Levisohn, S., Mikula, I., Manso-Silván, L., Lysnyansky, I., 2011. Characterization of in vivo-acquired resistance to macrolides of *Mycoplasma gallisepticum* strains isolated from poultry. Veterinary Research 42. https://doi.org/10.1186/1297-9716-42-90.

Gerrits, M.M., Berning, M., Van Vliet, A.H.M., Kuipers, E.J., Kusters, J.G., 2003. Effects of 16S rRNA gene mutations on tetracycline resistance in *Helicobacter pylori*. Antimicrobial Agents and Chemotherapy 47, 2984−2986. https://doi.org/10.1128/AAC.47.9.2984-2986.2003.

Gilleland, L.B., Gilleland, H.E., Gibson, J.A., Champlin, F.R., 1989. Adaptive resistance to aminoglycosides antibiotics in *Pseudomonas aeruginosa*. Journal of Medical Microbiology 29, 41−50. https://doi.org/10.1099/00222615-29-1-41.

Gowda, T., C., L., B., S., Van Damme, I., 2017. Occurrence and antibiotic susceptibility of *Listeria* species and *Staphylococcus aureus* in cattle slaughterhouses of Kerala, South India. Foodborne Pathogens and Disease 14, 573−579. https://doi.org/10.1089/fpd.2017.2293.

Grossman, T.H., 2016. Tetracycline antibiotics and resistance. Cold Spring Harbor Perspectives in Medicine 6, a025387. https://doi.org/10.1101/cshperspect.a025387.

Guénard, S., Muller, C., Monlezun, L., Benas, P., Broutin, I., Jeannot, K., et al., 2014. Multiple mutations lead to MexXY-OprM-dependent aminoglycoside resistance in clinical strains of *Pseudomonas aeruginosa*. Antimicrobial Agents and Chemotherapy 58, 221−228. https://doi.org/10.1128/AAC.01252-13.

Handzlik, J., Matys, A., Kieć-Kononowicz, K., 2013. Recent advances in Multi-Drug Resistance (MDR) efflux pump inhibitors of gram-positive bacteria *S. aureus*. Antibiotics 2, 28−45. https://doi.org/10.3390/antibiotics2010028.

Hansmann, Y., 2009. Treatment and prevention of lyme disease. Current Problems in Dermatology 37, 111−129. https://doi.org/10.1159/000213071.

Hedayatianfard, K., Akhlaghi, M., Sharifiyazdi, H., 2014. Detection of tetracycline resistance genes in bacteria isolated from fish farms using polymerase chain reaction. Veterinary Research Forum 5, 269−275.

Huang, J., Li, Y., Shang, K., Kashif, J., Qian, X., Wang, L., 2014. Efflux pump, methylation and mutations in the 23S rRNA genes contributing to the development of macrolide resistance in *Streptococcus suis* isolated from infected human and swine in China. Pakistan Veterinary Journal 34, 82−86. https://doi.org/10.1542/peds.110.6.1255.

Jackson, C.R., Davis, J.A., Frye, J.G., Barrett, J.B., Hiott, L.M., 2015. Diversity of plasmids and antimicrobial resistance genes in multidrug-resistant *Escherichia coli* isolated from healthy companion animals. Zoonoses *and* Public Health 62, 479−488. https://doi.org/10.1111/zph.12178.

Jo, J.T.H., Brinkman, F.S.L., Hancock, R.E.W., 2003. Aminoglycoside efflux in *Pseudomonas aeruginosa*: involvement of novel outer membrane proteins. Antimicrobial Agents and Chemotherapy 47, 1101−1111. https://doi.org/10.1128/AAC.47.3.1101-1111.2003.

Johnson, A.P., Burns, L., Woodford, N., Threlfall, E.J., Naidoo, J., Cooke, E.M., et al., 1994. Gentamicin resistance in clinical isolates of *Escherichia coli* encoded by genes of veterinary origin. Journal of Medical Microbiology 40, 221−226. https://doi.org/10.1099/00222615-40-3-221.

Kadlec, K., Michael, G.B., Sweeney, M.T., Brzuszkiewicz, E., Liesegang, H., Daniel, R., et al., 2011. Molecular basis of macrolide, triamilide, and lincosamide resistance in *Pasteurella multocida* from bovine respiratory disease. Antimicrobial Agents and Chemotherapy 55, 2475−2477. https://doi.org/10.1128/AAC.00092-11.

Kamionka, A., Sehnal, M., Scholz, O., Hillen, W., 2004. Independent regulation of two genes in *Escherichia coli* by tetracyclines and tet repressor variants. Journal of Bacteriology 186, 4399−4401. https://doi.org/10.1128/JB.186.13.4399-4401.2004.

Khan, J.A., Rathore, R.S., Abulreesh, H.H., Qais, F.A., Ahmad, I., 2018. Prevalence and antibiotic resistance profiles of *Campylobacter jejuni* isolated from poultry meat and related samples at retail shops in northern India. Foodbourne Pathogens and Disease 15, 218−225. https://doi.org/10.1089/fpd.2017.2344.

Kirst, H.A., 2005. Macrolide antibiotics in food-animal health. Expert Opinion on Investigational Drugs 6, 103−118. https://doi.org/10.1517/13543784.6.2.103.

Kogure, T., Shimada, R., Ishikawa, J., Yazawa, K., Brown, J.M., Mikami, Y., et al., 2010. Homozygous triplicate mutations in three 16S rRNA genes responsible for high-level aminoglycoside resistance in *Nocardia farcinica* clinical isolates from a Canada-wide bovine mastitis epizootic. Antimicrobial Agents and Chemotherapy 54, 2385−2390. https://doi.org/10.1128/AAC.00021-10.

Kondo, S., Hotta, K., 1999. Semisynthetic aminoglycoside antibiotics: development and enzymatic modifications. Journal of Infection and Chemotherapy 5, 1−9. https://doi.org/10.1007/s101560050001.

Kong, L.-C., Gao, D., Jia, B.-Y., Wang, Z., Gao, Y.-H., Pei, Z.-H., et al., 2016. Antimicrobial susceptibility and molecular characterization of macrolide resistance of *Mycoplasma bovis* isolates from multiple provinces in China. Journal of Veterinary Medical Science 78, 293−296. https://doi.org/10.1292/jvms.15-0304.

Krause, K.M., Serio, A.W., Kane, T.R., Connolly, L.E., 2016. Aminoglycosides: an overview. Cold Spring Harbor Perspectives in Medicine 6, a027029. https://doi.org/10.1101/cshperspect.a027029.

Kyselkov, M., Jirout, J., Vrchotov, N., Schmitt, H., Elhottov, D., 2015. Spread of tetracycline resistance genes at a conventional dairy farm. Frontiers in Microbiology 6. https://doi.org/10.3389/fmicb.2015.00536.

Labby, K.J., Garneau-Tsodikova, S., 2013. Strategies to overcome the action of aminoglycoside-modifying enzymes for treating resistant bacterial infections. Future Medicinal Chemistry 5, 1285−1309. https://doi.org/10.4155/fmc.13.80.

Lan, Y.F., Li, K., Zhang, H., Huang, S.C., Rehman, M.U., Zhang, L.H., et al., 2016. Prevalence of high-level aminoglycoside resistant *Enterococci* isolated from Tibetan pigs. Pakistan Veterinary Journal 36, 503−505.

Leener, E De, Decostere, A., De Graef, E.M., Moyaert, H., Haesebrouck, F., 2005. Presence and mechanism of antimicrobial resistance among *Enterococci* from cats and dogs. Microbial Drug Resistance 11, 395−403. https://doi.org/10.1089/mdr.2005.11.395.

Lerner, U., Amram, E., Ayling, R.D., Mikula, I., Gerchman, I., Harrus, S., et al., 2014. Acquired resistance to the 16-membered macrolides tylosin and tilmicosin by mycoplasma bovis. Veterinary Microbiology 168, 365−371. https://doi.org/10.1016/j.vetmic.2013.11.033.

Li, W., Atkinson, G.C., Thakor, N.S., Allas, Ü., Lu, C., Chan, K.-Y., et al., 2013. Mechanism of tetracycline resistance by ribosomal protection protein Tet(O). Nature Communications 4, 1477. https://doi.org/10.1038/ncomms2470.

Lioy, V.S., Goussard, S., Guerineau, V., Yoon, E.-J., Courvalin, P., Galimand, M., et al., 2014. Aminoglycoside resistance 16S rRNA methyltransferases block endogenous methylation, affect translation efficiency and fitness of the host. RNA 20, 382−391. https://doi.org/10.1261/rna.042572.113.

Lüthje, P., Schwarz, S., 2006. Antimicrobial resistance of coagulase-negative staphylococci from bovine subclinical mastitis with particular reference to macrolide-lincosamide resistance phenotypes and genotypes. Journal of Antimicrobial Chemotherapy 57, 966−969. https://doi.org/10.1093/jac/dkl061.

Markley, J.L., Wencewicz, T.A., 2018. Tetracycline-inactivating enzymes. Frontiers in Microbiology 9. https://doi.org/10.3389/fmicb.2018.01058.

Matsuoka, M., Inoue, M., Endo, Y., Nakajima, Y., 2003. Characteristic expression of three genes, msr (A), mph (C) and erm (Y), that confer resistance to macrolide antibiotics on *Staphylococcus aureus*. FEMS Microbiology Letters 220, 287−293. https://doi.org/10.1016/S0378-1097(03)00134-4.

Maynard, C., Fairbrother, J.M., Bekal, S., Sanschagrin, F., Levesque, R.C., Brousseau, R., et al., 2003. Antimicrobial resistance genes in enterotoxigenic *Escherichia coli* O149:K91 isolates obtained over a 23-year period from pigs. Antimicrobial Agents and Chemotherapy 47, 3214−3221. https://doi.org/10.1128/AAC.47.10.3214-3221.2003.

Maynard, C., Bekal, S., Sanschagrin, F., Levesque, R.C., Brousseau, R., Masson, L., et al., 2004. Heterogeneity among virulence and antimicrobial resistance gene profiles of extraintestinal *Escherichia coli* isolates of animal and human origin. Journal of Clinical Microbiology 42, 5444−5452. https://doi.org/10.1128/JCM.42.12.5444-5452.2004.

Melano, R., 2003. Multiple antibiotic-resistance mechanisms including a novel combination of extended-spectrum -lactamases in a *Klebsiella pneumoniae* clinical strain isolated in Argentina. Journal of Antimicrobial Chemotherapy 52, 36−42. https://doi.org/10.1093/jac/dkg281.

Michael, G.B., Eidam, C., Kadlec, K., Meyer, K., Sweeney, M.T., Murray, R.W., et al., 2012. Increased MICs of gamithromycin and tildipirosin in the presence of the genes erm(42) and msr(E)-mph(E) for bovine *Pasteurella multocida* and *Mannheimia haemolytica*. Journal of Antimicrobial Chemotherapy 67, 1555−1557. https://doi.org/10.1093/jac/dks076.

Mima, T., Schweizer, H.P., 2010. The BpeAB-OprB efflux pump of *Burkholderia pseudomallei* 1026b does not play a role in quorum sensing, virulence factor production, or extrusion of aminoglycosides but is a broad-spectrum drug efflux system. Antimicrobial Agents and Chemotherapy 54, 3113−3120. https://doi.org/10.1128/AAC.01803-09.

Moore, R.A., Deshazer, D., Reckseidler, S., Weissman, A., Woods, D.E., 1999. Efflux-mediated aminoglycoside and macrolide resistance in *Burkholderia pseudomallei*. Antimicrobial Agents and Chemotherapy 43, 465−470.

Morita, Y., Tomida, J., Kawamura, Y., 2012. MexXY multidrug efflux system of *Pseudomonas aeruginosa*. Frontiers in Microbiology 3. https://doi.org/10.3389/fmicb.2012.00408.

Ng, L.-K., Martin, I., Alfa, M., Mulvey, M., 2001. Multiplex PCR for the detection of tetracycline resistant genes. Molecular and Cellular Probes 15, 209−215. https://doi.org/10.1006/mcpr.2001.0363.

Nguyen, F., Starosta, A.L., Arenz, S., Sohmen, D., Dönhöfer, A., Wilson, D.N., 2014. Tetracycline antibiotics and resistance mechanisms. Biological Chemistry 395, 559−575. https://doi.org/10.1515/hsz-2013-0292.

Oka, A., Sugisaki, H., Takanami, M., 1981. Nucleotide sequence of the kanamycin resistance transposon Tn903. Journal of Molecular Biology 147, 217−226. https://doi.org/10.1016/0022-2836(81)90438-1.

Olsen, A.S., Warrass, R., Douthwaite, S., 2015. Macrolide resistance conferred by rrna mutations in field isolates of *Mannheimia haemolytica* and *Pasteurella multocida*. Journal of Antimicrobial Chemotherapy 70, 420−423. https://doi.org/10.1093/jac/dku385.

Ouoba, L.I.I., Lei, V., Jensen, L.B., 2008. Resistance of potential probiotic lactic acid bacteria and bifidobacteria of African and European origin to antimicrobials: determination and transferability of the resistance genes to other bacteria. International Journal of Food Microbiology 121, 217−224. https://doi.org/10.1016/j.ijfoodmicro.2007.11.018.

Pang, Z., Raudonis, R., Glick, B.R., Lin, T.-J., Cheng, Z., 2019. Antibiotic resistance in *Pseudomonas aeruginosa*: mechanisms and alternative therapeutic strategies. Biotechnology Advances 37, 177−192. https://doi.org/10.1016/j.biotechadv.2018.11.013.

Poole, K., 2005. Aminoglycoside resistance in *Pseudomonas aeruginosa*. Antimicrobial Agents and Chemotherapy 49, 479−487. https://doi.org/10.1128/AAC.49.2.479-487.2005.

Poole, K., 2012. Efflux-Mediated Antimicrobial Resistance. Antibiot. Discov. Dev. Springer US, Boston, MA, pp. 349−395. https://doi.org/10.1007/978-1-4614-1400-1_10.

Pyörälä, S., Baptiste, K.E., Catry, B., van Duijkeren, E., Greko, C., Moreno, M.A., et al., 2014. Macrolides and lincosamides in cattle and pigs: use and development of antimicrobial resistance. The Veterinary Journal 200, 230−239. https://doi.org/10.1016/j.tvjl.2014.02.028.

Rahmani, M., Peighambari, S.M., Svendsen, C.A., Cavaco, L.M., Agersø, Y., Hendriksen, R.S., 2013. Molecular clonality and antimicrobial resistance in *Salmonella enterica* serovars *Enteritidis* and *Infantis* from broilers in three Northern regions of Iran. BMC Veterinary Research 9. https://doi.org/10.1186/1746-6148-9-66.

Ramirez, M., Tolmasky, M., 2017. Amikacin: uses, resistance, and prospects for inhibition. Molecules 22, 2267. https://doi.org/10.3390/molecules22122267.

Rich, M., Deighton, L., Roberts, L., 2005. Clindamycin-resistance in methicillin-resistant *Staphylococcus aureus* isolated from animals. Veterinary Microbiology 111, 237–240. https://doi.org/10.1016/j.vetmic.2005.09.011.

Roberts, M.C., 1996. Tetracycline resistance determinants: mechanisms of action, regulation of expression, genetic mobility, and distribution. FEMS Microbiology Reviews 19, 1–24. https://doi.org/10.1016/0168-6445(96)00021-6.

Rodriguez, M.B., Costa, S.O.P., 1999. Spontaneous kanamycin-resistant *Escherichia coli* mutant with altered periplasmic oligopeptide permease protein (OppA) and impermeability to aminoglycosides. Revista De Microbiologia 30, 153–156. https://doi.org/10.1590/S0001-37141999000200013.

Rose, S., Desmolaize, B., Jaju, P., Wilhelm, C., Warrass, R., Douthwaite, S., 2012. Multiplex PCR to identify macrolide resistance determinants in *Mannheimia haemolytica* and *Pasteurella multocida*. Antimicrobial Agents and Chemotherapy 56, 3664–3669. https://doi.org/10.1128/AAC.00266-12.

Rosenberg, E.Y., Ma, D., Nikaido, H., 2000. AcrD of *Escherichia coli* is an aminoglycoside efflux pump. Journal of Bacteriology 182, 1754–1756. https://doi.org/10.1128/JB.182.6.1754-1756.2000.

Scholz, P., Haring, V., Wittmann-Liebold, B., Ashman, K., Bagdasarian, M., Scherzinger, E., 1989. Complete nucleotide sequence and gene organization of the broad-host-range plasmid RSF1010. Gene 75, 271–288. https://doi.org/10.1016/0378-1119(89)90273-4.

Schwarz, S., Blobel, H., 1990. Isolation of a plasmid from 'canine' *Staphylococcus epidermidis* mediating constitutive resistance to macrolides and lincosamides. Comparative Immunology, Microbiology and Infectious Diseases 13, 209–216. https://doi.org/10.1016/0147-9571(90)90090-G.

Schwarz, S., Roberts, M.C., Werckenthin, C., Pang, Y., Lange, C., 1998. Tetracycline resistance in *Staphylococcus* spp. from domestic animals. Veterinary Microbiology 63, 217–227.

Serpersu, E.H., Ozen, C., Wright, E., 2008. Studies of enzymes that cause resistance to aminoglycosides antibiotics. Methods in Molecular Medicine 142, 261–271. https://doi.org/10.1007/978-1-59745-246-5_20.

Shin, S.W., Shin, M.K., Jung, M., Belaynehe, K.M., Yoo, H.S., 2015. Prevalence of antimicrobial resistance and transfer of tetracycline resistance genes in *Escherichia coli* isolates from beef cattle. Applied and Environmental Microbiology 81, 5560–5566. https://doi.org/10.1128/AEM.01511-15.

Silva, AP da, Schmidt, C., Vargas, AC de, Maboni, G., Rampelotto, C., Schwab, M.L., et al., 2014. Antimicrobial susceptibility of *Staphylococcus* spp. isolated from canine superficial pyoderma. Pesquisa Veterinária Brasileira 34, 355–361.

Smith, C.A., Baker, E.N., 2005. Aminoglycoside antibiotic resistance by enzymatic deactivation. Current Drug Targets - Infectious Disorders 2, 143–160. https://doi.org/10.2174/1568005023342533.

Stipkovits, L., Kempf, I., 1996. Mycoplasmoses in poultry. Science and Technology Review 15, 1495–1525. https://doi.org/10.20506/rst.15.4.986.

Taylor, D.E., Jerome, L.J., Grewal, J., Chang, N., 2009. Tet(O), a protein that mediates ribosomal protection to tetracycline, binds, and hydrolyses GTP. Canadian Journal of Microbiology 41, 965–970. https://doi.org/10.1139/m95-134.

Tschudin-Sutter, S., Fosse, N., Frei, R., Widmer, A.F., 2018. Combination therapy for treatment of *Pseudomonas aeruginosa* bloodstream infections. PLoS One 13. https://doi.org/10.1371/journal.pone.0203295.

Turutoglu, H., Hasoksuz, M., Ozturk, D., Yildirim, M., Sagnak, S., 2009. Methicillin and aminoglycoside resistance in *Staphylococcus aureus* isolates from bovine mastitis and sequence analysis of their mecA genes. Veterinary Research Communications 33, 945–956. https://doi.org/10.1007/s11259-009-9313-5.

Urumova, V., Lyutskanov, M., Petrov, V., 2015. Investigations on the resistance of commensal swine Escherichia coli to some Aminoglycosides-Aminocyclitols. Arhiv Veterinarske Medicine 8 (1), 13–26.

Vakulenko, S.B., Mobashery, S., 2003. Versatility of aminoglycosides and prospects for their future. Clinical Microbiology Reviews 16, 430–450. https://doi.org/10.1128/CMR.16.3.430-450.2003.

van Duijkeren, E., Schwarz, C., Bouchard, D., Catry, B., Pomba, C., Baptiste, K.E., et al., 2019. The use of aminoglycosides in animals within the EU: development of resistance in animals and possible impact on human and animal health: a review. Journal of Antimicrobial Chemotherapy. https://doi.org/10.1093/jac/dkz161.

Vliegenthart, J.S., Ketelaar-van Gaalen, P.A., van de Klundert, J.A., 1989. Nucleotide sequence of the aacC2 gene, a gentamicin resistance determinant involved in a hospital epidemic of multiply resistant members of the family *Enterobacteriaceae*. Antimicrobial Agents and Chemotherapy 33, 1153–1159. https://doi.org/10.1128/AAC.33.8.1153.

Wagner, M., Loy, A., Report, P.A., Board, M.E., Ptc, A.G., Meka, V.G., et al., 2014. Bioresource technology removal of pharmaceuticals in microcosm constructed wetlands using *Typha* spp. and LECA. Environment International 40, 42–51. https://doi.org/10.1007/s00216-015-9075-6.

Wei, D.-D., Wan, L.-G., Yu, Y., Xu, Q.-F., Deng, Q., Cao, X.-W., et al., 2014. Characterization of extended-spectrum beta-lactamase, carbapenemase, and plasmid quinolone determinants in *Klebsiella pneumoniae* isolates carrying distinct types of 16S rRNA methylase genes, and their association with mobile genetic elements. Microbial Drug Resistance 21, 186–193. https://doi.org/10.1089/mdr.2014.0073.

Weisblum, B., 1998. Macrolide resistance. Drug Resistance Updates 1, 29–41. https://doi.org/10.1016/S1368-7646(98)80212-4.

Wipf, J.R.K., Riley, M.C., Kania, S.A., Bemis, D.A., Andreis, S., Schwendener, S., et al., 2017. New macrolide-lincosamide-streptogramin B resistance gene erm (48) on the novel plasmid pJW2311 in *Staphylococcus xylosus*. Antimicrobial Agents and Chemotherapy 61. https://doi.org/10.1128/AAC.00066-17.

Yamane, K., Wachino, J.I., Suzuki, S., Shibata, N., Kato, H., Shibayama, K., et al., 2007. 16S rRNA methylase-producing, gram-negative pathogens, Japan. Emerging Infectious Diseases 13, 642–646. https://doi.org/10.3201/eid1304.060501.

Yaǧci, B.B., Ural, K., Öcal, N., Haydardedeoǧlu, A.E., 2008. Azithromycin therapy of papillomatosis in dogs: a prospective, randomized, double-blinded, placebo-controlled clinical trial. Veterinary Dermatology 19, 194−198. https://doi.org/10.1111/j.1365-3164.2008.00674.x.

Yeh, J.-C., Lo, D.-Y., Chang, S.-K., Chou, C.-C., Kuo, H.-C., 2017. Antimicrobial susceptibility, serotypes and genotypes of *Pasteurella multocida* isolates associated with swine pneumonia in Taiwan. The Veterinary Record 181, 323. https://doi.org/10.1136/vr.104023.

YuanTing, Z., HaiMei, L., LiKou, Z., Sheng, Y., ChengTao, W., XinFeng, H., et al., 2017. Antimicrobial resistance and resistance genes in *Salmonella* strains isolated from broiler chickens along the slaughtering process in China. International Journal of Food Microbiology 259, 43−51. https://doi.org/10.1016/j.ijfoodmicro.2017.07.023.

Zacharczuk, K., Piekarska, K., Szych, J., Jagielski, M., Hidalgo, L., Millán, Á.S., et al., 2011. Plasmid-borne 16s rRNA methylase ArmA in aminoglycoside-resistant *Klebsiella pneumoniae* in Poland. Journal of Medical Microbiology 60, 1306−1311. https://doi.org/10.1099/jmm.0.024026-0.

Zaheer, R., Cook, S.R., Klima, C.L., Stanford, K., Alexander, T., Topp, E., et al., 2013. Effect of subtherapeutic vs. therapeutic administration of macrolides on antimicrobial resistance in *Mannheimia haemolytica* and *Enterococci* isolated from beef cattle. Frontiers in Microbiology 4. https://doi.org/10.3389/fmicb.2013.00133.

Zechini, B., Versace, I., 2009. Inhibitors of multidrug resistant efflux systems in bacteria. Recent Patents on Anti-Infective Drug Discovery 4, 37−50. https://doi.org/10.2174/157489109787236256.

Zehra, A., Singh, R., Kaur, S., Gill, J.P.S., 2017. Molecular characterization of antibiotic-resistant *Staphylococcus aureus* from livestock (bovine and swine). Veterinary World 10, 598−604. https://doi.org/10.14202/vetworld.2017.598-604.

Zhang, T., Wang, C.G., Jiang, G.E., Lv, J.C., Zhong, X.H., 2012. Molecular epidemiological survey on aminoglycoside antibiotics-resistant genotype and phenotype of avian *Escherichia coli* in North China. Poultry Science 91, 2482−2486. https://doi.org/10.3382/ps.2012-02400.

Zygner, W., Jaros, D., GojskaZygner, O., Wedrychowicz, H., Gojska-Zygner, O., 2008. Azithromycin in the treatment of a dog infected with giardia intestinalis. Polish Journal of Veterinary Sciences 11, 231−234.

Chapter 10

Colistin resistance

Chapter outline

Overview

Colistin belongs to a class of antibiotic more commonly referred as polymyxins (Loho and Dharmayanti, 2015). Polymyxins encompass different class of compound of which polymyxins B and E (colistin) are used as antibiotic. They contain cyclic nonprotein polypeptide chains and fall under peptide antibiotic like many other antimicrobial and antitumour compounds such as actinomycin and bacitracin.

Colistin is synthesized from certain strains of Gram-positive nitrogen-fixing bacteria, *Paenibacillus polymyxa* (also known as *Bacillus polymyxa*). It is a decade-old drug and used in clinical practices since 1950s. In 1949 it was first isolated from a fermenting strain of bacteria in Japan (*B. polymyxa* subspecies *colistinus* Koyama). Both colistin and polymyxin B are the secondary metabolite of nonribosomal protein of these bacteria. Since 1959 with the advent of colistimethate sodium (CMS), a much less toxic and inactive form of the drug, injectable colistin became available for treatment of many infectious diseases caused by Gram-negative bacteria (GNB) in Japan, Europe and the United States. Following parental administration, CMS is converted to colistin to exhibit antibacterial activity (Biswas et al., 2012; Dijkmans et al., 2015).

However, with introduction of aminoglycosides, the use of colistin was considerably reduced and fell out of favour during 1980s because of nephrotoxicity (Falagas and Rafailidis, 2009) and neurotoxicity of the drug (Loho and Dharmayanti, 2015; Velkov et al., 2018; Kelesidis and Falagas, 2015). With the emergence of multidrug-resistant bacteria and long void in discovery of novel antibiotics, colistin is again getting popularity for treatment of refractory infection caused by multiple drug–resistant pathogens since early 1990s (Jacobs et al., 2017; Karaiskos et al., 2017; Paul et al., 2018; Wang et al., 2018a). Colistin based combination treatments were found effective for the infections caused by carbapenemase-producing strains (Paul et al., 2018; Wang et al., 2018a; Balkan et al., 2014).

Colistin exhibits the antibacterial property by acting on the bacterial cell membrane. It is a polycationic peptide having both the hydrophilic and hydrophobic moieties. It binds with the lipopolysaccharides (LPS) and phospholipid of the bacterial outer cell membrane and competitively dislodges the divalent cations such as calcium and magnesium (Ca^{2+} and Mg^{2+}) from the phosphate group of LPS. Divalent cations are important to stabilize the negatively charged component of LPS. This ultimately leads to leakage of cell membrane, complete disruption of the cell membrane and cellular structural integrity. There is complete loss of essential ingredients from cellular environment ultimately leading to cell death. In addition, colistin binds with the lipid A moiety of LPS and thus neutralizes the LPS. It substantially reduces the chances of sepsis owing to endotoxin.

Colistin resistance mechanism

Bacteria resort to several mechanisms to get resistant to colistin. Many GNB are naturally and intrinsically resistant to polymyxin or colistin. Among them important are *Serratia* spp., *Edwardsiella tarda* and *Burkholderia cepacia*, *Proteus* spp., *Providencia* spp., *Morganella morganii* and most of them have their LPS modified with L-Ara4N (Olaitan et al., 2014).

One of the main avenues they employ is to modify the target of colistin — LPS (Chen and Groisman, 2013). The overall charge of LPS is negative and that is stabilized by the divalent cations. On the other hand, colistin/polymyxins are positively charged and they bind with negatively charged phosphate groups of the lipid A of bacterial LPS via electrostatic interaction. Bacteria usually make such alteration by covalent modification of the lipid A moiety of LPS to reduce the overall charge of LPS. This is most commonly done by addition of 4-amino-4-deoxy-L-arabinose (L-Ara4N) or phosphoethanolamine (pEtN) to lipid A. Cationic substitution by L-Ara4N is very effective to reduce the overall charge of LPS. Such alteration ultimately reduces the affinity of LPS towards colistin (Chen and Groisman, 2013).

Such kind of alteration in bacteria is governed by pleiotropic two-component regulatory system (Ly et al., 2012). This helps the bacteria survive in stress situation by modifying the LPS to evade host defence mechanism and bactericidal agents (Chen and Groisman, 2013). One of such systems is PhoP-PhoQ system that responds to environmental cues or stimulation like extracytoplasmic divalent cations — Mg^{2+}, Ca^{2+} and Mn^{2+} (Groisman, 2001). Another such two-component regulator is PmrA/PmrB system (Chen and Groisman, 2013; Ly et al., 2012) which responds to extracellular accumulation of cations like Fe^{3+}. The activation of PhoP-PhoQ or PmrA/PmrB system is usually responsible for overexpression of genes leading to LPS alteration. There is increased synthesis and transfer of L-Ara4N and pEtN to lipid A of LPS resulting in decreased binding affinity of LPS to colistin (Fig. 10.1) (Olaitan et al., 2014; Lee et al., 2014).

In addition to such regulatory system, disruption of mgrB gene (a negative feedback regulator of PhoP-PhoQ system) was also reported to cause colistin resistance among *Klebsiella pneumoniae* (Simon et al., 2017; Cannatelli et al., 2013, 2014). The gene mgrB is a conserved one consisting of 141 nucleotides and it exerts negative feedback on PhoP/PhoQ system via encoding a short transmembrane protein of 47 amino acids. Disruption of mgrB gene was reported to be caused by nonsense or missense mutation, premature termination of mgrB transmembrane protein or formation of peptides with substituted amino acids. Such disruption was also recorded to be caused by insertional inactivation of mgrB gene by elements such as IS5-like, IS903B, IS1F-like and ISKpn14 leading to truncation of mgrB gene (Cannatelli et al., 2014). Moreover, in few strains of colistin-resistant *Escherichia coli*, small deletion or complete deletion of mgrB locus was reported. Furthermore, Bernasconi et al. (2018) also reported on unusual colistin-resistant *K. pneumoniae* with complete deletion of mgrB locus (Bernasconi et al., 2018). Mutations in pmrA/pmrB TCS were observed to provide colistin resistance among *Acinetobacter baumannii* (Dahdouh et al., 2017).

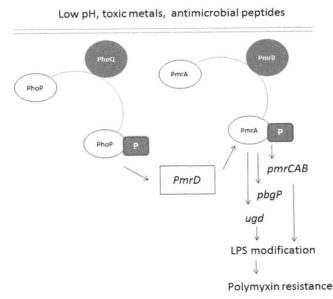

FIGURE 10.1 Two-component regulatory system and their relation with colistin resistance. Low pH, toxic metals and antimicrobial peptides may upregulate this two-component regulatory system.

There are other events involving modification of LPS which can cause polymyxin resistance. Ample evidences have suggested that activation of lpxR gene may cause removal of 3-acyloxy acyl residue from lipid A leading to polymyxin resistance. Similarly mutation involving the genes such as microcin transporter, a putative membrane protein, a putative transport protein and the methyl viologen-resistance protein SmvA or the genes involved in synthesis of outer membrane proteins such as waaL, rfbA and vacJ were found to cause colistin resistance (Olaitan et al., 2014). In *A. baumannii*, such polymyxin/colistin resistance was observed because of mutation, deletion or insertional inactivation of lipid A biosynthesis genes such as *lpxA, lpxC* and *lpxD* (Moffatt et al., 2010). Similar instances were found among *Pseudomonas aeruginosa* where mutation or disruption of genes involved in biosynthesis of LPS such as *galU, lptC, wapR* and *ssg* was found to cause colistin resistance (Fernández et al., 2013). Overexpression of outer membrane protein *OrpH* also results in polymyxin resistance in *P. aeruginosa*. *OrpH* is a relatively small 21.0 Kda protein, which is slightly basic in nature and in low Mg^{2+} concentration this OrpH binds with divalent cation-binding sites of the outer membrane/LPS to stabilize them and confer polymyxin resistance (Fernández et al., 2013; Young et al., 1992). Additionally, two novel two-component regulatory systems — ColR/ColS and CprR/CprS — were described in polymyxin-resistant *P. aeruginosa* (Olaitan et al., 2014).

Capsules also play a significant role in polymyxin or colistin resistance as observed in *K. pneumoniae*. It has been observed that *K. pneumoniae* isolates can shed capsular polysaccharides, which can comfortably entrap polymyxin or colistin molecules via electrostatic interactions and thereby reduce the drag transport and interaction with bacterial cell membranes (Zhou et al., 2016). In addition, changes in efflux pumps such as AcrAB and KpnEF may also mediate such resistance (Li et al., 2015).

Lately, a plasmid-mediated colistin resistance gene mcr-1 has been identified in *Enterobacteriaceae* including *E. coli*. The gene mcr-1 encodes for an enzyme phosphoethanolamine transferases, which catalyses the modification of lipid A of bacterial LPS (Gao et al., 2016; Wang et al., 2017). This gene has been so far detected among five species — five species: *E. coli, Salmonella enterica, K. pneumonia, Enterobacter aerogenes* and *Enterobacter cloacae*. Such kind of resistance mechanism was detected among various livestock/animal species such as cattle, poultry, pigs and dogs apart from human. Because of presence and carriage of the gene via mobile genetic element, this kind of resistance may spread rapidly and thus has been detected in food chain, animal products and even in healthy human microbiome across the globe (Wang et al., 2017; Xu et al., 2018). Other resistance mechanisms were also found to co-exist with *mcr-1* like carbapenem resistance and extended-spectrum β-lactamases. Furthermore, other alleles/variants of this gene were found in animals and human beings, viz., mcr-2, mcr-3 mcr-4 and mcr-5 (Yin et al., 2017; Borowiak et al., 2017; Fukuda et al., 2018).

Spread and status in animals

First instance of plasmid-mediated colistin resistance was reported from People Republic of China where the workers noticed an *E coli* strain, SHP45 of porcine origin, possessing colistin resistance that could be transferred to another strain (Liu et al., 2016). Based on their findings using sequence comparisons, homology modeling and electrospray ionization mass spectrometry, plasmid-mediated mcr-1 gene was found singularly responsible for colistin resistance. The workers identified mcr-1 gene in 78 (15%) of 523 samples of raw meat and 166 (21%) of 804 animals during the survey conducted for 4 years (2011−14). Furthermore, the gene mcr-1 was detected in ESBL (extended spectrum β-lactamase)-producing *E. coli* strains isolated from rectal swab of pigs and large areas of the pig slaughterhouses located in the Hoai Duc region of the Hanoi province, Vietnam (Malhotra-Kumar et al., 2016). Plasmid sequencing showed presence of multiple resistance genes encoding resistance to trimethoprim (dfrA12), tetracycline (tet (A)), aminoglycoside (aadA3, aph(3′)-IA), phenicol (cmlA1), quinolone (qnrS1, oqxA), lincosamide (lnu(F)), sulphonamide (sul2, sul3) and β-lactam (extended-spectrum β-lactamase $bla_{CTX-M55}$) antibiotics. However, none of the isolates from human patients with symptomatic urinary tract infection harboured mcr-1 gene. But evidence of its presence in human gut microbiome was established from China and Laos (Ruppé et al., 2016; Hu et al., 2016). Furthermore, it was reported from human blood stream infections and imported chicken meat (Hasman et al., 2015). Lima Barbieri et al. (2017) screened 1200 *E. coli* isolates consisting of 980 avian Pathogenic *E. coli* (APEC) from diseased birds and 220 avian fecal *E. coli* (AFEC) from healthy birds for the presence of mcr-1 and mcr-2 mediated colistin resistance. Although none of the AFEC isolates from healthy birds was positive for mcr-1/2, 12 isolates recovered from diseased production birds from China and Egypt possessed mcr-1 (Lima Barbieri et al., 2017). Plasmid-mediated colistin resistance was reported in the isolates from chicken and pig from Brazil and recently, Palmeira et al. (2018) reported ESBL producing mcr-1-mediated plasmid-mediated colistin-resistant *E. coli* isolate from bovine (Palmeira et al., 2018). The ESBL and mcr-1 gene(s) were located in two different plasmids of the isolate (mcr-1 on an IncX4 plasmid and blaCTX-M-2 on an IncF plasmid). Such co-existence of ESBL gene(s) — blaCTX-M-14 or blaCTX-M-55 and mcr-1 — was also noted in the *E. coli* isolates from Japanese travellers who have recently visited Vietnam

(Nakayama et al., 2018). A retrospective study conducted with 1611 *E. coli* isolates of chicken origin, collected for a period of five decades, 1974−2014, showed incremental increase of *mcr-1* positive isolates from 2009 to 2014 (Shen et al., 2016). This was correlated with use of colistin as animal feed additive during this 5-year period. However, the workers also identified 3 *E. coli* strains of 1980 with *mcr-1*. Of late, plasmid-mediated colistin resistance − mcr-1 − was reported in human clinical isolate from Egypt (Elnahriry et al., 2016). In another retrospective study at Great Romagna Hub Laboratory, Italy, a total of 19,053 isolates belonging to *Enterobacteriaceae* were analysed for colistin resistance. Of them, 90 were colistin-resistant. The gene mcr-1 was detected in 26 *E. coli* with an overall prevalence of 0.14% (Del Bianco et al., 2018). Brennan et al. (2016) have done an exhaustive study for a period of 7 years (2004−10) to screen 150 *E. coli* strains from fecal samples from cattle with suspected enteric infection or milk aliquots from cattle with suspected mastitis in France and Germany of which three exhibited higher MIC (minimum inhibitory concentration) towards colistin − *E. coli* 22134 O9:H9 U/ST10, *E. coli* 11-1896 O9:H12 U/ST58 and *E. coli* 29957 O101:H9 A or C/ST167. All the three had several nonsynonymous amino acid substitutions in genes associated with two-component regulatory systems such as *pmrA*, *pmrB*, *phoP* and *eptB*. The gene mcr-1 was identified only in the isolate − *E. coli* 29957 (Brennan et al., 2016). A new variant, plasmid-mediated *mcr-2*, was reported in *E. coli* isolates of porcine and bovine origin and the same was found 1617 bp long, 9 bases shorter than mcr-1 (1626 bp) with approximately 76% similarity (Xavier et al., 2016). Again, another allelic variant *mcr-3* was detected in a porcine *E. coli* with about 45.0% and 47.0% nucleotide sequence identity to *mcr-1* and *mcr-2*, respectively (Yin et al., 2017). The gene mcr-4 was reported in *Salmonella typhimurium* from pigs in Italy and in *E. coli* strains isolated from piglet diarrhoea in Spain and Belgium (Cannatelli et al., 2014). Very recently, another plasmid-mediated colistin resistance − mcr-5, a novel phosphoethanolamine transferase, was detected in association with transposon of the Tn3 family located in a multicopy ColE-type plasmid of a *S. enterica* subsp. enterica serovar Paratyphi B isolate and the study suggested that colistin resistance mediating phosphoethanolamine transferase genes were probably transferred from bacterial chromosome to its plasmid (Borowiak et al., 2017). Chromosomal association of mcr-5 was further noted in a colistin-resistant *P. aeruginosa* isolate (Snesrud et al., 2018). However, plasmid-mediated mcr-5 was detected in an *Aeromonas hydrophila* isolate (Ma et al., 2018) and the plasmid had about 80% similarity with ColE-type plasmids previously reported by Borowiak et al. (2017). Apart from poultry, pigs seem to be potent reservoir of plasmid-mediated colistin resistance. Fukuda et al. (2018) reported high prevalence of mcr-1, mcr-3 and mcr-5 in diseased pigs from Japan. Newly identified mcr gene(s) mcr-4 and mcr-5 were also detected from the upper and lower alimentary tracts of pigs and poultry in China (Chen et al., 2018).

Co-occurrence of two plasmid-mediated colistin resistance gene(s) − mcr-1 and mcr-3 − in one isolate of *E. coli* of bovine origin was reported from Spain (Hernández et al., 2017). Again such co-occurrence of mcr-1, mcr-4 and mcr-5 genes in multidrug-resistant ST10 enterotoxigenic and shiga toxin-producing *E. coli* from pigs was reported in Spain (García et al., 2018). Lately, Wang et al. (2018a,b) reported the occurrence of mcr-1 in other *Enterobacteriaceae* such as *Providencia alcalifaciens* and a mcr-1 variant, named mcr-1.3, in *Raoultella planticola*. Both of the mcr-1-carrying plasmids in these two isolates belong to IncI2 type of plasmids. Additionally, the workers detected the mcr-1 gene in one *E. cloacae* isolate (Wang et al., 2018b). Such findings indicated the widespread dissemination of plasmid-mediated colistin resistance determinants across the GNB.

Detection of colistin resistance

Because of inherent cationic properties of colistin, detection of colistin resistance is little complicated. Unlike many of the antibiotics, colistin resistance cannot be determined by routine disc diffusion assay because colistin cannot diffuse well in the agar and therefore broth microdilution assay is preferred and recommended. The broth microdilution is usually conducted in cation-adjusted Mueller Hinton broth and growth of the organism is tested against colistin sulphate over a range of dilutions (0.12−128 µg/mL). As colistin readily adheres or gets captured in the plastic or polystyrene, many workers recommended the use of surfactants such as polysorbate − 80 (Tween − 80 @ 0.002% par well) either to MHA (Mueller Hinton Agar) broth or to the inoculum suspension. Following overnight incubation, plates are observed for growth and MICs are noted.

For *Enterobacteriaceae*, the interpretation is generally based on the values given by European Committee on Antimicrobial Susceptibility Testing (EUCAST). In general, isolates with MICs < 2 µg/mL are categorized as susceptible, whereas isolates with MICs more than 4 µg/mL are categorized as resistant. *E. coli* ATCC 25922 is generally used as a referral or control strain.

In recent times, a rapid test was developed by a group of workers for detection of polymyxin resistance. The said test is associated with glucose uptake and metabolism by the bacteria in presence of defined concentration of colistin/polymyxin. The resistant bacteria can grow and utilize the glucose leading to formation of acid metabolites and change the pH.

Such change in pH can be visually interpreted because of colorimetric changes in the presence of pH indicator like phenol red. The test was found to have sensitivity and specificity of 99.3% and 95.4%, respectively, and could be performed within 2 h (Nordmann et al., 2016).

Detection of molecular mechanism of colistin resistance

As transmissible colistin resistance is a cause of great concern because of its rapid emergence and reports in animals, food and human worldwide, it is crucial to screen the isolates for plasmid-mediated colistin resistance genes such as *mcr-1*. Furthermore, other plasmid-mediated colistin resistance genes such as *mcr-2, mcr-3, mcr-4* and *mcr-5* were recently reported. Briefly, one loopful culture of overnight growth is resuspended in 100 µL of TE buffer and boiled at for 5−10 min and snap cooled. Following centrifugation at 6000*g* for 5 min the supernatant can be used as template at 1:10 dilution in Tris-HCL for using in PCR stated below.

Details regarding the primers, amplicon size and PCR condition are deliberated in table 10.1.

The *mgrB* inactivation leading to upregulation of the Pmr LPS modification system is also a common mechanism for colistin resistance. Therefore, screening of *mgrB* is an important task for exploring the cause of colistin resistance. Following PCR amplification and sequencing of *mgr*B coding region, different kinds of alterations such as insertions of different types of mobile elements (IS5-like, IS1F-like or ISKpn14), nonsilent point mutations and small intragenic deletions can be detected. Entire sequence information of the *mgrB* locus may be examined taking *K. pneumonia* HS11286 chromosome as reference (GenBank accession no. CP000649). Likewise, mutations (deletion/substitution) in *pmrA, pmrB, phoP* and *phoQ* genes were screened as responsible factors leading to colistin resistance. Single amino acid change (Asp191Tyr) in PhoP was reported to cause alteration of the secondary structure of the protein and disregulation of the two-component regulatory system PhoPQ leading to colistin resistance. The amplified sequences should be compared with a wild colistin susceptible strain (ATCC 53153).

Details of oligonucleotides and PCR conditions are stated in table 10.2.

Therapeutic strategy

Colistin is usually preferred for treating cases caused by pan-drug-resistant strains especially the carbapenemase producers. However, nephrotoxic effect of colistin is a strong contraindication which needs to be considered when colistin is advocated in such ailing patients. Prolong colistin therapy may have an adverse impact over the health condition and vital organ function of such patients. On the other hand, effective drug regimen is an essential prerequisite to prevent the spread of infection and impending septicaemia. Therefore, treatment protocol must be initiated keeping all these factors in mind. However, colistin resistance in carbapenemase producers put significant threat over the life of ailing patients, and the previous study by Capone et al. (2013) indicated that almost 36% of the carbapenem-resistant strains may also be colistin-resistant. In such cases, colistin plus rifampin was found effective in treating the infections caused by colistin-resistant carbapenemase producers as indicated in a study conducted in Italy (Tascini et al., 2013). The authors pointed out that

TABLE 10.1 Oligonucleotides and PCR conditions for the detection of plasmid-mediated colistin resistance

Target	Oligonucleotides	PCR conditions	Amplicon size	Reference
mcr-1	F: AGTCCGTTTGTTCTTGTGGC R: AGATCCTTGGTCTCGGCTTG	94°C 15 min +25X (94°C 30 s +58°C 90 s +72°C 60 s) + 72°C 10min	309 bp	(Borowiak et al., 2017; Rebelo et al., 2018)
mcr-2	F: CAAGTGTGTTGGTCGCAGTT R: TCTAGCCCGACAAGCATACC		715 bp	
mcr-3	F: AAATAAAAATTGTTCCGCTTATG R: AATGGAGATCCCCGTTTTT		929 bp	
mcr-4	F: TCACTTTCATCACTGCGTTG R: TTGGTCCATGACTACCAATG		1116 bp	
mcr-5	F: ATGCGGTTGTCTGCATTTATC R: TCATTGTGGTTGTCCTTTTCTG		1664 bp	

TABLE 10.2 Oligonucleotides and PCR conditions for detection of deletion or mutation of the two-component regulatory system involved in colistin resistance.

Target	Oligonucleotides (5'-3')	PCR conditions	Amplicon size	Reference
mgrB	F: AAGGCGTTCATTCTACCACC R: TTAAGAAGGCCGTGCTATCC	Initial denaturation 3 min at 95°C; 30 cycles of 30 s at 95°C, 30 s at 54°C and 105 s at 72°C; and finally, 5 min at 72°C.	253 bp	Cannatelli et al. (2014)
mgrB	F: GGCTATGGCGAGGATAATGAG R: GCTGTGATGTAAGCGTCTGGTG		1057 bp	
mgrB locus	F: CGGTGGGTTTTACTGATAGTCA R: ATAGTGCAAATGCCGCTGA		110 bp	
pmrA	F: CATTTCCGCGCACTGTCTGC R: CAGGTTTCAGTTGCAAACAG	Initial denaturation 5 min at 95°C; 30 cycles of 30 s at 95°C, 30 s at 55°C and 1 min at 72°C; and finally, 5 min at 72°C.	850 bp	Jayol et al. (2014) *K. pneumoniae* ATCC 53153
pmrB	F: ACCTACGCGAAAAGATTGGC R: GATGAGGATAGCGCCCATGC		1274 bp	
phoP	F: GAGCTTCAGACTACTATCGA R: GGGAAGATATGCCGCAACAG		739 bp	
phoQ	F: ATACCCACAGGACGTCATCA R: CAGGTGTCTGACAGGGATTA		1597 bp	

colistin—rifampin combination may be effective in the treatment of multidrug-resistant *K. pneumoniae* and such treatment regimen may considerably slow down the selection of heteroresistant subpopulations during colistin therapy. Again, Oliva et al., 2015 reported successful treatment of such bloodstream infection using a combination of colistin and double carbapenem (ertapenem and meropenem). Synergistic effect of colistin and carbapenem or rifampicin was previously indicated by other workers in experimental model also (Lee et al., 2013; Deris et al., 2012). A study conducted by Nordqvist et al. (2016) reported that combined use of colistin and rifampicin completely inhibited the growth of all colistin-resistant subpopulations and significantly lowered the mutant prevention concentration of colistin for *A. baumannii*. Thus, such combined regimen may be effective intervention to prevent the emergence of colistin-resistant strains (Nordqvist et al., 2016).

In experimental model of murine thigh and bacteraemia infection induced by plasmid-mediated colistin-resistant *K. pneumonia* (mcr-1), colistin and clarithromycin combination therapy was found effective (MacNair et al., 2018). The *in vitro* and *ex vivo* experiments conducted by the workers revealed that the use of colistin in combination with antibiotics acting on Gram-positive bacteria such as rifampicin, rifabutin, clarithromycin, minocycline and novobiocin may provide a better alternative for treating the highly drug-resistant Gram-negative pathogens with mcr-1.

References

Balkan, I.I., Aygün, G., Aydın, S., Mutcalı, S.I., Kara, Z., Kuşkucu, M., et al., 2014. Blood stream infections due to OXA-48-like carbapenemase-producing *Enterobacteriaceae*: treatment and survival. International Journal of Infectious Diseases 26, 51—56. https://doi.org/10.1016/j.ijid.2014.05.012.

Bernasconi, O.J., Donà, V., Pires, J., Kuenzli, E., Hatz, C., Luzzaro, F., et al., 2018. Deciphering the complete deletion of the mgrB locus in an unusual colistin-resistant *Klebsiella pneumoniae* isolate colonising the gut of a traveller returning from India. International Journal of Antimicrobial Agents 51, 529—531. https://doi.org/10.1016/j.ijantimicag.2017.09.014.

Biswas, S., Brunel, J.-M., Dubus, J.-C., Reynaud-Gaubert, M., Rolain, J.-M., 2012. Colistin: an update on the antibiotic of the 21st century. Expert Review of Anti-infective Therapy 10, 917—934. https://doi.org/10.1586/eri.12.78.

Borowiak, M., Fischer, J., Hammerl, J.A., Hendriksen, R.S., Szabo, I., Malorny, B., 2017. Identification of a novel transposon-associated phosphoethanolamine transferase gene, mcr-5, conferring colistin resistance in d-tartrate fermenting *Salmonella enterica* subsp. enterica serovar Paratyphi B. Journal of Antimicrobial Chemotherapy 72, 3317—3324. https://doi.org/10.1093/jac/dkx327.

Brennan, E., Martins, M., McCusker, M.P., Wang, J., Alves, B.M., Hurley, D., et al., 2016. Multidrug-resistant *Escherichia coli* in bovine animals, Europe. Emerging Infectious Diseases 22, 1650—1652. https://doi.org/10.3201/eid2209.160140.

Cannatelli, A., D'Andrea, M.M., Giani, T., Di Pilato, V., Arena, F., Ambretti, S., et al., 2013. In vivo emergence of colistin resistance in *Klebsiella pneumoniae* producing KPC-type carbapenemases mediated by insertional inactivation of the PhoQ/PhoP mgrB regulator. Antimicrobial Agents and Chemotherapy 57, 5521—5526. https://doi.org/10.1128/AAC.01480-13.

Cannatelli, A., Giani, T., D'Andrea, M.M., Di Pilato, V., Arena, F., Conte, V., et al., 2014. MgrB inactivation is a common mechanism of colistin resistance in KPC-producing *Klebsiella pneumoniae* of clinical origin. Antimicrobial Agents and Chemotherapy 58, 5696−5703. https://doi.org/10.1128/AAC.03110-14.

Capone, A., Giannella, M., Fortini, D., Giordano, A., Meledandri, M., Ballardini, M., et al., 2013. High rate of colistin resistance among patients with carbapenem-resistant *Klebsiella pneumoniae* infection accounts for an excess of mortality. Clinical Microbiology and Infections 19, E23−E30. https://doi.org/10.1111/1469-0691.12070.

Chen, H.D., Groisman, E.A., 2013. The biology of the PmrA/PmrB two-component system: the major regulator of lipopolysaccharide modifications. Annual Review of Microbiology 67, 83−112. https://doi.org/10.1146/annurev-micro-092412-155751.

Chen, L., Zhang, J., Wang, J., Butaye, P., Kelly, P., Li, M., et al., 2018. Newly identified colistin resistance genes, mcr-4 and mcr-5, from upper and lower alimentary tract of pigs and poultry in China. PLoS One 13, e0193957. https://doi.org/10.1371/journal.pone.0193957.

Dahdouh, E., Gómez-Gil, R., Sanz, S., González-Zorn, B., Daoud, Z., Mingorance, J., et al., 2017. A novel mutation in pmrB mediates colistin resistance during therapy of *Acinetobacter baumannii*. International Journal of Antimicrobial Agents 49, 727−733. https://doi.org/10.1016/j.ijantimicag.2017.01.031.

Del Bianco, F., Morotti, M., Pedna, M.F., Farabegoli, P., Sambri, V., 2018. Microbiological surveillance of plasmid mediated colistin resistance in human *Enterobacteriaceae* isolates in Romagna (Northern Italy): August 2016−July 2017. International Journal of Infectious Diseases 69, 96−98. https://doi.org/10.1016/j.ijid.2018.02.006.

Deris, Z.Z., Yu, H.H., Davis, K., Soon, R.L., Jacob, J., Ku, C.K., et al., 2012. The combination of colistin and doripenem is synergistic against *Klebsiella pneumoniae* at multiple inocula and suppresses colistin resistance in an in vitro pharmacokinetic/pharmacodynamic model. Antimicrobial Agents and Chemotherapy 56, 5103−5112. https://doi.org/10.1128/AAC.01064-12.

Dijkmans, A.C., Wilms, E.B., Kamerling, I.M.C., Birkhoff, W., Ortiz-Zacarías, N.V., van Nieuwkoop, C., et al., 2015. Colistin. Therapeutic Drug Monitoring 37, 419−427. https://doi.org/10.1097/FTD.0000000000000172.

Elnahriry, S.S., Khalifa, H.O., Soliman, A.M., Ahmed, A.M., Hussein, A.M., Shimamoto, T., et al., 2016. Emergence of plasmid-mediated colistin resistance gene mcr-1 in a clinical *Escherichia coli* isolate from Egypt. Antimicrobial Agents and Chemotherapy 60, 3249−3250. https://doi.org/10.1128/AAC.00269-16.

Falagas, M.E., Rafailidis, P.I., 2009. Nephrotoxicity of colistin: new insight into an old antibiotic. Clinical Infectious Diseases 48, 1729−1731. https://doi.org/10.1086/599226.

Fernández, L., Álvarez-Ortega, C., Wiegand, I., Olivares, J., Kocíncová, D., Lam, J.S., et al., 2013. Characterization of the polymyxin B resistome of *Pseudomonas aeruginosa*. Antimicrobial Agents and Chemotherapy 57, 110−119. https://doi.org/10.1128/AAC.01583-12.

Fukuda, A., Sato, T., Shinagawa, M., Takahashi, S., Asai, T., Yokota, S.-I., et al., 2018. High prevalence of mcr-1, mcr-3 and mcr-5 in *Escherichia coli* derived from diseased pigs in Japan. International Journal of Antimicrobial Agents 51, 163−164. https://doi.org/10.1016/j.ijantimicag.2017.11.010.

Gao, R., Hu, Y., Li, Z., Sun, J., Wang, Q., Lin, J., et al., 2016. Dissemination and mechanism for the MCR-1 colistin resistance. PLoS Pathogens 12, e1005957. https://doi.org/10.1371/journal.ppat.1005957.

García, V., García-Meniño, I., Mora, A., Flament-Simon, S.C., Díaz-Jiménez, D., Blanco, J.E., et al., 2018. Co-occurrence of mcr-1, mcr-4 and mcr-5 genes in multidrug-resistant ST10 Enterotoxigenic and Shiga toxin-producing *Escherichia coli* in Spain (2006-2017). International Journal of Antimicrobial Agents. https://doi.org/10.1016/j.ijantimicag.2018.03.022.

Groisman, E.A., 2001. The pleiotropic two-component regulatory system PhoP-PhoQ. Journal of Bacteriology 183, 1835−1842. https://doi.org/10.1128/JB.183.6.1835-1842.2001.

Hasman, H., Hammerum, A.M., Hansen, F., Hendriksen, R.S., Olesen, B., Agersø, Y., et al., 2015. Detection of mcr-1 encoding plasmid-mediated colistin-resistant *Escherichia coli* isolates from human bloodstream infection and imported chicken meat, Denmark 2015. Euro Surveillance 20, 30085. https://doi.org/10.2807/1560-7917.ES.2015.20.49.30085.

Hernández, M., Iglesias, M.R., Rodríguez-Lázaro, D., Gallardo, A., Quijada, N., Miguela-Villoldo, P., et al., 2017. Co-occurrence of colistin-resistance genes mcr-1 and mcr-3 among multidrug-resistant *Escherichia coli* isolated from Cattle, Spain, September 2015. Euro Surveillance 22, 30586. https://doi.org/10.2807/1560-7917.ES.2017.22.31.30586.

Hu, Y., Liu, F., Lin, I.Y.C., Gao, G.F., Zhu, B., 2016. Dissemination of the mcr-1 colistin resistance gene. The Lancet Infectious Diseases 16, 146−147. https://doi.org/10.1016/S1473-3099(15)00533-2.

Jacobs, D.M., Safir, M.C., Huang, D., Minhaj, F., Parker, A., Rao, G.G., 2017. Triple combination antibiotic therapy for carbapenemase-producing *Klebsiella pneumoniae*: a systematic review. Annals of Clinical Microbiology and Antimicrobials 16, 76. https://doi.org/10.1186/s12941-017-0249-2.

Jayol, A., Poirel, L., Brink, A., Villegas, M.-V., Yilmaz, M., Nordmann, P., 2014. Resistance to colistin associated with a single amino acid change in protein PmrB among *Klebsiella pneumoniae* isolates of worldwide origin. Antimicrobial Agents and Chemotherapy 58, 4762−4766. https://doi.org/10.1128/AAC.00084-14.

Karaiskos, I., Antoniadou, A., Giamarellou, H., 2017. Combination therapy for extensively-drug resistant gram-negative bacteria. Expert Review of Anti-infective Therapy 15, 1123−1140. https://doi.org/10.1080/14787210.2017.1410434.

Kelesidis, T., Falagas, M.E., 2015. The safety of polymyxin antibiotics. Expert Opinion on Drug Safety 14, 1687−1701. https://doi.org/10.1517/14740338.2015.1088520.

Lee, H.J., Bergen, P.J., Bulitta, J.B., Tsuji, B., Forrest, A., Nation, R.L., et al., 2013. Synergistic activity of colistin and rifampin combination against multidrug-resistant *Acinetobacter baumannii* in an in vitro pharmacokinetic/pharmacodynamic model. Antimicrobial Agents and Chemotherapy 57, 3738−3745. https://doi.org/10.1128/AAC.00703-13.

Lee, J.-Y., Chung, E.S., Na, I.Y., Kim, H., Shin, D., Ko, K.S., 2014. Development of colistin resistance in pmrA-, phoP-, parR- and cprR-inactivated mutants of *Pseudomonas aeruginosa*. Journal of Antimicrobial Chemotherapy 69, 2966–2971. https://doi.org/10.1093/jac/dku238.

Li, X.-Z., Plésiat, P., Nikaido, H., 2015. The challenge of efflux-mediated antibiotic resistance in gram-negative bacteria. Clinical Microbiology Reviews 28, 337–418. https://doi.org/10.1128/CMR.00117-14.

Lima Barbieri, N., Nielsen, D.W., Wannemuehler, Y., Cavender, T., Hussein, A., Yan, S., et al., 2017. mcr-1 identified in Avian Pathogenic *Escherichia coli* (APEC). PLoS One 12, e0172997. https://doi.org/10.1371/journal.pone.0172997.

Liu, Y.-Y., Wang, Y., Walsh, T.R., Yi, L.-X., Zhang, R., Spencer, J., et al., 2016. Emergence of plasmid-mediated colistin resistance mechanism MCR-1 in animals and human beings in China: a microbiological and molecular biological study. The Lancet Infectious Diseases 16, 161–168. https://doi.org/10.1016/S1473-3099(15)00424-7.

Loho, T., Dharmayanti, A., 2015. Colistin: an antibiotic and its role in multiresistant Gram-negative infections. Acta Medica Indonesiana 47, 157–168.

Ly, N.S., Yang, J., Bulitta, J.B., Tsuji, B.T., 2012. Impact of two-component regulatory systems PhoP-PhoQ and PmrA-PmrB on colistin pharmacodynamics in *Pseudomonas aeruginosa*. Antimicrobial Agents and Chemotherapy 56, 3453–3456. https://doi.org/10.1128/AAC.06380-11.

Ma, S., Sun, C., Hulth, A., Li, J., Nilsson, L.E., Zhou, Y., et al., 2018. Mobile colistin resistance gene mcr-5 in porcine *Aeromonas hydrophila*. Journal of Antimicrobial Chemotherapy 73, 1777–1780. https://doi.org/10.1093/jac/dky110.

MacNair, C.R., Stokes, J.M., Carfrae, L.A., Fiebig-Comyn, A.A., Coombes, B.K., Mulvey, M.R., et al., 2018. Overcoming mcr-1 mediated colistin resistance with colistin in combination with other antibiotics. Nature Communications 9, 458. https://doi.org/10.1038/s41467-018-02875-z.

Malhotra-Kumar, S., Xavier, B.B., Das, A.J., Lammens, C., Hoang, H.T.T., Pham, N.T., et al., 2016. Colistin-resistant *Escherichia coli* harbouring mcr-1 isolated from food animals in Hanoi, Vietnam. The Lancet Infectious Diseases 16, 286–287. https://doi.org/10.1016/S1473-3099(16)00014-1.

Moffatt, J.H., Harper, M., Harrison, P., Hale, J.D.F., Vinogradov, E., Seemann, T., et al., 2010. Colistin resistance in *Acinetobacter baumannii* is mediated by complete loss of lipopolysaccharide production. Antimicrobial Agents and Chemotherapy 54, 4971–4977. https://doi.org/10.1128/AAC.00834-10.

Nakayama, T., Kumeda, Y., Kawahara, R., Yamaguchi, T., Yamamoto, Y., 2018. Carriage of colistin-resistant, extended-spectrum β-lactamase-producing *Escherichia coli* harboring the mcr-1 resistance gene after short-term international travel to Vietnam. Infection and Drug Resistance 11, 391–395. https://doi.org/10.2147/IDR.S153178.

Nordmann, P., Jayol, A., Poirel, L., 2016. Rapid detection of polymyxin resistance in *Enterobacteriaceae*. Emerging Infectious Diseases 22, 1038–1043. https://doi.org/10.3201/eid2206.151840.

Nordqvist, H., Nilsson, L.E., Claesson, C., 2016. Mutant prevention concentration of colistin alone and in combination with rifampicin for multidrug-resistant *Acinetobacter baumannii*. European Journal of Clinical Microbiology and Infectious Diseases 35, 1845–1850. https://doi.org/10.1007/s10096-016-2736-3.

Olaitan, A.O., Diene, S.M., Kempf, M., Berrazeg, M., Bakour, S., Gupta, S.K., et al., 2014. Worldwide emergence of colistin resistance in *Klebsiella pneumoniae* from healthy humans and patients in Lao PDR, Thailand, Israel, Nigeria and France owing to inactivation of the PhoP/PhoQ regulator mgrB: an epidemiological and molecular study. International Journal of Antimicrobial Agents 44, 500–507. https://doi.org/10.1016/j.ijantimicag.2014.07.020.

Oliva, A., Mascellino, M.T., Cipolla, A., D'Abramo, A., De Rosa, A., Savinelli, S., et al., 2015. Therapeutic strategy for pandrug-resistant *Klebsiella pneumoniae* severe infections: short-course treatment with colistin increases the in vivo and in vitro activity of double carbapenem regimen. International Journal of Infectious Diseases 33, 132–134. https://doi.org/10.1016/J.IJID.2015.01.011.

Palmeira, J.D., Ferreira, H., Madec, J.-Y., Haenni, M., 2018. Draft genome of a ST443 mcr-1 – and bla CTX-M-2 -carrying *Escherichia coli* from cattle in Brazil. The Journal of Global Antimicrobial Resistance 13, 269–270. https://doi.org/10.1016/j.jgar.2018.05.010.

Paul, M., Daikos, G.L., Durante-Mangoni, E., Yahav, D., Carmeli, Y., Benattar, Y.D., et al., 2018. Colistin alone versus colistin plus meropenem for treatment of severe infections caused by carbapenem-resistant Gram-negative bacteria: an open-label, randomised controlled trial. The Lancet Infectious Diseases 18, 391–400. https://doi.org/10.1016/S1473-3099(18)30099-9.

Rebelo, A.R., Bortolaia, V., Kjeldgaard, J.S., Pedersen, S.K., Leekitcharoenphon, P., Hansen, I.M., et al., 2018. Multiplex PCR for detection of plasmid-mediated colistin resistance determinants, mcr-1, mcr-2, mcr-3, mcr-4 and mcr-5 for surveillance purposes. Euro Surveillance 23. https://doi.org/10.2807/1560-7917.ES.2018.23.6.17-00672.

Ruppé, E., Chatelier, E Le, Pons, N., Andremont, A., Ehrlich, S.D., 2016. Dissemination of the mcr-1 colistin resistance gene. The Lancet Infectious Diseases 16, 290–291. https://doi.org/10.1016/S1473-3099(16)00066-9.

Shen, Z., Wang, Y., Shen, Y., Shen, J., Wu, C., 2016. Early emergence of mcr-1 in *Escherichia coli* from food-producing animals. The Lancet Infectious Diseases 16, 293. https://doi.org/10.1016/S1473-3099(16)00061-X.

Simon, M., Melzl, H., Hiergeist, A., Richert, K., Falgenhauer, L., Pfeifer, Y., et al., 2017. Colistin- and carbapenem-resistant *Klebsiella oxytoca* harboring blaVIM-2 and an insertion in the mgrB gene isolated from blood culture. International Journal of Medical Microbiology 307, 113–115. https://doi.org/10.1016/j.ijmm.2017.01.001.

Snesrud, E., Maybank, R., Kwak, Y.I., Jones, A.R., Hinkle, M.K., Mc Gann, P., 2018. Chromosomally encoded mcr-5 in colistin non-susceptible *Pseudomonas aeruginosa*. Antimicrobial Agents and Chemotherapy. https://doi.org/10.1128/AAC.00679-18. AAC.00679-18.

Tascini, C., Tagliaferri, E., Giani, T., Leonildi, A., Flammini, S., Casini, B., et al., 2013. Synergistic activity of colistin plus rifampin against colistin-resistant KPC-producing *Klebsiella pneumoniae*. Antimicrobial Agents and Chemotherapy 57, 3990–3993. https://doi.org/10.1128/AAC.00179-13.

Velkov, T., Dai, C., Ciccotosto, G.D., Cappai, R., Hoyer, D., Li, J., 2018. Polymyxins for CNS infections: pharmacology and neurotoxicity. Pharmacology and Therapeutics 181, 85–90. https://doi.org/10.1016/j.pharmthera.2017.07.012.

Wang, Q., Sun, J., Li, J., Ding, Y., Li, X.-P., Lin, J., et al., 2017. Expanding landscapes of the diversified mcr-1-bearing plasmid reservoirs. Microbiome 5, 70. https://doi.org/10.1186/s40168-017-0288-0.

Wang, J., He, J.-T., Bai, Y., Wang, R., Cai, Y., 2018. Synergistic activity of colistin/fosfomycin combination against carbapenemase-producing *Klebsiella pneumoniae* in an in vitro pharmacokinetic/pharmacodynamic model. BioMed Research International 2018, 5720417. https://doi.org/10.1155/2018/5720417.

Wang, X., Wang, Y., Wang, Y., Zhang, S., Shen, Z., Wang, S., 2018. Emergence of the colistin resistance gene mcr-1 and its variant in several uncommon species of *Enterobacteriaceae* from commercial poultry farm surrounding environments. Veterinary Microbiology 219, 161—164. https://doi.org/10.1016/j.vetmic.2018.04.002.

Xavier, B.B., Lammens, C., Ruhal, R., Malhotra-Kumar, S., Butaye, P., Goossens, H., et al., 2016. Identification of a novel plasmid-mediated colistin-resistance gene, mcr-2, in *Escherichia coli*, Belgium, June 2016. Euro Surveillance 21, 30280. https://doi.org/10.2807/1560-7917.ES.2016.21.27.30280.

Xu, Y., Wei, W., Lei, S., Lin, J., Srinivas, S., Feng, Y., 2018. An evolutionarily conserved mechanism for intrinsic and transferable polymyxin resistance. mBio 9. https://doi.org/10.1128/mBio.02317-17 e02317-17.

Yin, W., Li, H., Shen, Y., Liu, Z., Wang, S., Shen, Z., et al., 2017. Novel plasmid-mediated colistin resistance gene mcr-3 in *Escherichia coli*. mBio 8. https://doi.org/10.1128/mBio.00543-17 e00543-17.

Young, M.L., Bains, M., Bell, A., Hancock, R.E., 1992. Role of *Pseudomonas aeruginosa* outer membrane protein OprH in polymyxin and gentamicin resistance: isolation of an OprH-deficient mutant by gene replacement techniques. Antimicrobial Agents and Chemotherapy 36, 2566—2568.

Zhou, K., Cattoir, V., Xiao, Y., 2016. Intrinsic colistin resistance. The Lancet Infectious Diseases 16, 1227—1228. https://doi.org/10.1016/S1473-3099(16)30394-2.

Chapter 11

Antifungal resistance

Chapter outline

Overview

Since the beginning of 20th century, bacterial diseases were recorded to cause significant mortality with the onset of the First World War. Fungal diseases did not achieve the same magnitude. However, the picture started changing in the early 60s when fungal diseases began to gear up, thanks to the exuberant use of antibiotics causing the destruction of commensals and use of corticosteroids and chemotherapeutics leading to immunosuppression in patients with organ transplants, cancer or other systemic or metabolic diseases. Currently, invasive fungal (IF) disease has been recorded to cause a significant burden of human illness with more than 1.5 million annual death being attributed to fungal diseases caused by *Candida*, *Aspergillus*, *Pneumocystis* and *Cryptococcus* spp. (Bongomin et al., 2017). In systemic fungal diseases, mortality may reach up to 50% in bloodstream candidiasis and invasive aspergillosis, which has emerged as a cause of concern across the globe (Hahn-Ast et al., 2010).

In spite of extensive research, the available therapeutic armamentarium against IF diseases is limited, and like bacteria, some fungi also develop resistance against antifungal agents. Thus, the emergence of antifungal resistance has become a major problem in managing systemic or invasive mycosis. Although antibiotic resistance is largely known to medical/veterinary doctors, public health personnel and technical persons, information on antifungal resistance are rather limited.

Presently, four groups of antifungal agents are used in clinical practice; fluoropyrimidine analogues, polyenes, azoles and echinocandins. From the antifungal group, fluoropyrimidine analogue, 5-fluorocytosine (5-FC) is mainly used in human clinical practice. These compounds are basically synthetic structural analogues of pyrimidine—cytosine. Initially known for its antitumor property, 5-FC has a broad range of antifungal activity including against *Candida* and *Cryptococcus* genera. The compound can be effectively distributed all over the body for its high water solubility and small size. Entering the fungi cell, 5-FC is metabolized into fluorinated pyrimidine, which destabilizes the fungal replication machinery and causes cell cycle arrest after being incorporated in the nucleic acid (DNA/RNA).

Antifungals of the polyenes group, also known as polyene antimycotic or polyene antibiotic, are obtained from *Streptomyces* group of bacteria and include the antifungals such as amphotericin B, deoxycholate, natamycin and nystatin and other analogues. Polyenes by their irreversible binding with the ergosterol moiety of the mycotic cell membrane cause loss of transmembrane potential with the formation of pores and leakage of monovalent ions and important cellular components leading to death (Groll and Walsh, 2009; Ghannoum and Rice, 1999).

Azoles inhibit the cytochrome P450-dependent enzyme lanosterol 14-α-demethylase (also known as 14α-sterol demethylase or P-450$_{DM}$), which is responsible for converting lanosterol to ergosterol, the main sterol component of fungal cell membrane. The enzyme is also crucial for the synthesis of cholesterol in mammals. However, in therapeutic concentration, antifungal agents show more affinity towards the fungal enzyme. With the depletion of ergosterol and accumulation of 14-α methylated sterols, there is a complete disruption in the structure and function of the fungal cell membrane with loss of nutrient transport (Sheehan et al., 1999). Furthermore, ergosterol possesses

Antimicrobial Resistance in Agriculture. https://doi.org/10.1016/B978-0-12-815770-1.00011-0

hormone-like activity to stimulate the growth and function of mycotic cells; thus, ergosterol loss causes an overall depression in the activities of fungus cells. Clinically important azoles include imidazoles (ketoconazole and miconazole, clotrimazole) or triazoles (itraconazole and fluconazole). Although imidazoles (except ketoconazole) are mostly used in superficial mycoses, triazoles are used in both superficial and systemic mycoses (Sheehan et al., 1999; Zavrel and White, 2015). New generation triazoles such as voriconazole and isavuconazole are being used with more efficacy and potency against complicated fungal infections especially in IF infections (Bagshaw et al., 2018; Elewa et al., 2015).

Echinocandins are more effective against *Candida* and *Aspergillus;* however, they have little activity against Zygomycetes or against *Cryptococcus, Trichosporon, Scedosporium* and *Fusarium* species. Echinocandins that includes semisynthetic compounds such as caspofungin, micafungin and anidulafungin noncompetitively inhibits the enzyme 1,3 β-glucan synthase and thereby the synthesis of β-1-3-D glucan, the essential component for the structural and functional integrity of the cell wall. Thus it leads to disruption of the cell wall structure, formation of the defective cell wall and malformed hyphal growth in moulds. Just because echinocandins act on the fungal cell wall in a manner similar to what penicillin causes on the bacterial cell wall, echinocandins are also known as 'penicillin of antifungals' (Chen et al., 2011; Denning, 2003).

Mechanism of antifungal resistance

Depending on the classes of antifungal agents and their mode of action, mechanism of resistance differs significantly. In general, resistance towards antifungal drugs evolves following three distinct categories — (1) decrease in effective intracellular drug concentration, (2) alteration in drug target molecules and (3) metabolic bypass (White et al., 1998; Kontoyiannis and Lewis, 2002; Vanden Bossche et al., 1998). Decreased drug concentration is usually achieved by drugs being expelled out under active mediation of drug efflux pumps. In fungal pathogens, such kind of drug efflux pumps belongs to ATP-binding cassette (ABC) transporters and transporters of the major facilitator superfamily (MFS). Genomic analysis of fungal pathogens revealed the presence of a number of transporters of ABC and MFS families. Of several classes of ABC transporters, transporters of pleiotropic drug resistance (PDR) class are relevant to antifungal drug resistance. In *C. albicans,* CDR1 and CDR2 (*Candida* drug resistance) are the most commonly found ABC transporters responsible for azole resistance (Chen et al., 2010). Such ABC transporters were also detected in *C. glabrata* (CgCDR1, CgCDR2, CgSNQ2 genes), *C. dubliniensis* (CdMDR1 and CdCDR2) and *C. neoformans* (AFR1) (Sionov et al., 2010). Several workers reported upregulation of such kind of ABC transporter genes —*AfuMDR3* and *AfuMDR-4* in azole-resistant *A. fumigatus* (Da Silva Ferreira et al., 2004; Nascimento et al., 2003).

Alteration of the target site is another mechanism involved in the development of antifungal resistance. The target site for the azole group of the drug is lanosterol C14α-demethylase enzyme and mutation in *ERG11*, the gene encoding the enzyme may prevent efficient binding of azole compounds. Although a number of mutations were reported in *ERG11*, only a few of them such as Y132F/H and G464S/D were found responsible for azole resistance in *Candida* (Flowers et al., 2015). In few circumstances, mutation in *ERG11* may be combined with a mutation in *ERG3*, the gene encoding for the another enzyme involved in the ergosterol biosynthesis. Such simultaneous mutation in two genes was previously reported in *C. albicans* and *C. tropicalis* (Whaley et al., 2017; Eddouzi et al., 2013).

The third possible mechanism for antifungal resistance is the increased concentration of the target enzyme. It has been noticed that increased expression of *ERG11* and production of lanosterol C14α-demethylase enzyme substantially exhausts the antifungal compound (azoles) and thereby the azoles in therapeutic concentration become ineffective. Such increased production of target enzyme can be modulated by increased genetic expression, augmented transcription factors (UPC 2) and decreased degradation of the genes.

Modification of the target site or its overexpression was also noticed in azole-resistant *A. fumigatus*. Point mutation of cyp51A has been found the main mechanism involving triazole resistance of *A. fumigatus*. However, depending upon the site of point mutation and amino acid supplementation, the resistance profile of the isolates may differ. Strains with a mutation at the position of glycine 54 were found resistant to itraconazole and posaconazole but not to voriconazole. Likewise, a mutation at methionine 220 was found exhibit resistance to posaconazole, voriconazole and ravuconazole. Substitution or mutation like G464S was found to show resistance towards voriconazole and moderate resistance to itraconazole and posaconazole. Moreover, multiple azole resistance was reported in an isolate with a G138C substitution (Nascimento et al., 2003; Alanio et al., 2011; Warris, 2015; Lelièvre et al., 2013; Vermeulen et al., 2013; Diaz-Guerra et al., 2003).

TABLE 11.1 Breakpoints for determination of antifungal susceptibility testing.

Antifungal agents (mg/L)		Fluconazole		Itraconazole		Voriconazole		Micafungin		Anidulafungin	
Pathogens	Standards	S ≤	R >	S	R	S	R	S	R	S	R
C. albicans	EUCAST	2	4	0.064	0.064	0.1255	0.1255	0.016	0.016	0.032	0.032
	CLSI	2	4	0.125	0.5	0.125	0.5	0.25	0.5	0.25	0.5
C. glabrata	EUCAST	0.002	32					0.032	0.032	0.064	0.064
	CLSI	32 (SDD)	32	0.125	0.5			0.06	0.12	0.12	0.25
C. krusei	EUCAST									0.064	0.064
	CLSI			0.125	0.5	0.5	1	0.25	0.5	0.25	0.5
C. parapsilosis	EUCAST	2	4	0.125	0.125	0.1255	0.1255	0.002	2	0.002	4
	CLSI			0.125	0.5	0.125	0.5	2	4	2	4
C. tropicalis	EUCAST	2	4	0.125	0.125	0.1255	0.1255			0.064	0.064
	CLSI			0.125	0.5	0.125	0.5	0.25	0.5	0.25	0.5

Detection techniques

Like antibacterial susceptibility testing, antifungal susceptibility testing (AFST) is generally conducted to detect antifungal resistance and find out therapeutic option for fungal diseases. Microdilution AFST is the gold standard and both CLSI and EUCAST have defined their own breakpoints for AFST — which are followed worldwide. However, the method is time-consuming and labour-intensive. Breakpoints referred by CLSI and EUCAST (Alastruey-Izquierdo et al., 2015) are depicted in Table 11.1 below. CLSI has recommended following concentration ranges of the different antifungal drugs to be tested for MIC determination - amphotericin B - 0.0313—16 µg/mL; flucytosine - 0.125—64 µg/mL; ketoconazole - 0.0313—16 µg/mL; itraconazole - 0.0313—16 µg/mL; fluconazole - 0.125—64 µg/mL; and new triazoles - 0.0313—16 µg/ mL. Most of these antifungal agents such as amphotericin B, ketoconazole and itraconazole are not water soluble and need to be dissolved in organic diluents - dimethyl sulfoxide (DMSO), ethyl alcohol, polyethylene glycol and carboxymethyl cellulose at least 100 times higher than the highest desired test concentration. RPMI 1640 (with glutamine, without bicarbonate and with phenol red as a pH indicator) buffered to a pH of 7.0 ± 0.1 at 25°C using MOPS [3-(N-morpholino) propanesulfonic acid] is generally preferred medium for conducting AFST using broth dilution method. Pure and viable culture obtained from an overnight culture in Sabouraud dextrose agar or potato dextrose agar is used for the preparation of inoculum. Following incubation, at 35°C for 24 h (for Candida) or 48 h (for C. neoformans) 5-6 one-mm colonies are suspended in 0.85% normal saline solution for 0.5 McFarland standard for inoculation. The inoculated tubes should be incubated for 46—50 h at 35°C and in case of C. neoformans incubation period should be extended to 70—74 h. In general, for testing the susceptibility of the yeast, an inoculum containing 0.5 to 2.5 × 10³ CFU/mL should be used in RPMI-1640 and incubated at 35°C for 48 h to decide over the MIC level. EUCAST had recommended adding dextrose to facilitate the growth of yeast so as to reduce the incubation period up to 24 h (Fothergill et al., 2006) in addition to reduce the incubation temperature to 30°C in case the control fails to achieve optimum growth point (OD: 0.2) at 35°C (Alastruey-Izquierdo et al., 2015).

With regard to MIC of Candida for amphotericin B, the break-points are well defined in EUCAST. According to EUCAST, all the Candida sp (C. albicans, C. glabrata, C. krusei, C. parapsilosis and C. tropicalis) with MIC <1 µg/mL are categorized as susceptible whereas those with MIC >1 µg/mL are classified as resistant (Lass-Flörl et al., 2011). The interpretative criteria for amphotericin B has not been defined in the CLSI and Pfaller and Diekema, 2012 fixed 2 µg/ml as the epidemiological cutoff value for amphotericin B in all species of Candida; the isolates with MIC >2 µg/mL were designated as wild type and those with MIC ≤2 µg/mL were categorized as non-wild type (Pfaller and Diekema, 2012); another group of workers suggested that the isolates with MICs <1 µg/mL for amphotericin B to be considered as susceptible while isolates with MICs ≥2 µg/mL as resistant (Yenisehirli et al., 2015). Previously CLSI had recommended single interpretive breakpoints for azole and echinocandins. However, it was revised later and species-specific breakpoints were established based on clinical studies. Details are described in Table 11.1. No breakpoints for ketoconazole are suggested by CLSI. However, Yenisehirli et al., 2015 recommended that *Candida albicans* isolates with MIC ≤ 0.125 μg/mL for ketoconazole to be considered susceptible, isolates with MICs from 0.25 μg/mL to 0.5 μg/mL dose-dependently susceptible and isolates with MICs ≥ 1 μg/mL as resistant (Yenisehirli et al., 2015). Similarly, for posaconazole for which also no CLSI breakpoint is available, the workers mentioned isolates with MICs ≤ 0.125 μg/mL susceptible, isolates with $\leq 0.25 - 0.5$ μg/mL intermediate and isolates with ≥ 1 μg/mL resistant.

Although, EUCAST breakpoints are available for the micafungin and anidulafungin, such breakpoints are not established for caspofungin due to significant inter-laboratory variation. A study from India suggested the following breakpoints for caspofungin; however, it was a mere reflection of their observation with 60 preserved *Candida* isolates from a tertiary care teaching hospital — isolates with MICs ≤ 0.25 μg/mL for *C. albicans* and *C. tropicalis*, MICs ≤ 0.12 μg/mL for *C. glabrata* and MICs ≤ 2 μg/mL for *Candida parapsilosis* were determined susceptible; isolates with MICs 0.5 μg/mL for *C. albicans* and *C. tropicalis*, MIC of 0.25 μg/mL for *C. glabrata* and MIC of 4 μg/mL for *C. parapsilosis* were considered intermediate; finally, the isolates with MICs ≥ 1 μg/mL for *C. albicans* and *C. tropicalis*, MIC ≥ 0.5 μg/mL for *C. glabrata* MIC ≥ 8 μg/mL for *C. parapsilosis* were categorized resistant (Yenisehirli et al., 2015). Previously, CLSI recommended the same clinical breakpoints for caspofungin, micafungin and anidulafungin. However, based on their observation in relation to MICs for different echinocandins of wild and mutated strains of *Candia*, Pfaller et al., 2011 laid down species-specific CBPs as follows - in *C. albicans*, *C. tropicalis* and *C. krusei*, isolates with MIC for caspofungin/micafungin/anidulafungin ≤ 0.25 mcg/mL to be interpreted as sensitive, isolates with MIC of 0.5 mcg/mL to be categorized intermediate and isolates with MIC of ≥ 1 mcg/mL to be taken resistant; in *C. parapsilosis*, MIC of ≤ 2 mcg/mL, MIC of 4 mcg/mL and MIC of ≥ 8 mcg/mL to be treated as breakpoints for sensitive, intermediate and resistant isolates, respectively; for *C. glabrata*, the recommended CBPs for anidulafungin and caspofungin were ≤ 0.12 mcg/mL (S), 0.25 mcg/mL (I) and ≥ 0.5 mcg/mL (R), whereas those for micafungin were ≤ 0.06 mcg/mL (S), 0.12 mcg/mL (I) and ≥ 0.25 mcg/mL (R).

Disk tests are easy to perform and inexpensive. However, disk test has limited scope except in evaluating the effectiveness of azoles and echinocandins for *Candida* spp. isolates. MH agar containing 2% glucose and 0.5 mg/L methylene blue dye with a pH of 7.2−7.4 is usually recommended for performing disk tests. The agar should have a thickness of at least 4 cm. Following inoculation with 0.5 McFarland of inoculum, the plates should be incubated for a period of 24 h at 35°C. In case of insufficient growth, incubation may be extended for another 24 h. Results obtained from disk test was found 90% in agreement with MIC values for azole (fluconazole and voriconazole) in case of *Candida* and *Cryptococcus* spp. The disk diffusion test was reported to detect the fluconazole-resistance in *Candida* using a 25 mg fluconazole disk after 24 h of incubation (Kirkpatrick et al., 1998).

One major drawback of AFST is the time and labour it involves; isolation, harvesting and MIC determination for fungus may altogether take a long period which can compromise the clinical outcome the patients due to delay in appropriate therapeutic intervention. In this context, genotypic tools may be alternatively used in sophisticated laboratories in such cases, where the utility of genetic tools in determining antifungal resistance is unequivocally established. The genetic machinery was successfully employed in detection of mutant *Aspergillus fumigatus* strains which had become azole (itraconazole)-resistant due the point mutations in the 14α-sterol demethylases (*cyp51A* and *cyp51B*) genes; the mutation and thereby the azole resistance can be easily captured by amplifying and sequencing of full coding region of *cyp*51A and *cyp*51B (Diaz-Guerra et al., 2003). The PCR should be carried out for 32 cycles consisting of 1 cycle of 5 min at 94°C, 45 s at 58°C and 2 min at 72°C, and then 30 cycles of 30 s at 94°C, 45 s at 58°C and 2 min at 72°C, followed by one final cycle similar to the previous one but with 10 min at 72°C. Workers found molecular tools useful in the detection of fluconazole/azole resistance in *Candida* sp, most commonly driven by point mutation in *ERG5* or *ERG11* genes encoding C22-desaturase and lanosterol demethylase (14α-demethylase) enzymes, or by increased expression of ERG11 (Warnock, 1992). Entire ERG11 open reading frame can be amplified using the primers −ERG11-1F and ERG11-1R (Perea et al., 2002). The PCR is carried out in a 100-μL volume containing 100 ng of genomic DNA; each primer at a concentration of 300 nM; dATP, dGTP, dCTP and dTTP, each at a concentration of 350 μM; 1.75 mM PCR buffer with $MgCl_2$; and 0.75 μL of an enzyme mixture (Thermo stable *Taq* and *Pwo* polymerases) as suggested, previously. PCR cycle is consisted of 1 cycle of 4 min at 94°C and then for 30 cycles (30 s at 94°C, 1 min at 54°C and 2 min at 68°C) and this is to be followed by 1 final cycle for 7 min at 68°C. The PCR products can be purified and sequenced for mutation detection. For amplification of ERG 5 and ERG 11, other sets of primers were also described by a separate group of workers (Martel et al., 2010) to amplify the entire length of the respective

TABLE 11.2 Oligonucleotides used for detection of azole-resistant fungus.

Sl No	Genes	Oligonucleotides (5'-3')	Reference
1	ERG11-1F	GCG GAT CCT TAA AAC ATA CAA GTT TCT CTT TT	Perea et al. (2002)
	ERG11-1R	ACG CGT CGA CAA TAT GGC TAT TGT TGA AAC TGT C	
2	ERG11-2F	ATGGATATCGTACTAGAA	Martel et al. (2010)
	ERG11-2R	TCATTGTTCAACATATTC	
3	ERG5-F	ATGAATTCAACAGAGGTC	
	ERG-5R	CTATAAACTCTTTAATGG	
4	cyp51A P450-F	ATGGTGCCGATGCTATGG	Diaz-Guerra et al. (2003)
	cyp51A P450-F	CTGTC-TCACTTGGATGTG	
5	cyp51B P450-F	ATGGGTCTCATCGCGTTC	
	cyp51B P450-R	TCAGGCTTTGGTAGCGG	
6	CDR1F	AAGAGAACCATTACCAGG	Monroy-Pérez et al. (2016)
	CDR1R	AGGAATCGACGGATCAC	
7	MDR1F	GGAGTTTAGGTGCTGT	
	MDR1R	CGGTGATGGCTCTCAA	
8	C albicans *cpy51*F	AGATCATAACTCAATATGGC	Asai et al. (1999)
	C albicans *cpy51*R	GTTGAGCAAATGAACGGTCA	

genes (Table 11.2). As was described previously, mutation in the CPY-51 gene is known to cause azole-resistance in *C albicans* also and Asai et al., 1999 described a protocol to amplify a 673-bp fragment covering the potential polymorphic region of the gene using the specific primers (Table 11.2) and subsequent restriction-analysis or sequencing can determine mutation/polymorphism (Asai et al., 1999).

In addition, overexpression of ABC-transporter-family genes such as CDR1, CDR2 and MDR1 is responsible for azole resistance in *Candida* spp; thus, monitoring the expression profile of these gene(s) can provide an important clue as described by others (Monroy-Pérez et al., 2016). Following synthesis of cDNA, PCR is to be carried out using the primers described in Table 11.2 in 25 μL final volume consisting of 12.5 μL of SYBR Green Master Mix, 1 μL of forward primer (1 μM), 1 μL of reverse primer (1 μM), 2 μL of cDNA (~20 ng) and 8.5 μL RNase-free water.

Status present

Till date, limited information is available regarding antifungal resistance in the veterinary sector, although it is not uncommon in human. The invasive fungal infection, a common nuisance at healthcare settings, is known to cause substantial morbidity and mortality and can only be managed following aggressive and expensive treatment protocol. In the USA, invasive candidiasis (IC) is recognized as one of the most common causes for hospital-borne bloodstream infection with 46,000 new cases being reported each year (Anonymous, 2019). Interestingly among IC, non-*albicans* species are being recorded more frequently than *C. albicans*; it includes *C. glabrata, C. parapsilosis, C. tropicalis, C. krusei, C. lusitaniae, C. guilliermondii* and *C. dubliniensis* especially in haematological malignancies (Mikulska et al., 2011; Sabino et al., 2010; Uzun and Anaissie, 2000; Pfeiffer, 2001). It is a cause of further concern that many of the non-*albicans* species - especially *C. glabrata* and *C. krusei* were recorded to exhibit resistance to first and second line antifungal drugs - fluconazole and echinocandins (Garnacho-Montero et al., 2010; Forastiero et al., 2015; Perlin, 2015; Berkow and Lockhart, 2017). Reports from the CDC revealed that almost 7% of the *Candida*-associated blood stream infections mostly caused by *C. glabrata* were found fluconazole-resistant. However, the proportion of fluconazole-resistant *Candida* has remained fairly constant for the past 20—25 year, whereas echinocandin resistance is on the rise, with approximately 3% of *C. glabrata* isolates being resistant to echinocandins. Such emerging trend of echinocandin resistance was also reiterated by another group of workers, as well (Beyda et al., 2012; Alexander et al., 2013); this is quite alarming, as echinocandin still remains the frontline remedy for *C. glabrata* infection. It is not uncommon to notice simultaneous resistance to fluconazole and echinocandin — a cause of concern for the critically ill patients for whom clinicians would prefer not to use drugs such as amphotericin B because of toxicity (Arendrup and Patterson, 2017). Information regarding fungal resistance is limited and only based on a few systemic epidemiological studies most of which were conducted in the USA and European countries. One of such large surveillance programme, conducted with 256882 *Candida* isolates of 31 different species from 41 countries for a period of 11 years (1997—2007), revealed that 90.2% of the isolates tested were fluconazole-susceptible, but around 13 of the 31 species identified in this survey exhibit decreased fluconazole susceptibility-which included *C. parapsilosis, C. guilliermondii, C. lusitaniae, C. sake* and *C. pelliculosa, C. glabrata* and *C. krusei* — a clear indication of growing fluconazole-resistance among the non-*albicans* (Pfaller et al., 2010). In a separate study conducted in Spain involving 773 cases of IC revealed that almost 21% of the *Candida* was fluconazole-non-susceptible, while about 0.3% of *C. albicans* and 3.4% of *C. glabrata* was reported echinocandin-resistant (Puig-Asensio et al., 2014). Decreased fluconazole susceptibility among the *Candida* isolates also came up in another surveillance study in Denmark covering 303 cases of IC (Arendrup et al., 2005).

In recent years, several studies reported the frequent occurrence of invasive (IA) and pulmonary aspergillosis (caused by *A. fumigatus*) in human with critically ill patients with profound neutropenia and those with the pulmonary obstructive disease are at high risk (Gamson et al., 2014; Kousha et al., 2011). Increasing evidence of antifungal resistance among filamentous fungi/moulds such as *A. fumigatus* associated with IFD has emerged as a grave problem particularly among the recipients of haematopoietic stem cell transplant (HSCT) and solid organ transplant (SOT) because of prolonged immunosuppressive treatment — a condition that favours the aspergillus spores to invade and multiply (Trnacevic et al., 2018). Azole-resistance linked to a point mutation of the gene CYP51A, that encodes 14α-sterol demethylase, was noted among *A. fumigatus* - the most common cause of invasive aspergillosis (Lelièvre et al., 2013). The real incidence of azole-resistant *A. fumigatus* is not known. Yet azole resistance has been observed to increase over time since its first detection from the UK in 1997 and spread beyond the European countries to the Middle East, China and India (Warris, 2015; Lelièvre et al., 2013; Chowdhary et al., 2013). In the Netherland, the prevalence of azole-resistant aspergillosis was found to vary from below 2% to more than 12% depending on the geographical region and the hospitals included in the study (Buil et al., 2019). In the UK the prevalence of itraconazole-resistant *Aspergillus* gradually increased to 20% in 2009 from 5% in 2004. In one of the recent studies conducted at a specialized cardio-thoracic centre in London revealed the presence of triazole-resistant *Aspergillus fumigatus* from 18 of the 135 (13.3%) patients, including 12 of the 74 (16.2%) patients with cystic fibrosis (CF), the patient between 11 and 20 years being at the highest risk (Abdolrasouli et al., 2018). Sporadic azole resistance was reported from various other European countries — Germany, France, Belgium, Denmark, Spain and other parts of the world like Iran, China and India (Vermeulen et al., 2013; Chowdhary et al., 2012).

Little is known about the resistance of the fungal pathogens of animal origin. Recent investigation carried out on the azole-resistance pattern of *C. albicans* isolates of animal origin by Rocha et al., 2017 indicated high degree of fluconazole and itraconazole -resistance mediated by increased efflux pump activity (CDR1/2; MDR1 and EGR11) and the overexpression of different genes (Rocha et al., 2017). Such fluconazole resistance was also reported in *Candida parapsilosis* complex isolated from animals in recent past where most of the isolates were found bio-film producing (Brilhante et al., 2014). The paucity of literature on antifungal resistance in animals does not indicate that the gravity of the problem is less in veterinary sector by any means and previous exposure to antifungal drug in the form of therapy may not be the sole precondition for recovery of a resistant fungus from a particular animal; the recovery of azole-resistant *C. albicans* from a wild Brazilian porcupine (*Coendou prehensilis*) is the evidence of it (Castelo-Branco et al., 2013). Again *Candida tropicalis* isolated from diverse aquatic and terrestrial animals (goat, sheep, horse, psittacines etc) exhibited high rate of azole-resistance (De Aguiar Cordeiro et al., 2015). A multi-resistant *Lecythophora hoffmannii* (*Coniochaeta hoffmannii*), an ascomycete fungus — that is rarely known to cause serious infection was isolated from a 2-year-old spayed female mongrel dog with osteomyelitis. The isolate was found resistant to amphotericin B, 5-FC, fluconazole, itraconazole, miconazole and micafungin (Sakaeyama et al., 2007).

A brief illustration of animal mycotic diseased is desiderated in Table 11.3.

TABLE 11.3 Mycotic disease of food and pet animals (Joseph, 2019).

Sl No	Diseases	Pathogenic agent	Hosts	Clinical symptoms	Pathological changes	Treatment
1	Blastomycosis	*Blastomyces dermatitidis*	Dogs and cats apart from human being	Mostly pulmonary form with fever, severe cough, weight loss, dyspnoea and lymphadenopathy. Ocular and cutaneous form may be also seen. Formation of granulomatous lesion over skin and discharge of serosanguineous fluid from ulcerative lesions. Dysuria and haematuria in urogenital form.	Nodular pyogranulomas in various organ.	Itraconazole (5 mg/kg/day) for 6–8 weeks. In severe form, combination treatment with amphotericin B may be given
2	Rhinosporidiosis	*Rhinosporidium seeberi*	Cattle, horse and other pet animals	Severe dyspnoea, hemorrhagic nasal discharge. Cutaneous lesions may be developed.	Large polyps in the nasal cavity and posterior nares.	Surgical excision is recommended. Itraconazole and amphotericin B may be tried.
3	Candidiasis	Mostly by *Candida albicans*. Non–*C. albicans* may be also involved.	Cattle, pigs, sheep, foals, birds, dogs and cats	Cattle with gastrointestinal (GI) candidiasis mostly suffer from diarrhoea, dehydration, inappetence and gradual emaciation. Likewise, pigs with oral or gastric candidiasis also suffer from diarrhoea and weight loss. Loss of condition with poor growth rate is observed in chicks. Intestinal forms are also seen in horses.	Lesions may involve GI tract, especially tongue, oesophagus and forestomach with hyperkeratinization and destruction of mucosal layer.	Topical application of amphotericin B, nystatin and iodine solution are effective. Systematic application of amphotericin B and fluconazole was also indicated.
4	Epizootic lymphangitis (Pseudoglanders/equine cryptococcosis) (Al-Ani, 1999)	*Histoplasmosis farciminosi*	Equines Rarely among camels, cattle and humans	Formation of subcutaneous hard nodules, which may subsequently enlarge and rupture. The infection usually spreads through lymphatic vessels forming cord-like lesion. Surrounding tissues are usually painful and oedematous. Keratoconjunctivitis and arthritis may be seen in a few cases.	Nodular lesions are formed across the lymphatic duct.	Treatment is not successful. Surgical intervention may be adopted along with the application of amphotericin B.

Continued

TABLE 11.3 Mycotic disease of food and pet animals (Joseph, 2019).—cont'd

SI No	Diseases	Pathogenic agent	Hosts	Clinical symptoms	Pathological changes	Treatment
5	Sporotrichosis	*Sporothrix schenckii*	Various domestic, pet and wild animals	Generally, three forms are observed: lymphocutaneous, cutaneous and disseminated forms. There is formation of subcutaneous or dermal nodules, which may rupture with serosanguineous discharges. It may spread to distant organs such as the bone, lungs, liver, spleen, testes, GI tract or brain via haematogenous or tissue routes to establish disseminated forms.	Formation of hard ulcerating nodules in the dermal or subcutaneous layers in visceral organs.	Itraconazole at 10 mg/kg/day to be continued for 3–4 weeks. Other alternatives include terbinafine and potassium iodide.
6	Coccidioidomycosis	*Coccidioides immitis*	Primarily dogs, cat, nonhuman primates. Other animals may be affected	Respiratory illness, infection of bones and joints, ophthalmic and cutaneous infection. Infection may be asymptomatic. However, the disseminated fatal form may result in chronic persistent cough, pulsating temperature, dyspnoea, anorexia, diarrhoea, weight loss, swelling of the joints, anaemia, oedema of legs and peripheral lymphadenopathy. In cutaneous form, chronic indurated ulceration with thick mucopurulent discharges may be observed over the skin (Beaudin et al., 2005). Cats often present cutaneous form of the disease. Death may occur due to sudden rupture of liver.	Formation of nodules in various organs especially in the lung, thoracic cavity and mediastinal or thoracic lymph nodes. Pericarditis may be also observed in dogs (Shubitz et al., 2001). Marked leucocytosis.	Fluconazole (2.5–10 mg/kg/day) is known to be the most effective remedy for chronic and disseminated respiratory form of the disease. Other drugs include ketoconazole (10–30 mg/kg/day) and itraconazole (10 mg/kg/day), although they are bit expensive options. Amphotericin B is known to be highly effective. However, its severe nephrotoxicity limits use. In any case, long-term antifungal therapy is warranted for the patients. Recently, nikkomycin Z was found effective for treatment of respiratory coccidioidomycosis in naturally infected dogs (Shubitz et al., 2013).
7	Histoplasmosis	*Histoplasma capsulatum*	Dogs and cats	No typical symptom can be noted. Symptoms may involve diarrhoea, chronic weight loss, anorexia and protracted fever.	Diffuse pulmonary and peritoneal effusion, lymphadenopathy, hepatosplenomegaly, anaemia, leucocytosis and thrombocytopenia may be noted depending on the spread of infection (Duse et al., 2016; Lau et al., 1978; VanSteenhouse and DeNovo, 1986; Clinkenbeard et al., 1988).	Itraconazole (10 mg/kg/day) or ketoconazole 10–15 mg/kg bid may be given for a long period, i.e., 4–6 months.

#	Disease	Organism	Animals affected	Clinical signs	Lesions	Treatment
8	Dermatophytosis	*Microsporum canis, Trichophyton mentagrophytes, Microsporum gypseum.*	Dogs, cats, horses, cows and other mammals	Generally circular patches of alopecia with red circular inflammation in a ring shape. Itching	Generally, superficial layer of skin, hairs and nails are affected.	Infection may be complicated and refractory and may not respond to the topical application. Griseofulvin and alternately ketoconazole, itraconazole and fluconazole can be used.
9	Cryptococcosis	*Cryptococcus neoformans, Cryptococcus gattii*	Generally in cats. But dogs, cattle, horses, sheep, goats, birds and wild animals are also affected	Generally known to appear in four forms – cutaneous, ocular, nasal and cerebral forms. In cats, nasal forms appear with chronic nasal discharge which may be hemorrhagic, sneezing and polyps-like growth in the nasal cavity. The cerebral form appears with stiffness, hyperaesthesia, incoordination, convulsion, high prostration, change in behaviour, depression, paralysis or paresis, circling and blindness. Ocular forms include panophthalmitis, optic neuritis, retinal abnormality and blindness. Mastitis in cows with thick watery milk and enlarged supramammary lymph nodes	Lesions in nasal mucosa, pulmonary abscess, pneumonia, peripheral lymphadenopathy, lymphadenitis, placentitis, lymphocutaneous and abortion.	Fluconazole (2.5–10 mg/kg/day) or itraconazole (10 mg/kg/day) is the first line of treatment. Amphotericin B can be given SC (0.5–0.8 mg/kg) diluted in dextrose saline solution can be given. Flucytosine can be used alone or in combination with amphotericin B to avoid resistance.

Continued

TABLE 11.3 Mycotic disease of food and pet animals (Joseph, 2019).—cont'd

Sl No	Diseases	Pathogenic agent	Hosts	Clinical symptoms	Pathological changes	Treatment
10	Rhinosporidiosis	*Rhinosporidium seeberi*	Horses, cattle, dogs and cats	Usually, large growth develops in the nasal mucosa or in the skin. Masses may be large enough to occlude the nasal cavity or passage.	Lesions are characterized by granulomatous reactions in the nasal mucosa and skin.	Surgical excision is recommended.
11	Pythiosis	*Pythium insidiosum*	Horse and dogs	Large fistulas with nodules are developed in several parts of the body of horses such as the abdomen, chest and genitalia. Subcutaneous oedema may be noted. In dogs, GI tract involvement is more common.	In the horse, the nodules are usually characterized by firm fibrous tissue with necrotic foci and coagulative necrosis. Pyogranulomatous lesions with infiltration of PMN cells and giant cells.	Surgical excision of the masses is required. Long-term therapy includes the application of itraconazole (10 mg/kg/day) and terbinafine (5–10 mg/kg/day) or amphotericin B depending on the severity.

References

Abdolrasouli, A., Scourfield, A., Rhodes, J., Shah, A., Elborn, J.S., Fisher, M.C., et al., 2018. High prevalence of triazole resistance in clinical *Aspergillus fumigatus* isolates in a specialist cardiothoracic centre. International Journal of Antimicrobial Agents 52, 637–642. https://doi.org/10.1016/j.ijantimicag.2018.08.004.

Al-Ani, F.K., 1999. Epizootic lymphangitis in horses: a review of literature. Revue Scientifique et Technique (l'OIE) 18, 691–699. https://doi.org/10.20506/rst.18.3.1186.

Alanio, A., Cordonnier, C., Bretagne, S., 2011. Azole resistance in *Aspergillus fumigatus*—current epidemiology and future perspectives. Current Fungal Infection Reports 5, 168–178. https://doi.org/10.1007/s12281-011-0061-y.

Alastruey-Izquierdo, A., Melhem, M.S.C., Bonfietti, L.X., Rodriguez-Tudela, J.L., 2015. Susceptibility test for fungi: clinical and laboratorial correlations in medical mycology. Revista do Instituto de Medicina Tropical de Sao Paulo 57 (Suppl. 1), 57–64. https://doi.org/10.1590/S0036-46652015000700011.

Alexander, B.D., Johnson, M.D., Pfeiffer, C.D., Jiménez-Ortigosa, C., Catania, J., Booker, R., et al., 2013. Increasing echinocandin resistance in candida glabrata: clinical failure correlates with presence of FKS mutations and elevated minimum inhibitory concentrations. Clinical Infectious Diseases 56, 1724–1732. https://doi.org/10.1093/cid/cit136.

Anonymous, 2019. Statistics | Invasive Candidiasis | Candidiasis | Types of Diseases | Fungal Diseases | CDC. https://www.cdc.gov/fungal/diseases/candidiasis/invasive/statistics.html.

Arendrup, M.C., Patterson, T.F., 2017. Multidrug-resistant *Candida*: epidemiology, molecular mechanisms, and treatment. The Journal of Infectious Diseases 216, S445–S451. https://doi.org/10.1093/infdis/jix131.

Arendrup, M.C., Fuursted, K., Gahrn-Hansen, B., Jensen, I.M., Knudsen, J.D., Lundgren, B., et al., 2005. Seminational surveillance of fungemia in Denmark: notably high rates of fungemia and numbers of isolates with reduced azole susceptibility. Journal of Clinical Microbiology 43, 4434–4440. https://doi.org/10.1128/JCM.43.9.4434-4440.2005.

Asai, K., Tsuchimori, N., Okonogi, K., Perfect, J.R., Gotoh, O., Yoshida, Y., 1999. Formation of azole-resistant *Candida albicans* by mutation of sterol 14- demethylase P450. Antimicrobial Agents and Chemotherapy 43, 1163–1169.

Bagshaw, E., Enoch, D., Blackney, M., Posthumus, J., Kuessner, D., 2018. Economic impact of treating invasive mold disease with isavuconazole compared with liposomal amphotericin B in the UK. Future Microbiology. https://doi.org/10.2217/fmb-2018-0119 fmb-2018-0119.

Beaudin, S., Rich, L.J., Meinkoth, J.H., Cowell, R.L., 2005. Draining skin lesion from a desert poodle. Veterinary Clinical Pathology 34, 65–68.

Berkow, E., Lockhart, S., 2017. Fluconazole resistance in *Candida* species: a current perspective. Infection and Drug Resistance 10, 237–245. https://doi.org/10.2147/IDR.S118892.

Beyda, N.D., Lewis, R.E., Garey, K.W., 2012. Echinocandin resistance in *Candida* species: mechanisms of reduced susceptibility and therapeutic approaches. The Annals of Pharmacotherapy 46, 1086–1096. https://doi.org/10.1345/aph.1R020.

Bongomin, F., Gago, S., Oladele, R., Denning, D., 2017. Global and multi-national prevalence of fungal diseases—estimate precision. Journal of Fungi 3, 57. https://doi.org/10.3390/jof3040057.

Brilhante, R.S.N., Rodrigues, T. d. JS., Castelo-Branco, D. d. SCM., Teixeira, C.E.C., Macedo, R. d. B., Bandeira, S.P., et al., 2014. Antifungal susceptibility and virulence attributes of animal-derived isolates of Candida parapsilosis complex. Journal of Medical Microbiology 63, 1568–1572. https://doi.org/10.1099/jmm.0.076216-0.

Buil, J.B., Snelders, E., Denardi, L.B., Melchers, W.J.G., Verweij, P.E., 2019. Trends in azole resistance in *Aspergillus fumigatus*, The Netherlands, 1994–2016. Emerging Infectious Diseases 25, 176–178. https://doi.org/10.3201/eid2501.171925.

Castelo-Branco, D.S.C.M., Brilhante, R.S.N., Paiva, M.A.N., Teixeira, C.E.C., Caetano, E.P., Ribeiro, J.F., et al., 2013. Azole-resistant Candida albicans from a wild Brazilian porcupine (*Coendou prehensilis*): a sign of an environmental imbalance? Medical Mycology 51, 555–560. https://doi.org/10.3109/13693786.2012.752878.

Chen, L.M., Xu, Y.H., Zhou, C.L., Zhao, J., Li, C.Y., Wang, R., 2010. Overexpression of CDR1 and CDR2 genes plays an important role in fluconazole resistance in *Candida albicans* with G487T and T916C mutations. Journal of International Medical Research 38, 536–545. https://doi.org/10.1177/147323001003800216.

Chen, S.C.A., Slavin, M.A., Sorrell, T.C., 2011. Echinocandin antifungal drugs in fungal infections. Drugs 71, 11–41. https://doi.org/10.2165/11585270-000000000-00000.

Chowdhary, A., Kathuria, S., Xu, J., Sharma, C., Sundar, G., Singh, P.K., et al., 2012. Clonal expansion and emergence of environmental multiple-triazole-resistant *Aspergillus fumigatus* strains carrying the TR34/L98H mutations in the cyp51A gene in India. PLoS One 7, e52871. https://doi.org/10.1371/journal.pone.0052871.

Chowdhary, A., Kathuria, S., Xu, J., Meis, J.F., 2013. Emergence of azole-resistant *Aspergillus fumigatus* strains due to agricultural azole use creates an increasing threat to human health. PLoS Pathogens 9, e1003633. https://doi.org/10.1371/journal.ppat.1003633.

Clinkenbeard, K.D., Cowell, R.L., Tyler, R.D., 1988. Identification of *Histoplasma* organisms in circulating eosinophils of a dog. Journal of the American Veterinary Medical Association 192, 217–218.

Da Silva Ferreira, M.E., Luiz Capellaro, J., Dos Reis Marques, E., Malavazi, I., Perlin, D., Park, S., et al., 2004. In vitro evolution of itraconazole resistance in *Aspergillus fumigatus* involves multiple mechanisms of resistance. Antimicrobial Agents and Chemotherapy 48, 4405–4413. https://doi.org/10.1128/AAC.48.11.4405-4413.2004.

De Aguiar Cordeiro, R., De Oliveira, J.S., De Souza Collares Maia Castelo-Branco, D., Teixeira, C.E.C., De Farias Marques, F.J., Bittencourt, P.V., et al., 2015. *Candida tropicalis* isolates obtained from veterinary sources show resistance to azoles and produce virulence factors. Medical Mycology 53, 145–152. https://doi.org/10.1093/mmy/myu081.

Denning, D.W., 2003. Echinocandin antifungal drugs. Lancet 362, 1142−1151. https://doi.org/10.1016/S0140-6736(03)14472-8.

Diaz-Guerra, T.M., Mellado, E., Cuenca-Estrella, M., Rodriguez-Tudela, J.L., 2003. A point mutation in the 14 -sterol demethylase gene cyp51A contributes to itraconazole resistance in *Aspergillus fumigatus*. Antimicrobial Agents and Chemotherapy 47, 1120−1124. https://doi.org/10.1128/AAC.47.3.1120-1124.2003.

Duse, A., Persson Waller, K., Emanuelson, U., Ericsson Unnerstad, H., Persson, Y., Bengtsson, B., 2016. Occurrence and spread of quinolone-resistant *Escherichia coli* on dairy farms. Applied and Environmental Microbiology 82, 3765−3773. https://doi.org/10.1128/AEM.03061-15.

Eddouzi, J., Parker, J.E., Vale-Silva, L.A., Coste, A., Ischer, F., Kelly, S., et al., 2013. Molecular mechanisms of drug resistance in clinical *Candida* species isolated from Tunisian hospitals. Antimicrobial Agents and Chemotherapy 57, 3182−3193. https://doi.org/10.1128/AAC.00555-13.

Elewa, H., El-Mekaty, E., El-Bardissy, A., Ensom, M.H.H., Wilby, K.J., 2015. Therapeutic drug monitoring of voriconazole in the management of invasive fungal infections: a critical review. Clinical Pharmacokinetics 54, 1223−1235. https://doi.org/10.1007/s40262-015-0297-8.

Flowers, S.A., Colón, B., Whaley, S.G., Schuler, M.A., Rogers, P.D., 2015. Contribution of clinically derived mutations in ERG11 to azole resistance in *Candida albicans*. Antimicrobial Agents and Chemotherapy 59, 450−460. https://doi.org/10.1128/AAC.03470-14.

Forastiero, A., Garcia-Gil, V., Rivero-Menendez, O., Garcia-Rubio, R., Monteiro, M.C., Alastruey-Izquierdo, A., et al., 2015. Rapid development of *Candida krusei* echinocandin resistance during caspofungin therapy. Antimicrobial Agents and Chemotherapy 59, 6975−6982. https://doi.org/10.1128/AAC.01005-15.

Fothergill, A.W., Rinaldi, M.G., Sutton, D.A., 2006. Antifungal susceptibility testing. Infectious Disease Clinics of North America 20, 699−709. https://doi.org/10.1016/j.idc.2006.06.008.

Gamson, K., Ding, Y., Aronowitz, P., 2014. Invasive aspergillosis. Journal of General Internal Medicine 29, 686−687. https://doi.org/10.1007/s11606-013-2584-0.

Garnacho-Montero, J., Diaz-Martin, A., Garcia-Cabrera, E., Ruiz Perez de Pipaon, M., Hernandez-Caballero, C., Aznar-Martin, J., et al., 2010. Risk factors for fluconazole-resistant candidemia. Antimicrobial Agents and Chemotherapy 54, 3149−3154. https://doi.org/10.1128/AAC.00479-10.

Ghannoum, M.A., Rice, L.B., 1999. Antifungal agents: mode of action, mechanisms of resistance, and correlation of these mechanisms with bacterial resistance. Clinical Microbiology Reviews 12, 501−517.

Groll, A.H., Walsh, T.J., 2009. Antifungal polyenes. *Aspergillus fumigatus* and aspergillosis. American Society of Microbiology 391−415. https://doi.org/10.1128/9781555815523.ch30.

Hahn-Ast, C., Glasmacher, A., Mückter, S., Schmitz, A., Kraemer, A., Marklein, G., et al., 2010. Overall survival and fungal infection-related mortality in patients with invasive fungal infection and neutropenia after myelosuppressive chemotherapy in a tertiary care centre from 1995 to 2006. Journal of Antimicrobial Chemotherapy 65, 761−768. https://doi.org/10.1093/jac/dkp507.

Joseph, T., 2019. Overview of Fungal Infections. MSD Veterinary manual.

Kirkpatrick, W.R., Turner, T.M., Fothergill, A.W., McCarthy, D.I., Redding, S.W., Rinaldi, M.G., et al., 1998. Fluconazole disk diffusion susceptibility testing of *Candida* species. Journal of Clinical Microbiology 36, 3429−3432.

Kontoyiannis, D.P., Lewis, R.E., 2002. Antifungal drug resistance of pathogenic fungi. Lancet 359, 1135−1144. https://doi.org/10.1016/S0140-6736(02)08162-X.

Kousha, M., Tadi, R., Soubani, A.O., 2011. Pulmonary aspergillosis: a clinical review. European Respiratory Review 20, 156−174. https://doi.org/10.1183/09059180.00001011.

Lass-Flörl, C., Arendrup, M.C., Rodriguez-Tudela, J.-L., Cuenca-Estrella, M., Donnelly, P., Hope, W., 2011. EUCAST technical note on amphotericin B. Clinical Microbiology and Infections 17, E27−E29. https://doi.org/10.1111/j.1469-0691.2011.03644.x.

Lau, R.E., Kim, S.N., Pirozok, R.P., 1978. *Histoplasma capsulatum* infection in a metatarsal of a dog. Journal of the American Veterinary Medical Association 172, 1414−1416.

Lelièvre, L., Groh, M., Angebault, C., Maherault, A.-C., Didier, E., Bougnoux, M.-E., 2013. Azole resistant *Aspergillus fumigatus*: an emerging problem. Medecine et Maladies Infectieuses 43, 139−145. https://doi.org/10.1016/j.medmal.2013.02.010.

Lupetti, A., Danesi, R., Campa, M., Del Tacca, M., Kelly, S., 2002 Feb 1. Molecular basis of resistance to azole antifungals. Trends in molecular medicine 8 (2), 76−81.

Martel, C.M., Parker, J.E., Bader, O., Weig, M., Gross, U., Warrilow, A.G.S., et al., 2010. A clinical isolate of *Candida albicans* with mutations in ERG11 (encoding sterol 14 -demethylase) and ERG5 (encoding C22 desaturase) is cross resistant to azoles and amphotericin B. Antimicrobial Agents and Chemotherapy 54, 3578−3583. https://doi.org/10.1128/AAC.00303-10.

Mikulska, M., Bassetti, M., Ratto, S., Viscoli, C., 2011. Invasive candidiasis in non-hematological patients. Mediterranean Journal of Hematology and Infectious Diseases 3, e2011007. https://doi.org/10.4084/mjhid.2011.007.

Monroy-Pérez, E., Paniagua-Contreras, G.L., Rodríguez-Purata, P., Vaca-Paniagua, F., Vázquez-Villaseñor, M., Díaz-Velásquez, C., et al., 2016. High virulence and antifungal resistance in clinical strains of *Candida albicans*. The Canadian Journal of Infectious Diseases and Medical Microbiology 2016, 1−7. https://doi.org/10.1155/2016/5930489.

Nascimento, A.M., Goldman, G.H., Park, S., Marras, S.A.E., Delmas, G., Oza, U., et al., 2003. Multiple resistance mechanisms among *Aspergillus fumigatus* mutants with high-level resistance to itraconazole. Antimicrobial Agents and Chemotherapy 47, 1719−1726. https://doi.org/10.1128/AAC.47.5.1719-1726.2003.

Perea, S., Lopez-Ribot, J.L., Wickes, B.L., Kirkpatrick, W.R., Dib, O.P., Bachmann, S.P., et al., 2002. Molecular mechanisms of fluconazole resistance in *Candida dubliniensis* isolates from human immunodeficiency virus-infected patients with oropharyngeal candidiasis. Antimicrobial Agents and Chemotherapy 46, 1695−1703. https://doi.org/10.1128/AAC.46.6.1695-1703.2002.

Perlin, D.S., 2015. Echinocandin resistance in *Candida*. Clinical Infectious Diseases 61, S612−S617. https://doi.org/10.1093/cid/civ791.

Pfaller, M.A., Diekema, D.J., 2012. Progress in antifungal susceptibility testing of *Candida* spp. by use of clinical and laboratory standards institute broth microdilution methods, 2010 to 2012. Journal of Clinical Microbiology 50, 2846–2856. https://doi.org/10.1128/JCM.00937-12.

Pfaller, M.A., Diekema, D.J., Gibbs, D.L., Newell, V.A., Ellis, D., Tullio, V., et al., 2010. Results from the artemis disk global antifungal surveillance study, 1997 to 2007: a 10.5-year analysis of susceptibilities of candida species to fluconazole and voriconazole as determined by CLSI standardized disk diffusion. Journal of Clinical Microbiology 48, 1366–1377. https://doi.org/10.1128/JCM.02117-09.

Pfeiffer, N., 2001. Crucial question in candidemia. Oncology Times 23, 65–67. https://doi.org/10.1097/01.COT.0000315764.04172.67.

Puig-Asensio, M., Padilla, B., Garnacho-Montero, J., Zaragoza, O., Aguado, J.M., Zaragoza, R., et al., 2014. Epidemiology and predictive factors for early and late mortality in *Candida* bloodstream infections: a population-based surveillance in Spain. Clinical Microbiology and Infections 20, O245–O254. https://doi.org/10.1111/1469-0691.12380.

Rocha, M.F.G., Bandeira, S.P., de Alencar, L.P., Melo, L.M., Sales, J.A., de Paiva, M.A.N., et al., 2017. Azole resistance in *Candida albicans* from animals: highlights on efflux pump activity and gene overexpression. Mycoses 60, 462–468. https://doi.org/10.1111/myc.12611.

Sabino, R., Veríssimo, C., Brandão, J., Alves, C., Parada, H., Rosado, L., et al., 2010. Epidemiology of candidemia in oncology patients: a 6-year survey in a Portuguese central hospital. Medical Mycology 48, 346–354. https://doi.org/10.3109/13693780903161216.

Sakaeyama, S.I., Sano, A., Murata, Y., Kamei, K., Nishimura, K., Hatai, K., 2007. *Lecythophora hoffmannii* isolated from a case of canine osteomyelitis in Japan. Medical Mycology 45, 267–272. https://doi.org/10.1080/13693780601188602.

Sheehan, D.J., Hitchcock, C.A., Sibley, C.M., 1999. Current and emerging azole antifungal agents. Clinical Microbiology Reviews 12, 40–79.

Shubitz, L.F., Matz, M.E., Noon, T.H., Reggiardo, C.C., Bradley, G.A., 2001. Constrictive pericarditis secondary to *Coccidioides immitis* infection in a dog. Journal of the American Veterinary Medical Association 218, 537–540, 526.

Shubitz, L.F., Roy, M.E., Nix, D.E., Galgiani, J.N., 2013. Efficacy of Nikkomycin Z for respiratory coccidioidomycosis in naturally infected dogs. Medical Mycology 51, 747–754. https://doi.org/10.3109/13693786.2013.770610.

Sionov, E., Lee, H., Chang, Y.C., Kwon-Chung, K.J., 2010. *Cryptococcus neoformans* overcomes stress of azole drugs by formation of disomy in specific multiple chromosomes. PLoS Pathogens 6, e1000848. https://doi.org/10.1371/journal.ppat.1000848.

Trnacevic, S., Mujkanovic, A., Nislic, E., Begic, E., Karasalihovic, Z., Cickusic, A., et al., 2018. Invasive aspergillosis after kidney transplant - treatment approach. Medical Archives 72, 456. https://doi.org/10.5455/medarh.2018.72.456-458.

Uzun, O., Anaissie, E.J., 2000. Predictors of outcome in cancer patients with candidemia. Annals of Oncology 11, 1517–1521. https://doi.org/10.1023/A:1008308923252.

Vanden Bossche, H., Dromer, F., Improvisi, I., Lozano-Chiu, M., Rex, J.H., Sanglard, D., 1998. Antifungal drug resistance in pathogenic fungi. Medical Mycology 36 (Suppl. 1), 119–128.

VanSteenhouse, J.L., DeNovo, R.C., 1986. Atypical *Histoplasma capsulatum* infection in a dog. Journal of the American Veterinary Medical Association 188, 527–528.

Vermeulen, E., Lagrou, K., Verweij, P.E., 2013. Azole resistance in *Aspergillus fumigatus*. Current Opinion in Infectious Diseases 26, 493–500. https://doi.org/10.1097/QCO.0000000000000005.

Warnock, D.W., 1992. Azole drug resistance in *Candida* species. Journal of Medical Microbiology 37, 225–226. https://doi.org/10.1099/00222615-37-4-225.

Warris, A., 2015. Azole-resistant aspergillosis. Journal of Infection 71, S121–S125. https://doi.org/10.1016/j.jinf.2015.04.023.

Whaley, S.G., Berkow, E.L., Rybak, J.M., Nishimoto, A.T., Barker, K.S., Rogers, P.D., 2017. Azole antifungal resistance in *Candida albicans* and emerging non-albicans *Candida* species. Frontiers in Microbiology 7. https://doi.org/10.3389/fmicb.2016.02173.

White, T.C., Marr, K.A., Bowden, R.A., 1998. Clinical, cellular, and molecular factors that contribute to antifungal drug resistance. Clinical Microbiology Reviews 11, 382–402.

Yenisehirli, G., Bulut, N., Yenisehirli, A., Bulut, Y., 2015. In vitro susceptibilities of *Candida albicans* isolates to antifungal agents in Tokat, Turkey. Jundishapur Journal of Microbiology 8, e28057. https://doi.org/10.5812/jjm.28057.

Zavrel, M., White, T.C., 2015. Medically important fungi respond to azole drugs: an update. Future Microbiology 10, 1355–1373. https://doi.org/10.2217/FMB.15.47.

Chapter 12

Biofilm formation and persister cells

Chapter outline

Background

Bacteria get stick to each other on the surface in an encapsulation formed by the extracellular polymeric substances (EPS) released by the bacteria in their sessile aggregate form and this stage is known as biofilm (De Lancey Pulcini and Pulcini, 2001). Biofilms are ubiquitous in nature and can be detected on biotic or abiotic surface. On liquid surface biofilm may appear as floating or submerge mass. Biofilm may appear as homogenous or heterogeneous mass of bacteria adhered together with the EPS, which is mainly composed of polysaccharides along with other biomolecules such as proteins, lipids and nucleic acids (Neu and Lawrence, 2010; Vu et al., 2009). It was as early as 1684 when Antoni van Leeuwenhoek gave the initial idea of biofilm on dental plaque in a report to the Royal Society of London (Slavkin, 1997). Later on, Characklis (1973) studied on the formation of biofilm in industrial water and showed the resistance of such biofilms to the chemical disinfectant such as chlorine. It was Costerton JW who first coined the term biofilm in 1978 and explained how the bacterial adherence is developed with living and nonliving substances for the development of biofilm (Høiby, 2014; Costerton and Wilson, 2004). Various complex carbohydrate and lipid molecules entrapped in the biofilm may be suitably used by the bacteria as their food. Moreover, the water molecules are also present in the biofilm with hydrophilic polysaccharides. The biofilm is mostly composed of water ($\sim 97\%$), microbial cells ($\sim 2\%-5\%$), polysaccharide ($\sim 1\%-2\%$), protein ($<1\%-2\%$), DNA and RNA ($<1\%-2\%$) (Jamal et al., 2015). In general, biofilm has two layers — in one layer, there lies the water channel which facilitates the transfer of nutrients and macromolecules, whereas the internal layer contains densely packed bacterial cells. Biofilm is instrumental to evade the host immunity with change in the expression of surface protein possibly mediated by genetic alteration. Moreover, the impenetrable nature of biofilm and differential gene expression are responsible for increased drug resistance feature of the microbial population in the biofilm. In addition, the entrapped organisms in the biofilm are also resistant to bacteriophages and chemical biocides. The viscoelastic behavior of biofilm gives it much strength to survive under impending mechanical stress. Thus biofilm is a major problem for bacterial adherence and growth over medical implants or devices causing long-standing or recalcitrant infections (Gupta et al., 2016). There are some beneficial effects of biofilm as well when environmental perspective is taken into account. Microbial population in biofilm is responsible for production and degradation of the organic substances and bioremediation of environmental pollutants.

Formation of biofilm

Biofilm formation is a complex process that depends on biochemical, nutritional and environmental condition where the pathogens are growing and at the same time the process requires physical, physiological and biochemical changes of the

Antimicrobial Resistance in Agriculture. https://doi.org/10.1016/B978-0-12-815770-1.00012-2

pathogens. There are five steps involved in formation of biofilm — reversible attachment, irreversible attachment, maturation stage I and II and finally dispersion (Gupta et al., 2016; Stoodley et al., 2002).

Initially when bacteria come in contact with a surface or support, there is an abrupt decrease in their motion to facilitate their settling on contact point. This is usually the first process to make a reversible adherence with the surface or attachment with other microbes already adhered to the surface. A solid—liquid interface provides an ideal environment for such adherence (Donlan, 2002). Biofilm formation is a complex process which depends on various factors such as temperature, pressure, availability of nutrients and other physiochemical properties of the contact surface and the process is facilitated by bacterial appendages such as fimbriae and pili (Marić and Vraneš, 2007). Rough, hydrophilic coated surfaces provide better environment for adhesion. Various bonds and interactions such as van der Waals forces, steric and electrostatic (double layer) interactions are known to play. While the bacterial colonization and settling to contact surface is known as adhesion, the bacterial attachment with each other is known as cohesion. Both processes are involved during reversible attachment. This adherence and attachment become strong and irreversible when the cells overcome the repulsive force of the contact surface and this is usually mediated by the appendages such as fimbriae and pili and hydrophobic interaction between the bacterial cells and the contact surface. Thus the cells strongly adhered with the contact surface and ultimately get immobilized (Garrett et al., 2008). Finally at the end of stage 2, strong and specific adhesions are established. In the third phase, maturation phase 1, bacteria release autoinducer signals for communication among them, which in turn facilitates the expression of biofilm formation gene(s). Thus the EPS are released from the bacterial cells which act as a scaffold to form the binding network of the bacteria. The thickness of biofilm may be increased up to 10 μm. Furthermore, with subsequent adherence, the thickness grows into 100 μm and there may be accumulation of diverse species, which usually depend on each other for nutrient supply and clearance of metabolic waste and toxic elements. Final stage is known as dispersion stage where the bacteria usually detach from the biofilm adherence and return back to the sessile stage/planktonic phase. This is usually a natural phenomenon which can be triggered by mechanical stress and helped with release of certain saccharolytic enzymes which are instrumental in breaking the biofilm stabilizing polysaccharides (Kaplan, 2010). In this process, such biofilm producers usually stop to produce EPS and there is increased expression of the gene(s) responsible for flagella proteins which can help the bacteria to be motile and relocate into new sites. Although the dispersed cells are back to planktonic phase, they usually retain some of the properties of biofilm population, most remarkably the reduced susceptibility towards antibiotics.

There are several signaling systems that are operational in biofilm formation, of which quorum sensing has been studied a lot. It is a bacterial communication process where autoinducer signals are being employed. In case of GNB, N-acyl homoserine lactones are the autoinducer (Kim et al., 2011; Steindler and Venturi, 2007), whereas in GPB, oligopeptides act as autoinducer (Monnet and Gardan, 2015). Whenever the bacterial population or density reaches an optimum level, these molecules which are being accumulated outside the cells began to regulate the expression of the gene(s) associated with biofilm formation and virulence. This phenomenon has been well studied in case of *Staphylococcus aureus* where it is regulated by *agr* (accessory gene regulator) operon with an autoinducer peptide. In general, agr is instrumental to control the expression of a series of toxins and virulence factors and their interaction with the innate immune system among *S. aureus* and *Staphylococcus epidermidis*. However, another key function regulated by agr operon is to enhance biofilm detachment by upregulation of the expression of detergent-like peptides. Furthermore, another gene, AI-2 synthase *luxS*, also reduces cell-to-cell adhesion by downregulating expression of biofilm EPS (Kong et al., 2006). In addition to biofilm, quorum sensing is also useful for communication among the bacteria with regard to their exposure to environmental stressor, disinfectants, antibiotics and nutritional shortage. Many of the pathogenic bacteria also use this phenomenon for collective expression of virulence gene(s). There are some other signal pathways which were also recorded to be involved in biofilm formation — two-component systems and extracytoplasmic function signaling pathway (Prüß and Prüß, 2017).

Types of biofilm

Depending on the types of interaction between bacterial cells and surface, biofilm may be monolayer or multilayer (Gupta et al., 2016). In case of single-layer biofilm, the interaction of the constituent cells with the surface is more intense rather than the interaction of cells among themselves. Thus the kind of interaction and the adhesive molecules are the most important factors to determine whether a biofilm will be monolayer or multilayer. In case of monolayer biofilm when the interaction is transient, bacterial cell components such as pilus and flagellum compose the major component, whereas the interaction becomes more rigid and permanent with formation of microbial adhesion. The multilayer biofilm requires more intense interaction between the constituent cells. The surface charge characteristics of the cells often drive a repulsive force to prevent the close interaction of the cells. For example, the presence of O-antigen makes the surface of the Gram-negative bacteria negatively charged. Thus GNB pathogens need to overcome the repulsive force because of their uniform negatively charged surface for attachment with one another and formation of multilayer biofilm. A series of factors are known to neutralize such negatively charged cell surface like downregulation or silencing of the gene(s) of O surface antigen, formation of adhesive agents such as EPS and aggregation of divalent cations.

Biofilm and drug resistance

The exact reason behind development of drug resistance in biofilm is still under ambiguity and how the bacteria established biofilm evading the host immune response is not clear. It is important to note that while host immune system is effective against the planktonic phase of the bacteria; its efficacy is substantially reduced against biofilm. The extracellular bacteria establish its strong foothold in the form of biofilm by gradual adaptation that often leads to evasion from innate immunity of the host. The possible reason behind antibiotic resistance associated with biofilm has been tried to be explained by different hypothesis.

Poor penetration of the antibiotic molecules is often regarded as one of the important mechanism for failure to deliver antibiotic in sufficient concentration to the sites of biofilm and bacterial infection (Hall-Stoodley et al., 2004; Davies, 2003; Fux et al., 2005). Bacterial EPS, which act as physical barrier against the passage of antibiotic molecules and high molecular weight substances such as lysozymes, are unable to move in. Sometimes antibiotics (such as aminoglycosides) get adsorbed in high amount in the EPS molecules of the biofilm (Khan et al., 2010; Wilton et al., 2016). Positively charged antibiotics get entrapped in the negatively charged EPS of the biofilms. Such phenomenon has been detected in case of slow or insufficient passage of fluoroquinolones and aminoglycosides through the biofilm matrix of *Pseudomonas aeruginosa* mostly made up of anionic alginate exopolysaccharide. A recent study conducted in diverse bacterial species emphasized that although penetration barrier contributed to bacterial biofilm associated resistance in case of certain antibacterial compounds such as vancomycin and chloramphenicol, for resistance to β-lactams, aminoglycosides, tetracyclines, fluoroquinolones and some other factors are operational (Singh et al., 2016).

It is also not impossible for the antibiotics being degraded during their passage through the biofilms. Different enzymes released by the bacteria in the biofilm may cause degradation or inactivation of antibiotics. In case of biofilm with cystic fibrosis caused by *P. aeruginosa* AmpC type cephalosporinase may cause such degradation of cephalosporins (Chalhoub et al., 2018; Aghazadeh et al., 2014). Moreover, the acidic waste or metabolic products formed in the biofilm may also be responsible for inactivation of several antibiotic molecules in acidic pH. Deeper layers of biofilms do not contain sufficient amount of consumable oxygen and some antibiotics such as aminoglycosides cannot act in such anaerobic atmosphere. Again, osmotic stress in biofilm also reduces the porin channels to reduce the intracellular entry of antibiotics. In addition, reduced expression or absence of porin channel OprF could be associated with increased resistance in biofilm and production of the Pel exopolysaccharide as revealed in a recent study (Bouffartigues et al., 2015). Similarly, deletion of the ompQ gene for outer membrane porin protein attenuated the ability of *Bordetella bronchiseptica*, an aerobic Gram-negative bacterium to form a mature biofilm (Cattelan et al., 2016). Biological waste and metabolic toxic products which are gradually accumulated in biofilm are responsible for metabolic slowdown of the bacteria making many of the antibiotics ineffective, especially those which act over the metabolic pathways or over the metabolically active growing bacterial population. Oxygen limitation and metabolic slowdown in the interior of the biofilm were found responsible for antibiotic tolerance of *P. aeruginosa* biofilm system against aminoglycosides (tobramycin) and fluoroquinolones (ciprofloxacin) (Walters et al., 2003). Another hypothesis with regard to bacterial resistance in biofilm expounds about development of a small population of bacterial cells which forms a protective layer and becomes insensitive to antibiotics, and these cells are known as biofilm phenotype. Such cells are similar to the bacterial subpopulation which readily transforms to spore-forming phenotype. Besides, differential gene expression and overexpression of efflux pumps as recorded in *P. aeruginosa* may also be responsible for antibiotic resistance in bacterial cells established in biofilm (Alav et al., 2018; Yamasaki et al., 2015).

Biofilm and infection

Biofilm formation is an ancient method used by the bacteria to protect themselves from any kind of adversities and assaults such as UV irradiation, enzymatic degradation, heat inactivation, chemical treatment, pH changes and dehydration apart from antibiotic treatment. Bacteriological contamination and colonization is known to be an important determining factor for retarded healing of infected wound, and biofilm is known to play an important role there. Besides, implanted medical devices also get infected by bacteria and thus infection may be established in the host via such implants. Thus medical devices pose the highest rate of biofilm-related infections (Hughes and Webber, 2017). In most of the cases, *Staphylococcus* and *Pseudomonas* were recorded in biofilm associated with medical device—related infections (Gupta et al., 2016).

TABLE 12.1 Details of biofilm-related infection in medical implants and devices.

SI No	Description	Pathogens involved	References
1	Endocarditis	*Staphylococcus, Streptococcus*, GNB, *Candida*	Gupta et al., 2016
2	Periodontitis	*Fusobacterium nucleatum* and *Pseudomonas* sp, some anaerobic bacteria and protozoa	Chen, 2001; Schaudinn et al., 2009; Park et al., 2014
3	Cystic fibrosis	*Pseudomonas aeruginosa*	Beloin et al., 2014; Høiby et al., 2010
4	Rhinosinusitis	*Staphylococcus aureus, Streptococcus pneumoniae, Haemophilus influenza* and *Moraxella catarrhalis*.	Leid et al., 2011; Zhang et al., 2011; Prince et al., 2008
5	Osteomyelitis	*S. aureus*	Gomes et al., 2013; Brady et al., 2008
6	Catheter infection	Multiple pathogens such as *S. epidermis, S. aureus, C. albicans, P. aeruginosa, Klebsiella pneumoniae*	Gupta et al., 2016
7	Urinary catheter infection	Mostly GNB - *Escherichia coli, Proteus mirabilis, P. aeruginosa, K. pneumonia*. Besides, *S epidermidis* and *Enterococcus faecalis* may be involved.	Holá and Růžička, 2008; Sabir et al., 2017; Trautner and Darouiche, 2004
8	Prosthetic heart valve infection	*S. aureus, Streptococcus* spp, Gram-negative bacilli, *Candida* spp, *Enterococci* and diptheroids	Silverstein and Donatucci, 2003; Talpaert et al., 2015

Different biofilm-related systemic and medical device—related infection and the associated causative bacterial pathogens are illustrated in the Table 12.1 below.

Overview of persistence/drug tolerance

Biofilm formation and development of multidrug-tolerant persister cells is an age old problem and thought to contribute to the development of majority of the recalcitrant chronic infections.

Persister cells or the antibiotic-tolerant cells are the bacterial subpopulation that is not responsive to antibiotic, and unlike the commonly known resistant bacteria, tolerant population does not undergo any genetic change or mutation. While the resistant bacteria are able to survive and grow in presence of antimicrobials, the tolerant population can hardly grow (Lewis, 2005, 2007, 2010a; Wood et al., 2013). The tolerant bacteria comprise of about 0.01% of exponentially growing bacterial population. However, in stationary phase this proportion reaches about 1%. In stationary phase, *P. aeruginosa* exhibits large number of persister cells (10^2-10^3). Such phenomenon has also been found in case of stationery phase culture of *S. aureus* and *Escherichia coli* (Bjarnsholt, 2011). In presence of antibiotic, the tolerant population which constitutes only a small proportion becomes metabolically inactive with a stage of dormancy and thus remains unaffected with antimicrobial therapy. Once the antibiotic is withdrawn, the tolerant cells proliferate and reestablish the infection. Persister cells use such metabolic inactivity as a strategy to ensure their survival in presence of antibiotics. Persistence is not a problem when the bacterial cells are in planktonic or free-floating state as selected antibiotic usually destroy the bulk of susceptible population, while immune system clears out the persisters. However, persistence becomes challenge with formation of biofilms that contribute to most of all the chronic infections and the infections associated with indwelling medical devices and medical implants. As discussed, biofilm is an aggregate of microbial population that are self-adherent and entrapped within protective shield or capsule formed by extracellular matrix or EPS produced by them. Persistence or antibiotic tolerance is almost an inherent phenomenon of biofilm with considerable population of tolerant cells which are entrapped within the safe haven of biofilm with the protective shield of EPS. Although the bulk of bacterial pathogen in biofilm is unremarkable, it is the minority — i.e., the persisters remain untouched and unaffected with antimicrobial therapy and can repopulate and reinitiate the infection once antimicrobial therapy is over or the concentration of antimicrobial drops to a certain level. Therefore, persisters are a subpopulation of bacterial cell which become highly tolerant or invulnerable to antibiotics and attain this stage without any obvious genetic change (Gupta et al., 2016; Fux et al., 2005; Lewis, 2007; Wood et al., 2013; Wood, 2016). Persisters may not exhibit elevated MIC towards antibiotics as commonly seen with case of fairly resistant bacterial population. Moreover, unlike resistant bacteria, they do not grow in presence of antibiotic. But neither do they die. This ability to avert killing is the most significant feature of persistence. In a wide number of bacteria, *E. coli* (where they are best studied), *P. aeruginosa, S. aureus, Lactobacillus acidophilus* and *Gardnerella vaginalis*, such persistence phenomenon have been demonstrated (Lewis, 2005, 2007; Wood, 2016, 2017; Möker et al., 2010; Conlon, 2014; Lechner et al., 2012; Law et al., 2015; Keren et al., 2004).

Mechanism of persistence or drug tolerance

The mechanism of multidrug tolerance or persistence is largely unknown. In general, it is presumed that persistent cells are generated in passive manner stochastically with genetic switch in a growing cell population. However, several inducing factors were also proposed in such phenomenon. In contrast to resistant bacteria which usually prevents the drug to bind the target (either by deactivating the drug or by preventing its entry or with change of drug targets), tolerant bacteria shut down or slow down their metabolic activity and thereby the availability of drug targets like protein and nucleic acid are reduced considerably.

Modulation of toxin—antitoxin pair system is considered as the main avenue for formation of persister cell with induction of metabolic shut down and dormancy. The system consists of a toxin — usually a protein that interferes with the essential cellular functions (such as transcription or translation) — and a labile antitoxin — usually RNA or a protein that acts as an inhibitor of the toxin molecule (Wood et al., 2013). Depending on their modus operandi and biochemical nature, antitoxin may fall into five categories, type I—type V. Type I is RNA antitoxin that acts as antisense RNA and inhibits the translation of toxin mRNA. Another RNA antitoxin inhibits the toxin by directly binding to it and is referred as type II antitoxin. Similarly type III antitoxin is protein molecule and directly binds to antitoxin to inactivate it. However, type IV antitoxin, which is also a protein molecule, prevents the toxin to bind its target. On the other hand, type V protein antitoxin acts by cleaving toxin mRNA specifically (Deter et al., 2017; Fasani and Savageau, 2013). It was in 1983 when TA system was first linked to persistence when high persistence (hip) mutants of *E. coli* were detected. Mutation of HipA7 toxin gene leads to the formation of a toxin which can poorly interact with antitoxin; thus, its overactivity was proposed to cause persistence (Li et al., 2016; Kaspy et al., 2013). However, this proposition was not fully convincing to the scientists. Later on, several other toxin—antitoxin systems were linked to persistence such as YafQ/DinJ, RelE/RelB, MazF/MazE, MqsR/MqsA and TisB/IstR-1 of which overproduction of the toxin RelE was seen to substantially increase in persistence. On the other hand, while MqsR toxin renders the cell dormant by diminishing translation, the TisB toxin is known to decrease the proton-motive force and ATP levels to slow down the metabolic activity of the cells to become dormant (Dörr et al., 2010; Sun et al., 2017). Bacterial cells producing such kind of TisB toxin are usually persistent to several antibiotics of diverse groups including ampicillin, ciprofloxacin and streptomycin. However, the mechanism of persistence involves multifarious ways and the process is too complicated. For example, overexpression of the toxin TisB can cause induction of persistence in the exponential phase but not in the stationary phase. Thus persistence was explained with cellular response to the stress signals with activation of the genes to manage the impending stress and gradual halting of metabolic activity so that the cells can survive through inactivity. In addition, alarmone guanosine tetraphosphate (ppGpp) is another factor which is thought to carry the stress response to the toxin/antitoxin system such as MazF and HipA.

Dormancy and persistence

In general, one group of workers hypothesized that reduced metabolic activity and substantially reduced growth rate in persister cells in biofilms are the main reasons for reduced antimicrobial susceptibility. Augmented intracellular toxins with overexpression of genes such as MqsR or RelE as detected in many persisters usually repress their own protein translation and thus these cells can easily escape the effect of antibiotics that target protein translation. To mimic such situation, the bacterial cells were pretreated with drugs such as rifampin, tetracycline or other bacteriostatic compounds which have inhibitory effect on protein synthesis and workers were able to induce persistence (Kudrin et al., 2017; Kwan et al., 2013). Similarly, pretreatment with carbonyl cyanide m-chlorophenyl hydrazine, which blocks ATP synthesis, was also shown to induce persistence and thereby diminishes antimicrobial susceptibility. Reduced metabolic activity was also linked to persistence as demonstrated in PhoU mutant *E. coli* and catabolic repressor protein deleted *P. aeruginosa* strains (Li and Zhang, 2007). Taken together, these studies pointed out that metabolic slow down showing growth rate along with dormancy in the inner subpopulation of the biofilm is the main triggering factor for persistence (Lewis, 2005, 2007, 2010a, 2010b; Keren et al., 2004; Wood, 2017; Simões et al., 2011). Although dormancy is proposed for development of persistence since long, the issue is still shrouded under controversy. Many workers suggested that the persisters are in fact metabolically more active and respond genetically to modulate themselves to respond to the impending stress to become tolerant (Wood et al., 2013). Wakamoto et al. (2013) suggested such kind of metabolically hyperactive *Mycobacterium smegmatis* strains tolerant to isoniazid. Still, such kind of evidence is insufficient to exclude out the possibility of metabolic inactivity responsible for antibiotic tolerance.

Present status

Like in human diseases, the role of biofilm-forming pathogens in animal infection cannot be undermined especially in case of refractory infections as observed in bovine mastitis, pyometra or canine pyoderma. Formation of microbial biofilm was reiterated as one of the major causes for refractory cases of bovine mastitis (Melchior, 2011; Melchior et al., 2006). Presence of polysaccharide intercellular adhesion, a component of *S. aureus*—associated biofilm, was demonstrated in several cases of bovine intramammary infection (Schönborn et al., 2016). Furthermore, Notcovich et al. (2018) showed that the majority of the *S. aureus* isolates of bovine mastitis origin were biofilm-forming, although they were devoid of biofilm-forming genes such as intercellular adhesion (*icaA* and icaD) and biofilm-associated protein (*bap*) (Notcovich et al., 2018). Similarly, biofilm-forming *Streptococcus uberis* and *Streptococcus agalactiae* were also recorded in bovine mastitis (Miranda et al., 2018; Reinoso, 2017). In dogs, biofilm-forming uropathogenic *E. coli* were evident to cause recurrent urinary tract infection and its recalcitrance to fluoroquinolone therapy (Lewis, 2005; Wood, 2017). Biofilm-forming bacteria such as *Staphylococcus intermedius*, *S. epidermidis* and *Streptococcus canis* were implicated in chronic nonhealing pressure wounds over both elbow regions of a 4-year-old spayed female Mastiff (Swanson et al., 2014). In addition, biofilm-forming bacteria in oral cavity of dogs (Zambori et al., 2013) and dental tartar such as *Pseudomonas fragi*, *Citrobacter koseri*, *Streptococcus mutans* and *Malassezia pachydermatis* (Manuel et al., 2014) and possibility of their zoonotic transfer to human being through dog bites were reported. Besides, role of biofilm-forming pathogens (such as streptococci, enterococci, *E. coli*, *Pseudomonas*, coryneforms) in clinical complication of diseases such as otitis and pyometra was also recorded in dogs (Nuttall, 2016; Albright). A high prevalence of the biofilm-associated gene(s) (*icaA* and *icaD*) was recorded in *Staphylococcus pseudintermedius* isolates from canine pyoderma (Casagrande Proietti et al., 2015). Similar observation was noticed by Stefanetti et al. (2017) in a separate study carried out in Italy (Stefanetti et al., 2017). Besides, the other biofilm-forming veterinary/animal pathogens, which are frequently encountered, include *Listeria monocytogenes*, *Staphylococcus pettenkoferi*, *Pasteurella multocida*, *Mycobacterium avium* subsp. *paratuberculosis*, *Corynebacterium pseudotuberculosis* and *Fusobacterium necrophorum* (Rodríguez-Melcón et al., 2018; Petruzzi et al., 2018; Dutta et al., 2018; Abdullahi et al., 2016).

Detection of biofilm formation

Various methods that are used to detect biofilm production include tissue culture plate (TCP) assay, tube method (TM), Congo red agar method (CRA), bioluminescent assay, piezoelectric sensors and fluorescent microscopic examination. Of these, first three are cost-effective and can be employed in routine laboratory tests. TCP assay is often considered as a gold standard for detection of biofilm formation (Christensen et al., 1985). In TCP assay, following 18—24 h incubation in trypticase soy broth with 1% glucose or brain heart infusion with 2% sucrose in tissue culture plates, the test organisms are washed with PBS to remove the planktonic or free-floating bacteria, and the biofilm-forming adherent 'sessile' organisms in plate are fixed with sodium acetate (2%) and stained with crystal violet (0.1% w/v). After removing the excess stain, the colour intensity is measured to detect the quantity of biofilm formation. In TM, the same principal is used to measure qualitative assessment of biofilm formation and the assay is conducted in tube (Christensen et al., 1982). In CRA method, organisms (generally *Staphylococcus*) are incubated for 24—48 h in brain heart infusion broth (BHI) supplemented with 5% sucrose and Congo red and biofilm formation is indicated by presence of black colonies with a dry crystalline consistency (Freeman et al., 1989).

Therapeutic strategies in biofilm

It is indeed challenging to treat the infection associated with biofilm. But to ensure the survivability of the patients and their welfare, it is imperative to control and treat biofilm-associated infection as bacteria increases their virulence and pathogenicity in the chronic persisting infection. The conventional therapeutic regimen is often ineffective and thus the strategies against biofilm encompasses three different approaches, particularly with regard to biofilm in the medical devices — (1) prevention of attachment of the bacterial cells; (2) disruption of the transiently attached bacterial population; (3) disruption and dissolution of the formed biofilms.

As medical devices such as catheter and prosthetics often invites biofilm, large doses of antibiotics are often advocated either to coat the devices or for systematic administration. Anti-staphylococcal antimicrobials are often given as *S. aureus* or related CoNS infections are involved in most of the biofilm. Penicillin and related compounds are effective as first-line therapy. In case of colonization of MRSA, vancomycin is truly effective; however, repeated and prolonged vancomycin therapy may lead to secondary anaerobic infection with *Clostridium difficile* and toxicity (Gupta et al., 2016). There are also evidences that vancomycin may induce biofilm formation in certain circumstances (He et al., 2017). To avoid such scenario, linezolid, fosfomycin and daptomycin may be used with safer and effective outcome (Chai et al., 2016; Meije et al., 2014). Again rifampicin is another suitable alternative which is not only effective against sessile bacteria for removal of biofilm-associated infections but also has very negligible side effects. Better efficacy of rifampicin was observed *in vitro* when used in combination with tigecycline against biofilm-forming *S. haemolyticus* (Szczuka et al., 2015). Such kind of combined therapy - imipenem—rifampicin and colistin—rifampicin were also found effective against biofilm production of carbapenem-resistant *Acinetobacter baumannii* (Song et al., 2015).

Devices or bone implants are often coated with different antibiotics to prevent biofilm, and gentamicin (Neut et al., 2011) and tobramycin (Scott and Higham, 2003) are the most frequently prescribed antibiotics in such cases. Sometimes aminoglycosides are used in combination with other antibiotics such as fusidic acid and clindamycin to increase the spectrum and antibacterial efficacy (Neut et al., 2006). Calcium sulphate beads coated with antibiotics are often used in such cases of bone implants. These are inert and get easily dissolved in the body without any severe side effect. Owing to persistent and prolonged release, proper concentration of antibiotics are usually achieved and sustained to prevent biofilm formation. Antibiotic lock technique was also devised to instill proper concentration of antibiotic to coat the catheter before implantation for prevention of biofilm formation (Justo and Bookstaver, 2014). Again iron chelating agents (2,2′-dipyridyl, acetohydroxamic acid and EDTA) when coupled with aminoglycosides were found effective in treatment of biofilm associated with *P. aeruginosa* infection (Liu et al., 2010; O'May et al., 2009). Although several approaches were made to reduce the biofilm-associated infection in the catheter, devices or implants, it is always difficult often to control such infection (Gupta et al., 2016; Holá and Růžička, 2008; Abdullahi et al., 2016). With continued presence of foreign bodies in the system, it often becomes difficult to control biofilm-associated infection because of suppression and diminution of phagocytic killing and clearance by polymorphonuclear cells. Thus removal or exchange of indwelling catheter is a prerequisite to control and exterminate the biofilm formation. Presence of infected central venous catheter or dialysis catheter may cause intermittent bacteremia and thus the infected catheters need to be changed with short-term intravenous antibiotic therapy to remove the bacteria released from infected catheter in the circulation (Michalopoulos and Geroulanos, 1996). When such change is not possible, instillation of large dosage of antimicrobial compounds in the catheter and lock therapy are effective. Usually clinicians recommend vancomycin (1 mg/mL) or gentamicin (2 mg/mL) for Gram-positive and GNB infection, respectively. Daptomycin may also be an alternative in Gram-positive infection (Meije et al., 2014; Justo and Bookstaver, 2014). Instead, 70% ethanol or 2 mol/L HCL may be given in the lumen of the catheter as lock therapy (Orman and Brynildsen, 2013). Infection of urinary catheter often leads to urosepsis and septicaemia; thus, timely change of urinary catheter is important. Otherwise, the newly implanted catheter may get infected with residual bacteria in the bladder or ureter. Usually, the catheters are replaced only after treating with effective antibiotic for at least 48 h to clear off the residual bacteria.

Agents other than antibiotics, which have been tried with promising results, include proinflammatory Th2 cytokine IL-12, nitric oxide, silver nanoparticle and bacteriophages as alternative therapeutics in biofilm-associated infection (Barraud et al., 2006; Freire et al., 2017; Abedon, 2016). Manganin is another nonantibiotic but antiinfective material obtained from *Xenopus laevis* and when covalently linked to mercapto undecanoic acid and 6-mercaptohexanol could be used to prevent bacterial adhesion. Its antibacterial and antibiofilm activity was reported against drug-resistant *Acinetobacter baumannii* (Kim et al., 2018). Nisin is another antibacterial peptide which shows its antibacterial property by causing pores in the bacterial cell membrane. Nisin and lysostaphin were found to have potential effect on biofilm-forming *S. aureus* of bovine mastitis origin (Ceotto-Vigoder et al., 2016). Furanone, one novel compound synthesized by red algae *Delisea pulchra,* was reported to disrupt the biofilm formation (Baveja et al., 2004). Several bioactive compounds and polymers were also found efficacious against biofilm infections such as bioactive arginyl-glycyl-aspartic acid (RGD), cis-2-decanoic acid (from *P. aeruginosa*) and amino acids from bacteria (like *N*-acetyl cysteine).

Modulation of cell signalling is an important way to prevent or disrupt the biofilm formation. Thus the agents which can inhibit the biosynthesis of di-c-GMP can be advocated against biofilm (Antoniani et al., 2010). In case of *E. coli* such kind of di-c-GMP biosynthesis inhibition with the help of a sulphonamide compound − sulphathiazole was tried with much success. Besides, coating of the medical devices with anti-infective agents is another way to prevent biofilm formation. Titanium prosthetic coated with silver or silicon devices coated with triclosan substantially reduce the infection rate and biofilm formation (Devlin-Mullin et al., 2017; Mcbride et al., 2009). Silicone rubber coated with quaternary ammonium compounds were found effective against staphylococcal growth (Gottenbos et al., 2002). Similarly, resin beads coated with polyethylene oxide (Jang et al., 2015) and antimicrobial peptide can reduce the biofilm formation.

Enzymatic disruption of biofilm is one of the possible ways which has been targeted by many researchers (Wood, 2017; Wu et al., 2015). Proteases like trypsin and proteinase K were regarded as important molecules to degrade the extracellular matrix of biofilm produced by *S. aureus*. Similarly, DNAse I enzyme can also be used to breakdown the EPS of biofilm as most of the GPB such as *Staphylococcus* use DNA to build the biofilm. Interestingly, alginate lyase, one enzyme released by *P. aeruginosa*, is helpful to clear its own biofilm when used in combination of antibiotics. Dispersin B is another compound produced by the GNB like *Actinobacillus actinomycetemcomitans* to clear the biofilms produced by *S. epidermidis*. In addition, novel molecules (A-861) like sesquiterpene lactone and benxoquinone derivative may also disrupt the amyloid protein molecules associated with bacterial biofilm of *Bacillus subtilis*. Besides, Esp, a serine protease from *S. epidermidis*, was reported to exhibit efficacy against the biofilms of *S. aureus*. Again, ultrasound guided micro-bubble destruction was documented to improve the antibacterial efficacy of vancomycin against *S. epidermidis* biofilm.

Rosmarinic acid produced from *Ocimum basilicum* can be used to inhibit quorum sensing and this has been tried by many researchers to inhibit biofilm (Slobodníková et al., 2013). Such property was also observed in a compound - ajeone (allyl sulphide) against *P. aeruginosa*. This ajeone in combination with tobramycin can be used to control pulmonary infection. Bioactive compounds (like catechin) extracted from leaves and bark of *Combretum albiflorum* (Tul.) Jongkind (Combretaceae) were found to quench the production of QS-dependent factors in *P. aeruginosa*. The authors also documented that the catechin reduced pyocyanin and elastase productions and biofilm formation, possibly by down regulation of expression of the QS-regulated genes (Vandeputte et al., 2010). Again, ellagic acid derivatives from *Terminalia chebula* were reported to down-regulate the expression of quorum sensing genes in *P. aeruginosa* (Sarabhai et al., 2013). Furanones as described before are also known to modulate QS to inhibit biofilm.

How to overcome persistence

In general, three different kind of approaches may be taken for treating the persister cells like, - 1. Preventing the formation of persisters 2. Killing the persisters when they are in dormancy, 3. Converting the persisters in active stage and killing them with conventional antibiotics.

Quite a large number of experiments and research trials were conducted to overcome the problem of persistence. Conventional antimicrobials which mostly attack the growing cells are unable to attack persister cells, as the machineries that are usually targeted by conventional antibiotics are inactive in dormancy. Therefore, the agents that may act independently without any help of cell machinery may be effective against the persisters. Such agents must be able to enter the cells passively without any help of active transport pumps (Wood, 2017). One such agent is mitomycin C, which can enter the bacterial cell passively without any help of active transport or proton pumps and cause the cross-linking of DNA of the bacteria irrespective their growth status. Mitomycin is effective for the cells that are growing exponentially as well as against the cells which are in stationary phase. The efficacy of mitomycin have been seen against a broad range of bacteria including *E. coli*, *S. aureus*, *P. aeruginosa* and even against the persister cells of the spirochete *Borrelia burgdorferi* causing Lyme disease. Its potentiality against viable but nonculturable bacteria (VBNC) has established mitomycin as a suitable alternative for treating the persister cells. The only limiting factor for mitomycin is its inherent toxicity and thus large oral dose for treating refractory infection of persister may cause problem (Wood, 2017). However, topical application of mitomycin is without such limitation. Acyldepsipeptide ADEP4 is another agent which was documented to cause protein degradation in *S. aureus* persisters in murine model and cause the death of persisters when combined with antibiotics like rifampicin (Lewis, 2010a). Pyrazinamide is another important drug which is often used in the chemotherapy of tuberculosis in combination with isoniazid, ethambutol, and rifampicin. Pyrazinamide is effective in killing the sleeping persister *Mycobacterium*. Similarly, daptomycin exhibited its efficacy against the *B. burgdorferi* persisters. However, owing to its limited potentiality against the growing cell population, it is given in combination with other drugs like tetracycline (doxycycline) and β-lactam (cefoperazone) to effectively eradicate the *B. burgdorferi* infection (Rahmani-Badi et al., 2015; Marques et al., 2015; Davies and Marques, 2009). Cationic antimicrobial peptide is another option which can directly act over the cell membrane and thus can annihilate the majority of the dormant microbial population in biofilm. Antibiotic−antimicrobial peptide conjugate has also been tried to destroy the rigid cell population under persistence. Such hybrid compound was developed by conjugating the AMP with aminoglycoside like tobramycin. The hybrid compound was found effective to significantly destroy the persister cells of *E. coli* and *S. aureus* due to combined antibacterial effect of both the AMP and antibiotic (Janssens et al., 2008; Yujie et al., 2013). One group of workers have tried to break the dormancy by addition of glycolysis intermediates such as pyruvate which normally acts by generating proton-motive force making the cells susceptible to antibiotics such as aminoglycosides. The glycolysis intermediates such as mannitol glucose, fructose and pyruvate can activate the metabolic activity and break the physiological silence of the dormant cells. Other than these nutritional intermediates, some other compounds may also be used to break such dormancy such as cis-2-decenoic acid (Kim et al., 2011), brominated furanones (Starkey et al., 2014), 3-(4-[4methoxyphenyl] piperazin-1-yl) piperidin-4-yl biphenyl-4-carboxylate (Melchior et al., 2006). Attenuation of quorum sensing was employed by another group of workers using benzimidazole compounds to prevent the transformation of cells into persisters (Miranda et al., 2018; Reinoso, 2017).

References

Abdullahi, U.F., Igwenagu, E., Mu'azu, A., Aliyu, S., Umar, M.I., 2016. Intrigues of biofilm: a perspective in veterinary medicine. Veterinary World 9, 12−18. https://doi.org/10.14202/vetworld.2016.12-18.

Abedon, S.T., 2016. Bacteriophage exploitation of bacterial biofilms: phage preference for less mature targets? FEMS Microbiology Letters 363, fnv246. https://doi.org/10.1093/femsle/fnv246.

Aghazadeh, M., Hojabri, Z., Mahdian, R., Nahaei, M.R., Rahmati, M., Hojabri, T., et al., 2014. Role of efflux pumps: MexAB-OprM and MexXY(-OprA), AmpC cephalosporinase and OprD porin in non-metallo-β-lactamase producing *Pseudomonas aeruginosa* isolated from cystic fibrosis and burn patients. Infection, Genetics and Evolution 24, 187−192. https://doi.org/10.1016/j.meegid.2014.03.018.

Alav, I., Sutton, J.M., Rahman, K.M., 2018. Role of bacterial efflux pumps in biofilm formation. Journal of Antimicrobial Chemotherapy 73, 2003−2020. https://doi.org/10.1093/jac/dky042.

Albright S., n.d. Understanding the Role of *E. Coli* Biofilm in Canine Pyometra. https://www.akc.org/expert-advice/dog-breeding/canine-pyometra-e-coli-biofilm/.

Antoniani, D., Bocci, P., Maciag, A., Raffaelli, N., Landini, P., 2010. Monitoring of diguanylate cyclase activity and of cyclic-di-GMP biosynthesis by whole-cell assays suitable for high-throughput screening of biofilm inhibitors. Applied Microbiology and Biotechnology 85, 1095−1104. https://doi.org/10.1007/s00253-009-2199-x.

Barraud, N., Hassett, D.J., Hwang, S.-H., Rice, S.A., Kjelleberg, S., Webb, J.S., 2006. Involvement of nitric oxide in biofilm dispersal of *Pseudomonas aeruginosa*. Journal of Bacteriology 188, 7344−7353. https://doi.org/10.1128/JB.00779-06.

Baveja, J., Willcox, M.D., Hume, E.B., Kumar, N., Odell, R., Poole-Warren, L., 2004. Furanones as potential anti-bacterial coatings on biomaterials. Biomaterials 25, 5003−5012. https://doi.org/10.1016/j.biomaterials.2004.02.051.

Beloin, C., Renard, S., Ghigo, J.M., Lebeaux, D., 2014. Novel approaches to combat bacterial biofilms. Current Opinion in Pharmacology 18, 61−68. https://doi.org/10.1016/j.coph.2014.09.005.

Bjarnsholt, T., 2011. Introduction to biofilms. Biofilm Infections 1−9. https://doi.org/10.1007/978-1-4419-6084-9_1.

Bouffartigues, E., Moscoso, J.A., Duchesne, R., Rosay, T., Fito-Boncompte, L., Gicquel, G., et al., 2015. The absence of the *Pseudomonas aeruginosa* OprF protein leads to increased biofilm formation through variation in c-di-GMP level. Frontiers in Microbiology 6. https://doi.org/10.3389/fmicb.2015.00630.

Brady, R.A., Leid, J.G., Calhoun, J.H., Costerton, J.W., Shirtliff, M.E., 2008. Osteomyelitis and the role of biofilms in chronic infection. FEMS Immunology and Medical Microbiology 52, 13−22. https://doi.org/10.1111/j.1574-695X.2007.00357.x.

Casagrande Proietti, P., Stefanetti, V., Hyatt, D.R., Marenzoni, M.L., Capomaccio, S., Coletti, M., et al., 2015. Phenotypic and genotypic characterization of canine pyoderma isolates of *Staphylococcus pseudintermedius* for biofilm formation. Journal of Veterinary Medical Science 77, 945−951. https://doi.org/10.1292/jvms.15-0043.

Cattelan, N., Villalba, M., Parisi, G., Arnal, L., Serra, D.O., Aguilar, M., et al., 2016. Outer membrane protein OmpQ of *Bordetella bronchiseptica* is required for mature biofilm formation. Microbiology (United Kingdom) 162, 351−363. https://doi.org/10.1099/mic.0.000224.

Ceotto-Vigoder, H., Marques, S.L.S., Santos, I.N.S., Alves, M.D.B., Barrias, E.S., Potter, A., et al., 2016. Nisin and lysostaphin activity against preformed biofilm of *Staphylococcus aureus* involved in bovine mastitis. Journal of Applied Microbiology 121, 101−114. https://doi.org/10.1111/jam.13136.

Chai, D., Liu, X., Wang, R., Bai, Y., Cai, Y., 2016. Efficacy of linezolid and fosfomycin in catheter-related biofilm infection caused by methicillin-resistant *Staphylococcus aureus*. BioMed Research International 2016, 1−7. https://doi.org/10.1155/2016/6413982.

Chalhoub, H., Sáenz, Y., Nichols, W.W., Tulkens, P.M., Van Bambeke, F., 2018. Loss of activity of ceftazidime-avibactam due to MexAB-OprM efflux and overproduction of AmpC cephalosporinase in *Pseudomonas aeruginosa* isolated from patients suffering from cystic fibrosis. International Journal of Antimicrobial Agents 52, 697−701. https://doi.org/10.1016/j.ijantimicag.2018.07.027.

Characklis, W.G., 1973. Attached microbial growths—II. Frictional resistance due to microbial slimes. Water Research 7, 1249−1258. https://doi.org/10.1016/0043-1354(73)90002-X.

Chen, C., 2001. Periodontitis as a biofilm infection. Journal of the California Dental Association 29, 362−369.

Christensen, G.D., Simpson, W.A., Bisno, A.L., Beachey, E.H., 1982. Adherence of slime-producing strains of Staphylococcus epidermidis to smooth surfaces. Infection and Immunity 37, 318−326. https://doi.org/10.1039/c4nr02231a.

Christensen, G.D., Simpson, W.A., Younger, J.J., Baddour, L.M., Barrett, F.F., Melton, D.M., et al., 1985. Adherence of coagulase-negative staphylococci to plastic tissue culture plates: a quantitative model for the adherence of staphylococci to medical devices. Journal of Clinical Microbiology 22, 996−1006.

Conlon, B.P., 2014. *Staphylococcus aureus* chronic and relapsing infections: evidence of a role for persister cells an investigation of persister cells, their formation and their role in *S. aureus* disease. BioEssays 36, 991−996. https://doi.org/10.1002/bies.201400080.

Costerton, W.J., Wilson, M., 2004. Introducing biofilms. Biofilms 1, 1−4. https://doi.org/10.1017/S1479050504001164.

Davies, D.G., Marques, C.N.H., 2009. A fatty acid messenger is responsible for inducing dispersion in microbial biofilms. Journal of Bacteriology 191, 1393−1403. https://doi.org/10.1128/JB.01214-08.

Davies, D., 2003. Understanding biofilm resistance to antibacterial agents. Nature Reviews Drug Discovery 2, 114–122. https://doi.org/10.1038/nrd1008.

De Lancey Pulcini, E., Pulcini, E., 2001. Bacterial biofilms: a review of current research. Nephrologie 22, 439–441.

Deter, H.S., Jensen, R.V., Mather, W.H., Butzin, N.C., 2017. Mechanisms for differential protein production in toxin–antitoxin systems. Toxins (Basel) 9. https://doi.org/10.3390/toxins9070211.

Devlin-Mullin, A., Todd, N.M., Golrokhi, Z., Geng, H., Konerding, M.A., Ternan, N.G., et al., 2017. Atomic layer deposition of a silver nanolayer on advanced titanium orthopedic implants inhibits bacterial colonization and supports vascularized de novo bone ingrowth. Advanced Healthcare Materials 6, 1700033. https://doi.org/10.1002/adhm.201700033.

Donlan, R.M., 2002. Biofilms: microbial life on surfaces. Emerging Infectious Diseases 8, 881–890. https://doi.org/10.3201/eid0809.020063.

Dörr, T., Vulić, M., Lewis, K., 2010. Ciprofloxacin causes persister formation by inducing the TisB toxin in *Escherichia coli*. PLoS Biology 8. https://doi.org/10.1371/journal.pbio.1000317.

Dutta, T.K., Chakraborty, S., Das, M., Mandakini, R., Vanrahmlimphuii, Roychoudhury, P., et al., 2018. Multidrug-resistant Staphylococcus pettenkoferi isolated from cat in India. Veterinary World 11, 1380–1384. https://doi.org/10.14202/vetworld.2018.1380-1384.

Fasani, R.A., Savageau, M.A., 2013. Molecular mechanisms of multiple toxin-antitoxin systems are coordinated to govern the persister phenotype. Proceedings of the National Academy of Sciences of the United States of America 110, E2528–E2537. https://doi.org/10.1073/pnas.1301023110.

Freeman, D.J., Falkiner, F.R., Keane, C.T., 1989. New method for detecting slime production by coagulase negative staphylococci. Journal of Clinical Pathology 42, 872–874. https://doi.org/10.1136/jcp.42.8.872.

Freire, P.L.L., Albuquerque, A.J.R., Sampaio, F.C., Galembeck, A., Flores, M.A.P., Stamford, T.C.M., et al., 2017. AgNPs: the new allies against S. Mutans biofilm - a pilot clinical trial and microbiological assay. Brazilian Dental Journal 28, 417–422. https://doi.org/10.1590/0103-6440201600994.

Fux, C.A., Costerton, J.W., Stewart, P.S., Stoodley, P., 2005. Survival strategies of infectious biofilms. Trends in Microbiology 13, 34–40. https://doi.org/10.1016/j.tim.2004.11.010.

Garrett, T.R., Bhakoo, M., Zhang, Z., 2008. Bacterial adhesion and biofilms on surfaces. Progress in Natural Science 18, 1049–1056. https://doi.org/10.1016/j.pnsc.2008.04.001.

Gomes, D., Pereira, M., Bettencourt, A.F., 2013. Osteomyelitis: an overview of antimicrobial therapy. Brazilian Journal of Pharmaceutical Sciences 49, 13–27. https://doi.org/10.1590/S1984-82502013000100003.

Gottenbos, B., van der Mei, H.C., Klatter, F., Nieuwenhuis, P., Busscher, H.J., 2002. In vitro and in vivo antimicrobial activity of covalently coupled quaternary ammonium silane coatings on silicone rubber. Biomaterials 23, 1417–1423. https://doi.org/10.1016/S0142-9612(01)00263-0.

Gupta, P., Sarkar, S., Das, B., Bhattacharjee, S., Tribedi, P., 2016. Biofilm, pathogenesis and prevention—a journey to break the wall: a review. Archives of Microbiology 198, 1–15. https://doi.org/10.1007/s00203-015-1148-6.

Hall-Stoodley, L., Costerton, J.W., Stoodley, P., 2004. Bacterial biofilms: from the Natural environment to infectious diseases. Nature Reviews Microbiology 2, 95–108. https://doi.org/10.1038/nrmicro821.

He, X., Yuan, F., Lu, F., Yin, Y., Cao, J., 2017. Vancomycin-induced biofilm formation by methicillin-resistant *Staphylococcus aureus* is associated with the secretion of membrane vesicles. Microbial Pathogenesis 110, 225–231. https://doi.org/10.1016/j.micpath.2017.07.004.

Høiby, N., Ciofu, O., Bjarnsholt, T., 2010. *Pseudomonas aeruginosa* biofilms in cystic fibrosis. Future Microbiology 5, 1663–1674. https://doi.org/10.2217/fmb.10.125.

Høiby, N., 2014. A personal history of research on microbial biofilms and biofilm infections. Pathogens and Disease 70, 205–211. https://doi.org/10.1111/2049-632X.12165.

Holá, V., Růžička, F., 2008. Urinary catheter biofilm infections. Epidemiologie, Mikrobiologie, Imunologie 57, 47–52.

Hughes, G., Webber, M.A., 2017. Novel approaches to the treatment of bacterial biofilm infections. British Journal of Pharmacology 174, 2237–2246. https://doi.org/10.1111/bph.13706.

Jamal, M., Tasneem, U., Hussain, T., Andleeb and, S., Andleeb, S., 2015. Bacterial biofilm: its composition, formation and role in human infections. Journal of Microbiology and Biotechnology 4, 1–14.

Jang, C.H., Cho, Y.B., Jang, Y.S., Kim, M.S., Kim, G.H., 2015. Antibacterial effect of electrospun polycaprolactone/polyethylene oxide/vancomycin nanofiber mat for prevention of periprosthetic infection and biofilm formation. International Journal of Pediatric Otorhinolaryngology 79, 1299–1305. https://doi.org/10.1016/j.ijporl.2015.05.037.

Janssens, J.C.A., Steenackers, H., Robijns, S., Gellens, E., Levin, J., Zhao, H., et al., 2008. Brominated furanones inhibit biofilm formation by *Salmonella enterica* serovar typhimurium. Applied and Environmental Microbiology 74, 6639–6648. https://doi.org/10.1128/AEM.01262-08.

Justo, J.A., Bookstaver, P.B., 2014. Antibiotic lock therapy: review of technique and logistical challenges. Infection and Drug Resistance 7, 343. https://doi.org/10.2147/IDR.S51388.

Kaplan, J.B.B., 2010. Biofilm dispersal: mechanisms, clinical implications, and potential therapeutic uses. Journal of Dental Research 89, 205–218. https://doi.org/10.1177/0022034509359403.

Kaspy, I., Rotem, E., Weiss, N., Ronin, I., Balaban, N.Q., Glaser, G., 2013. HipA-mediated antibiotic persistence via phosphorylation of the glutamyl-tRNA-synthetase. Nature Communications 4. https://doi.org/10.1038/ncomms4001.

Keren, I., Kaldalu, N., Spoering, A., Wang, Y., Lewis, K., 2004. Persister cells and tolerance to antimicrobials. FEMS Microbiology Letters 230, 13–18. https://doi.org/10.1016/S0378-1097(03)00856-5.

Khan, W., Bernier, S.P., Kuchma, S.L., Hammond, J.H., Hasan, F., O'Toole, G.A., 2010. Aminoglycoside resistance of *Pseudomonas aeruginosa* biofilms modulated by extracellular polysaccharide. International Microbiology 13, 207–212. https://doi.org/10.2436/20.1501.01.127.

Kim, J.-S., Heo, P., Yang, T.-J., Lee, K.-S., Cho, D.-H., Kim, B.T., et al., 2011. Selective killing of bacterial persisters by a single chemical compound without affecting normal antibiotic-sensitive cells. Antimicrobial Agents and Chemotherapy 55, 5380–5383. https://doi.org/10.1128/AAC.00708-11.

Kim, M., Kang, N., Ko, S., Park, J., Park, E., Shin, D., et al., 2018. Antibacterial and antibiofilm activity and mode of action of magainin 2 against drug-resistant *Acinetobacter baumannii*. International Journal of Molecular Sciences 19, 3041. https://doi.org/10.3390/ijms19103041.

Kong, K.-F., Vuong, C., Otto, M., 2006. Staphylococcus quorum sensing in biofilm formation and infection. International Journal of Medical Microbiology 296, 133—139. https://doi.org/10.1016/j.ijmm.2006.01.042.

Kudrin, P., Varik, V., Oliveira, S.R.A., Beljantseva, J., Del Peso Santos, T., Dzhygyr, I., et al., 2017. Subinhibitory concentrations of bacteriostatic antibiotics induce relA-dependent and relA-independent tolerance to β-lactams. Antimicrobial Agents and Chemotherapy 61. https://doi.org/10.1128/AAC.02173-16.

Kwan, B.W., Valenta, J.A., Benedik, M.J., Wood, T.K., 2013. Arrested protein synthesis increases persister-like cell formation. Antimicrobial Agents and Chemotherapy 57, 1468—1473. https://doi.org/10.1128/AAC.02135-12.

Law, W., Leatham-Jensen, M., Cohen, P., Camberg, J., 2015. Persister cell control mechanisms in uropathogenic *Escherichia coli*. The FASEB Journal 29. https://doi.org/10.1096/fasebj.29.1_supplement.575.5, 575.5.

Lechner, S., Lewis, K., Bertram, R., 2012. *Staphylococcus aureus* persisters tolerant to bactericidal antibiotics. Journal of Molecular Microbiology and Biotechnology 22, 235—244. https://doi.org/10.1159/000342449.

Leid, J.G., Cope, E.K., Parmenter, S., Shirtliff, M.E., Dowd, S., Wolcott, R., et al., 2011. The Importance of Biofilms in Chronic Rhinosinusitis. Biofilm Infect. Springer New York, New York, NY, pp. 139—160. https://doi.org/10.1007/978-1-4419-6084-9_8.

Lewis, K., 2005. Persister cells and the riddle of biofilm survival. Biochemistry 70, 267—274. https://doi.org/10.1007/s10541-005-0111-6.

Lewis, K., 2007. Persister cells, dormancy and infectious disease. Nature Reviews Microbiology 5, 48—56. https://doi.org/10.1038/nrmicro1557.

Lewis, K., 2010. Persister Cells and the Paradox of Chronic Infections Dormant Persister Cells Are Tolerant to Antibiotics and Are Largely Responsible for Recalcitrance of Chronic Infections, vol. 5, pp. 429—437.

Lewis, K., 2010. Persister cells. Annual Review of Microbiology 64, 357—372. https://doi.org/10.1146/annurev.micro.112408.134306.

Li, Y., Zhang, Y., 2007. PhoU is a persistence switch involved in persister formation and tolerance to multiple antibiotics and stresses in *Escherichia coli*. Antimicrobial Agents and Chemotherapy 51, 2092—2099. https://doi.org/10.1128/AAC.00052-07.

Li, T., Yin, N., Liu, H., Pei, J., Lai, L., 2016. Novel inhibitors of toxin HipA reduce multidrug tolerant persisters. ACS Medicinal Chemistry Letters 7, 449—453. https://doi.org/10.1021/acsmedchemlett.5b00420.

Liu, Y., Yang, L., Molin, S., 2010. Synergistic activities of an efflux pump inhibitor and iron chelators against *Pseudomonas aeruginosa* growth and biofilm formation. Antimicrobial Agents and Chemotherapy 54, 3960—3963. https://doi.org/10.1128/AAC.00463-10.

Manuel, A., Rao, J.V., John, K., Aranjani, J.M., 2014. Biofilm production and antibiotic susceptibility of planktonic and biofilm bacteria of canine dental tartar isolates. Acta Scientiae Veterinariae 42.

Marić, S., Vraneš, J., 2007. Characteristics and significance of microbial biofilm formation. Periodicum Biologorum 109, 115—121.

Marques, C.N.H., Davies, D.G., Sauer, K., 2015. Control of biofilms with the fatty acid signaling molecule cis-2-Decenoic acid. Pharmaceuticals 8, 816—835. https://doi.org/10.3390/ph8040816.

Mcbride, M., Malcolm, K., Woolfson, D., Gorman, S., 2009. Sustained release of triclosan from silicone elastomers modified with allyl monomethoxy poly(ethylene glycol). Journal of Pharmacy and Pharmacology 61. A12—3.

Meije, Y., Almirante, B., Del Pozo, J.L., Martín, M.T., Fernández-Hidalgo, N., Shan, A., et al., 2014. Daptomycin is effective as antibiotic-lock therapy in a model of *Staphylococcus aureus* catheter-related infection. Journal of Infection 68, 548—552. https://doi.org/10.1016/j.jinf.2014.01.001.

Melchior, M.B., Vaarkamp, H., Fink-Gremmels, J., 2006. Biofilms: a role in recurrent mastitis infections? The Veterinary Journal 171, 398—407. https://doi.org/10.1016/j.tvjl.2005.01.006.

Melchior, M.B., 2011. Bovine mastitis and biofilms. Biofilms and Veterinary Medicine 6, 205—221. https://doi.org/10.1007/978-3-642-21289-5.

Michalopoulos, A., Geroulanos, S., 1996. Central venous catheter-related infections. European Journal of Anaesthesiology 13, 445—455. https://doi.org/10.1097/00003643-199609000-00004.

Miranda, P.S.D., Lannes-Costa, P.S., Pimentel, B.A.S., Silva, L.G., Ferreira-Carvalho, B.T., Menezes, G.C., et al., 2018. Biofilm formation on different pH conditions by Streptococcus agalactiae isolated from bovine mastitic milk. Letters in Applied Microbiology 67, 235—243. https://doi.org/10.1111/lam.13015.

Möker, N., Dean, C.R., Tao, J., 2010. *Pseudomonas aeruginosa* increases formation of multidrug-tolerant persister cells in response to quorum-sensing signaling molecules. Journal of Bacteriology 192, 1946—1955. https://doi.org/10.1128/JB.01231-09.

Monnet, V., Gardan, R., 2015. Quorum-sensing regulators in Gram-positive bacteria: "cherchez le peptide". Molecular Microbiology 97, 181—184. https://doi.org/10.1111/mmi.13060.

Neu, T.R., Lawrence, J.R., 2010. Extracellular polymeric substances in microbial biofilms. Microbial Glycobiology 733—758. https://doi.org/10.1016/B978-0-12-374546-0.00037-7. Elsevier.

Neut, D., Hendriks, J.G.E., van Horn, J.R., Kowalski, R.S.Z., van der Mei, H.C., Busscher, H.J., 2006. Antimicrobial efficacy of gentamicin-loaded acrylic bone cements with fusidic acid or clindamycin added. Journal of Orthopaedic Research 24, 291—299. https://doi.org/10.1002/jor.20058.

Neut, D., Dijkstra, R.J.B., Thompson, J.I., Van Der Mei, H.C., Busscher, H.J., 2011. Antibacterial efficacy of a new gentamicin-coating for cementless prostheses compared to gentamicin-loaded bone cement. Journal of Orthopaedic Research 29, 1654—1661. https://doi.org/10.1002/jor.21433.

Notcovich, S., DeNicolo, G., Flint, S., Williamson, N., Gedye, K., Grinberg, A., et al., 2018. Biofilm-forming potential of *Staphylococcus aureus* isolated from bovine mastitis in New Zealand. Veterinary Sciences 5, 8. https://doi.org/10.3390/vetsci5010008.

Nuttall, T., 2016. Successful management of otitis externa. In Practice 38, 17—21. https://doi.org/10.1136/inp.i1951.

O'May, C.Y., Sanderson, K., Roddam, L.F., Kirov, S.M., Reid, D.W., 2009. Iron-binding compounds impair *Pseudomonas aeruginosa* biofilm formation, especially under anaerobic conditions. Journal of Medical Microbiology 58, 765—773. https://doi.org/10.1099/jmm.0.004416-0.

Orman, M.A., Brynildsen, M.P., 2013. Establishment of a method to rapidly assay bacterial persister metabolism. Antimicrobial Agents and Chemotherapy 57, 4398–4409. https://doi.org/10.1128/AAC.00372-13.

Park, J.H., Lee, J.K., Um, H.S., Chang, B.S., Lee, S.Y., 2014. A periodontitis-associated multispecies model of an oral biofilm. Journal of Periodontal and Implant Science 44, 79–84. https://doi.org/10.5051/jpis.2014.44.2.79.

Petruzzi, B., Dalloul, R.A., LeRoith, T., Evans, N.P., Pierson, F.W., Inzana, T.J., 2018. Biofilm formation and avian immune response following experimental acute and chronic avian cholera due to *Pasteurella multocida*. Veterinary Microbiology 222, 114–123. https://doi.org/10.1016/j.vetmic.2018.07.005.

Prince, A.A., Steiger, J.D., Khalid, A.N., Dogrhamji, L., Reger, C., Claire, S.E., et al., 2008. Prevalence of biofilm-forming bacteria in chronic rhinosinusitis. American Journal of Rhinology 22, 239–245. https://doi.org/10.2500/ajr.2008.22.3180.

Prüß, B.M., Prüß, B.M., 2017. Involvement of two-component signaling on bacterial motility and biofilm development. Journal of Bacteriology 199. https://doi.org/10.1128/JB.00259-17.

Rahmani-Badi, A., Sepehr, S., Babaie-Naiej, H., 2015. A combination of cis-2-decenoic acid and chlorhexidine removes dental plaque. Archives of Oral Biology 60, 1655–1661. https://doi.org/10.1016/j.archoralbio.2015.08.006.

Reinoso, E.B., 2017. Bovine mastitis caused by *Streptococcus uberis*: virulence factors and biofilm. Journal of Microbial and Biochemical Technology 9, 237–243. https://doi.org/10.4172/1948-5948.1000371.

Rodríguez-Melcón, C., Capita, R., Rodríguez-Jerez, J.J., Martínez-Suárez, J.V., Alonso-Calleja, C., 2018. Effect of low doses of disinfectants on the biofilm-forming ability of *Listeria monocytogenes*. Foodborne Pathogens and Disease. https://doi.org/10.1089/fpd.2018.2472.

Sabir, N., Ikram, A., Zaman, G., Satti, L., Gardezi, A., Ahmed, A., et al., 2017. Bacterial biofilm-based catheter-associated urinary tract infections: causative pathogens and antibiotic resistance. American Journal of Infection Control 45, 1101–1105. https://doi.org/10.1016/j.ajic.2017.05.009.

Sarabhai, S., Sharma, P., Capalash, N., 2013. Ellagic acid derivatives from *Terminalia chebula* Retz. Downregulate the expression of quorum sensing genes to attenuate *Pseudomonas aeruginosa* PAO1 virulence. PLoS One 8. https://doi.org/10.1371/journal.pone.0053441.

Schaudinn, C., Gorur, A., Keller, D., Sedghizadeh, P.P., Costerton, J.W., 2009. Periodontitis: an archetypical biofilm disease. Journal of the American Dental Association 140, 978–986. https://doi.org/10.14219/jada.archive.2009.0307.

Schönborn, S., Krömker, V., Schoenborn, S., Kroemker, V., 2016. Detection of the biofilm component polysaccharide intercellular adhesin in *Staphylococcus aureus* infected cow udders. Veterinary Microbiology 196, 126–128. https://doi.org/10.1016/j.vetmic.2016.10.023.

Scott, C.P., Higham, P.A., 2003. Antibiotic bone cement for the treatment of Pseudomonas aeruginosa in joint arthroplasty: comparison of tobramycin and gentamicin-loaded cements. Journal of Biomedical Materials Research Part B: Applied Biomaterials 64, 94–98. https://doi.org/10.1002/jbm.b.10515.

Silverstein, A., Donatucci, C.F., 2003. Bacterial Biofilms and implantable prosthetic devices. International Journal of Impotence Research 15. https://doi.org/10.1038/sj.ijir.3901093.

Simões, L.C., Lemos, M., Pereira, A.M., Abreu, A.C., Saavedra, M.J., Simões, M., 2011. Persister cells in a biofilm treated with a biocide. Biofouling 27, 403–411. https://doi.org/10.1080/08927014.2011.579599.

Singh, R., Sahore, S., Kaur, P., Rani, A., Ray, P., 2016. Penetration barrier contributes to bacterial biofilm-associated resistance against only select antibiotics, and exhibits genus-, strain- and antibiotic-specific differences. Pathogens and Disease 74, ftw056. https://doi.org/10.1093/femspd/ftw056.

Slavkin, S.H.C., 1997. Biofilms, microbial ecology and Antoni van Leeuwenhoek. Journal of the American Dental Association 128, 492–495. https://doi.org/10.14219/jada.archive.1997.0238.

Slobodníková, L., Fialová, S., Hupková, H., Grančai, D., 2013. Rosmarinic acid interaction with planktonic and biofilm *Staphylococcus aureus*. Natural Product Communications 8, 1747–1750.

Song, J.Y., Cheong, H.J., Noh, J.Y., Kim, W.J., 2015. In vitro comparison of anti-biofilm effects against carbapenem-resistant *Acinetobacter baumannii*: imipenem, colistin, tigecycline, rifampicin and combinations. Infection and Chemotherapy 47, 27. https://doi.org/10.3947/ic.2015.47.1.27.

Starkey, M., Lepine, F., Maura, D., Bandyopadhaya, A., Lesic, B., He, J., et al., 2014. Identification of anti-virulence compounds that disrupt quorum-sensing regulated acute and persistent pathogenicity. PLoS Pathogens 10. https://doi.org/10.1371/journal.ppat.1004321.

Stefanetti, V., Bietta, A., Pascucci, L., Marenzoni, M.L., Coletti, M., Franciosini, M.P., et al., 2017. Investigation of the antibiotic resistance and biofilm formation of Staphylococcus pseudintermedius strains isolated from canine pyoderma. Veterinaria Italiana 53, 289–296. https://doi.org/10.12834/VetIt.465.2275.6.

Steindler, L., Venturi, V., 2007. Detection of quorum-sensing N -acyl homoserine lactone signal molecules by bacterial biosensors. FEMS Microbiology Letters 266, 1–9. https://doi.org/10.1111/j.1574-6968.2006.00501.x.

Stoodley, P., Sauer, K., Davies, D.G., Costerton, J.W., 2002. Biofilms as complex differentiated communities. Annual Review of Microbiology 56, 187–209. https://doi.org/10.1146/annurev.micro.56.012302.160705.

Sun, C., Guo, Y., Tang, K., Wen, Z., Li, B., Zeng, Z., et al., 2017. MqsR/MqsA toxin/antitoxin system regulates persistence and biofilm formation in pseudomonas putida KT2440. Frontiers in Microbiology 8, 840. https://doi.org/10.3389/fmicb.2017.00840.

Swanson, E.A., Freeman, L.J., Seleem, M.N., Snyder, P.W., 2014. Biofilm-infected wounds in a dog. Journal of the American Veterinary Medical Association 244, 699–707. https://doi.org/10.2460/javma.244.6.699.

Szczuka, E., Grabska, K., Kaznowski, A., 2015. In vitro activity of rifampicin combined with daptomycin or tigecycline on Staphylococcus haemolyticus biofilms. Current Microbiology 71, 184–189. https://doi.org/10.1007/s00284-015-0821-y.

Talpaert, M.J., Balfour, A., Stevens, S., Baker, M., Muhlschlegel, F.A., Gourlay, C.W., et al., 2015. Candida biofilm formation on voice prostheses. Journal of Medical Microbiology 64, 199–208. https://doi.org/10.1099/jmm.0.078717-0.

Trautner, B.W., Darouiche, R.O., 2004. Role of biofilm in catheter-associated urinary tract infection. American Journal of Infection Control 32, 177–183. https://doi.org/10.1016/j.ajic.2003.08.005.

Vandeputte, O.M., Kiendrebeogo, M., Rajaonson, S., Diallo, B., Mol, A., Jaziri, M.E., et al., 2010. Identification of catechin as one of the flavonoids from combretum albiflorum bark extract that reduces the production of quorum-sensing-controlled virulence factors in pseudomonas aeruginosa PAQ1. Applied and Environmental Microbiology 76, 243−253. https://doi.org/10.1128/AEM.01059-09.

Vu, B., Chen, M., Crawford, R.J., Ivanova, E.P., 2009. Bacterial extracellular polysaccharides involved in biofilm formation. Molecules 14, 2535−2554. https://doi.org/10.3390/molecules14072535.

Wakamoto, Y., Dhar, N., Chait, R., Schneider, K., Signorino-Gelo, F., Leibler, S., et al., 2013. Dynamic persistence of antibiotic-stressed mycobacteria. Science (80-) 339, 91−95. https://doi.org/10.1126/science.1229858.

Walters, M.C., Roe, F., Bugnicourt, A., Franklin, M.J., Stewart, P.S., 2003. Contributions of antibiotic penetration, oxygen limitation, and low metabolic activity to tolerance of *Pseudomonas aeruginosa* biofilms to ciprofloxacin and tobramycin. Antimicrobial Agents and Chemotherapy 47, 317−323. https://doi.org/10.1128/AAC.47.1.317-323.2003.

Wilton, M., Charron-Mazenod, L., Moore, R., Lewenza, S., 2016. Extracellular DNA acidifies biofilms and induces aminoglycoside resistance in *Pseudomonas aeruginosa*. Antimicrobial Agents and Chemotherapy 60, 544−553. https://doi.org/10.1128/AAC.01650-15.

Wood, T.K., Knabel, S.J., Kwan, B.W., 2013. Bacterial persister cell formation and dormancy. Applied and Environmental Microbiology 79, 7116−7121. https://doi.org/10.1128/AEM.02636-13.

Wood, T.K., 2016. Combatting bacterial persister cells. Biotechnology and Bioengineering 113, 476−483. https://doi.org/10.1002/bit.25721.

Wood, T.K., 2017. Strategies for combating persister cell and biofilm infections. Microbial Biotechnology 10, 1054−1056. https://doi.org/10.1111/1751-7915.12774.

Wu, H., Moser, C., Wang, H.Z., Høiby, N., Song, Z.J., 2015. Strategies for combating bacterial biofilm infections. International Journal of Oral Science 7, 1−7. https://doi.org/10.1038/ijos.2014.65.

Yamasaki, S., Wang, L.-Y.Y., Hirata, T., Hayashi-Nishino, M., Nishino, K., 2015. Multidrug efflux pumps contribute to *Escherichia coli* biofilm maintenance. International Journal of Antimicrobial Agents 45, 439−441. https://doi.org/10.1016/j.ijantimicag.2014.12.005.

Yujie, L., Geng, X., Huang, Y.C., Li, Y., Yang, K., Ye, L., et al., 2013. The effect of brominated furanones on the formation of *Staphylococcus aureus* biofilm on PVC. Cell Biochemistry and Biophysics 67, 1501−1505. https://doi.org/10.1007/s12013-013-9652-2.

Zambori, C., Cumpanasoiu, C., Bianca, M., Tirziu, E., 2013. Biofilms in oral cavity of dogs and implication in zoonotic infections. Scientific Papers Animal Science and Biotechnologies/Lucrari Stiintifice Zootehnie Si Biotehnologii 46, 155−158.

Zhang, Z., Kofonow, J.M., Finkelman, B.S., Doghramji, L., Chiu, A.G., Kennedy, D.W., et al., 2011. Clinical factors associated with bacterial biofilm formation in chronic rhinosinusitis. Otolaryngology−Head and Neck Surgery 144, 457−462. https://doi.org/10.1177/0194599810394302.

Chapter 13

Characteristics of antimicrobial resistance among microorganisms of concern to animal, fish and human health: *Salmonella*

Chapter outline

In 19th century, etiology of typhoid fever was suspected, which later became confirmed as *Salmonella*. Salmon and Smith (1885) first isolated *Bacillus cholera suis* as a causative agent of hog cholera, an infection shattering swine industry. It was considered as a reason of 'hog cholera' until the discovery of the real causative virus. The nomenclature of '*Salmonella*' was done in memory of Salmon and now the bacterium is known as *Salmonella enterica* subspecies *enterica* serovar Choleraesuis. Gartner first isolated *Salmonella enteritidis* from meat poisoning case in a man in 1888. In 1889, Klein in the United Kingdom isolated *Salmonella gallinarum* from chicken suffering with a disease referred as 'fowl typhoid'. Rettger (1900) first described *Salmonella pullorum* from chicken suffering from severe diarrhoea.

Nontyphoidal *Salmonella* (NTS), *Campylobacter* and *Escherichia coli* are considered as most common zoonotic pathogens transmitted through food animals or food products to human (WHO, 2014). A global estimate revealed 93.8 million cases of salmonellosis each year and among them 80 million cases are considered as foodborne infections (Majowicz et al., 2010; Crim et al., 2015). In the United States, nontyphoidal *Salmonella* causes an estimated 1.2 million illnesses, 23,000 hospitalizations and 450 deaths (Scaallan et al., 2011; CDC, 2013). During the period 1997−2011, *Salmonella* infections increased from 13.6 to 16.4 cases per 100,000 people (17.1%, U.S. Department of Health and Human Services, 2014). The annual cost associated with salmonellosis in the United States alone has been estimated to be approximately 14.6 billion US dollar including 365 million US dollar as direct medical costs (Scharff, 2010; CDC, 2013). In sub-Saharan Africa, NTS are observed as the most common organism present in bloodstream of children and adults suffering with fever (Feasey et al., 2012).

Antimicrobial agents are frequently used in therapeutic and subtherapeutic doses in food animals and poultry for the treatment of infection and promotion of growth. The commensal present in food animals and exposed to the antimicrobial pressure develop survival strategies through evolutionary adaptations and thus the resistant bugs are generated (Mahanti et al., 2017). Although, use of antimicrobials in subtherapeutic dosage in food animals might not be the sole factor responsible for generation of antimicrobial resistance. Currently, *antimicrobial-resistant* nontyphoidal *Salmonella* raises concern with an estimated 100,000 annual domestic cases and 40 deaths in the United States alone (CDC, 2013). In Europe and North America, outbreaks of multidrug-resistant *Salmonella* are observed in people because of consumption of pork or beef products (Mindlin et al., 2013; Laufer et al., 2015). In African countries, incidence of NTS infection especially with *S. typhimurium* or *S. enteritidis* is increased in recent times with the acquisition of multidrug resistance (García et al., 2016).

Properties

Morphology: *Salmonella* are Gram negative short rods, 2–4 μm in length and 0.5 μm in width varying form coccoid shape to long filamentous forms. They are nonspore-forming and mostly motile by peritrichous flagella (except certain strains of *S. gallinarum* and *S. pullorum*). A few mucoid colony-forming strains are capsulated and are fimbriated.

Classification: The genus *Salmonella* belongs to the family *Enterobacteriaceae* under the order Enterobacteriales. There are two major species under the genus *Salmonella*, known as *Salmonella enterica* and *Salmonella bongori*. *S. enterica* is considered as type species of the genus and it has six subspecies (ssp): *salamae, arizonae, diarizonae, houtenae, indica* and *enterica*. Currently in total 2610 serovars of *Salmonella* has been identified. The serovars such as Typhi, Enteritidis, Typhimurium, Newport, Heidelberg, Dublin, Choleraesuis, Pullorum, Gallinarum and Abortusovis are considered as virulent serovars. The serovars Enteritidis, Typhimurium, Newport and Heidelberg are most commonly associated with human infections (Helke et al., 2017).

Serovar Dublin is highly host adapted to cattle and occasionally it causes human infection with high mortality (Mandal and Brennand, 1988). In a comprehensive study with various *Salmonella* serovars isolated from cattle during 2006–15 revealed the serovar Dublin as the most prevalent serovar in the United States (Valenzuela et al., 2017). Other serovars such as Newport, Kentucky, Montevideo, Anatum, Typhimurium, Cerro and 4,5,12:i are also common in cattle with or without producing any clinical symptoms (Cummings et al., 2010; Rao et al., 2010; Loneragan et al., 2012; Rodriguez-Rivera et al., 2014). Serovar Cerro is rarely associated with human infection, although in recent past, occurrence of Cerro has increased both in cattle and human in the United States (Tewari et al., 2012; CDC, 2014). Probably 'Dublin' specific vaccination in cattle has created selection pressure which favors the increased occurrence of Cerro (Valenzuela et al., 2017). In India, Typhimurium, Anatum, Dublin, Weltevreden, Newport, Enteritidis and Richmond serovars are common in cattle and buffalo (Gupta and Verma, 1993).

The serovars Cholerasuis var. Kunzendorf, Typhimurium, Typhimurium var.5, Derby and Heidelberg are currently circulating in swine population (Clothier et al., 2010; Deckert et al., 2010; Aslam et al., 2012; Schmidt et al., 2012; Arguello et al., 2013; Gantzhorn et al., 2014). In India, serovars Cholerae suis, Anatum, Stanley, Virginia, Litchfield, Poona and Weltevreden are detected in pigs (Gupta and Verma, 1993).

Salmonella enterica serovars such as Hadar, Kentucky, Enteritidis, Heidelberg and Typhimurium are common in poultry and in the farm environment, carcass rinsate and retail products (Melendez et al., 2010; M'Ikanatha et al., 2010; Aslam et al., 2012; Diarra et al., 2014; Sapkota et al., 2014). In the United States, nationwide microbiological baseline data collection program during 2007–08 revealed the presence of Kentucky, Heidelberg, Typhimurium and Typhimurium (*var* 5-) serovars in young chicken (Food Safety Inspection Service, 2008). The serovar Kentucky was most frequently detected in poultry carcass surveillance programs through FoodNet in the United States (Jones et al., 2008). In Asian countries such as in India, Typhimurium and Enteritidis are common in commercial poultry eggs (Suresh et al., 2006; Singh et al., 2013). Our own study with the samples collected from backyard poultry, their feed, drinking water, utensils, litter, dried manure under the house, soil and eggs also revealed the presence of *S. enteritidis* and *S. typhimurium* in India (Samanta et al., 2014). *Salmonella* Corvallis, originally isolated from poultry in 1949, is observed in Japan, Bulgaria, Denmark and Tunisia with higher frequency (Hamada and Tsuji, 2001; Archambault et al., 2006; Ben Aissa et al., 2007).

Among all these serovars present in food animals and birds, antimicrobial resistance is common in four serovars such as Typhimurium, Enteritidis, Newport and Heidelberg as observed in the United States (Medalla et al., 2013; Crim et al., 2015).

Susceptibility to disinfectants: Common disinfectants such as phenol, cresol and formaldehyde (during fumigation) are lethal to *Salmonella*. Disinfection is hampered in presence of faeces, mucus and organic substances. Faecal materials protect the bacteria from desiccation under the direct sunlight. *Salmonella* do not multiply at low temperature but can survive freezing. They can also survive in acidic foods (pH ≤ 4.6). *Salmonella dublin* can survive for months in organic matter such as slurry, manure and soil (Taylor and Burrows, 1971) and for years in dried-in faecal matter (Plym-Forshell and Ekesbo, 1996).

Natural habitat: All warm-blooded animals and human and a few cold-blooded animals can harbour *Salmonella* in their intestinal tract. It can survive approximately up to 9 months in moist soil, water and vegetables. The carrier animals or birds showing no clinical symptoms often shed the bacteria and act as a source of infection. Active carriers are formed after recovery from the *Salmonella* infection and the carriers can shed the bacteria for several months/years up to 10^5 cfu/g of faeces. Certain stress factors such as transportation, parturition, steroid administration and concurrent viral/protozoal infection may enhance the shedding.

Cold-blooded animals such as turtles, tortoises, snakes and lizards are common pets especially in European Union countries (Engler and Parry-Jones, 2007). Reptiles are considered as intermittent shedder of salmonellae in their faeces. Transmission of *Salmonella* into turtle or tortoise eggs takes place during the passage through the cloaca or while the eggs are buried in soil or sand (Feeley and Treger, 1969). In snakes, the bacteria can colonize the ovaries and it can cross the thin membrane surrounding the eggs (Schroter et al., 2006).

Genome

The genome size of *Salmonella* varies from 4659 to 4686 Mb. It carries several pseudogenes. The numbers of pseudogenes vary with *Salmonella* serovars. *Salmonella* has a major pathogenicity island in the genome, i.e., *Salmonella* pathogenicity island-7 (SPI-7) and several other minor islands. The SPI-7 is the largest genomic island (134 Kb) yet identified in *Salmonella*. It was first discovered as a large insertion in the genome of the human restricted pathogen such as *S. typhi* and *S. typhimurium*. Among the other islands, SPI-1 and 2 contain type III secretion system (T3SS). It is a protein complex that helps in virulence factor entry into the host cells. Recent advancement also detects type VI secretion system (T6SS) in many *Salmonella* strains. The T6SS is associated with biofilm formation, cytotoxicity and survival in the phagocytes. It is encoded by the *Salmonella* pathogenicity island 19 (SPI-19), present in serovar Enteritidis, Dublin, Weltevreden and Gallinarum.

The serovars such as Typhimurium, Enteritidis and Choleraesuis are known to harbour virulence plasmids, known as pSLT (94 kbp) and pSEV (60 kbp) for *S. typhimurium* and *S. enteritidis*, respectively. These kinds of plasmids have a genetic region called '*Salmonella* plasmid virulence' (spv, 8 kbp), which contains *spvR* gene as a positive activator and the *spvABCD* operon. These genes help in intracellular bacterial survival, replication and extraintestinal dissemination (Fierer and Guiney, 2001). The spvC has phosphothreonine lyase activity which can inactivate Erk, p38 and JNK mitogen-activated protein kinases (MAPKs). Inactivation of signaling can downregulate the cytokine release from infected cells. The SpvB can deplete F-actin filaments leading to cytotoxicity and apoptosis (Guiney and Fierer, 2011). Some of these virulence plasmids contain transfer (*tra*) genes that help in transfer of these plasmids into other compatible bacterial strain by conjugation.

Genomic organization of an antimicrobial-resistant *Salmonella* was described in a clinical strain of *S. enteritidis*, isolated from a child with gastroenteritis in Spain (CNM 4839/03) in 2003 (Rodríguez et al., 2008). The genome of the isolate contained a derivative of virulence plasmid (pSEV), known as pUO-SeVR1 (Rodríguez et al., 2011).The virulence plasmid DNA is distributed into five segments (I−V) within pUO-SeVR1. Each of the segments is demarcated with two copies of IS26 (IS26-2 to IS26-6), which plays a significant role in transmission of resistance genes among other Gram-negative bacteria (He et al., 2015). Two of the IS26 sequences, i.e., IS26-2 and IS26-3, are flanked by target site duplication sequences (8 bp) (TCGAAAAG and GGAGCTGG, respectively). The DNA located between IS26-1 and IS26-4 is highly homologous to DNA present in plasmids (IncM/IncL) encoding for carbapenemase and extended-spectrum β-lactamases in *Enterobacteriaceae* (Di Pilato et al., 2014; Carattoli et al., 2015). The genomic region starting from IS26-4 to remaining part contains kikA region (killing of *Klebsiella* phenotype), followed by a cluster of resistance genes such as tetracycline (*tetA*), chloramphenicol (catA2) and sulfonamides (*sul*) along with class 1 integron and transposons (Tn1721).

Antigenic characteristics

Motile *Salmonella* possesses two major types of antigens, i.e., somatic and flagellar antigens. On the basis of the variations and types of 'O' and 'H' antigens, Agbaje et al. (2011) developed an antigenic classification system. The isolates are identified by serotyping, with more than 2600 serovars (each a unique combination of O, H1 and H2 antigens) reported. All the serovars are designated by an antigenic formula containing O, H1 and H2 antigens. Currently, other typing systems such as phage typing, pulse-field gel electrophoresis, PCR ribotyping, antimicrobial resistance patterns and multilocus sequencing are also used for differentiation of *Salmonella* strains.

Vi-antigen

It is an additional antigen found in *S. typhi*, *S.* Paratyphi C, *S.* Hirschfeldii and some strains of *S.* Dublin. Structurally, it is a polymer of N-acetyl aminohexuronic acid. Two genetic loci, *viaA*-locus and *viaB*-locus, are required for the production of Vi antigen in *S. typhi* and *S.* Paratyphi C. It is associated with virulence of the organism in mice. It can also be used for Vi-typing of the isolates possessing the antigen. It is also used in Vi-based vaccine production against *Salmonella*.

Toxins and virulence factors produced

Toxins

(i) *Salmonella* Enterotoxin (Stn): It is a heat labile enterotoxin and is produced by *S. typhimurium*. It is functionally related with cholera toxin (CT) and heat labile toxin (LT) of *E. coli*. It binds with ganglioside receptor of host cell. It elevates cAMP level and diarrhoea in a similar way of LT/CT. It can elongate Chinese hamster ovary (CHO) cells in culture, induce fluid secretion in rabbit ligated ileal loop.

(ii) Cytotoxin: It is toxic for target cells due to inhibition of protein synthesis. Death of target cells may interfere absorption or secretion of fluid from intestinal lumen causing diarrhoea. Three kinds of cytotoxins have been detected. (a) Heat labile, trypsin sensitive cytotoxin which causes HeLa and Vero cell cytotoxicity. (b) Low molecular weight cytotoxin (a part of outer membrane protein). (c) Contact haemolysin (26 KDa) which is cytolytic for Vero and other cells.

(iii) Endotoxin (LPS): Lipid-A component of lipopolysaccharide is responsible for toxicity and it is released during bacterial disintegration. The LPS produces vascular damage and thrombosis in the intestine through the induction of inflammatory mediators and cytokines such as interferon, tumour necrosis factor, colony-stimulating factor and interleukin 1. Systemic changes observed in the infection like fever, circulatory collapse, disseminated intravascular coagulation, circulatory collapse characteristic for shock are attributed to the endotoxin action.

Virulence factors: Major virulence factors produced by *Salmonella* are described in Table 13.1.

Transmission

Faecal-oral route is the major transmission route of *Salmonella* in human. Other possible routes include inhalation and through conjunctiva. Carrier food animals and birds can excreate the organisms through the faeces (10^5 cfu/g) that contaminate the environment. Minimum infective dose of *Salmonella* in human is 10^4–10^6 cfu/mL, although low concentration (even in the range of 10–10^2 cfu/mL) can produce infection, if present in foods with higher fat content such as cheese, chocolate, butter, salami (Bell, 2002). Other than food animals, turtles and tortoises, snakes, lizards kept as pet and wild animals and birds can also act as source of infection. In United States, it is observed that 6% of sporadic salmonellosis and 11% of cases in young people below 21 years are caused by reptile and amphibian contact (Sauteur et al., 2013). United States Centers for disease control and prevention (CDC) has recommended to avoid the direct contact with reptiles for the children below the age of five (Vora et al., 2012). An increasing trend is noted for bidirectional transmission of *Salmonella* between wild and food animals (Thomas et al., 2017).For antimicrobial resistant *Salmonella* transmission in susceptible human population, industrial agriculture shares a major responsibility (Grace, 2015).

Among the food animals, poultry are considered as primarily responsible for *Salmonella* associated outbreaks in human. Analysis of *Salmonella* associated outbreak data occurred during 2006–11 in United States and Canada, affecting more than 6000 individuals, revealed that 10 out of 25 outbreaks were related to eggs, live birds or processed poultry products (Cosby et al., 2015). Poultry eggs are major sources of *Salmonella* infection (especially *S. enteritidis*) in consumers. *S. enteritidis* and Typhimurium are most common serovars associated with human outbreaks (Jones et al., 2008). The contamination of poultry houses with *Salmonella* occurs through human, sewage, rodents, or any other sources. The organisms survive and multiply in hen house environment and enter the birds thorough the oral route. The bacteria can penetrate the egg shell during or after oviposition in healthy birds through the faecal contamination. *Salmonella* can also enter into the eggs by direct contamination of yolk, albumen, egg shell before oviposition due to infection in the reproductive tract. Contaminated environment plays major role in transmission of *Salmonella* after laying, when the eggs come out. Other than eggs, undercooked meat or meat products, raw milk, contaminated pasteurized milk and milk products also act as source of infection to human.

Human to human transmission rarely occurs.

TABLE 13.1 Major virulence factors produced by *Salmonella*.

Virulence factors	Function
Acid tolerance response (ATR) regulatory factors/acid shock proteins (RpoS σ-factor, PhoPQ, and Fur proteins)	RpoS and PhoPQ proteins are important for the regulation of survival in the low pH environment created by inorganic acids, whereas Fur and RpoS are involved in the regulation of organic acid tolerance. Thus the organisms can survive in the acidic pH of the intestine.
Fimbriae [type 1 fimbriae (Fim), long polar fimbriae (Lpf), thin aggregative or curli fimbriae and plasmid-encoded fimbriae (Pef)]	Fimbriae help in adhesion of the bacteria with host cells. 'Fim-fimbriae' binds α—D-mannose containing receptor in many host cells. 'Lpf' binds to the surface of the Peyer's patches and M cells, 'Pef' binds to the villous intestine, and curli- fimbriae bind to the small intestine.
Salmonella pathogenicity island 1 (SP1) associated type III secreation system (T3SS)	Major T3SS associated virulence protein is 'SopB'. It causes alteration of ion balance within the cell. It leads to fluid secreation within the intestinal lumen & diarrhoea. Other proteins such as SipA, SopA, SopD, and SopE2 may also play a role in *Salmonella*-associated gastroenteritis. Other T3SS proteins like '*Salmonella* invasion protein' [SipA, SipC; encoded by 'invasin' gene (*inv*)], as well as SopB interact with the actin cytoskeleton causing cytoskeletal rearrangements leading to membrane ruffling. The organisms are trapped within these ruffles. Later they are up taken by these enterocytes. Membrane ruffling helps in internalization of the bacteria within the cells. Hil-A (hyperinvasion) protein either acts as invasion protein or an activator for expression of an invasion protein.
Salmonella pathogenicity island 2 (SP2) associated type III secretion system (T3SS)	Invasive *Salmonella* can express this T3SS associated proteins within 'salmonella containing vacuoles (SCV)' after internalization by the host cell. Major T3SS associated proteins are SifA, SseF, and SseG that interact with microtubule bundles and are involved in the formation of *Salmonella*-induced filaments (SIF) that extend from SCV. This SIF helps in the bacterial replication. Other protein like SpiC is translocated into the cytosol of host macrophages and disrupts the secreation of antimicrobial products like reactive oxygen intermediates (ROI). So intracellular survival depends on these T3SS proteins.
Salmonella pathogenicity island 3 (SP3) encoded proteins	These proteins also help in intracellular survival and are required for growth in Mg^+ deficient conditions.
Salmonella pathogenicity island 4 (SP4) encoded proteins	These proteins help in invasion of host cells
Salmonella pathogenicity island 5 (SP5) encoded proteins	Identified in *S.* Dublin, required for enteric form of the infection.
Salmonella pathogenicity island 7 (SP7)	Identified in *S. typhi, S. typhimurium*. SP7 is associated with the locus for production and export of Vi antigen (*viaB*-locus) and a type IV pilli.
Plasmid encoded virulence factors (a) *Salmonella* plasmid virulence (*spv*)gene encoded proteins (b) '*traT*' gene encoded protein (c) *mig-5* (macrophage-inducible gene) (d) *rck* (e) srgA (SdiA-regulated gene)	(a) These proteins help in intracellular bacterial replication specially during extra intestinal infection. (b) Serum resistance (c) Encodes a carbonic anhydrase expressed after ingestion of the bacteria by macrophages (d) It confers resistance to complement killing by inhibiting C9 polymerization and hence formation of the membrane attack complex (e) It encodes a putative disulphide bond oxido-reductase. Sdi-A is an a quorum sensing protein of the LuxR family
Iron acquisition system: Enterochelin (enterobactin)	It helps in acquisition of iron required for bacterial growth

Diagnosis

Sampling, storage of samples and other critical steps for detection of *Salmonella* from human foods, animal feeds, animal or bird faeces, dust, swabs and environment are described by international organization of standardization (ISO 6579:1-2017). Such guidelines are created to maintain the compatibility between the testing laboratories throughout the world. Several countries have developed their own guidelines such as European Union zoonoses monitoring directive (2003/99/EC), Food and Drug Administration (FDA) food code and Nordic Committee on Food Analysis code etc (EC, 2003; Lee et al., 2015).

Clinical samples include faeces, cloacal swabs of birds and affected tissues, like liver, spleen, reproductive tract, caeca etc. In case of a poultry farm, environmental samples, such as naturally pooled faeces, litter and dust or drag or boot swabs from floor surfaces should be examined in the laboratory to get idea about an outbreak. Specimens should be collected before antibiotic treatment from live animals. After death, the collection should be done immediately from fresh carcasses. In these faecal or environmental samples number of *Salmonella* is low. So for 'pre-enrichment', swabs should be collected in buffered peptone water to help isolation. Pre-enrichment in buffered peptone water helps in survival of *Salmonella* from freezing, heating and desiccation. The cold chain and care to prevent contamination should be maintained during transportation of the samples to the laboratory. Clinical and pathological signs are usually too unspecific to diagnose *Salmonella* infections in food animals and birds.

Presence of fat rich matrices creates hindrance in detection of *Salmonella* in food items. *Salmonella* is identified more easily in cat food and vegetable burgers than liquid eggs, peanut butter, baby oatmeal, cantaloupe etc. For pre-enrichment of food items, buffered peptone water, lactose broth, *Yersinia pestis* enrichment broth are effective.

Laboratory examinations

Direct examination

A smear can be prepared from swab/faecal sample/tissues and stained by Gram's Method. *Salmonella* appears as Gram-negative small rods with no distinct characteristics.

Isolation of Salmonella

Faecal culture specificity for *Salmonella* detection is usually 100%, but the sensitivity is low. Repeated faecal culture can be done for detection of carriers. Alternatively, serological screening followed by faecal culture is recommended (Veling et al., 2002). Minimum 100 cfu/g of the bacterial cell is required in the samples for efficient detection by faecal culture (Richardson and Fawcett, 1973). For efficient culture based detection faecal samples or swabs should be collected in buffered peptone water or lactose broth (pre-enrichment). Pre-enrichment helps in recovery of injured *Salmonella* cells and inhibits the growth of non-specific bacteria (Tietjen and Fung, 1995). Traditional isolation protocol of *Salmonella* includes enrichment of samples followed by isolation of pure colony in specific medium, biochemical, immunological or PCR based confirmation of isolated pure colonies. Current ISO protocol suggests the use of Rappaporte Vassiliadis (RV) and Muller-Kauffmann Tetrathionate-Novobiocin (MKTTn) media for enrichment (ISO, 2017). RappaporteVassiliadis (RV) medium and tetrathionate (TT) broth are also recommended for *Salmonella* enrichment by food emergency response network (FERN) of FDA. For determination of antimicrobial resistant *Salmonella*, specific antibiotics should be added in enrichment and specific isolation media.

The broth containing more than 10^4 cfu/mL of bacterial cells after enrichment can be inoculated into specific isolation media such as *Salmonella-Shigella* agar (SS), brilliant green agar (BGA), bismuth-sulfite agar (BSA), Hektoen enteric (HE), and xylose-lysine-deoxycholate agar (XLD). *S. typhi* produces colourless colonies with black center on SS agar. In BGA, non-fermentation of lactose by *Salmonella* produces alkaline pH. The phenol red indicator produces red coloured colony in this alkaline pH.

HE agar contains bile salts, lactose, salicin and iron salt. *Salmonella* does not ferment these sugars and alkaline pH is produced. The bromothymol blue indicator produces green colonies in alkaline pH. The center of the colony is black due to H_2S production that reacts with iron salt to produce iron sulphide.

XLD agar contains bile salt, xylose, lactose, sucrose, lysine and iron salt. The bile salts prevent the growth of Gram-positive bacteria. *Salmonella* ferments xylose and decarboxylates lysine. Ratio of xylose & lysine is such that decarboxylation always predominates producing alkaline pH. The phenol red indicator produces red colonies in this alkaline pH. The center of the colony is black due to H_2S production that reacts with iron salt to produce iron sulphide. The XLD agar shows higher recovery of *Salmonella* from food items than other selective plating media.

For biochemical confirmation, pure colonies obtained from selective media are inoculated into tripple sugar iron agar, lysine iron agar, urease agar with 40% urea. The whole procedure may require 5−6 days and false positive results are sometimes produced due to presence of contaminant such as *Proteus* spp. (Lee et al., 2015).

Immunological tests

Immunological tests can detect *Salmonella* antigens in the samples and confirm their presence more rapidly than the cultural method. Immunological tests has several loopholes such as prolonged enrichment time for production of optimum numbers of bacterial cells, cross-reactions with related group of bacteria, variations in antigenic structure, erroneous results due to some sample matrices and presence of stressed bacterial cells (Uyttendaele et al., 2003).

Antigen capture ELISA is developed for detection of *Salmonella* in food samples which is commercially validated and is available in the market. It can detect *Salmonella* concentration at the level of $10^4−10^5$ cfu/mL (Lee et al., 2015). Latex agglutination assay uses latex particles coated with anti-*Salmonella* antibodies which react with the bacterial antigens to produce visible aggregates. Several latex based kits are available in the market which is used for confirmation of *Salmonella* in the samples (Eijkelkamp et al., 2009). Presence of motile *Salmonella* in the samples can be detected by immunodiffusion technique (*Salmonella* one to two test system) which produces three-dimensional immunodiffusion band after 14 h incubation (D'Aoust and Sewell, 1988). Immunochromatography or dipstick assay can rapidly detect *Salmonella* in the food samples. However, it requires pre-enrichment and enrichment of samples before conducting the test (Van Beurden, 1992).

Serological tests

ELISAs have developed to detect *S. enteritidis* and *S. typhimurium* in egg yolk, *S.* Dublin in bulk milk or serum of cattle, *Salmonella* in sera or tissue fluid samples of pigs. In Denmark, bulk tank milk is collected in every fourth month from all dairy farms for detection of *S.* Dublin, bovine viral diarrhoea and infectious bovine rhinotracheitis viruses under national surveillance programme. Using bulk tank milk has certain limits such as dilution of high titer milk samples with low titer ones and the dilution rate varies with numbers of cows present in a herd (Nielsen and Ersbøll, 2005). Serum ELISA for detection of *S.* Dublin antibodies in cattle is performed in 3−10 months old animals. Serum ELISA can indicate the presence of *Salmonella* in cattle which might not be a persistent shedder, so detected negative in faecal culture (Nielsen, 2013). Indirect ELISA using LPS antigen can be done for detection of *S. pullorum/gallinarum* in poultry serum or egg yolk.

Molecular biology

Molecular biology based methods can produce reliable results within a few hours to a day which reduce storage space of conventional chemicals and increase the throughput of samples. The sensitivity of PCR based method is 10^4 cfu/mL after enrichment. Processing of food samples require prior treatment to reduce contaminants, non-culturable cells and PCR inhibitory materials such as antibiotics, organic compounds, fat, protein, sugars, and heavy metals (Alakomi and Saarela, 2009). Conventional PCR based diagnostic methods of *Salmonella* target 16S rRNA or *invA* genes (Trkov and Avguštin, 2003). The BAX system is the first commercially available PCR based kit for confirmation of *Salmonella* in food samples (Bennett et al., 1998). Cross-reaction with other related group of bacteria can be reduced with DNA probe hybridization assays specific for *Salmonella* which can give positive results within 48 h. Enrichment of the samples is required to produce higher bacterial concentration for generation of optimum signal (Agron et al., 2001).

Typing of *Salmonella* strains can be done by pulsed field gel electrophoresis (PFGE), multilocus variable tandem repeat analysis (MLVA) and whole genome sequencing (WGS). The PFGE is considered as gold standard typing method specially for searching the sources of foodborne outbreaks. United States CDC initiated typing of bacterial isolates originated from foodborne outbreaks in four state public health laboratories during 1996. The network expanded later and became 'PulseNet international' which included 88 countries from Africa, Asia Pacific, Canada, Europe, Latin America and the Caribbean, Middle East and United States. 'PulseNet' central database still depends on PFGE fingerprints of the isolates from which the database concludes whether the outbreak is 'new' or part of existing circulating bacteria and regarding the origin of the outbreak. For PFGE of *Salmonella* isolates, *XbaI* (50U/sample) *BlnI/AvrII* (30U/sample) and *SpeI* (30U/sample) enzymes are recommended by 'PulseNet' (PulseNet, 2017). MLVA can be used as a complementary technique to PFGE to establish minor differences between the isolates having same PFGE profile. WGS provides more precise data than PFGE by comparing millions of nucleotides present in a bacterial genome.

Nanobiosensor technology

Nano particle based biosensor technology shows potential for detection of *Salmonella* in food items. In an experimental study, sensitivity of quantum dot nanoparticles was detected as 10^3 cfu *Salmonella* cells/mL in food extracts (Kim et al., 2013).

Characteristics of antimicrobial resistance

Multidrug resistant *Salmonella* isolates confer phenotypical resistance against penicillin/ampicillin, chloramphenicol, aminoglycosides (streptomycin), sulfonamides/trimethoprim, tetracycline, cephalosporins and even against relatively fresh antibiotic such as tigecycline (Foley and Lynne, 2008; Sun et al., 2013).Antimicrobial resistance in *Salmonella* isolates is attributed to modification or inactivation of drugs or their target molecules, activation of efflux pumps or increased cell membrane permeability for removal of drugs from bacterial cells (Walsh, 2000). All of these mechanisms are mediated by horizontal transfer of resistance genes and clonal spread of resistant isolates. Plasmids and integrons (class I and class II) containing different types of resistance genes (within gene cassette) play a significant role in horizontal transfer. The role of IncA/C plasmid was elucidated in *Salmonella* strains showing multi drug resistance isolated from food animals (Glenn et al., 2011). Class I and class II integrons are detected in *Salmonella* genomic islands and in the transposon (TN7), respectively (Fluit, 2005; Cosby et al., 2015). *Salmonella* may receive resistance genes either from similar or different types of bacteria such as *E. coli* (Hamada et al., 2003). Global dissemination of the multidrug-resistant *Salmonella typhimurium* DT104 and *S. typhi* (through a specific lineage H58) is example of clonal spread (Davis et al., 2002; Wong et al., 2015).

Tetracycline resistance

The most prevalent phenotypical resistance of *Salmonella* isolates from food animals in United States, Canada and Denmark was detected against tetracycline (Louden et al., 2012). Removal of drug from bacterial cells by an energy-dependent efflux pump is the major mechanism of tetracycline resistance of *Salmonella* isolates. Among different genes conferring tetracycine resistance, *tet(A)*, *tet(B)*, *tet(C)*, *tet(D)*, *tet(G)*, and *tet(H)* are detected in *Salmonella* (Chopra and Roberts, 2001). Among them, *tet(A)* and *tet(B)*, present in mobile genetic elements, are most commonly observed in *Salmonella* isolates (Carattoli et al., 2002).

Aminoglycoside and chloramphenicol resistance

Like other Gram-negative bacteria, resistance to aminoglycosides is produced in non-typhoidal *Salmonella* by reduced uptake of the antibiotic, modification of the antibiotic or ribosomal target of the drug (Alcaine et al., 2007). Resistance to chloramphenicol is generated by enzymatic lysis (chloramphenicol O-acetyl-transferase) or activation of efflux pump to drain out the drug from the bacterial cell (Cannon et al., 1990). Few chloramphenicol associated resistance genes such as *cmlA* and *cmlB* were identified in *Salmonella* isolates (Schwarz and Chaslus-Dancla, 2001). Such kind of resistance was not detected against florfenicol, a similar kind of drug (Keys et al., 2000). Florfenicol was approved by United States Food and Drug Administration (FDA) for veterinary use and was banned for human use to avoid resistance issue (White et al., 2000).

Sulfonamide resistance

Sul gene expressing dihydrofolate synthetase was found responsible for sulfonamide and trimethoprim resistance in *Salmonella* strains (Antunes et al., 2005).

Quinolone resistance

Resistance or reduced susceptibility to quinolones is a common feature of *Salmonella* observed in Korea, Brazil, and other countries (Piddock, 2002; Ferrari et al., 2011; Kim et al., 2013). Animal *Salmonella* isolates showing quinolone resistance was first described in 1990 (Piddock et al., 1990). Ciprofloxacin resistant *S.* Copenhagen strains were isolated from cattle in Germany which showed similarity with human isolates (Heisig, 1993). Mutation in chromosomal genes (*gyrA*, *gyrB* etc.) specially C $\rightarrow$ T transition resulting Ser83 $\rightarrow$ Phe amino acid substitution can produce quinolone resistance in *Salmonella*/*E. coli*. The loss of hydrogen bond forming capacity of serine due to loss of hydroxyl group, and replacement of serine with a hydrophobic residue causes decrease in binding of quinolones with DNA gyrase (Griggs et al., 1996). In mutant bacterial strains, increased expression of certain transcriptional activators (MarA and SoxS) alters the production of the proteins such as OmpF and acrAB. Reduced production of OmpF inhibits the entry of quinolones within bacterial cells and increased production of acrAB activates proton motive force driven efflux pump which evacuate the drug from the bacterial cell (Okusu et al., 1996). Over expression of MarA and SoxS is induced by quinolones and also by tetracycline, chloramphenicol and certain disinfectants such as pine oil, dinitrophenol, menadione, paraquat, benzoate and sodium salicylate (Cohen et al., 1993). Cross resistance of quinolone resistant *Salmonella* strains against tetracycline, chloramphenicol and disinfectants is common (Piddock, 2002). Recent study in Brazil explored *S.* Corvallis strains in poultry carcasses exhibiting reduced susceptibility to quinolone along with production of extended spectrum β-lactamases conferring resistance against higher generation of cephalosporins (Yamatogi et al., 2015). As quinolone resistance is mediated through chromosomal genes, selection and spread of quinolone-resistant *Salmonella* strains depend on exposure of human or animals to quinolones or transmission of bacteria between the animals and human. Initially six fluoroquinolones were approved for animal use in the United States from which sarafloxacin and enrofloxacin were removed due to increased resistance against them observed in *Salmonella* strains isolated from human patients (Nelson et al., 2007).

Colistin resistance

Colistin was considered as a last resort antibiotic during emergence of resistant organisms. Recently phenotypical colistin resistance and associated resistance gene (*mcr-1*) was detected in *Salmonella* Derby, Paratyphi B, 1,4 [5],12:i:, isolated from sausage, guinea fowl pie, chicken breast, environmental samples from chicken farms in France (Webb et al., 2016).
    Characteristics of antimicrobial resistance in *Salmonella* isolates observed in different livestock, poultry, wildlife, fishes as well as in human are discussed in the following section.

Cattle

In a comprehensive study with bovine *Salmonella* strains isolated during 2006—15 in United States, susceptibility against enrofloxacin, gentamicin, neomycin and trimethoprim sulfamethoxazole was detected probably due to restricted use of fluoroquinolones and sulfonamides in food animals during this period. Comparative study revealed a changing resistance pattern in bovine *Salmonella* isolates with increased resistance against macrolides, specially tulathromycin, currently used in bovine respiratory infections (Valenzuela et al., 2017).Bovine respiratory tract bacteria (*Pasteurella* spp., *Mannheimia* spp.) circulating in United States and Canada (not in European Union) also showed increased resistance against macrolides, associated with increasing use of macrolides in livestock (Pyorala et al., 2014). Manure management practices in livestock farm also play a significant role in development of resistance in *Salmonella* isolates (Habing et al., 2012). Higher stocking rate (numbers of animals present in farm, kg/m^2) was detected to be positively correlated with faecal shedding of resistant *Salmonella* (Farzan et al., 2010). In Europe, in 2002, responsibility for homogenous interpretation of antimicrobial resistance data was submitted to The European Food Safety Authority (EFSA). The EFSA developed a standard protocol for interpretation of data and all national laboratories of different member countries routinely monitor the samples following the standard protocol and report the data to EFSA. As a part of this curriculum, highest proportion of *S. typhimurium* with ampicillin resistance was observed in cattle in Sweden in 2008. The resistance reduced to 0% in 2009 and further increased to 10% in 2011 (Garcia-Migura et al., 2014).

Pigs

As a part of EFSA curriculum in Spain, a decreasing trend in prevalence of third generation cephalosporin resistant *S. typhimurium* was detected in pigs during the period 2008—11 (11%—5.3%). In Denmark also a similar kind of reducing trend of ceftiofur resistance was noted during 2006—08 (<1%—0.2%) in swine industry (Garcia-Migura et al., 2014).

Horses

Heidelberg, Newport, Typhimurium serovars and phage type DT104 of *Salmonella* were common in horse faeces showing antimicrobial resistance (Amavisit et al., 2001; Weese et al., 2001; Niwa et al., 2009; Dallap Schaer et al., 2010). Extended-spectrum β-lactamase genes such as *bla*$_{CTX-M-1}$, *bla*$_{CTX-M-15}$, *bla*$_{SHV-12}$, plasmid-mediated *ampC*, sulfonamide and trimethoprim resistance genes were identified in *Salmonella* isolates from the horses (Rankin et al., 2005; Vo et al., 2007; Fischer et al., 2014). Resistance genes associated with integrons were detected in *Salmonella* phage type DT 104

(Niwa et al., 2009). A comprehensive study with *Salmonella* isolates from foals with sepsis revealed reduced susceptibility to gentamicin and ceftizoxime (Theelen et al., 2014).

Poultry

Use of antibiotics as growth promoter (bambermycin, avilamycin, efrotomycin) or therapeutic solution (bacitracin, chlortetracycline, erythromycin, penicillin) in poultry farms is still common in some countries (Butaye et al., 2003; Kilonzo-Nthenge et al., 2008). Use of antibiotics as growth promoter is based on certain hypothesis such as efficient conversion of feed to animal products, increase in growth rate and decrease in morbidity/mortality rate (Adzitey, 2015). Use of antibiotics can clear the population of commensal bacteria present in birds or animals. Presence of commensal can trigger immune response and most of the provided feed is wasted to generate the immune response in place of muscle development. Moreover, antibiotics are also used to treat animals or birds during sufferings. In general, poultry are considered as the major reservoir of *S. typhimurium* resistant to fluoroquinolones among all the domestic animals and birds (Garcia-Migura et al., 2014). *Salmonella* isolates from chicken carcasses in Vietnam, live chicken and guinea fowls kept in experimental farms of Tennessee State University, chicken carcasses in central Anatolia region of Turkey showed high resistance to tetracycline, ampicillin, streptomycin, penicillin, oxacillin, clindamycin, vancomycin, erythromycin (Kilonzo-Nthenge et al., 2008; Yildirim et al., 2011; Ta et al., 2012). In India, *Salmonella* (22/360, 6.1%) were isolated from cloacal swabs, feed, drinking water and eggs of the birds (Rhode Island Red breed) reared in backyard system. Although the isolates were found to be phenotypically resistant to chloramphenicol, ciprofloxacin, gentamicin, levofloxacin, norfloxacin, and oxytetracycline, none of the isolates possessed genes for major extended spectrum β-lactamases (ESBL). Third generation cephalosporins and ampicillin were apparently never used by the farmers in the backyard birds due to either higher cost or lack of poultry preparation of the medicine which could be the reason for ESBL-gene free birds (Samanta et al., 2014, 2018). In another study in northeastern India, phenotypical resistance of *Salmonella* isolated from broiler poultry against tetracycline and chloramphenicol was detected (Murugkar et al., 2005).

Wildlife

Cent percent prevalence of antimicrobial resistance genes is observed in *Salmonella* strains isolated from wildlife in California, Italy and other countries (Smith et al., 2002; Botti et al., 2013). A recent whole-genome sequencing-based study of *Salmonella* strains isolated from wild birds (wild turkey, ratite, chicken, pigeon, emu, quail, rhea), reptiles (alligator, python, boa) and mammals (giraffe, hedgehog, snow leopard, antelope) during 1998–2003 in Oklahoma revealed that 50% of the isolates were resistant to at least one antibiotic. Phenotypical resistance was highest against aminoglycoside and streptomycin. Genes encoding aminoglycoside and beta-lactam antibiotic resistance, *csg* operons, type 1 fimbriae, type III secretion system (T3SS) were detected in most of the isolates (Thomas et al., 2017).

Aquaculture

Aquaculture farms specially present in the Eastern and South-Eastern Asia (China, Hong Kong, Macau, Korea, Taiwan, Russia) are detected as source of antimicrobial resistant *Salmonella* strains (DT104) (Marshall and Levy, 2011).

Human

Regular use of ampicillin, chloramphenicol and co-trimoxazole has lead to the emergence and global spread of resistant *Salmonella* Typhi strains during 1970–80 (Wain et al., 2003). WHO recommended the use of third-generation cephalosporins and fluoroquinolones against typhoid fever which caused emergence of ciprofloxacin and third-generation cephalosporin-resistant *S. typhi* in Asian countries during last decade (WHO, 2003; Menezes et al., 2011; Kumarasamy and Krishnan, 2012). In a recent study in India, conducted with *S. typhi* strains isolated during 1998–2012 from typhoid fever patients, a stable reduction in resistance against ampicillin, chloramphenicol and co-trimoxazole (46.4%–15.6%) and increased resistance against nalidixic acid (60.7%–93.8%) and ciprofloxacin (0%–25%) were observed (Das et al., 2017). Resistance to azithromycin, an empirical treatment of typhoid fever, was also reported sporadically (Hassing et al., 2014). Multidrug resistance in *S. typhi* is due to the existence of resistance genes either on a specific locus in bacterial chromosome or on the IncHI1 plasmids (Holt et al., 2011; Wong et al., 2015). In a comprehensive study with 19,410 non-typhoidal *Salmonella* strains isolated from human during 2004–12 in different states of USA, 2320 (12%) isolates showed overall resistance. The study was conducted by 'national antimicrobial resistance monitoring system (NARMS), a working group under US centers for disease control and prevention (CDC). Ampicillin (6.5% isolates) was the most common antimicrobial agent against which the resistance was observed, followed by ceftriaxone/ampicillin (3.1% isolates) and non-susceptibility to ciprofloxacin (2.4% isolates). Most common resistant serovars were Enteritidis (18%), Typhimurium (17%), Newport (11%), and Heidelberg (4%). Indeed during this study period (2004−12), occurrence of ceftriaxone-resistant serovar Heidelberg was increased from 9% to 22% (Medalla et al., 2013). Use of third generation cephalosporins in poultry was considered as a contributing factor for generation of ceftriaxone resistant Heidelberg serovars in human (Angulo et al., 2004; Dutil et al., 2010; Folster et al., 2012). Similarly, consumption of contaminated ground beef or exposure to infected cattle was detected as a root cause of outbreaks associated with serovar Typhimurium resistant to ampicillin (Dechet et al., 2006; Krueger et al., 2014) and serovar Newport resistant to ceftriaxone (Gupta et al., 2003; Varma et al., 2006). Extended spectrum beta-lactamase genes specially bla_{CMY} was detected in many serovars of *Salmonella* isolated from human in United States (Folster et al., 2010).

Raising food animals without addition of antibiotics in feed did not prevent the occurrence of antimicrobial resistant *Salmonella* spp. in animals or food products. Although, prevalence of resistant *Salmonella* was comparatively lower in chicken or poultry meat raised in antibiotic free husbandry systems (Alali et al., 2010; M'Ikanatha et al., 2010; Mazengia et al., 2014; Samanta et al., 2014). Some authors identified core feed components, not the feed additives, as major responsible agents for generation of resistant *Salmonella* spp. (Alali et al., 2010; Molla et al., 2010). Moreover, transmission of antimicrobial resistant *Salmonella* in human from the food animals is not always validated. In a study during human salmonellosis outbreak in Scotland, *Salmonella* DT104 were isolated from both affected human and suspected cattle with or without any syndrome. Whole genome sequencing of the both kinds of isolates revealed the existence of distinct clades circulating among the human and cattle (Mather et al., 2013). Diversity of *Salmonella* serovars was noted in different species of animals and geographical regions (Hoelzer et al., 2010). National antimicrobial resistance monitoring system (a collaboration among the US Food and Drug Administration, Centers for Disease Control and Prevention and US Department of Agriculture) data revealed similarity of only 50% serovars present in both animals and human (FDA, 2015).It seems that generation of resistant *Salmonella* spp. in food animals is a multifactorial issue where host-parasite interaction and environment may play a significant role other than use of antimicrobials in animals (Helke et al., 2017). The role of crops where manure from animal farms is used for fertilization remains to be elucidated. Sometimes, drugs effective in vitro, may not act properly in vivo due to inaccessibility of privileged sites, dormant non-replicative status of the bacteria and lack of harmony between body defense system and antimicrobials.

References

Adzitey, F., 2015. Antibiotic classes and antibiotic susceptibility of bacterial isolates from selected poultry; a mini review. World's Veterinary Journal 5 (3), 36−41.

Agbaje, M., Begum, R.H., Oyekunle, M.A., Ojo, O.E., Adenubi, O.T., 2011. Evolution of Salmonella nomenclature: a critical note. Folia microbiologica 56 (6), 497−503.

Agron, P.G., Walker, R.L., Kinde, H., Sawyer, S.J., Hayes, D.C., Wollard, J., et al., 2001. Identification by subtractive hybridization of sequences specific for *Salmonella enterica* serovar Enteritidis. Applied and Environmental Microbiology 67, 4984−4991.

Alakomi, H.L., Saarela, M., 2009. *Salmonella* importance and current status of detection and surveillance methods. Quality Assurance and Safety of Crops and Foods 1, 142−152.

Alali, W.Q., Thakur, S., Berghaus, R.D., Martin, M.P., Gebreyes, W.A., 2010. Prevalence and distribution of *Salmonella* in organic and conventional broiler poultry farms. Foodborne Pathogens and Disease 7 (11), 1363−1371.

Alcaine, S.D., Warnick, L.D., Wiedmann, M., 2007. Antimicrobial resistance in nontyphoidal *Salmonella*. Journal of Food Protection 70, 780−790.

Amavisit, P., Markham, P.F., Lightfoot, D., Whithear, K.G., Browning, G.F., 2001. Molecular epidemiology of *Salmonella* Heidelberg in an equine hospital. Veterinary Microbiology 80, 85−98.

Angulo, F.J., Nargund, V.N., Chiller, T.C., 2004. Evidence of an association between use of anti-microbial agents in food animals and anti-microbial resistance among bacteria isolated from humans and the human health consequences of such resistance. Journal of Veterinary Medicine. B, Infectious Diseases and Veterinary Public Health 51, 374−379.

Antunes, P., Machado, J., Sousa, J.C., Peixe, L., 2005. Dissemination of sulfonamide resistance genes (sul1, sul2, and sul3) in Portuguese *Salmonella enterica* strains and relation with integrons. Antimicrobial Agents and Chemotherapy 49 (2), 836−839.

Archambault, M., Petrov, P., Hendriksen, R.S., Asseva, G., Bangtrakulnonth, A., Hasman, H., Aarestrup, F.M., 2006. Molecular characterization and occurrence of extended-spectrum beta-lactamase resistance genes among *Salmonella enterica* serovar Corvallis from Thailand, Bulgaria, and Denmark. Microbial Drug Resistance 12, 192−198.

Arguello, H., Sørensen, G., Carvajal, A., Baggesen, D.L., Rubio, P., Pedersen, K., 2013. Prevalence, serotypes and resistance patterns of *Salmonella* in Danish pig production. Research in Veterinary Science 95 (2), 334−342.

Aslam, M., Checkley, S., Avery, B., Chalmers, G., Bohaychuk, V., Gensler, G., Reid-Smith, R., Boerlin, P., 2012. Phenotypic and genetic characterization of antimicrobial resistance in *Salmonella* serovars isolated from retail meats in Alberta, Canada. Food Microbiology 32 (1), 110−117.

Bell, C., 2002. Salmonella. In: Blackburn, C.W., McClure, P.J. (Eds.), Foodborne Pathogens: Hazards, Risk Analysis and Control. CRC, Boca Raton, FL, pp. 307−334.

Ben Aissa, R., Al-Gallas, N., Troudi, H., Bethadj, N., Belhadj, A., 2007. Trends in *Salmonella enterica* serotypes isolated from human, food, animal, and environment in Tunisia, 1994-2004. Journal of Infection 55, 324−339.

Bennett, A.R., Greenwood, D., Tennant, C., Banks, J.G., Betts, R.P., 1998. Rapid and definitive detection of *Salmonella* in foods by PCR. Letters in Applied Microbiology 26, 437−441.

Botti, V., Navillod, F.V., Domenis, L., Orusa, R., Pepe, E., Robetto, S., Guidetti, C., 2013. *Salmonella* spp. and antibiotic-resistant strains in wild mammals and birds in north-western Italy from 2002 to 2010. Veterinaria Italiana 49 (2), 195−202.

Butaye, P., Devriese, L.A., Haesebrouck, F., 2003. Antimicrobial growth promoters used in animal feed: effects of less well known antibiotics on gram-positive bacteria. Clinical Microbiology Reviews 16, 175−188.

Cannon, M., Harford, S., Davies, J.A., 1990. A comparative study on the inhibitory actions of chloramphenicol, thiamphenicol and some fluorinated derivatives. Journal of Antimicrobial Chemotherapy 26, 307−317.

Carattoli, A., Filetici, E., Villa, L., Dionisi, A.M., Ricci, A., Luzzi, L., 2002. Antibiotic resistance genes and *Salmonella* genomic island 1 in *Salmonella enterica* serovar Typhimurium isolated in Italy. Antimicrobial Agents and Chemotherapy 46, 2821−2828.

Carattoli, A., Seiffert, S.N., Schwendener, S., Perreten, V., Endimiani, A., 2015. Differentiation of IncL and IncM plasmids associated with the spread of clinically relevant antimicrobial resistance. PLoS One 10, e0123063.

CDC, 2013. Antibiotic Resistance Threats in the United States. Available from: http://www.cdc.gov/drugresistance/pdf/ar-threats-2013-508.pdf.

CDC, 2014. Multiple-Serotype *Salmonella* Outbreaks in Two State Prisons—Arkansas, August 2012. Morbidity Mortality Weekly Report (MMWR). http://www.cdc.gov/mmwr/preview/mmwrhtml/mm6308a2.htm.

Chopra, I., Roberts, M., 2001. Tetracycline antibiotics: mode of action, applications, molecular biology, and epidemiology of bacterial resistance. Microbiology and Molecular Biology Reviews 65 (2), 232−260.

Clothier, K.A., Kinyon, J.M., Frana, T.S., 2010. Comparison of *Salmonella* serovar isolation and antimicrobial resistance patterns from porcine samples between 2003 and 2008. Journal of Veterinary Diagnostic Investigation 22 (4), 578−582.

Cohen, S.P., Levy, S.B., Foulds, J., Rosner, J.L., 1993. Salicylate induction of antibiotic resistance in *Escherichia coli*: activation of the mar operon and a mar-independent pathway. Journal of Bacteriology 175 (24), 7856−7862.

Cosby, D.E., Cox, N.A., Harrison, M.A., Wilson, J.L., Buhr, R.J., Fedorka-Cray, P.J., 2015. *Salmonella* and antimicrobial resistance in broilers: a review. The Journal of Applied Poultry Research 24 (3), 408−426.

Crim, S.M., Griffin, P.M., Tauxe, R., Marder, E.P., Gilliss, D., Cronquist, A.B., et al., 2015. Preliminary incidence and trends of infection with pathogens transmitted commonly through food -Foodborne Diseases Active Surveillance Network, 10 U.S. sites, 2006−2014. Morbidity and Mortality Weekly Report 64, 495−499.

Cummings, K.J., Warnick, L.D., Elton, M., Rodriguez-Rivera, L.D., Siler, J.D., Wright, E.M., Gröhn, Y.T., Wiedmann, M., 2010. *Salmonella enterica* serotype cerro among dairy cattle in New York: an emerging pathogen? Foodborne Pathogens and Disease 7 (6), 659−665.

Dallap Schaer, B.L., Aceto, H., Rankin, S.C., 2010. Outbreak of salmonellosis caused by *Salmonella enterica* serovar Newport MDR AmpC in a large animal veterinary teaching hospital. Journal of Veterinary Internal Medicine 24, 1138−1146.

D'Aoust, J.Y., Sewell, A.M., 1988. Reliability of the immunodiffusion 1-2 Test™ system for detection of *Salmonella* in foods. Journal of Food Protection 51, 853−856.

Das, S., Samajpati, S., Ray, U., Roy, I., Dutta, S., 2017. Antimicrobial resistance and molecular subtypes of *Salmonella enterica* serovar Typhi isolates from Kolkata, India over a 15 years period 1998−2012. International Journal of Medical Microbiology 307 (1), 28−36.

Davis, M.A., Hancock, D.D., Besser, T.E., 2002. Multi-resistant clones of *Salmonella enterica*: the importance of dissemination. The Journal of Laboratory and Clinical Medicine 140 (3), 135−141.

Dechet, A.M., Scallan, E., Gensheimer, K., Hoekstra, R., Gunderman- King, J., Lockett, J., et al., 2006. Outbreak of multidrug-resistant *Salmonella enterica* serotype Typhimurium definitive type 104 infection linked to commercial ground beef, northeastern United States, 2003−2004. Clinical Infectious Diseases 42, 747−752.

Deckert, A., Gow, S., Rosengren, L., Léger, D., Avery, B., Daignault, D., Dutil, L., Reid-Smith, R., Irwin, R., 2010. Canadian integrated program for antimicrobial resistance surveillance (CIPARS) farm program: results from finisher pig surveillance. Zoonoses Public Health 57 (Suppl. 1), 71−84.

Di Pilato, V., Arena, F., Giani, T., Conte, V., Cresti, S., Rossolini, G.M., 2014. Characterization of pFOX-7a, a conjugative IncL/M plasmid encoding the FOX-7 AmpC-type β-lactamase, involved in a large outbreak in a neonatal intensive care unit. Journal of Antimicrobial Chemotherapy 69, 2620−2624.

Diarra, M.S., Delaquis, P., Rempel, H., Bach, S., Harlton, C., Aslam, M., Pritchard, J., Topp, E., 2014. Antibiotic resistance and diversity of *Salmonella enterica* serovars associated with broiler chickens. Journal of Food Protection 77 (1), 40−49.

Dutil, L., Irwin, R., Finley, R., Ng, L.K., Avery, B., Boerlin, P., et al., 2010. Ceftiofur resistance in *Salmonella enterica* serovar Heidelberg from chicken meat and humans, Canada. Emerging Infectious Diseases 16, 48−54.

Eijkelkamp, J.M., Aarts, H.J.M., van der Fels-Klerx, H.J., 2009. Suitability of rapid detection methods for *Salmonella* in poultry slaughterhouses. Food Analytical Methods 2, 1−13.

Engler, M., Parry-Jones, R., 2007. Opportunity or Threat: The Role of the European Union in Global Wildlife Trade. Traffic Europe, Brussels.

European Commission (EC), 2003. Regulation no. 2160/2003 of the European Parliament and of the Council of 17 November 2003 on the control of *Salmonella* and other specified food-borne zoonotic agents. Official Journal of the European Union L325, 1e15.

Farzan, A., Friendship, R.M., Dewey, C.E., Poppe, C., Funk, J., 2010. Evaluation of the risk factors for shedding *Salmonella* with or without antimicrobial resistance in swine using multinomial regression method. Zoonoses and Public Health 57 (s1), 85—93.

FDA, 2015. National Antimicrobial Resistance Monitoring System (NARMS) - 2012 NARMS Retail Meat Report. http://www.fda.gov/downloads/AnimalVeterinary/SafetyHealth/Antimicrobial Resistance/NationalAntimicrobialResistanceMonitoringSystem/UCM442212.pdf.

Feasey, N.A., Dougan, G., Kingsley, R.A., Heyderman, R.S., Gordon, M.A., 2012. Invasive non-typhoidal *Salmonella* disease: an emerging and neglected tropical disease in Africa. Lancet 379, 2489—2499.

Feeley, J.C., Treger, M.D., 1969. Penetration of turtle eggs by *Salmonella* braenderup. Public Health Reports 84 (2), 156—158.

Ferrari, R., Galiana, A., Cremades, R., Rodriguez, J.C., Magnani, M., Tognim, M.C.B., Oliveira, T.C.R.M., Royo, G., 2011. Plasmid-mediated quinolone resistance by genes *qnr*A1 and *qnr*B19 in *Salmonella* strains isolated in Brazil. The Journal of Infection in Developing Countries 5, 496—498.

Fierer, J., Guiney, D.G., 2001. Diverse virulence traits underlying different clinical outcomes of *Salmonella* infection. Journal of Clinical Investigation 107, 775—780.

Fischer, J., Rodr_iguez, I., Baumann, B., Guiral, E., Beutin, L., Schroeter, A., Kaesbohrer, A., Pfeifer, Y., Helmuth, R., Guerra, B., 2014. *bla*$_{CTX-M-15}$-carrying *Escherichia coli* and *Salmonella* isolates from livestock and food in Germany. Journal of Antimicrobial Chemotherapy 69, 2951—2958.

Fluit, A.C., 2005. Towards more virulent and antibiotic-resistant *Salmonella*? Pathogens and Disease 43 (1), 1—11.

Foley, S.L., Lynne, A.M., 2008. Food animal-associated *Salmonella* challenges: pathogenicity and antimicrobial resistance. Journal of Animal Science 86 (14 Suppl. l), E173—E187.

Folster, J.P., Pecic, G., Bolcen, S., Theobald, L., Hise, K., Carattoli, A., Zhao, S., McDermott, P.F., Whichard, J.M., 2010. Characterization of extended-spectrum cephalosporin—resistant *Salmonella enterica* serovar heidelberg isolated from humans in the United States. Foodborne Pathogens and Disease 7 (2), 181—187.

Folster, J.P., Pecic, G., Singh, A., Duval, B., Rickert, R., Ayers, S., et al., 2012. Characterization of extended-spectrum cephalosporin-resistant *Salmonella enterica* serovar Heidelberg isolated from food animals, retail meat, and humans in the United States 2009. Foodborne Pathogens and Disease 9, 638—645.

Food Safety Inspection Service, 2008. The Nationwide Microbiological Baseline Data Collection Program: Young Chicken Survey. http://www.fsis.usda.gov/PDF/Baseline_Data_Young_Chicken_2007-200/.pdf.

Gantzhorn, M.R., Pedersen, K., Olsen, J.E., Thomsen, L.E., 2014. Biocide and antibiotic susceptibility of *Salmonella* isolates obtained before and after cleaning at six Danish pig slaughterhouses. International Journal of Food Microbiology 181, 53—59.

García, V., García, P., Rodríguez, I., Rodicio, R., Rodicio, M.R., 2016. The role of IS26 in evolution of a derivative of the virulence plasmid of *Salmonella enterica* serovar Enteritidis which confers multiple drug resistance. Infection, Genetics and Evolution 45, 246—249.

Garcia-Migura, L., Hendriksen, R.S., Fraile, L., Aarestrup, F.M., 2014. Antimicrobial resistance of zoonotic and commensal bacteria in Europe: the missing link between consumption and resistance in veterinary medicine. Veterinary Microbiology 170 (1), 1—9.

Gartner, 1888. Correspond. d. allgemein. drztl. Vereins Thiuringen. Ref. BRUCE WHITE, Med. Res. Counc. System of Bact. 1929, p. 4.

Glenn, L.M., Lindsey, R.L., Frank, J.F., Meinersmann, R.J., Englen, M.D., Fedorka-Cray, P.J., Frye, J.G., 2011. Analysis of antimicrobial resistance genes detected in multidrug-resistant *Salmonella enterica* serovar Typhimurium isolated from food animals. Microbial Drug Resistance 17 (3), 407—418.

Grace, D., 2015. Review of Evidence on Antimicrobial Resistance and Animal Agriculture in Developing Countries. Evidence on Demand, UK. https://doi.org/10.12774/eod_cr.june2015.graced.

Griggs, D.J., Gensberg, K., Piddock, L.J.V., 1996. Mutations in the *gyrA* gene of quinolone-resistant *Salmonella* serotypes isolated from man and animals. Antimicrobial Agents and Chemotherapy 40 (4), 1009—1013.

Guiney, D.G., Fierer, J., 2011. The role of the spv genes in *Salmonella* pathogenesis. Frontiers in Microbiology 2, 129.

Gupta, B.R., Verma, J.C., 1993. In: Monograph on Animal Salmonellosis. Communication Centre, Indian Veterinary Research Institute, Izatnagar, Bareilly, UP, India.

Gupta, A., Fontana, J., Crowe, C., Bolstorff, B., Stout, A., Van Duyne, S., et al., 2003. Emergence of multidrug-resistant *Salmonella enterica* serotype Newport infections resistant to expanded-spectrum cephalosporins in the United States. The Journal of Infectious Diseases 188, 1707—1716.

Habing, G.G., Lombard, J.E., Kopral, C.A., Dargatz, D.A., Kaneene, J.B., 2012. Farm-level associations with the shedding of *Salmonella* and antimicrobial-resistant *Salmonella* in U.S. dairy cattle. Foodborne Pathogens and Disease 9, 815—821.

Hamada, K., Tsuji, H., 2001. *Salmonella* Brandenburg and *S.* Corvallis involved in a food poisoning outbreak in a hospital in Hyogo Prefecture. Japanese Journal of Infectious Diseases 54, 195—196.

Hamada, K., Oshima, K., Tsuji, H., 2003. Chromosomal transferable multidrug resistance genes of *Salmonella enterica* serovar Infantis. Japanese Journal of Infectious Diseases 56 (5/6), 216—218.

Hassing, R.J., Goessens, W.H.F., Pelt, W., Mevius, D.J., Stricker, B.H., Molhoek, N., Verbon, A., Genderen, P.J.J., 2014. *Salmonella* subtypes with increased MICs inazithromycin in travelers returned to Netherlands. Emerging Infectious Diseases 20, 705—710.

He, S., Hickman, A.B., Varani, A.M., Siguier, P., Chandler, M., Dekker, J.P., Dyda, F., 2015. Insertion sequence IS26 reorganizes plasmids in clinically isolated multidrug-resistant bacteria by replicative transposition. mBio 6, e00762.

Heisig, P., 1993. High-level fluoroquinolone resistance in *Salmonella typhimurium* isolate due to alterations in both *gyrA* and *gyrB* genes. Journal of Antimicrobial Chemotherapy 32, 367—377.

Helke, K.L., McCrackin, M.A., Galloway, A.M., Poole, A.Z., Salgado, C.D., Marriott, B.P., 2017. Effects of antimicrobial use in agricultural animals on drug-resistant foodborne salmonellosis in humans: a systematic literature review. Critical Reviews in Food Science and Nutrition 57 (3), 472—488.

Hoelzer, K., Soyer, Y., Rodriguez-Rivera, L.D., Cummings, K.J., McDonough, P.L., Schoonmaker-Bopp, D.J., Root, T.P., Dumas, N.B., Warnick, L.D., Gröhn, Y.T., Wiedmann, M., Baker, K.N.K., Besser, T.E., Hancock, D.D., Davis, M.A., 2010. The prevalence of multidrug resistance is higher among bovine than human *Salmonella enterica* serotype Newport, Typhimurium, and 4,5,12:i:- isolates in the United States but differs by serotype and geographic region. Applied and Environmental Microbiology 76 (17), 5947–5959.

Holt, K.E., Phan, M.D., Baker, S., Duy, P.T., Nga, T.V.T., Nair, S., Turner, A.K., Walsh, C., Fanning, S., Farrell-Ward, S., Dutta, S., Kariuki, S., Weill, F.X., Parkhill, J., Dougan, G., Wain, J., 2011. Emergence of a globally dominant IncHI1 plasmidtype associated with multiple drug resistant typhoid. PLOS Neglected Tropical Diseases 5, e1245.

ISO, 2017. Microbiology of the Food Chain- Horizontal Method for the Detection, Enumeration and Serotyping of *Salmonella*- Part 1: Detection of *Salmonella* spp. https://www.iso.org/standard/56712.html.

Jones, T.F., Ingram, L.A., Cieslak, P.R., Vugia, D.J., Tobin-D'Angelo, M., Hurd, S., Medus, C., Cronquist, A., Angulo, F.J., 2008. Salomonellosis outcomes differ substantially by serotype. The Journal of Infectious Diseases 198, 109–114.

Keys, K., Hudson, C., Maurer, J.J., Thayer, S., White, D.G., Lee, M.D., 2000. Detection of florfenicol resistance genes in *Escherichia coli* isolated from sick chickens. Antimicrobial Agents and Chemotherapy 44, 421–424.

Kilonzo-Nthenge, A., Nahashon, S.N., Chen, F., Adefope, N., 2008. Prevalence and antimicrobial resistance of pathogenic bacteria in chicken and guinea fowl. Poultry Science 87, 1841–1848.

Kim, J.H., Cho, J.K., Kim, K.S., 2013. Prevalence and characterization of plasmid-mediated quinolone resistance genes in *Salmonella* isolated from poultry in Korea. Avian Pathology 42, 221–229.

Klein, E., 1889. Über eine epidemische Krankheit der Hühner, verursacht durch einer Bacillus-*Bacillus gallinarum*. Zentralblatt Bakteriologie und Parasitenkunde 5, 689–693. Abt I Orig.

Krueger, A.L., Greene, S.A., Barzilay, E.J., Henao, O., Vugia, D., Hanna, S., et al., 2014. Clinical outcomes of nalidixic acid, ceftriaxone, and multidrug-resistant nontyphoidal *salmonella* infections compared with pansusceptible infections in FoodNet sites, 2006–2008. Foodborne Pathogens and Disease 11, 335–341.

Kumarasamy, K., Krishnan, P., 2012. Report of a *Salmonella* enterica serovar typhi isolate from India producing CMY-2 AmpC β-lactamase. Journal of Antimicrobial Chemotherapy 67, 775–776.

Laufer, A.S., Grass, J., Holt, K., Whichard, J.M., Griffin, P.M., Gould, L.H., 2015. Outbreaks of *Salmonella* infections attributed to beef –United States, 1973–2011. Epidemiology and Infection 143, 2003–2013.

Lee, K.M., Runyon, M., Herrman, T.J., Phillips, R., Hsieh, J., 2015. Review of *Salmonella* detection and identification methods: aspects of rapid emergency response and food safety. Food Control 47, 264–276.

Loneragan, G.H., Thomson, D.U., McCarthy, R.M., Webb, H.E., Daniels, A.E., Edrington, T.S., Nisbet, D.J., Trojan, S.J., Rankin, S.C., Brashears, M.M., 2012. *Salmonella* diversity and burden in cows on and culled from dairy farms in the Texas high plains. Foodborne Pathogens and Disease 9 (6), 549–555.

Louden, B.C., Haarmann, D., Han, J., Foley, S.L., Lynne, A.M., 2012. Characterization of antimicrobial resistance in *Salmonella enterica* serovar Typhimurium isolates from food animals in the US. Food Research International 45 (2), 968–972.

Mahanti, A., Ghosh, P., Samanta, I., Joardar, S.N., Bandyopadhyay, S., Bhattacharyya, D., Banerjee, J., Batabyal, S., Sar, T.K., Dutta, T.K., 2017. Prevalence of CTX-M-producing *Klebsiella* spp. in broiler, kuroiler, and indigenous poultry in West Bengal state, India. Microbial Drug Resistance. https://doi.org/10.1089/mdr.2016.0096.

Majowicz, S.E., Musto, J., Scallan, E., Angulo, F.J., Kirk, M., O'Brien, S.J., Jones, T.F., Fazil, A., Hoekstra, R.M., Studies, I.C.o.E.D.B.o.I., 2010. The global burden of nontyphoidal *Salmonella* gastroenteritis. Clinical Infectious Diseases 50, 882–889.

Mandal, B.K., Brennand, J., 1988. Bacteraemia in salmonellosis: a 15 year retrospective study from a regional infectious diseases unit. BMJ 297, 1242–1243.

Marshall, B.M., Levy, S.B., 2011. Food animals and antimicrobials: impacts on human health. Clinical Microbiology Reviews 24, 718–733.

Mather, A.E., Reid, S.W.J., Maskell, D.J., Parkhill, J., Fookes, M.C., Harris, S.R., Brown, D.J., Coia, J.E., Mulvey, M.R., Gilmour, M.W., Petrovska, L., De Pinna, E., Kuroda, M., Akiba, M., Izumiya, H., Connor, T.R., Suchard, M.A., Lemey, P., Mellor, D.J., Haydon, D.T., Thomson, N.R., 2013. Distinguishable epidemics of multi drug resistant *Salmonella* typhimurium DT104 in different hosts. Science 341 (6153), 1514–1517.

Mazengia, E., Samadpour, M., Hill, H.W., Greeson, K., Tenney, K., Liao, G., Huang, X., Meschke, J.S., 2014. Prevalence, concentrations, and antibiotic sensitivities of salmonella serovars in poultry from retail establishments in Seattle, Washington. Journal of Food Protection 77 (6), 885–893.

Medalla, F., Hoekstra, R.M., Whichard, J.M., Barzilay, E.J., Chiller, T.M., Joyce, K., et al., 2013. Increase in resistance to ceftriaxone and non-susceptibility to ciprofloxacin and decrease in multidrug resistance among *Salmonella* strains, United States, 1996–2009. Foodborne Pathogens and Disease 10, 302–309.

Melendez, S.N., Hanning, I.B., Han, J., Nayak, R., Clement, A.R., Wooming, A., Hererra, P., Jones, F.T., Foley, S.L., Ricke, S.C., 2010. *Salmonella enterica* isolates from pasture-raised poultry exhibit antimicrobial resistance and class I integrons. Journal of Applied Microbiology 109 (6), 1957–1966.

Menezes, G.A., Harish, B.N., Khan, M.A., Goessens, W.H., Hays, J.P., 2011. Antimicrobial resistance trends in blood culture positive *Salmonella* Typhi isolates from Pondicherry, India, 2005–2009. Clinical Microbiology and Infections 18, 239–245.

M'Ikanatha, N.M., Sandt, C.H., Localio, A.R., Tewari, D., Rankin, S.C., Whichard, J.M., Altekruse, S.F., Lautenbach, E., Folster, J.P., Russo, A., Chiller, T.M., Reynolds, S.M., McDermott, P.F., 2010. Multidrug- resistant salmonella isolates from retail chicken meat compared with human clinical isolates. Foodborne Pathogens and Disease 7 (8), 929.

Mindlin, M.J., Lang, N., Maguire, H., Walsh, B., Verlander, N.Q., Lane, C., Taylor, C., Bishop, L.A., Crook, P.D., 2013. Outbreak investigation and case-control study: penta-resistant *Salmonella* Typhimurium DT104 associated with biltong in London in 2008. Epidemiology and Infection 141, 1920–1927.

Molla, B., Sterman, A., Mathews, J., Artuso-Ponte, V., Abley, M., Farmer, W., Rajala-Schultz, P., Morrow, W.E.M., Gebreyes, W.A., 2010. *Salmonella enterica* in commercial swine feed and subsequent isolation of phenotypically and genotypically related strains from fecal samples. Applied and Environmental Microbiology 76 (21), 7188–7193.

Murugkar, H.V., Rahman, H., Kumar, A., Bhattacharyya, D., 2005. Isolation, phage typing and antibiogram of *Salmonella* from man and animals in northeastern India. Indian Journal of Medical Research 122, 237–242.

Nelson, J.M., Chiller, T.M., Powers, J.H., Angulo, F.J., 2007. Fluoroquinolone-resistant Campylobacter species with the withdrawal of fluoroquinolones from use in poultry: a public health success story. Clinical Infectious Diseases 44, 977–980.

Nielsen, L.R., Ersbøll, A.K., 2005. Factors associated with variation in bulk-tank-milk *Salmonella* Dublin ELISA ODC% in dairy herds. Preventive Veterinary Medicine 68, 165–179.

Nielsen, L.R., 2013. Review of pathogenesis and diagnostic methods of immediate relevance for epidemiology and control of *Salmonella* Dublin in cattle. Veterinary Microbiology 162 (1), 1–9.

Niwa, H., Anzai, T., Izumiya, H., Morita-Ishihara, T., Watanabe, H., Uchida, I., Tozaki, T., Hobo, S., 2009. Antimicrobial resistance and genetic characteristics of *Salmonella typhimurium* isolated from horses in Hokkaido, Japan. Journal of Veterinary Medical Science 71, 1115–1119.

Okusu, H., Ma, D., Nikaido, H., 1996. AcrAB efflux pump plays a major role in the antibiotic resistance phenotype of *Escherichia coli* multiple-antibiotic-resistance (Mar) mutants. Journal of Bacteriology 178 (1), 306–308.

Piddock, L.J.V., Wray, C., MacClaren, I., Wise, R., 1990. Quinolone resistance in *Salmonella* spp.: veterinary pointers. Lancet 336, 125.

Piddock, L.J., 2002. Fluoroquinolone resistance in *Salmonella* serovars isolated from humans and food animals. FEMS Microbiology Reviews 26, 3–16.

Plym-Forshell, L., Ekesbo, I., 1996. Survival of Salmonellas in urine and dry faeces from cattle - an experimental study. Acta Veterinaria Scandinavica 37, 127–131.

PulseNet, 2017. https://www.cdc.gov/pulsenet/index.html.

Pyorala, S., Baptiste, K.E., Catry, B., van Duijkere, E., Greko, C., Moreno, M.A., Pomba, M.C., Rantala, M., Ružauskas, M., Sanders, P., Threlfall, E.J., Torren-Endo, J., Torneke, K., 2014. Macrolides and lincosamides in cattle and pigs: use and development of antimicrobial resistance. The Veterinary Journal 200, 230–239.

Rankin, S.C., Whichard, J.M., Joyce, K., Stephens, L., O'Shea, K., Aceto, H., Munro, D.S., Benson, C.E., 2005. Detection of a *bla$_{SHV}$* extended-spectrum beta-lactamase in *Salmonella enterica* serovar Newport MDR-AmpC. Journal of Clinical Microbiology 43, 5792–5793.

Rao, S., Van Donkersgoed, J., Bohaychuk, V., Besser, T., Song, X.-M., Wagner, B., Hancock, D., Renter, D., Dargatz, D., Morley, P.S., 2010. Antimicrobial drug use and antimicrobial resistance in enteric bacteria among cattle from Alberta feedlots. Foodborne Pathogens and Disease 7 (4), 449–457.

Rettger, L.F., 1900. Septicemia among young chickens. The New York Medical Journal 71, 803–805.

Richardson, A., Fawcett, A.R., 1973. *Salmonella* Dublin infection in calves – the value of rectal swabs in diagnosis and epidemiological studies. British Veterinary Journal 129, 151–156.

Rodríguez, I., Rodicio, M.R., Herrera-León, S., Echeita, A., Mendoza, M.C., 2008. Class 1 integrons in multidrug-resistant non-typhoidal *Salmonella enterica* isolated in Spain between 2002 and 2004. International Journal of Antimicrobial Agents 32, 158–164.

Rodríguez, I., Guerra, B., Mendoza, M.C., Rodicio, M.R., 2011. pUO-SeVR1 is an emergent virulence-resistance complex plasmid of *Salmonella enterica* serovar Enteritidis. Journal of Antimicrobial Chemotherapy 66, 218–220.

Rodriguez-Rivera, L.D., Wright, E.M., Siler, J.D., Elton, M., Cummings, K.J., Warnick, L.D., Wiedmann, M., 2014. Subtype analysis of *Salmonella* isolated from subclinically infected dairy cattle and dairy farm environments reveals the presence of both human- and bovine associated subtypes. Veterinary Microbiology 170 (3–4), 307–316.

Salmon, D.E., Smith, T., 1885. Report on Swine Plague. USDA Bureau of Animal Ind. 2nd Annual Report. USDA, Washington, DC.

Samanta, I., Joardar, S.N., Das, P.K., Sar, T.K., Bandyopadhyay, S., Dutta, T.K., Sarkar, U., 2014. Prevalence and antibiotic resistance profiles of *Salmonella* serotypes isolated from backyard poultry flocks in West Bengal, India. The Journal of Applied Poultry Research 23 (3), 536–545.

Samanta, I., Joardar, S.N., Das, P.K., 2018. Biosecurity strategies for backyard poultry: a controlled way for safe food production. In: Grumezescu, A., Maria Holban, A. (Eds.), Food Control and Biosecurity, first ed., vol. 16. Academic Press, The Netherlands.

Sapkota, A.R., Kinney, E.L., George, A., Hulet, R.M., Cruz-Cano, R., Schwab, K.J., Zhang, G., Joseph, S.W., 2014. Lower prevalence of antibiotic-resistant *Salmonella* on large-scale U.S. conventional poultry farms that transitioned to organic practices. The Science of the Total Environment 2014 (476–477), 387–392.

Sauteur, P.M.M., Relly, C., Hug, M., Wittenbrink, M.M., Berger, C., 2013. Risk factors for invasive reptile-associated salmonellosis in children. Vector Borne and Zoonotic Diseases 13, 419–421.

Scaallan, E., Hoekstra, R.M., Angulo, F.J., Tauxe, R.V., Widdowson, M.-A., Roy, S.L., Jones, J.L., Griffin, P.M., 2011. Foodborne illness acquired in the United States – major pathogens. Emerging Infectious Diseases 17, 7–15.

Scharff, R.L., 2010. Health-Related Cost from Foodborne Illness in the United States. http://www.pewtrusts.org/en/research-and-analysis/reports/0001/01/01/healthrelated-costs-from-foodborne-illness-in-the-united-states.

Schmidt, J.W., Brichta-Harhay, D.M., Kalchayanand, N., Bosilevac, J.M., Shackelford, S.D., Wheeler, T.L., Koohmaraie, M., 2012. Prevalence, enumeration, serotypes, and antimicrobial resistance phenotypes of *Salmonella enterica* isolates from carcasses at two large United States pork processing plants. Applied and Environmental Microbiology 78 (8), 2716–2726.

Schroter, M., Speicher, A., Hofmann, J., Roggentin, P., 2006. Analysis of the transmission of *Salmonella* spp. through generations of pet snakes. Environmental Microbiology 8 (3), 556–559.

Schwarz, S., Chaslus-Dancla, E., 2001. Use of antimicrobials in veterinary medicine and mechanisms of resistance. Veterinary Research 32, 201–225.

Singh, R., Yadav, A.S., Tripathi, V., Singh, R.P., 2013. Antimicrobial resistance profile of *Salmonella* present in poultry and poultry environment in north India. Food Control 33, 545–548.

Smith, W.A., Mazet, J.A., Hirsh, D.C., 2002. *Salmonella* in California wildlife species: prevalence in rehabilitation centers and characterization of isolates. Journal of Zoo and Wildlife Medicine 33 (3), 228–235.

Sun, Y., Cai, Y., Liu, X., Bai, N., Liang, B., Wang, R., 2013. The emergence of clinical resistance to tigecycline. International Journal of Antimicrobial Agents 41 (2), 110–116.

Suresh, T., Hatha, A.A.M., Sreenivasan, D., Sangeetha, N., Lashmanaperumalsamy, P., 2006. Prevalence and antimicrobial resistance of *Salmonella* Enteritidis and other salmonellas in the eggs and egg-storing trays from retails markets of Coimbatore, South India. Food Microbiology 23, 294–299.

Ta, Y.T., Nguyen, T.T., To, P.B., Pham, D.X., Le, H.T.H., Alali, W.Q., Walls, I., Lo Fo Wong, D.M., Doyle, M.P., 2012. Prevalence of *Salmonella* on chicken carcasses from retail markets in Vietnam. Journal of Food Protection 75 (10), 1851–1854.

Taylor, R.J., Burrows, M.R., 1971. The survival of *Escherichia coli* and *Salmonella* Dublin in slurry on pasture and the infectivity of S. Dublin for grazing calves. British Veterinary Journal 127, 536–542.

Tewari, D., Sandt, C.H., Miller, D.M., Jayarao, B.M., M'Ikanatha, N.M., 2012. Prevalence of *Salmonella* cerro in laboratory-based submissions of cattle and comparison with human infections in Pennsylvania, 2005–2010. Foodborne Pathogens and Disease 9 (10), 928–933.

Theelen, M.J.P., Wilson, W.D., Edman, J.M., Magdesian, K.G., Kass, P.H., 2014. Temporal trends in in vitro antimicrobial susceptibility patterns of bacteria isolated from foals with sepsis: 1979-2010. Equine Veterinary Journal 46, 161–168.

Thomas, M., Fenske, G.J., Ghimire, S., Welsh, R., Ramachandran, A., Scaria, J., 2017. Whole Genome Sequencing-Based Detection of Antimicrobial Resistance and Virulence in Non-Typhoidal *Salmonella enterica* Isolated from Wildlife. BioRxiv, p. 155192.

Tietjen, M., Fung, D.Y.C., 1995. Salmonellae and food safety. Critical Reviews in Microbiology 21, 53e83.

Trkov, M., Avguštin, G., 2003. An improved 16S rRNA based PCR method for the specific detection of *Salmonella enterica*. International Journal of Food Microbiology 80 (1), 67–75.

U.S. Department of Health and Human Services, 2014. Food Safety. Available from: https://www.healthypeople.gov/2020/topics-objectives/topic/food-safety/national-snapshot.

Uyttendaele, M., Vanwildemeersch, K., Debevere, J., 2003. Evaluation of realtime PCR vs automated ELISA and a conventional culture method using a semi-solid medium for detection of *Salmonella*. Letters in Applied Microbiology 37, 386–391.

Valenzuela, J.R., Sethi, A.K., Aulik, N.A., Poulsen, K.P., 2017. Antimicrobial resistance patterns of bovine *Salmonella enterica* isolates submitted to the Wisconsin Veterinary Diagnostic Laboratory: 2006–2015. Journal of Dairy Science 100 (2), 1319–1330.

Van Beurden, R., 1992. PATH-STIK rapid *Salmonella* test - a new immunoassay to detect foodborne pathogens. Scandinavian Dairy Information (Sweden) 6, 52–54.

Varma, J.K., Marcus, R., Stenzel, S.A., Hanna, S.S., Gettner, S., Anderson, B.J., et al., 2006. Highly resistant *Salmonella* Newport-MDRAmpC transmitted through the domestic US food supply: a FoodNet case–control study of sporadic *Salmonella* Newport infections, 2002–2003. The Journal of Infectious Diseases 194, 222–230.

Veling, J., Barkema, H.W., van der Schans, J., van Zijderveld, F., Verhoeff, J., 2002. Herd-level diagnosis for *Salmonella enterica* subsp. enterica Serovar Dublin infection in bovine dairy herds. Preventive Veterinary Medicine 53, 31–42.

Vo, A.T.T., van Duijkeren, E., Fluit, A.C., Gaastra, W., 2007. A novel *Salmonella* genomic island 1 and rare integron types in *Salmonella typhimurium* isolates from horses in The Netherlands. Journal of Antimicrobial Chemotherapy 59, 594–599.

Vora, N.M., Smith, K.M., Machalaba, C.C., Karesh, W.B., 2012. Reptile-and amphibian-associated salmonellosis in childcare centers, United States. Emerging Infectious Diseases 18, 2092–2094.

Wain, J., Diem Nga, L.T., Kidgell, C., James, K., Fortune, S., Diep, S.T., Ali, T., Gaora, P.O., Parry, C., Parkhill, J., Farrar, J., White, N.J., Dougan, G., 2003. Molecular analysis of incHI1 antimicrobial resistance plasmids from *Salmonella* serovars Typhi strains associated with typhoid fever. Antimicrobial Agents and Chemotherapy 47, 2732–2739.

Walsh, C., 2000. Molecular mechanisms that confer antibacterial drug resistance. Nature 406 (6797), 775–781.

Webb, H.E., Granier, S.A., Marault, M., Millemann, Y., den Bakker, H.C., Nightingale, K.K., Bugarel, M., Ison, S.A., Scott, H.M., Loneragan, G.H., 2016. Dissemination of the mcr-1 colistin resistance gene. The Lancet Infectious Diseases 16 (2), 144–145.

Weese, J.S., Baird, J.D., Poppe, C., Archambault, M., 2001. Emergence of *Salmonella typhimurium* definitive type 104 (DT104) as an important cause of salmonellosis in horses in Ontario. Canadian Veterinary Journal 42, 788–792.

White, D.G., Hudson, C., Maurer, J.J., Ayers, S., Zhao, S., Lee, M.D., Bolton, L., Foley, T., Sherwood, J., 2000. Characterization of chloramphenicol and florfenicol resistance in *Escherichia coli* associated with bovine diarrhea. Journal of Clinical Microbiology 38, 4593–4598.

WHO, 2014. Antimicrobial Resistance Global Report on Surveillance. WHO, Geneva.

Wong, V.K., Baker, S., Pickard, D.J., Parkhill, J., Page, A.J., Feasey, N.A., Kingsley, R.A., Thomson, N.R., Keane, J.A., Weill, F.X., Edwards, D.J., Hawkey, J., Harris, S.R., Mather, A.E., Cain, A.K., Hadfield, J., Hart, P.J., Nga, T.V.T., Klemm, E.J., Glinos, D.A., Breiman, R.F., Watson, C.H., Kariuki, S., Gordon, M.A., Heyderman, R.S., Okoro, C., Jacobs, J., Lunguya, O., Edmunds, W.J., Msefula, C., Chabalgoity, J.A., Kama, M., Jenkins, K., Dutta, S., Marks, F., Campos, J., Thompson, C., Obaro, S., MacLennan, C.A., Dolecek, C., Keddy, K.H., Smith, A.M., Parry, C.M., Karkey, A., Mulholland, E.K., Campbell, J.I., Dongol, S., Basnyat, B., Dufour, M., Bandaranayake, D., Naseri, T.T., Singh, S.P., Hatta, M., Newton, P., Onsare, R.S., Isaia, L., Dance, D., Davong, V., Thwaites, G., Wijedoru, L., Crump, J.A., Pinna, E.D., Nair, S., Nilles, E.J., Thanh, D.P., Turner, P., Soeng, S., Valcanis, M., Powling, J., Dimovski, K., Hogg, G., Farrar, J., Holt, K.E., Dougan, G., 2015. Phylogeographical analysis of the dominant multidrug-resistant H58 clade of *Salmonella* Typhi identifies inter and intra continental transmission events. Nature Genetics 47, 632−639.

World Health Organization, 2003. Background Document: The Diagnosis, Treatment and Prevention of Typhoid Fever. WHO Document. WHO, Geneva (WHO/V and B/03.07).

Yamatogi, R.S., Oliveira, H.C., Camargo, C.H., Fernandes, S.A., Hernandes, R.T., Pinto, J.P., Rall, V.L.M., Araújo Júnior, J.P., 2015. Clonal relatedness and resistance patterns of *Salmonella* Corvallis from poultry carcasses in a Brazilian slaughterhouse. Journal of Infection in Developing Countries 9 (10), 1161−1165.

Yildirim, Y., Gonulalan, Z., Pamuk, S., Ertas, N., 2011. Incidence and antibiotic resistance of *Salmonella* spp. on raw chicken carcasses. Food Research International 44 (3), 725−728.

Chapter 14

Klebsiella

Chapter outline

Klebsiella, especially *Klebsiella pneumoniae* and to a lesser degree *Klebsiella oxytoca*, are pathogenic bacteria causing a variety of infections in human ranging from community and nosocomial pneumonia, bacteraemia and urinary tract infections (UTIs) (Broberg et al., 2014). In last decades, 'pyogenic liver abscess' (PLA), another major complication associated with *K. pneumoniae* infection, was emerged in Asian countries (Hong Kong, Singapore, Korea and Taiwan) with possible metastatic complications such as endophthalmitis, meningitis and necrotizing meningitis (Keller et al., 2013). Later, PLA was also reported from non-Asian countries among the people having no Asian lineage (Moore et al., 2013). Prolonged stay in hospitals or nursing facilities favour *Klebsiella*-associated pneumonia and subsequent septicaemia in the patients (Kuehn, 2013).

K. pneumoniae is also present in gut of healthy animals and acts as indicator of environmental pollution (Tzouvelekis et al., 2012). In animals, *K. pneumoniae* is associated with mastitis in cattle, bacteraemia in calves, cervicitis and metritis in mares, pneumonia and septicaemia in foals, pneumonia, UTI and septicaemia in dogs (Roberts et al., 2000; Samanta, 2013).

Recent documentation indicated increased drug resistance among the nosocomial isolates, for example, 18% of long-term acute care facilities reported carbapenem-resistant *Enterobacteriaceae* (CRE) infections in human patients (Jacob et al., 2013). Approximately 600 deaths occur each year in the United States alone from two most common types of CRE infections, carbapenem-resistant *Klebsiella* and carbapenem-resistant *Escherichia coli* (CDC, 2013). Sequence type 258 (ST258) is the leading clonal type of CRE, disseminated throughout the globe (Bowers et al., 2015). Increased age of the population is directly correlated with increased occurrence and carriage of *Klebsiella* organisms which might be considered as a major contributing factor for spread of resistance determinants, as the population matures

Antimicrobial Resistance in Agriculture. https://doi.org/10.1016/B978-0-12-815770-1.00014-6

(Al-Hasan et al., 2010). In recent years, extended-spectrum β-lactamase (ESBL)—producing *Enterobacteriaceae* are also detected in asymptomatic human carriers (Nüesch-Inderbinen et al., 2013). In animal kingdom, healthy food animals (Carattoli, 2008) and feral animals (birds and fish) (Abgottspon et al., 2014; Zurfluh et al., 2013a; Mahanti et al., 2018) can also carry ESBL-producing *Enterobacteriaceae* including *Klebsiella* species. ESBL- and carbapenemase-producing *Enterobacteriaceae* were also detected in contaminated waterbodies such as rivers and lakes (Zurfluh et al., 2013b).

Properties

Morphology

Klebsiella are Gram-negative thick rods, $1-3 \times 0.5-1$ μm in measurement. They occur singly or in pair. They possess polysaccharide capsule both in vivo and in vitro. They are nonspore forming and nonmotile. Some strains are fimbriated.

Classification

The genus *Klebsiella* is classified under the family *Enterobacteriaceae* that belongs to the order Enterobacteriales. The important species currently under the genus *Klebsiella* are *K. pneumoniae*, *K. oxytoca*, *K. granulomatis*, *K. terrigena*, *K. planticola* (*K. trevisanii*) and *K. ornithinolytica*. *K. pneumoniae* causes 75%—86% of clinical infections in human followed by *K. oxytoca* causing 13%—25% of infections (Hansen et al., 2004). *K. pneumoniae* has several subspecies such as *pneumoniae*, *ozaenae* and *rhinoscleromatis*. Among them, *K. pneumoniae* ssp. *pneumoniae* and *K. oxytoca* are documented animal pathogens.

Susceptibility to disinfectants

Klebsiella may survive for months in dust, water, faeces of animal and poultry houses. They are susceptible to drying and common disinfectants such as phenol, cresol, etc. Increased resistance of *Klebsiella* to disinfectants was noted recently, for example, against chlorhexidine, an antiseptic used in hospitals to decontaminate floors and surfaces (Naparstek et al., 2012).

Natural habitat

Majority of these organisms are found in soil, surface water, sewage and plants as saprophytes. In animal sheds, it is commonly found in the sawdust beddings. Some strains of *Klebsiella* can live in respiratory, intestinal tract, penis exterior (horse) of healthy animals and may cause infection during alteration of normal bacterial flora. In human, the rate of carrier state varies from 5% (respiratory tract) to 38% (stool). The carriage increases with prolonged stay in hospitals or nursing facilities (Podschun and Ullmann, 1998).

Genome

Comparative genomic study of different *Klebsiella* strains isolated from clinical patient, healthy human and environment revealed a core set of 3631 genes comprising about 65%—75% of the genome. A large amount of genomic variability exists among the strains (Kumar et al., 2011). Another similar kind of study also detected different regions of genome plasticity (13 in numbers) comprising transposon or phage genes (Ramos et al., 2014). In addition to antibiotic resistance genes, metabolic pathway genes previously found in nitrogen fixers are also observed in some *Klebsiella* isolates (Hazen et al., 2014). The genome of tissue invasive *K. pneumoniae* strains possesses a 20 kb chromosomal region comprising of an iron uptake system (kfu) and a phosphoenolpyruvate sugar phosphotransferase system (PTS) (Ma et al., 2005). The kfu/PTS system helps in acquisition of iron even in deficient condition within the host.

Dissemination of resistance genes is most often associated with horizontal gene transfer via plasmids. Plasmids are classified into several replicon types, among which the incompatibility (Inc) groups F, A/C, L/M, I1, HI2 and N commonly possess antibiotic resistance genes (Carattoli, 2009). Most of the multidrug-resistant plasmids carrying β-lactamase genes belong to the IncA/C incompatibility group. The IncA/C plasmids are 131—195 kb in size and are detected in several *Enterobacteriaceae* members including *K. pneumoniae* (Doublet et al., 2012). More than 30 plasmids (3—270 Kbp) were identified in *K. pneumoniae* during the last decade (Bai et al., 2013). Different studies explored the characteristics of plasmids possessed by antibiotic-resistant *K. pneumoniae* strains. *K. pneumoniae* isolated from a neonate with meningitis possessed a plasmid (pJHCMW1), which contained transposon (Tn1331) with *aac(6′)-Ib*, *aadA1*, *bla*$_{OXA-9}$ and *bla*$_{TEM-1}$ genes (Sarno et al., 2002). Complete nucleotide sequencing of *K. pneumoniae* plasmids (pKP96, pK245) explored the quinolone resistance (*qnr*) and β-lactamase genes (*bla*$_{SHV-2}$) in China (Chen et al., 2006; Shen et al., 2008). The studies also revealed the genetic similarities between the antibiotic resistance gene containing regions of *K. pneumoniae* plasmids with plasmids of other bacteria such as *Salmonella* Virchow, *Salmonella* Infantis, *Shigella flexneri* and *Yersinia pestis* suggesting about horizontal transfer (Bistué et al., 2008). A recent study also reported the mosaic pattern of sequences detected in a *K. pneumoniae* plasmid (pKF3-140) indicating its origin from *E. coli* and the plasmid acquired the resistance genes from other enteric bacteria such as *Salmonella* (Bai et al., 2013).

Complete sequence of a *fosA3*-carrying plasmid (pKP1034) was determined in China, which was extracted from a fosfomycin-resistant carbapenemase-producing *K. pneumoniae* strain (ST 11 clonal type). The plasmid was multireplicon in nature, 136,848 bp in size with an average GC content of 54.5%, and it possessed 191 open reading frames. Three genetically distinct modules were identified in the studied plasmid, i.e., a composite transposon carrying *catA2* (chloramphenicol resistance) module; a 49.1 kb module homologous to another *fosA3*-carrying plasmid (pHN7A8), epidemic in Mainland China; and a 77.7 kb module homologous to *bla*$_{KPC}$-carrying plasmid (pKPC-LK30), prevalent in Taiwan. The mosaic pattern indicated horizontal transfer of different genetic constituents to create the chimeric plasmid. The 49.1 kb module possessed regulatory genes for plasmid stability and different resistance genes (Xiang et al., 2016). The plasmid pHN7A8 was originally described from a dog in Mainland China. Recently, dissemination of pHN7A8-like plasmids has been detected in food animals and pets in China associated with dissemination of different resistance genes (Hou et al., 2012; He et al., 2013).

Whole-genome sequencing (WGS) of FOX-AmpC-β-lactamase encoding *K. pneumoniae* and *K. oxytoca* strains isolated from a single health care facility in the United States was performed. The study suggested the possibility of FOX-IncA/C plasmid transfer between *Klebsiella* and other bacteria such as *E. coli* (Hazen et al., 2014).

Antigenic characteristics

Three kinds of antigens are present in *Klebsiella*, i.e., somatic (O), rough (R) and capsular (K). There are total 12 and 82 types of somatic and capsular antigens, respectively. The somatic antigens cannot be used for serotyping of the isolates because the heat-stable capsules hinder the detection of somatic antigens. Typing of the isolates is dependent on 77 capsular types recognized throughout the world. The capsule typing shows good reproducibility and is capable of differentiating most clinical isolates. The limitation is the serological cross-reactions that occur among the 77 capsule types. Individual sera have to be absorbed with the cross-reacting K-antigens. Capsular types K1 and K2 are the major virulent types of *K. pneumoniae*.

Toxins and virulence factors produced

Toxins

(i) Endotoxin [lipopolysaccharide (LPS)]: It is responsible for fever, neutropenia, petechiae, shock, pulmonary oedema, vascular collapse.

(ii) Enterotoxin: Some strains of *K. pneumoniae* produce an enterotoxin having structural similarity with stable enterotoxin of *E. coli* (ST). The toxin abnormally activates guanylate cyclase of the intestinal epithelial cells causing hypersecretion of fluid into the lumen and diarrhoea.

Virulence factors

Major virulence factors produced by *Klebsiella* are described in Table 14.1.

Transmission

Asymptomatic human beings can act as potential reservoir of *Klebsiella* with a considerable carriage rate (5%−38%). Hospital environment including fomites may play a significant role in nosocomial transmission of *Klebsiella* in human. Because of their ubiquitous presence, contaminated soil and water are also contributing factors in transmission of *Klebsiella*.

TABLE 14.1 Virulence factors and genes produced by *Klebsiella*.

Virulence factors	Function
Capsule	1. Capsules are the most significant virulence determinant of *Klebsiella*. It prevents phagocytosis. 2. Serum resistance: Serum acts as first line of defence against invading bacteria through complement activation. Most commensal Gram-negative bacteria are sensitive to the bactericidal effect of serum, whereas pathogenic strains often exhibit serum resistance properties. Capsule may hide the bacterial surface and prevent complement activation. 3. It inhibits the differentiation and functional capacity of macrophages in vitro.
Mucoviscosity-associated gene A (*magA*)/*wzyKpK1*	A chromosomal gene which is located in cps (capsular polysaccharide synthesis) operon. It helps in capsular polysaccharide formation and it is associated with *K. pneumoniae* strains causing primary liver abscess.
rmpA	The *rmpA* is a transcriptional activator of the cps genes and it functions as a positive regulator of extracapsular polysaccharide synthesis. It is associated with hypermucoid strains causing pyogenic liver abscess (PLA).
Pili/fimbriae (a) Type I pili (b) Type III pili (c) KPF-28 fimbriae	The pili help in binding of the bacteria to mucus or the epithelial cells of the urogenital, respiratory and intestinal tracts. Type 1 fimbriae were found to be associated with experimental urinary tract infection in mice. Type 3 fimbriae were detected to promote biofilm formation.
Adhesin: CF 29K (R-plasmid-encoded) of *K. pneumoniae*	It helps to mediate adherence to the human intestinal cell lines.
Lipopolysaccharide (LPS)	In some strains, O-side chain of LPS produces steric hindrance of lytic complement action (MAC formation) and promotes serum resistance.
Enterobactin, aerobactin, yersiniabactin, Kfu/phosphoenolpyruvate sugar phosphotransferase system (PTS), haemin and transferrin transporters	Acts as siderophore to help in iron acquisition. Enterobactin is necessary for penetration to deeper tissues. Yersiniabactin allows the growth of bacteria in the airways.
celB	The gene encodes putative cellobiose-specific PTS. It is associated with PLA-causing *K. pneumonia* strains. It plays role in biofilm formation also.
allS	It is detected in K1 strains of *K. pneumoniae*. It helps in anaerobic metabolism of allantoin which acts as the source of carbon, nitrogen and energy under aerobic or anaerobic condition.

In cattle, teat canal is the portal of entry of *Klebsiella* into the mammary gland. Coliform infections are usually associated with unsanitary environment; while *Klebsiella* are found in bedding materials of cattle shed containing sawdust. In horse, *K. pneumoniae* often utilise venereal route of transmission such as coitus, insemination with infected semen and genital manipulations.

Mobile genetic elements such as plasmids and transposons are responsible for carriage and spread of antibiotic resistance determinants between different strains of *Klebsiella*, environment and the bacteria or vice versa. Integrons, present in plasmids or transposons, contain specific genes for site-specific recombination and are capable of mobilizing antibiotic resistance genes and others. Integrons are broadly classified into two categories such as superintegrons and antibiotic resistance integrons (ARIs). ARIs are further subdivided into four classes (class 1, 2, 3, 4) based on their respective integrase (*intI*) genes (Cambray et al., 2010). Class 1 integrons are more commonly associated with clinical bacterial isolates, especially ESBL-producing *Enterobacteriaceae* including ESBL-producing *K. pneumoniae* (Machado et al., 2007). Class 2 and 3 integrons are rarely expressed by clinical isolates of extended-spectrum cephalosporinase-producing *K. pneumoniae* (Correia et al., 2003; Bhattacharjee et al., 2010). Carriage of integrons (class 1) was found to be associated with increased resistance against β-lactams, aminoglycosides and greater expression of multiple antibiotic-resistant phenotypes in *K. pneumoniae* isolates (Yao et al., 2007). Resistance against streptomycin and nitrofurantoin was inversely associated with integron carriage (Mobarak-Qamsari et al., 2013).

Diagnosis

Blood and stools are essential clinical samples for isolation or detection of *Klebsiella* from human patients. From animals, mastitic milk, faeces, urine, vaginal exudates, uterine secretions and ear exudates can be collected.

Laboratory examinations

Direct examination

A smear can be prepared from centrifuged deposit of collected urine or exudate samples and stained by Gram's Method. *Klebsiella* appears as Gram-negative small rods with capsules. The capsule can be demonstrated by India ink/nigrosin stain.

Radiographic imaging

In human patients, PLA can be diagnosed by pulmonary X-ray, which reveals right-sided pulmonary infiltrates with pleural effusion (Morii et al., 2012). The abdominal X-rays can also diagnose the infection on the basis of air-fluid levels (Tatsuta et al., 2011).

Ultrasonography and computed tomography scan

Ultrasonography (US) and computed tomography scanning (CT scan) are sensitive diagnostic techniques (96% and 100%, respectively) used in detection of PLA in human patients (Malik et al., 2010). In positive cases, US images of liver show hypoechoic nodules and solid mass depending on the pathological conditions. The CT scan images showed solitary abscess in the right lobe of liver in PLA patients (Li et al., 2010).

Isolation of Klebsiella

Klebsiella can grow in ordinary isolation media such as blood agar, MacConkey's agar. The incubation requires 37°C temperature for 24 h. The colonies in blood agar, after 24 h growth, are 2—3 mm in diameter, nonhaemolytic, mucoid and viscous. Large mucoid sometimes dome-shaped colonies are formed because of abundant capsule production. After subculture, the capsules are lost and small colonies are formed. In MacConkey's agar, lactose fermenting pink coloured colonies is found. Certain pathogenic *Klebsiella* (K1 and K2 serotypes) produce 'hypermucoviscous phenotype' in solid media. Colonies can also be confirmed by tube biochemical tests or commercial system (API system).

Serological tests

Enzyme-linked immunosorbent assay (ELISA) is developed to detect the capsular antigens and antibodies against *K. pneumoniae* (Trautmann et al., 1991).

Molecular biology

Polymerase chain reaction (PCR) has been developed for detection of K. *pneumoniae* based on identification of 16—23S internal transcribed spacer region. Capsular types (K1, K2) and putative virulence factors such as *rmpA* (regulator of mucoid phenotype A) are also confirmed by PCR. Molecular biology—based typing of *Klebsiella* isolates include plasmid profiling, ribotyping, multilocus enzyme analyses, pulsed-field gel electrophoresis and variable number tandem repeat analysis (Turton et al., 2010).

Early detection of multidrug-resistant *K. pneumoniae* (epidemic clonal type) in human or animals is considered as critical factor for effective control. Culture-based methods for detection of resistant organisms have several restrictions such as extended time and labour and lack of sensitivity and specificity (Viau et al., 2016). PCR-based methods have gained popularity for detection of resistant *Klebsiella* species with certain loopholes such as dependency on culture and chances of missing novel resistance genes (Dhar et al., 2016). WGS, microbiome sequencing (16S rRNA gene) and metagenomic sequencing are current methods of choice for detection of outbreaks associated with multidrug-resistant *Klebsiella*, sources of transmission, virulence factors and all possible resistance genes present in the isolates (Snitkin et al., 2012; Millares et al., 2015; Iqbal and Quigley, 2016). Recently, an amplicon sequencing—based tool ('KlebSeq') is described for detection of *Klebsiella* from complex samples such as wound, nasal swabs or faecal samples without culture (Bowers et al., 2016).

Characteristics of antimicrobial resistance

β-Lactam resistance

β-Lactam antibiotics (penicillin) are most commonly used in treatment of bacterial infections. Resistance to these antibiotics is developed in the bacteria through the production of β-lactamase enzyme that lyses the β-lactam ring structure present in these antibiotics. Extended spectrum of these antibiotics is developed later such as cephalosporins, which are resistant to the β-lactamase enzyme. Unfortunately, this time also the bacteria started to produce a new class of enzymes named as 'ESBLs' that can lyse cephalosporins (e.g., ceftazidime, cefotaxime and ceftriaxone), monobactams (e.g., aztreonam) and penicillins. First described in Germany (1983) and France (1985) among *Klebsiella* spp., ESBLs exist in every region of the world and in most genera of *Enterobacteriaceae* family (Knothe et al., 1983; Sirot et al., 1987). Three types of ESBLs, i.e., TEM, SHV and CTX-M, are most prevalent (Table 14.2).

AmpC *β*-lactamase-producing organisms can produce resistance against many β-lactams, including cephalosporins, penicillins, cephamycins, monobactams and also against *β*-lactamase inhibitors such as clavulanic acid (EFSA Panel on Biological Hazards, 2011). Presence of AmpC-*β*-lactamases is confirmed in *K. pneumoniae* from humans earlier (Bradford et al., 1997). FOX-encoding β-lactamases were identified as most prevalent AmpC β-lactamases in the United States. FOX-1-AmpC β-lactamases were first identified in *K. pneumoniae* strains isolated from human patients in Argentina in 1989 (Gonzalez-Leiza et al., 1994). The FOX-1 enzyme is encoded by plasmid-associated bla_{FOX} gene having 10 alleles detected so far (Hazen et al., 2014).

TABLE 14.2 Types of β-lactamases/carbapenemase enzymes produced by *Klebsiella pneumoniae* and their substrates.

Class	Gene	Geographical distribution	Substrates
Ambler class A	TEM-1 β-lactamase (temoneira, a patient)	Worldwide	Penicillin (ampicillin)
	SHV (sulfhydryl variant)	Worldwide	Penicillin, oxyimino β-lactams, aztreonam
	CTX-M (cefotaxime hydrolysing ESBL)	Worldwide	Higher generation cephalosporins, monobactams (except cephamycin and carbapenem)
	KPC (*K. pneumoniae* carbapenemase)	United States, Greece, South America, Israel, Europe, China	Penicillin, carbapenem, aztreonam
Ambler class B	Verona integrin encoded metallo-β-lactamase (VIM)	Greece, Asia (India, Australia, Phillipines, Japan, China)	All β-lactams (except aztreonam)
	Imipenemase (IMP)	–	All β-lactams (except aztreonam)
	New Delhi metallo-β-lactamase (NDM)	India, Pakistan, Bangladesh, United Kingdom, Balkan	All β-lactams (except aztreonam)
Ambler class D (serine β-lactamase)	Oxacillinase (OXA-48)	Turkey, Europe (Spain, The Netherlands), Africa, Eastern Mediterranean, North America, Australia, India and China	Penicillin, lower generation cephalosporins, carbapenems

Carbapenem resistance

Carbapenems are considered as the first-line drug of choice for treating *Klebsiella* infections because of presence of aminoglycoside-modifying enzymes, macrolide esterase, efflux system and other resistance factors against several common antibiotics. Since 2001, the picture started to alter with the emergence of carbapenem-resistant *K. pneumoniae* (CRKP) isolates from North Carolina (Yigit et al., 2001). Within the next 10 years, incidence of carbapenem-resistant *Klebsiella* increased from 1.6% to 10.4% (Jacob et al., 2013). The major enzyme identified for generation of carbapenem resistance was *K. pneumoniae* carbapenemase (KPC-1), a kind of β-lactamase that produced acylation of most carbapenems (Table 14.2, Markogiannakis et al., 2013). KPC-2 and their variants were detected later in the United States, Europe, South America, Israel and Far East (Nordmann et al., 2009; Cuzon et al., 2010; Saidel-Odes and Borer, 2013). However, a few scientific workers claimed KPC-1 and 2 as a same enzyme (Yigit et al., 2001a; Nordmann et al., 2009). Mutations in the *bla*$_{KPC-2}$ structural gene have generated two variants namely *bla*$_{KPC-3}$ (Woodford et al., 2004) and *bla*$_{KPC-4}$ (Palepou et al., 2005). A novel KPC variant (*bla*$_{KPC-5}$) was later detected in carbapenem-resistant *Pseudomonas aeruginosa* isolate from Puerto Rico (Wolter et al., 2009). Clinically significant *K. pneumoniae* clonal types (ST 258) harbour KPC genes on transposons (Tn3 based) and plasmids of various sizes and incompatibility groups (Cuzon et al., 2010).

Other than KPCs, metallo-β-lactamase, imipenemase (IMP), New Delhi, metallo-β-lactamase (NDM-1) were also identified as integrin/plasmid-encoded carbapenemases which can hydrolyse all β-lactams except aztreonam (Table 14.2; Walsh et al., 2005; Yong et al., 2009). International clonal types (ST 11, ST 37) of *K. pneumoniae* were mostly reported to produce carbapenemase (NDM-1), ESBL and AmpC (Netikul et al., 2014; Ma et al., 2015; Guo et al., 2016). The NDM-1 was named for New Delhi, the capital of India, as it was first detected in a Swedish patient who had undergone a surgery in New Delhi (Yong et al., 2009). The gene encoding NDM-1 was detected in a transferable plasmid and it produced resistance against multiple numbers of antibiotics including carbapenem. Environmental studies conducted in New Delhi (India) further confirmed NDM-1 producing isolates in drinking and seepage water which raised concern (Walsh et al., 2011).

Oxacillinase was described as another group of carbapenemase which can hydrolyse penicillins and carbapenems, but not the broad-spectrum cephalosporins. Clinically significant oxacillinase (OXA-48) was originated in *Shewanella* spp. and was harboured by a composite transposon (Tn1999) on IncL/M plasmid. Because of high conjugative nature of the plasmid, the oxacillinase spreads easily throughout the world (Potron et al., 2011). In *K. pneumoniae* isolates, OXA-48 was first detected in Turkey and later oxacillinase-producing *K. pneumoniae* was disseminated into Europe (Spain, the Netherlands, Germany), Africa, Eastern Mediterranean, North America, Australia and China (Pfeifer et al., 2012; Espedido et al., 2013; Wang et al., 2013; Lascols et al., 2013). Several OXA-48 variants such as OXA-162, OXA-181, OXA-204 and OXA-232 were also detected in *K. pneumoniae* isolates (Poirel et al., 2012). In Southeastern Asia, OXA-48-producing *K. pneumoniae* was detected in human patients from Singapore (OXA-181) and Thailand (ST 11 and ST 37 clonal types) (Koh et al., 2012; Lunha et al., 2016).

Among all the enzymes produced by *Klebsiella* and other *Enterobacteriaceae*, KPC, NDM and OXA-48 are most prevalent throughout the world (Lunha et al., 2016). Most of these enzymes producing carbapenem resistance are region- or country-specific, although they can spread throughout the world (Table 14.2).

To detect the underlying molecular mechanism for carbapenem resistance, a proteome-associated study was conducted with *bla*$_{KPC-2}$-carrying multidrug-resistant clinical *K. pneumoniae* strain which was exposed to meropenem (a carbapenem analogue) with a concentration lower than minimum inhibitory concentration. The meropenem exposure produced overexpression of certain stress-associated enzymes (phosphoglycerate kinase, fructose-bisphosphate aldolase class II, phosphoglyceromutase, alcohol dehydrogenase and malate dehydrogenase), stress-induced proteins such as chaperonin GroEL (60 kDa) and small heat shock protein and a probable resistance-associated protein (LysM domain/BON super-family). Development of stress in the meropenem-exposed bacteria occurred due to excess consumption of energy, utilized to repair damaged proteins and DNA or to activate the efflux pumps for removal of meropenem (Khan et al., 2017). Poor expression or mutation of outer membrane proteins (OmpK35, OmpK36) was also detected as contributing factor in carbapenem resistance other than the production of carbapenemase enzyme. Substitution of glycine (Gly) by a negatively charged aspartic acid (Asp) in the PEFXG motif of the Omp36 was noted as responsible for loss of pore conductance resulting in limited access of antibiotics (Dé et al., 2001; Lunha et al., 2016). Insertion of Asp-Gly or Gly-Asp at the end of the PEFGG motif (OmpK36) detected in KPC-producing *K. pneumoniae* isolates produced high-level carbapenem resistance (Partridge et al., 2015).

CRKP isolates are multidrug-resistant except a few aminoglycosides, tigecycline and colistin. In a study with CRKP strains isolated from human patients in the United Kingdom during 2006−09, susceptibility to one or more aminoglycosides was detected such as apramycin, isepamicin, and next-generation aminoglycosides (ACHN-490/plazomicin)

(Livermore et al., 2010). Blocking the transmission route and treatment of clinical infection based on sensitivity report are the ways to control CRKP. Disinfectants are effective tools to control the transmission route in hospital environment such as hands of attendants or physicians, desktops and medical devices and in livestock farms, which is considered as one of the potent sources of infection. Unfortunately, recent study explored the resistance of the CRKP strains to the common disinfectants such as chlorhexidine acetate (78%), iodophor (74%), iodine tincture (67%), benzalkonium bromide (63%), glutaraldehyde (59%) and ethyl alcohol (52%) and indicated a possible linkage between antibiotic resistance genes and tolerance to disinfectants (Guo et al., 2015).

Aminoglycoside resistance

Aminoglycosides control Gram-negative pathogens including *Klebsiella* by inhibition of protein synthesis after binding with aminoacyl site (A-site) of 16S rRNA present within the bacterial 30S ribosomal subunit. The enzymes such as acetyl transferases, nucleotidyl transferases and phosphotransferases are responsible for enzymatic inactivation of aminoglycosides. Defective cellular permeability, activation of efflux pumps and mutation of the target molecule are other resistance mechanisms against aminoglycosides (Magnet and Blanchard, 2005). *Actinomycetes* are intrinsically resistant to the aminoglycosides due to methylation of nucleotides present within A-site of 16S rRNA, which prevents binding of aminoglycosides with 30S subunit (Cundliffe, 1989). Clinical strains of *K. pneumoniae* were also reported to produce 16S rRNA methylase which produced increased resistance of the isolates against amikacin, tobramycin and gentamicin (Galimand et al., 2003). *ArmA* and *rmtA* were detected as major genes, encoding 16S rRNA methylase in clinical isolates of *K. pneumoniae* and *E. coli* (Yan et al., 2004). Higher GC content of 16S rRNA methylase genes (*ArmA*) suggests its origin from environmental saprophytes probably through horizontal gene transfer. *ArmA*- or *RmtA*-producing *K. pneumoniae* were reported from Europe (France, Spain, Bulgaria, Belgium) and Asian countries (Taiwan, South Korea) (Doi and Arakawa, 2007).

Colistin/polymyxin resistance

Cationic antimicrobial peptides (CAPs) such as colistin, polymyxin, and many others can destroy the bacteria by disrupting their cytoplasmic membrane. Mutation in two-component regulatory system (PhoPQ-PmrAB) can alter the negative charge of LPS molecule, present in the bacterial surface as O-antigen. Alteration in negative charge can prevent effective binding of CAPs (positively charged) with the bacterial surface and promote the development of resistance (Falagas et al., 2010). A recent study described a new two-component system (CrrAB) associated with colistin resistance (Wright et al., 2015). European Antimicrobial Resistance Surveillance Network (EARS-Net), under European Centre for Disease Prevention and Control, conducted a surveillance study and reported resistance pattern of *K. pneumoniae* against polymyxins. Overall, 8.8% of *K. pneumoniae* strains isolated from human patients residing in Greece, Italy, Romania and Hungary were resistant against polymyxins (Giske, 2015). Colistin was considered as a typical drug of choice for CRKP isolates. Currently, CRKP isolates showing resistance to colistin is an emerging concern in several countries such as Taiwan (Chiu et al., 2013). A linkage of polymyxin and carbapenem resistance was detected among *K. pneumoniae* isolates from human in Italy and Spain (Pena et al., 2014; Giske, 2015).

Temocillin resistance

Temocillin (ticarcillin derivative) is active against ESBL- and ampC-producing *Enterobacteriaceae* as the α-methoxy group present in the drug can prevent the entry of water molecule and activation of β-lactamase enzymes (Rodriguez-Villalobos et al., 2006). A Swedish study revealed considerable rate of resistance to temocillin (24%) among ESBL-producing *K. pneumoniae* isolates specially associated with CTX-M-1 production (Titelman et al., 2011).

Tigecycline resistance

Increased resistance of *K. pneumoniae* strains against tigecycline was detected in Greece (Neonakis et al., 2011), India (Arya and Agarwal, 2010) and Saudi Arabia (Al-Qadheeb et al., 2010). Resistance to tigecycline was associated with upregulation of *rarA*, *marA* and *ramA*, which activates bacterial efflux systems such as pump AcrAB and OqxAB (Veleba and Schneiders, 2012).

Fosfomycin resistance

Fosfomycin is preferred for KPC-producing *K. pneumoniae* and *E. coli* associated with UTIs as a primary drug or as an adjunct therapy (Michalopoulos et al., 2010). Recent studies noted emergence of fosfomycin resistance especially among the KPC-producing *K. pneumoniae* in Asian countries. The fosfomycin resistance was associated with plasmid-encoded *fosA3* gene, disseminated by IS26 composite transposon. FosA3 inactivates fosfomycin by glutathione *S*-transferase activity (Wachino et al., 2010). Another study indicated about the role of a common plasmid carrying both *fosA3* and *bla*$_{KPC-2}$ genes in clonal dissemination of resistant *K. pneumoniae* between different hospitals in China (Jiang et al., 2015). Two clonal types (ST11, ST494) and five pulse types (PTA, PTB, PTC, PTD, PTE) of *K. pneumoniae* were detected in China associated with fosfomycin resistance (Xiang et al., 2016).

Association of *bla*$_{CTX-M}$ and sometimes *rmtB* with *fosA3* was also reported (Xiang et al., 2016). Since initial description of fosA3 in CTX-M-producing *E. coli* in Japan, several workers reported the existence of fosA3 in food animals, companion animals, human patients and healthy persons in Asian countries (Hou et al., 2012; Ho et al., 2013; Sato et al., 2013).

Quinoxaline resistance

Quinoxaline is a kind of antibiotic having structural similarity with quinolone derivatives. Resistance to quinoxaline is mediated by an efflux pump (OqxAB) which can extrude the quinoxaline derivatives as well as chloramphenicol and fluoroquinolones from the bacterial cell (Hansen et al., 2007).OqxAB encoding gene was originated in chromosome of *K. pneumoniae* which later disseminated into *E. coli* and *Salmonella*. Clinical isolates of OqxAB-producing *K. pneumoniae* were reported from human patients in China, South Korea and Spain (Park et al., 2102; Yuan et al., 2012; Rodriguez-Martinez et al., 2013). Prevalence of *OqxAB* varied from 71% to 100% in KPC-producing *K. pneumoniae* strains isolated from paediatric long-term care facility, acute care hospitals and other hospitals in Ohio, New York, Taiwan, Australia, Argentina, Belgium, Turkey and South Africa (Perez et al., 2013).

Characteristics of antimicrobial resistance in *Klebsiella* isolates observed in different livestock, poultry, wildlife and environment as well as in human are discussed in the following section. In contrast to the human studies, where epidemic clones of *K. pneumoniae* showing resistance is well-characterized, the population biology of antimicrobial-resistant *Klebsiella* spp. is explored scarcely in livestock and wildlife.

Ruminants

Transfer of antibiotic resistance between bacterial species present in the rumen was first documented in sheep (Smith, 1975). Rumen is considered as a major site of resistance gene exchange or transfer between compatible bacteria since long time ago. Rumen protozoa engulfing the compatible bacteria favoured conjugation, the preliminary step for gene transfer (Schlimme et al., 1997). Engulfment by rumen protozoa helped in transfer of *bla*$_{CMY-2}$ from a *K. pneumoniae* donor to *Salmonella* recipient under experimental conditions (McCuddin et al., 2006).

Bovine mastitis is an economically significant menace affecting the dairy industry throughout the world. *K. pneumoniae* is considered as a major etiological factor for bovine mastitis. In a study for detection of antimicrobial resistance in Gram-negative bacteria associated with bovine mastitis during 1994—2000, conducted at Michigan State University, USA, *K. pneumoniae* isolates were detected as phenotypically resistant against tetracycline (33%), ampicillin (15.7%), ceftiofur (14.1%), cephalothin (4.2%) and sulfa trimethoprim (3.7%) (Erskine et al., 2002). *Klebsiella* isolated from cattle and horses in the United States was also detected to possess *intI* (Goldstein et al., 2001). Studies in the United Kingdom (Timofte et al., 2014), France (Locatelli et al., 2010) and Japan (Saishu et al., 2014) have reported the occurrence of ESBL-producing *K. pneumoniae* associated with mastitis in cattle. In India, ESBL-producing *K. pneumoniae* were isolated from milk samples of healthy cows and cows with subclinical and clinical mastitis. The isolates were more frequently detected in mastitis cattle than healthy ones. The isolates also possessed quinolone and sulfonamide resistance genes along with class 1 integrons. Clonal relationship was detected among the isolates from distant places indicating cross-transmission between the places (Koovapra et al., 2016).

Companion/pet animals

High occurrence rate of CTX-M-15-producing *K. pneumoniae* was reported from companion animals in France. Most of these isolates belonged to sequence type ST274 and were resistant to tetracycline, gentamicin, nalidixic acid, sulfonamides and trimethoprim/sulfamethoxazole (Poirel et al., 2013). Occurrence of CTX-M-15 is alarming as it is the most common ESBL identified worldwide in humans (Carattoli, 2008). Another recent study also detected OXA-48 carbapenemase and CTX-M-15 producing *K. pneumoniae* (ST 15 clonal type) from clinical samples such as faeces, urine, skin and soft tissues collected from dogs admitted in a veterinary clinic in Germany. Carbapenems are not licenced to use in livestock or companion animals in Germany. *K. pneumoniae* ST15 isolates possessing *bla*$_{OXA-48}$ are considered as an epidemic clone in human, especially in Copenhagen, Hungary, New Zealand and Asian countries (China, Finland and Thailand). The German study suggested about the nosocomial spread of ST15 clones from human or environment to the companion animals (Stolle et al., 2013). In another comprehensive study conducted with clinical samples (skin and soft tissues, urine, faeces, nasal swabs, eye swabs) from companion animals (dogs, cats, birds) received from Germany and few other European countries, CTX-M-15 was established as the predominant ESBL in *K. pneumoniae* isolates, mostly belonged to ST 15 clonal type. Plasmid typing detected IncFII, IncFIA and IncFIB as major replicons associated with *bla*$_{CTX-M-15}$ in *K. pneumoniae* isolates (Ewers et al., 2014). Future research will explore whether any parallel evolution has generated the CTM-15-producing *K. pneumoniae* ST 15 clones in companion animals from human isolates or they belong to uniform pool of the human isolates. However, the study conducted in Switzerland with cephalosporin-resistant *K. pneumoniae* isolates from companion animals and human did not find any epidemiological link. Most of the animal isolates belonged to *K. pneumoniae* ST11 clonal type producing plasmidic AmpC, whereas no specific clone was detected among the human isolates. Most of the animal isolates were resistant to quinolones and *bla*$_{DHA-1}$, *bla*$_{CTX-M-1}$ detected in the isolates was associated with nonconjugative R plasmids (Wohlwend et al., 2015).

In Italy, the study conducted with large numbers of pet dogs and cats, *K. pneumoniae* and *K. oxytoca* were isolated from clinical samples and necropsy specimens. Four major sequence types were detected by MLST, i.e., ST11, ST340, ST101 and ST15. Coexistence of the ESBL and AmpC gene was observed in a *K. pneumoniae* isolate (ST15) from a cat. Moreover, quinolone resistance associated with *qnrS*, *qnrA* and *aac(6_)-Ib-cr* genes was observed in *Klebsiella* isolates (Donati et al., 2014). Most of the ESBL gene carrying *K. pneumoniae* isolates from the pets possessed *Inc* plasmids (IncN, IncR) (Haenni et al., 2011; Donati et al., 2014). Association of ESBL genes (*bla*) and Inc replicons was reported as prevalent in zoonotic enterobacterial pathogens causing human infections (García-Fernández et al., 2009; Coelho et al., 2010).

Pigs

A study conducted with considerable numbers of faecal samples collected from swine finishing barns in Ohio, Kansas, Illinois, Michigan and Minnesota revealed the existence of *bla*$_{CTX-M-1}$ possessing *K. pneumoniae*. Antibiotics such as tetracyclines, lincosamides or macrolides were used in the feed and drinking water. No information was available regarding usage of higher generation cephalosporins in the studied pigs (Mollenkopf et al., 2013).

Horses

β-Lactamase gene possessing (*bla*$_{TEM-1}$, *bla*$_{SHV-1}$, *bla*$_{CTX-M-1}$) *K. pneumoniae* was detected in horses (including horses of 1-month old) in the Netherlands (Vo et al., 2007). In the Netherlands, third-generation cephalosporins are approved for treatment of respiratory tract and foot infections in cattle and pigs, not in horses. Ceftiofur is used in horses in the Netherlands for a clinical condition other than that for which it has been officially approved (off-label usage). In the United States, Australia and Europe (the United Kingdom, Belgium, the Netherland, France), *Enterobacteriaceae* possessing *bla*$_{CTX-M-15}$ harbouring plasmids (IncI1/ST31) was prevalent in horses, cattle and human (Zurfluh et al., 2015).

Poultry and Turkey

Multidrug-resistant (ampicillin, tetracycline, streptomycin, gentamicin, kanamycin) *K. pneumoniae* was isolated from a turkey farm and turkey products in Oklahoma, United States. Class 1 integrons and *bla*$_{SHV-1}$ were detected in most of the isolates, which was transferable as observed experimentally (Kim et al., 2005). In another study, *K. pneumoniae*, resistant to ampicillin, erythromycin, cefoxitin, streptomycin and nalidixic acid, were isolated from chicken and guinea fowl carcasses and environmental samples in Tennessee State University's poultry research facilities in the United States. *K. oxytoca* isolates from chickens were resistant to ampicillin and erythromycin (Kilonzo-Nthenge et al., 2008).

In India, a comprehensive study revealed the occurrence of CTX-M-producing *Klebsiella* spp. in healthy broilers, indigenous game birds (*Desi* and cross between Aseel and *Desi* breed) and Kuroilers (semisynthetic bird) either because of extensive use of third-generation cephalosporins (cefotaxime) in indigenous game birds or may be associated with high mobilization of the encoding genes from the contaminated environment. The game birds in this study were used in cock fighting and were often treated with costly antibiotics such as third-generation cephalosporins for both preventive and therapeutic purposes. Clonal relationship among the isolates from broilers and indigenous birds suggested possible cross-transmission (Mahanti et al., 2018).

Wildlife

Multidrug-resistant *K. pneumonia*e were isolated from Chinese hares (*Lepus sinensis*) suffering with pneumonia and diarrhoea in Hebei province of China. Notably the isolates were resistant to last resort antibiotics such as imipenem, meropenem and vancomycin, but were sensitive to cefepime, co-trimoxazole and enrofloxacin. The authors suggested role of contaminated environment, human activities and other wildlife in transmission of resistant *K. pneumoniae* to the studied hares (Du et al., 2014).

Environment

In Oklahoma (United States), *K. pneumoniae* were most commonly isolated from farm environments and retail products such as feathers of turkey, feeds, drinking water and faeces collected from a turkey farm and ground turkey products. The isolates were phenotypically resistant against ampicillin, streptomycin and tetracycline and possessed *aadA1* (streptomycin resistance) and *bla*$_{SHV-1}$ (ampicillin). Outer membrane proteins (OmpK35, OmpK36) were detected in isolates indicating that their β-lactam resistance was not associated with porin changes (Kim et al., 2005).

Plasmid typing of CTX-M-15-producing *Enterobacteriaceae* isolated from environment (rivers and lakes), livestock and human interface in Switzerland revealed the most frequent presence of IncF-type plasmids among the isolates. The IncF-type plasmid was detected as multireplicon type consisting of replicons such as IncFII, IncFIA and IncFIB. Other than IncF type, IncI1 type of plasmid (with *bla*$_{CTX-M-15}$) was also detected among the isolates which belonged to sequence types ST31, ST37, ST57, ST176 and ST177. The studied waterbodies in Switzerland acted as 'resistome' for different antibiotics along with transferable plasmids (Zurfluh et al., 2015).

Human

K. pneumoniae is considered as second most prevalent bacteria associated with UTIs in human patients, especially among the females. A study conducted with the UTI patients in Bangladesh revealed the resistance of *K. pneumoniae* isolates against ampicillin, amoxicillin, azithromycin, ciprofloxacin, nalidixic acid and cotrimoxazole. All the isolates were found susceptible to imipenem (Lina et al., 2007).

ESBL-producing *K. pneumoniae* were isolated from intensive care unit, neurosurgery, pulmonary internal medicine and general medicine wards of a human hospital in Republic of Korea. All isolates were resistant to common antibiotics such as penicillins, ceftazidime, cefotaxime, aztreonam, tobramycin, gentamicin and trimethoprim/sulfamethoxazole and the isolates showed reduced susceptibility to imipenem. Possession of *bla*$_{GES}$ of the isolates was found to be associated with reduced susceptibility to imipenem (Jeong et al., 2005).

In China, NDM-1-producing *K. pneumoniae* (ST 17, ST 20) was isolated from neonates associated with prematurity, low body weight and poor immunity. The isolates were phenotypically resistant against gentamicin and fosfomycin, although class 1 integrons were not associated with acquisition of the resistance genes (Jin et al., 2015).

K. pneumoniae and *K. oxytoca* isolated from human stool samples in Kenya (Africa) were detected to possess genes conferring resistance against β-lactamase, aminoglycosides, macrolides, tetracyclines, ansamycins, phenicols, fluoroquinolones, quaternary amines, streptothricin, sulfonamides and diaminopyrimidines. Extensive use of trimethoprim/sulfamethoxazole in HIV patients in African countries was identified as a contributor for selection pressure to carry the genes conferring resistance against trimethoprim and sulfonamides. The existence of selection pressure against tetracyclines and phenicols was also detected in Kenya (Taitt et al., 2017).

ESBL-producing *K. pneumoniae* were isolated from urine, trachea, wounds, blood and sputum of hospitalized patients in Iran. Significant correlations were observed between phenotypical resistance to aminoglycosides, fluoroquinolones and sulfonamides, and carriage of integrons (class 1, 2) and *bla*$_{SHV}$ gene. Role of integrons (class 1 and 2) in spreading *bla*$_{SHV}$ among nosocomial *K. pneumoniae* isolates was explored (Ashayeri-Panah et al., 2014).

References

Abgottspon, H., Nüesch-Inderbinen, M.T., Zurfluh, K., Althaus, D., Hächler, H., Stephan, R., 2014. *Enterobacteriaceae* with extended-spectrum- and pAmpC-type β-lactamase encoding genes isolated from freshwater fish from two lakes in Switzerland. Antimicrobial Agents and Chemotherapy 58, 2482–2484.

Al-Hasan, M.N., Lahr, B.D., Eckel-Passow, J.E., Baddour, L.M., 2010. Epidemiology and outcome of *Klebsiella* species bloodstream infection: a population-based study. Mayo Clinic Proceedings 85, 139–144.

Al-Qadheeb, N.S., Althawadi, S., Alkhalaf, A., Hosaini, S., Alrajhi, A.A., 2010. Evolution of tigecycline resistance in *Klebsiella pneumoniae* in a single patient. Annals of Saudi Medicine 30, 404–407.

Arya, S.C., Agarwal, N., 2010. Emergence of tigecycline resistance amongst multi-drug resistant gram negative isolates in a multi-disciplinary hospital. Journal of Infection 61, 358–359.

Ashayeri-Panah, M., Feizabadi, M.M., Eftekhar, F., 2014. Correlation of multi-drug resistance, integron and blaESBL gene carriage with genetic fingerprints of extended-spectrum β-lactamase producing *Klebsiella pneumoniae*. Jundishapur Journal of Microbiology 7 (2).

Bai, J., Liu, Q., Yang, Y., Wang, J., Yang, Y., Li, J., Li, P., Li, X., Xi, Y., Ying, J., Ren, P., 2013. Insights into the evolution of gene organization and multidrug resistance from *Klebsiella pneumoniae* plasmid pKF3-140. Gene 519 (1), 60–66.

Bhattacharjee, A., Sen, M.R., Prakash, P., Gaur, A., Anupurba, S., Nath, G., 2010. Observation on integron carriage among clinical isolates of *Klebsiella pneumoniae* producing extended spectrum β -lactamases. Indian Journal of Medical Microbiology 28, 207–210.

Bistué, A.J.S., Birshan, D., Tomaras, A.P., Dandekar, M., Tran, T., Newmark, J., Bui, D., Gupta, N., Hernandez, K., Sarno, R., Zorreguieta, A., 2008. *Klebsiella pneumoniae* multiresistance plasmid pMET1: similarity with the *Yersinia pestis* plasmid pCRY and integrative conjugative elements. PLoS One 3 (3), e1800.

Bowers, J.R., Kitchel, B., Driebe, E.M., MacCannell, D.R., Roe, C., Lemmer, D., de Man, T., Rasheed, J.K., Engelthaler, D.M., Keim, P., Limbago, B.M., 2015. Genomic analysis of the emergence and rapid global dissemination of the clonal group 258 *Klebsiella pneumoniae* pandemic. PLoS One 10.

Bowers, J.R., Lemmer, D., Sahl, J.W., Pearson, T., Driebe, E.M., Wojack, B., Saubolle, M.A., Engelthaler, D.M., Keim, P., 2016. KlebSeq, a diagnostic tool for surveillance, detection, and monitoring of *Klebsiella pneumoniae*. Journal of Clinical Microbiology 54 (10), 2582–2596.

Bradford, P.A., Urban, C., Mariano, N., Projan, S.J., Rahal, J.J., Bush, K., 1997. Imipenem resistance in *Klebsiella pneumoniae* is associated with the combination of ACT-1, a plasmid-mediated AmpC β-lactamase, and the loss of an outer membrane protein. Antimicrobial Agents and Chemotherapy 41, 563–569.

Broberg, C.A., Palacios, M., Miller, V.L., 2014. *Klebsiella*: a long way to go towards understanding this enigmatic jet-setter. F1000prime reports 6, 64.

Cambray, G., Guerout, A.M., Mazel, D., 2010. Integrons. Annual Review of Genetics 44, 141–166.

Carattoli, A., 2008. Animal reservoirs for extended-spectrum β-lactamase producers. Clinical Microbiology and Infections 14 (Suppl. 1), 117–123.

Carattoli, A., 2009. Resistance plasmid families in *Enterobacteriaceae*. Antimicrobial Agents and Chemotherapy 53, 2227–2238.

Centers for Disease Control and Prevention, April 2013. Office of Infectious Disease. Antibiotic Resistance Threats in the United States, 2013. Available at: http://www.cdc.gov/drugresistance/threat-report-2013.

Chen, Y.T., Shu, H.Y., Li, L.H., Liao, T.L., Wu, K.M., Shiau, Y.R., Yan, J.J., Su, I.J., Tsai, S.F., Lauderdale, T.L., 2006. Complete nucleotide sequence of pK245, a 98-kilobase plasmid conferring quinolone resistance and extended-spectrum-β-lactamase activity in a clinical *Klebsiella pneumoniae* isolate. Antimicrobial Agents and Chemotherapy 50 (11), 3861–3866.

Chiu, S.K., Wu, T.L., Chuang, Y.C., Lin, J.C., Fung, C.P., Lu, P.L., Wang, J.T., Wang, L.S., Siu, L.K., Yeh, K.M., 2013. National surveillance study on carbapenem non-susceptible *Klebsiella pneumoniae* in Taiwan: the emergence and rapid dissemination of KPC-2 carbapenemase. PLoS One 8, e69428.

Coelho, A., González-López, J.J., Miró, E., Alonso-Tarrés, C., Mirelis, B., Larrosa, M.N., Bartolomé, R.M., Andreu, A., Navarro, F., Johnson, J.R., Prats, G., 2010. Characterisation of the CTX-M-15-encoding gene in *Klebsiella pneumoniae* strains from the barcelona metropolitan area: plasmid diversity and chromosomal integration. International Journal of Antimicrobial Agents 36 (1), 73–78.

Correia, M., Boavida, F., Grosso, F., Salgado, M.J., Lito, L.M., Cristino, J.M., Mendo, S., Duarte, A., 2003. Molecular characterization of a new class 3 integron in *Klebsiella pneumoniae*. Antimicrobial Agents and Chemotherapy 47 (9), 2838–2843.

Cundliffe, E., 1989. How antibiotic-producing organisms avoid suicide. Annual Review of Microbiology 43, 207–233.

Cuzon, G., Naas, T., Truong, H., Villegas, M.V., Wisell, K.T., Carmeli, Y., Gales, A.C., Venezia, S.N., Quinn, J.P., Nordmann, P., 2010. Worldwide diversity of *Klebsiella pneumoniae* that produce beta-lactamase *bla*$_{KPC-2}$ gene. Emerging Infectious Diseases 16, 1349–1356.

Dé, E., Baslé, A., Jaquinod, M., Saint, N., Malléa, M., Molle, G., 2001. A new mechanism of antibiotic resistance in *Enterobacteriaceae* induced by a structural modification of the major porin. Molecular Microbiology 41 (1), 189–198.

Dhar, S., Martin, E.T., Lephart, P.R., McRoberts, J.P., Chopra, T., Burger, T.T., Tal-Jasper, R., Hayakawa, K., Ofer-Friedman, H., Lazarovitch, T., Zaidenstein, R., Perez, F., Bonomo, R.A., Kaye, K.S., Marchaim, D., 2016. Risk Factors and Outcomes for Carbapenem-Resistant *Klebsiella pneumoniae* Isolation.

Doi, Y., Arakawa, Y., 2007. 16S ribosomal RNA methylation: emerging resistance mechanism against aminoglycosides. Clinical Infectious Diseases 45 (1), 88–94.

Donati, V., Feltrin, F., Hendriksen, R.S., Svendsen, C.A., Cordaro, G., García-Fernández, A., Lorenzetti, S., Lorenzetti, R., Battisti, A., Franco, A., 2014. Extended-spectrum-beta-lactamases, AmpC beta-lactamases and plasmid mediated quinolone resistance in *Klebsiella* spp. from companion animals in Italy. PLoS One 9 (3), e90564.

Doublet, B., Boyd, D., Douard, G., Praud, K., Cloeckaert, A., Mulvey, M.R., 2012. Complete nucleotide sequence of the multidrug resistance IncA/C plasmid pR55 from *Klebsiella pneumoniae* isolated in 1969. Journal of Antimicrobial Chemotherapy 67, 2354–2360.

Du, Y., Luo, J., Wang, C., Wen, Q., Duan, M., Zhang, H., He, H., 2014. Detection of drug-resistant *Klebsiella pneumoniae* in Chinese hares (*Lepus sinensis*). Journal of Wildlife Diseases 50 (1), 109-112. e0133727.

EFSA Panel on Biological Hazards, 2011. Scientific opinion on the public health risks of bacterial strains producing extended-spectrum β-lactamases and/or AmpC β-lactamases in food and food-producing animals. EFSA Journal 9, 2322.

Erskine, R.J., Walker, R.D., Bolin, C.A., Bartlett, P.C., White, D.G., 2002. Trends in antibacterial susceptibility of mastitis pathogens during a seven-year period. Journal of Dairy Science 85 (5), 1111−1118.

Espedido, B.A., Steen, J.A., Ziochos, H., Grimmond, S.M., Cooper, M.A., Gosbell, I.B., van Hal, Sebastiaan, J., Jensen, S.O., 2013. Whole genome sequence analysis of the first Australian OXA-48-producing outbreak-associated *Klebsiella pneumoniae* isolates: the resistome and in vivo evolution. PLoS One 8, e59920.

Ewers, C., Stamm, I., Pfeifer, Y., Wieler, L.H., Kopp, P.A., Schønning, K., Prenger-Berninghoff, E., Scheufen, S., Stolle, I., Günther, S., Bethe, A., 2014. Clonal spread of highly successful ST15-CTX-M-15 *Klebsiella pneumoniae* in companion animals and horses. Journal of Antimicrobial Chemotherapy 69 (10), 2676−2680.

Falagas, M.E., Rafailidis, P.I., Matthaiou, D.K., 2010. Resistance to polymyxins: mechanisms, frequency and treatment options. Drug Resistance Updates 13, 132−138.

Galimand, M., Courvalin, P., Lambert, T., 2003. Plasmid-mediated high-level resistance to aminoglycosides in *Enterobacteriaceae* due to 16S rRNA methylation. Antimicrobial Agents and Chemotherapy 47, 2565−2571.

García-Fernández, A., Fortini, D., Veldman, K., Mevius, D., Carattoli, A., 2009. Characterization of plasmids harbouring qnrS1, qnrB2 and qnrB19 genes in *Salmonella*. Journal of Antimicrobial Chemotherapy 63, 274−281.

Giske, C.G., 2015. Contemporary resistance trends and mechanisms for the old antibiotics colistin, temocillin, fosfomycin, mecillinam and nitrofurantoin. Clinical Microbiology and Infections 21 (10), 899−905.

Goldstein, C., Lee, M.D., Sanchez, S., Hudson, C., Phillips, B., Register, B., Grady, M., Liebert, C., Summers, A.O., White, D.G., Maurer, J.J., 2001. Incidence of class 1 and 2 integrases in clinical and commensal bacteria from livestock, companion animals, and exotics. Antimicrobial Agents and Chemotherapy 45 (3), 723−726.

Gonzalez Leiza, M., Perez-Diaz, J.C., Ayala, J., Casellas, J.M., Martinez-Beltran, J., Bush, K., Baquero, F., 1994. Gene sequence and biochemical characterization of FOX-1 from *Klebsiella pneumoniae*, a new AmpC-type plasmid-mediated beta-lactamase with two molecular variants. Antimicrobial Agents and Chemotherapy 38, 2150−2157.

Guo, Q., Spychala, C.N., McElheny, C.L., Doi, Y., 2016. Comparative analysis of an IncR plasmid carrying armA, bla DHA-1 and qnrB4 from *Klebsiella pneumoniae* ST37 isolates. Journal of Antimicrobial Chemotherapy 71 (4), 882−886.

Guo, W., Shan, K., Xu, B., Li, J., 2015. Determining the resistance of carbapenem-resistant *Klebsiella pneumoniae* to common disinfectants and elucidating the underlying resistance mechanisms. Pathogens and Global Health 109 (4), 184−192.

Haenni, M., Ponsin, C., Métayer, V., Médaille, C., Madec, J.Y., 2011. Veterinary hospital-acquired infections in pets with a ciprofloxacin-resistant CTX-M-15-producing *Klebsiella pneumoniae* ST15 clone. Journal of Antimicrobial Chemotherapy 67, 770−771.

Hansen, D.S., Aucken, H.M., Abiola, T., Podschun, R., 2004. Recommended test panel for differentiation of *Klebsiella* species on the basis of a trilateral inter laboratory evaluation of 18 biochemical tests. Journal of Clinical Microbiology 42, 3665−3669.

Hansen, L.H., Jensen, L.B., Sorensen, H.I., Sorensen, S.J., 2007. Substrate specificity of the OqxAB multidrug resistance pump in *Escherichia coli* and selected enteric bacteria. Journal of Antimicrobial Chemotherapy 60, 145−147.

Hazen, T.H., Zhao, L., Boutin, M.A., Stancil, A., Robinson, G., Harris, A.D., Rasko, D.A., Johnson, J.K., 2014. Comparative genomics of an IncA/C multidrug resistance plasmid from *Escherichia coli* and *Klebsiella* isolates from intensive care unit patients and the utility of whole-genome sequencing in health care settings. Antimicrobial Agents and Chemotherapy 58 (8), 4814−4825.

He, L., Partridge, S.R., Yang, X., Hou, J., Deng, Y., Yao, Q., Zeng, Z., Chen, Z., Liu, J.H., 2013. Complete nucleotide sequence of pHN7A8, an F33:A-: B-type epidemic plasmid carrying $bla_{CTX-M-65}$, *fosA3*, and *rmtB* from China. Journal of Antimicrobial Chemotherapy 68, 46−50.

Ho, P.L., Chan, J., Lo, W.U., Law, P.Y., Chow, K.H., 2013. Plasmid-mediated fosfomycin resistance in *Escherichia coli* isolated from pig. Veterinary Microbiology 162, 964−967.

Hou, J., Huang, X., Deng, Y., He, L., Yang, T., Zeng, Z., Chen, Z., Liu, J.H., 2012. Dissemination of the fosfomycin resistance gene *fosA3* with CTX-M betalactamase genes and *rmtB* carried on IncFII plasmids among *Escherichia coli* isolates from pets in China. Antimicrobial Agents and Chemotherapy 56, 2135−2138.

Iqbal, S., Quigley, E.M., 2016. Progress in our understanding of the gut microbiome: implications for the clinician. Current Gastroenterology Reports 18, 49.

Jacob, J.T., Klein, G.E., Laxminarayan, R., Beldavs, Z., Lynfield, R., Kallen, A.J., Ricks, P., Edwards, J., Srinivasan, A., Fridkin, S., Rasheed, K.J., 2013. Vital signs: carbapenem-resistant *Enterobacteriaceae*. Morbidity and Mortality Weekly Report 62 (9), 165−169.

Jeong, S.H., Bae, I.K., Kim, D., Hong, S.G., Song, J.S., Lee, J.H., Lee, S.H., 2005. First outbreak of *Klebsiella pneumoniae* clinical isolates producing GES-5 and SHV-12 extended-spectrum β-lactamases in Korea. Antimicrobial Agents and Chemotherapy 49 (11), 4809−4810.

Jiang, Y., Shen, P., Wei, Z., Liu, L., He, F., Shi, K., Wang, Y., Wang, H., Yu, Y., 2015. Dissemination of a clone carrying a fosA3-harbouring plasmid mediates high fosfomycin resistance rate of KPC-producing *Klebsiella pneumoniae* in China. International Journal of Antimicrobial Agents 45 (1), 66−70.

Jin, Y., Shao, C., Li, J., Fan, H., Bai, Y., Wang, Y., 2015. Outbreak of multidrug resistant NDM-1-producing *Klebsiella pneumoniae* from a neonatal unit in Shandong Province, China. PLoS One 10 (3), e0119571.

Keller, J.J., Tsai, M., Lin, C., Lin, Y., Lin, H., 2013. Risk of infections subsequent to pyogenic liver abscess: a nationwide population-based study. Clinical Microbiology and Infections 19, 717–722.

Khan, A., Sharma, D., Faheem, M., Bisht, D., Khan, A.U., 2017. Proteomic analysis of a carbapenem-resistant *Klebsiella pneumoniae* strain in response to meropenem stress. Journal of Global Antimicrobial Resistance 8, 172–178.

Kilonzo-Nthenge, A., Nahashon, S.N., Chen, F., Adefope, N., 2008. Prevalence and antimicrobial resistance of pathogenic bacteria in chicken and Guinea fowl. Poultry Science 87 (9), 1841–1848.

Kim, S.H., Wei, C.I., Tzou, Y.M., An, H., 2005. Multidrug-resistant *Klebsiella pneumoniae* isolated from farm environments and retail products in Oklahoma. Journal of Food Protection 68 (10), 2022–2029.

Knothe, H., Shah, P., Krcmery, V., Antal, M., Mitsuhashi, S., 1983. Transferable resistance to cefotaxime, cefoxitin, cefamandole and cefuroxime in clinical isolates of Klebsiella pneumoniae and Serratia marcescens. Infection 11 (6), 315–317.

Koh, T.H., Cao, D.Y., Chan, K.S., Wijaya, L., Low, S.B., Lam, M.S., et al., 2012. bla$_{OXA}$-181-positive *Klebsiella pneumoniae*, Singapore. Emerging Infectious Diseases 18, 1524–1525.

Koovapra, S., Bandyopadhyay, S., Das, G., Bhattacharyya, D., Banerjee, J., Mahanti, A., Samanta, I., Nanda, P.K., Kumar, A., Mukherjee, R., Dimri, U., Singh, R.K., 2016. Molecular signature of extended spectrum β-lactamase producing *Klebsiella pneumoniae* isolated from bovine milk in eastern and north-eastern India. Infection, Genetics and Evolution 44, 395–402.

Kuehn, B.M., 2013. 'Nightmare' bacteria on the rise in US hospitals, long-term care facilities. Journal of the American Medical Association 309, 1573–1574.

Kumar, V., Sun, P., Vamathevan, J., Li, Y., Ingraham, K., Palmer, L., Huang, J., Brown, J.R., 2011. Comparative genomics of *Klebsiella pneumoniae* strains with different antibiotic resistance profiles. Antimicrobial Agents and Chemotherapy 55, 4267–4276.

Lascols, C., Peirano, G., Hackel, M., Laupland, K.B., Pitout, Johann, D.D., 2013. Surveillance and molecular epidemiology of *Klebsiella* pneumonia isolates that produce carbapenemases: first report of OXA-48-like enzymes in North America. Antimicrobial Agents and Chemotherapy 57, 130–136.

Li, J., Fu, Y., Wang, J.Y., Tu, C.T., Shen, X.Z., Li, L., Jiang, W., 2010. Early diagnosis and therapeutic choice of *Klebsiella pneumoniae* liver abscess. Frontiers of Medicine in China 4 (3), 308–316.

Lina, T.T., Rahman, S.R., Gomes, D.J., 2007. Multiple-antibiotic resistance mediated by plasmids and integrons in uropathogenic *Escherichia coli* and *Klebsiella pneumoniae*. Bangladesh Journal of Microbiology 24 (1), 19–23.

Livermore, D.M., Mushtaq, S., Warner, M., Zhang, J.C., Maharjan, S., Doumith, M., Woodford, N., 2010. Activity of aminoglycosides, including ACHN-490, against carbapenem-resistant *Enterobacteriaceae* isolates. Journal of Antimicrobial Chemotherapy 66 (1), 48–53.

Locatelli, C., Scaccabarozzi, L., Pisoni, G., Moroni, P., 2010. CTX-M-1 ESBL-producing *Klebsiella pneumoniae* subsp. *pneumoniae* isolated from cases of bovine mastitis. Journal of Clinical Microbiology 48, 3822–3823.

Lunha, K., Chanawong, A., Lulitanond, A., Wilailuckana, C., Charoensri, N., Wonglakorn, L., Saenjamla, P., Chaimanee, P., Angkititrakul, S., Chetchotisakd, P., 2016. High-level carbapenem-resistant OXA-48-producing *Klebsiella pneumoniae* with a novel OmpK36 variant and low-level, carbapenem-resistant, non-porin-deficient, OXA-181-producing *Escherichia coli* from Thailand. Diagnostic Microbiology and Infectious Disease 85 (2), 221–226.

Ma, L.C., Fang, C.T., Lee, C.Z., Shun, C.T., Wang, J.T., 2005. Genomic heterogeneity in *Klebsiella pneumoniae* strains is associated with primary pyogenic liver abscess and metastatic infection. The Journal of Infectious Diseases 192 (1), 117–128.

Ma, L., Wang, J.T., Wu, T.L., Siu, L.K., Chuang, Y.C., Lin, J.C., Lu, M.C., Lu, P.L., 2015. Emergence of OXA-48-producing *Klebsiella pneumoniae* in Taiwan. PLoS One 10 (9), e0139152.

Machado, E., Ferreira, J., Novais, A., Peixe, L., Cantón, R., Baquero, F., Coque, T.M., 2007. Preservation of integron types among *Enterobacteriaceae* producing extended-spectrum β-lactamases in a Spanish hospital over a 15-year period (1988 to 2003). Antimicrobial Agents and Chemotherapy 51, 2201–2204.

Magnet, S., Blanchard, J.S., 2005. Molecular insights into aminoglycoside action and resistance. Chemistry Review 105, 477–498.

Mahanti, A., Ghosh, P., Samanta, I., Joardar, S.N., Bandyopadhyay, S., Bhattacharyya, D., Banerjee, J., Batabyal, S., Sar, T.K., Dutta, T.K., 2018. Prevalence of CTX-M-Producing *Klebsiella* spp. in broiler, kuroiler, and indigenous poultry in West Bengal State, India. Microbial Drug Resistance 24 (3), 299–306.

Malik, A.A., Bari, S.U., Rouf, K.A., Wani, K.A., 2010. Pyogenic liver abscess: changing patterns in approach. World Journal of Gastrointestinal Surgery 2 (12), 395.

Markogiannakis, A., Tzouvelekis, L.S., Psichogiou, M., Petinaki, E., Daikos, G.L., 2013. Confronting carbapenemase-producing *Klebsiella pneumoniae*. Future Microbiology 8, 1147–1161, 2013.

McCuddin, Z.P., Carlson, S.A., Rasmussen, M.A., Franklin, S.K., 2006. *Klebsiella* to salmonella gene transfer within rumen protozoa: implications for antibiotic resistance and rumen defaunation. Veterinary Microbiology 114 (3), 275–284.

Michalopoulos, A., Virtzili, S., Rafailidis, P., Chalevelakis, G., Damala, M., Falagas, M.E., 2010. Intravenous fosfomycin for the treatment of nosocomial infections caused by carbapenem-resistant *Klebsiella pneumoniae* in critically ill patients : a prospective evaluation. Clinical Microbiology and Infections 16, 184–186.

Millares, L., Perez-Brocal, V., Ferrari, R., Gallego, M., Pomares, X., Garcia-Nunez, M., Monton, C., Capilla, S., Monso, E., Moya, A., 2015. Functional metagenomics of the bronchial microbiome in COPD. PLoS One 10, e0144448.

Mobarak-Qamsari, M., Ashayeri-Panah, M., Eftekhar, F., Feizabadi, M.M., 2013. Integron mediated multidrug resistance in extended spectrum beta-lactamase producing clinical isolates of *Klebsiella pneumoniae*. Brazilian Journal of Microbiology 44 (3), 849–854.

Mollenkopf, D.F., Mirecki, J.M., Daniels, J.B., Funk, J.A., Henry, S.C., Hansen, G.E., Davies, P.R., Donovan, T.S., Wittum, T.E., 2013. *Escherichia coli* and *Klebsiella pneumoniae* producing CTX-M cephalosporinase from swine finishing barns and their association with antimicrobial use. Applied and Environmental Microbiology 79 (3), 1052–1054.

Moore, R., O'Shea, D., Geoghegan, T., Mallon, P.W.G., Sheehan, G., 2013. Community-acquired *Klebsiella pneumoniae* liver abscess: an emerginginfectionin Ireland and Europe. Infection 41, 681–686.

Morii, K., Kashihara, A., Miura, S., Okuhin, H., Watanabe, T., Sato, S., Uesaka, K., Yuasa, S., 2012. Successful hepatectomy for intraperitoneal rupture of pyogenic liver abscess caused by *Klebsiella pneumoniae*. Clinical journal of gastroenterology 5 (2), 136–140.

Naparstek, L., Carmeli, Y., Chmelnitsky, I., Banin, E., Navon-Venezia, S., 2012. Reduced susceptibility to chlorhexidine among extremely drug-resistant strains of *Klebsiella pneumoniae*. Journal of Hospital Infection 81, 1–5.

Neonakis, I.K., Stylianou, K., Daphnis, E., Maraki, S., 2011. First case of resistance to tigecycline by *Klebsiella pneumoniae* in a European University hospital. Indian Journal of Medical Microbiology 29, 78–79.

Netikul, T., Sidjabat, H.E., Paterson, D.L., Kamolvit, W., Tantisiriwat, W., Steen, J.A., Kiratisin, P., 2014. Characterization of an IncN2-type bla NDM-1-carrying plasmid in *Escherichia coli* ST131 and *Klebsiella pneumoniae* ST11 and ST15 isolates in Thailand. Journal of Antimicrobial Chemotherapy 69 (11), 3161–3163.

Nordmann, P., Cuzon, G., Naas, T., 2009. The real threat of *Klebsiella pneumoniae* carbapenemase-producing bacteria. The Lancet Infectious Diseases 9, 228–236.

Nüesch-Inderbinen, M.T., Abgottspon, H., Zurfluh, K., Nüesch, H.J., Stephan, R., Hächler, H., 2013. Cross-sectional study on fecal carriage of *Enterobacteriaceae* with resistance to extended-spectrum cephalosporins in primary care patients. Microbial Drug Resistance 19, 362–369.

Palepou, M.F., Woodford, N., Hope, R., Colman, M., Glover, J., Kaufmann, M., Lafong, C., Reynolds, R., Livermore, D.M., 2005. Novel class A carbapenemase, KPC-4, in an *Enterobacter* isolate from Scotland. In: 15th Eur. Cong. Clin. Microbiol. Infect. Dis., Copenhagen, Denmark.

Park, K.S., Kim, M.H., Park, T.S., Nam, Y.S., Lee, H.J., Suh, J.T., 2012. Prevalence of the plasmid-mediated quinolone resistance genes, *aac(6=)-Ib-cr*, *qepA*, and *oqxAB* in clinical isolates of extended-spectrum beta-lactamase (ESBL)-producing *Escherichia coli* and *Klebsiella pneumoniae* in Korea. Annals of Clinical Laboratory Science 42, 191–197.

Partridge, S.R., Ginn, A.N., Wiklendt, A.M., Ellem, J., Wong, J.S., Ingram, P., Guy, S., Garner, S., Iredell, J.R., 2015. Emergence of bla KPC carbapeneme genes in Australia. International Journal of Antimicrobial Agents 45 (2), 130–136.

Pena, I., Picazo, J.J., Rodríguez-Avial, C., Rodríguez-Avial, I., 2014. Carbapenemase-producing *Enterobacteriaceae* in a tertiary hospital in Madrid, Spain: high percentage of colistin resistance among VIM-1-producing *Klebsiella pneumoniae* ST11 isolates. International Journal of Antimicrobial Agents 43, 460–464.

Perez, F., Rudin, S.D., Marshall, S.H., Coakley, P., Chen, L., Kreiswirth, B.N., Rather, P.N., Hujer, A.M., Toltzis, P., Van Duin, D., Paterson, D.L., 2013. OqxAB, a quinolone and olaquindox efflux pump, is widely distributed among multidrug-resistant *Klebsiella pneumoniae* isolates of human origin. Antimicrobial Agents and Chemotherapy 57 (9), 4602–4603.

Pfeifer, Y., Schlatterer, K., Engelmann, E., et al., 2012. Emergence of OXA-48-type carbapenemase-producing *Enterobacteriaceae* in German hospitals. Antimicrobial Agents and Chemotherapy 56, 2125–2128.

Podschun, R., Ullmann, U., 1998. Klebsiella spp. as nosocomial pathogens: epidemiology, taxonomy, typing methods, and pathogenicity factors. Clinical Microbiology Reviews 11, 589–603.

Poirel, L., Potron, A., Nordmann, P., 2012. OXA-48-like carbapenemases: the phantom menace. Journal of Antimicrobial Chemotherapy 67, 1597–1606.

Poirel, L., Nordmann, P., Ducroz, S., Boulouis, H.J., Arné, P., Millemann, Y., 2013. Extended-spectrum β-lactamase CTX-M-15-producing *Klebsiella pneumoniae* of sequence type ST274 in companion animals. Antimicrobial Agents and Chemotherapy 57 (5), 2372–2375.

Potron, A., Kalpoe, J., Poirel, L., Nordmann, P., 2011. European dissemination of a single OXA-48-producing *Klebsiella pneumoniae* clone. Clinical Microbiology and Infections 17, E24–E26.

Ramos, P.I.P., Picão, R.C., Almeida, LGP de, Lima, N.C.B., Girardello, R., Vivan, A.C.P., Xavier, D.E., Barcellos, F.G., Pelisson, M., Vespero, E.C., Médigue, C., Vasconcelos, ATR De, Gales, A.C., Nicolás, M.F., 2014. Comparative analysis of the complete genome of KPC-2-producing *Klebsiella pneumoniae* Kp13 reveals remarkable genome plasticity and a wide repertoire of virulence and resistance mechanisms. BMC Genomics 15, 54.

Roberts, D.E., McClain, H.M., Hansen, D.S., Currin, P., Howerth, E.W., 2000. An outbreak of *Klebsiella pneumoniae* infection in dogs with severe enteritis and septicemia. Journal of Veterinary Diagnostic Investigation 12, 168–173.

Rodriguez-Martinez, J.M., Diaz de Alba, P., Briales, A., Machuca, J., Lossa, M., Fernandez-Cuenca, F., Rodriguez Bano, J., Martinez-Martinez, L., Pascual, A., 2013. Contribution of OqxAB efflux pumps to quinolone resistance in extended-spectrum-beta-lactamase-producing *Klebsiella pneumoniae*. Journal of Antimicrobial Chemotherapy 68, 68–73.

Rodriguez-Villalobos, H., Malaviolle, V., Frankard, J., de Mendonça, R., Nonhoff, C., Struelens, M.J., 2006. In vitro activity of temocillin against extended spectrum β-lactamase-producing *Escherichia coli*. Journal of Antimicrobial Chemotherapy 57, 771–774.

Saidel-Odes, L., Borer, A., 2013. Limiting and controlling carbapenem resistant *Klebsiella pneumoniae*. Infection and Drug Resistance 7, 9–14.

Saishu, N., Ozaki, H., Murase, T., 2014. CTX-M-type extended-spectrum β-lactamase-producing *Klebsiella pneumoniae* isolated from cases of bovine mastitis in Japan. Journal of Veterinary Medical Science 76, 1153–1156.

Samanta, I., 2013. Klebsiella. In: Veterinary Bacteriology, first ed. New India Publishing Agency, New Delhi, India.

Sarno, R., McGillivary, G., Sherratt, D.J., Actis, L.A., Tolmasky, M.E., 2002. Complete nucleotide sequence of *Klebsiella pneumoniae* multiresistance plasmid pJHCMW1. Antimicrobial Agents and Chemotherapy 46, 3422–3427.

Sato, N., Kawamura, K., Nakane, K., Wachino, J., Arakawa, Y., 2013. First detection of fosfomycin resistance gene *fosA3* in CTX-M-producing *Escherichia coli* isolates from healthy individuals in Japan. Microbial Drug Resistance 19, 477–482.

Shen, P., Jiang, Y., Zhou, Z., Zhang, J., Yu, Y., Li, L., 2008. Complete nucleotide sequence of pKP96, a 67,850 bp multi resistance plasmid encoding qnrA1, aac(6′)-Ib-cr and blaCTX-M-24 from *Klebsiella pneumoniae*. Journal of Antimicrobial Chemotherapy 62, 1252−1256.

Sirot, D., Sirot, J., Labia, R., Morand, A., Courvalin, P., Darfeuille-Michaud, A., Perroux, R., Cluzel, R., 1987. Transferable resistance to third-generation cephalosporins in clinical isolates of Klebsiella pneumoniae: identification of CTX-1, a novel β-lactamase. Journal of Antimicrobial Chemotherapy 20 (3), 323−334.

Smith, M.G., 1975. In vivo transfer of R factors between *Escherichia coli* strains inoculated into the rumen of sheep. Journal of Hygiene 75, 363−370.

Snitkin, E.S., Zelazny, A.M., Thomas, P.J., Stock, F., NISC Comparative Sequencing Program Group, Henderson, D.K., Palmore, T.N., Segre, J.A., 2012. Tracking a hospital outbreak of carbapenem-resistant *Klebsiella pneumoniae* with whole-genome sequencing. Science Translational Medicine 4, 148ra116.

Stolle, I., Prenger-Berninghoff, E., Stamm, I., Scheufen, S., Hassdenteufel, E., Guenther, S., Bethe, A., Pfeifer, Y., Ewers, C., 2013. Emergence of OXA-48 carbapenemase-producing *Escherichia coli* and *Klebsiella pneumoniae* in dogs. Journal of Antimicrobial Chemotherapy 68 (12), 2802−2808.

Taitt, C.R., Leski, T.A., Erwin, D.P., Odundo, E.A., Kipkemoi, N.C., Ndonye, J.N., Kirera, R.K., Ombogo, A.N., Walson, J.L., Pavlinac, P.B., Hulseberg, C., 2017. Antimicrobial resistance of *Klebsiella pneumoniae* stool isolates circulating in Kenya. PLoS One 12 (6), e0178880.

Tatsuta, T., Wada, T., Chinda, D., Tsushima, K., Sasaki, Y., Shimoyama, T., Fukuda, S., 2011. A case of gas-forming liver abscess with diabetes mellitus. Internal Medicine 50 (20), 2329−2332.

Timofte, D., Maciuca, I.E., Evans, N.J., Williams, H., Wattret, A., Fick, J.C., Williams, N.J., 2014. Detection and molecular characterization of *Escherichia coli* CTX-M-15 and *Klebsiella pneumoniae* SHV-12 producing β-lactamases isolated from cases of bovine mastitis in the United Kingdom. Antimicrobial Agents and Chemotherapy 58, 789−794.

Titelman, E., Iversen, A., Kahlmeter, G., Giske, C.G., 2011. Antimicrobial susceptibility to parenteral and oral agents in a largely polyclonal collection of CTX-M-14 and CTX-M-15-producing *Escherichia coli* and *Klebsiella pneumoniae*. Acta Pathologica, Microbiologica et Immunologica Scandinavica 119, 853−863.

Turton, J.F., Perry, C., Elgohari, S., Hampton, C.V., 2010. PCR characterization and typing of *Klebsiella pneumoniae* using capsular type-specific, variable number tandem repeat and virulence gene targets. Journal of Medical Microbiology 59 (5), 541−547.

Trautmann, M., Ghandchi, A., Held, T., Cryz, S.J., Cross, A.S., 1991. An enzyme-linked immunosorbent assay for the detection of soluble *Klebsiella pneumoniae* capsular polysaccharide. Journal of Microbiological Methods 13 (4), 305−313.

Tzouvelekis, L.S., Markogiannakis, A., Psichogiou, M., Tassios, P.T., Daikos, G.L., 2012. Carbapenemases in *Klebsiella pneumoniae* and other *Enterobacteriaceae*: an evolving crisis of global dimensions. Clinical Microbiology Reviews 25, 682−707.

Veleba, M., Schneiders, T., 2012. Tigecycline resistance can occur independently of the ramA gene in *Klebsiella pneumoniae*. Antimicrobial Agents and Chemotherapy 56, 4466−4467.

Viau, R., Frank, K.M., Jacobs, M.R., Wilson, B., Kaye, K., Donskey, C.J., Perez, F., Endimiani, A., Bonomo, R.A., 2016. Intestinal carriage of carbapenemase-producing organisms: current status of surveillance methods. Clinical Microbiology Reviews 29, 1−27.

Vo, A.T., Van Duijkeren, E., Fluit, A.C., Gaastra, W., 2007. Characteristics of extended-spectrum cephalosporin-resistant *Escherichia coli* and *Klebsiella pneumoniae* isolates from horses. Veterinary Microbiology 124 (3), 248−255.

Wachino, J., Yamane, K., Suzuki, S., Kimura, K., Arakawa, Y., 2010. Prevalence of fosfomycin resistance among CTX-M-producing *Escherichia coli* clinical isolates in Japan and identification of novel plasmid-mediated fosfomycin-modifying enzymes. Antimicrobial Agents and Chemotherapy 54, 3061−3064.

Walsh, T.R., Toleman, M.A., Poirel, L., Nordmann, P., 2005. Metallo-beta lactamases: the quiet before the storm? Clinical Microbiology Reviews 18, 306−325.

Walsh, T.R., Weeks, J., Livermore, D.M., Toleman, M.A., 2011. Dissemination of NDM-1 positive bacteria in the New Delhi environment and its implications for human health: an environmental point prevalence study. The Lancet Infectious Diseases 11, 355−362.

Wang, Q., Li, B., Tsang, A.K.L., Yi, Y., Woo, P.C.Y., Liu, C.H., 2013. Genotypic analysis of *Klebsiella pneumoniae* isolates in a Beijing Hospital reveals high genetic diversity and clonal population structure of drug-resistant isolates. PLoS One 8, e57091.

Wohlwend, N., Endimiani, A., Francey, T., Perreten, V., 2015. Third generation-cephalosporin-resistant *Klebsiella pneumoniae* isolates from humans and companion animals in Switzerland: spread of a DHA-producing ST11 clone in the veterinary setting. Antimicrobial Agents and Chemotherapy 59 (5), 2949−2955. AAC-04408.

Wolter, D.J., Kurpiel, P.M., Woodford, N., Palepou, M.F.I., Goering, R.V., Hanson, N.D., 2009. Phenotypic and enzymatic comparative analysis of the novel KPC variant KPC-5 and its evolutionary variants, KPC-2 and KPC-4. Antimicrobial Agents and Chemotherapy 53 (2), 557−562.

Woodford, N., Tierno Jr., P.M., Young, K., Tysall, L., Palepou, M.F., Ward, E., Painter, R.E., Suber, D.F., Shungu, D., Silver, L.L., Inglima, K., Kornblum, J., Livermore, D.M., 2004. Outbreak of *Klebsiella pneumoniae* producing a new carbapenem-hydrolyzing class A beta-lactamase, KPC-3, in a New York Medical Center. Antimicrobial Agents and Chemotherapy 48, 4793−4799.

Wright, M.S., Suzuki, Y., Jones, M.B., Marshall, S.H., Rudin, S.D., van Duin, D., Kaye, K., Jacobs, M.R., Bonomo, R.A., Adams, M.D., 2015. Genomic and transcriptomic analyses of colistin-resistant clinical isolates of *Klebsiella pneumoniae* reveal multiple pathways of resistance. Antimicrobial Agents and Chemotherapy 59, 536−543.

Xiang, D.R., Li, J.J., Sheng, Z.K., Yu, H.Y., Deng, M., Bi, S., Hu, F.S., Chen, W., Xue, X.W., Zhou, Z.B., Doi, Y., 2016. Complete sequence of a novel IncR-F33: a−: B−plasmid, pKP1034, harboring fosA3, blaKPC-2, blaCTX-M-65, blaSHV-12, and rmtB from an epidemic *Klebsiella pneumoniae* sequence type 11 strain in China. Antimicrobial Agents and Chemotherapy 60 (3), 1343−1348.

Yan, J.J., Wu, J.J., Ko, W.C., Tsai, S.H., Chuang, C.L., Wu, H.M., Lu, Y.J., Li, J.D., 2004. Plasmid-mediated 16S rRNA methylases conferring high-level aminoglycoside resistance in *Escherichia coli* and *Klebsiella pneumoniae* isolates from two Taiwanese hospitals. Journal of Antimicrobial Chemotherapy 54 (6), 1007−1012.

Yao, F., Quian, Y., Chen, S., Wang, P., Huang, Y., 2007. Incidence of extended spectrum β -lactamases and characterization of integrons in extended spectrum β-lactamase producing *Klebsiella pneumoniae* isolated in Shantou, China. Acta Biochimica et Biophysica Sinica 39, 527−532.

Yigit, H., Queenan, A.M., Anderson, G.J., Domenech-Sanchez, A., Biddle, J.W., Steward, C.D., Alberti, S., Bush, K., Tenover, F.C., 2001. Novel carbapenem hydrolyzing beta-lactamase, KPC-1, from a carbapenem resistant strain of *Klebsiella pneumoniae*. Antimicrobial Agents and Chemotherapy 45, 1151−1161.

Yong, D., Toleman, M.A., Giske, C.G., Cho, H.S., Sundman, K., Lee, K., Walsh, T.R., 2009. Characterization of a new metallo-beta-lactamase gene, bla(NDM-1), and a novel erythromycin esterase gene carried on a unique genetic structure in *Klebsiella pneumoniae* sequence type 14 from India. Antimicrobial Agents and Chemotherapy 53, 5046−5054.

Yuan, J., Xu, X., Guo, Q., Zhao, X., Ye, X., Guo, Y., Wang, M., 2012. Prevalence of the oqxAB gene complex in *Klebsiella pneumoniae* and *Escherichia coli* clinical isolates. Journal of Antimicrobial Chemotherapy 67, 1655−1659.

Zurfluh, K., Nüesch-Inderbinen, M., Stephan, R., Hächler, H., 2013a. Higher-generation cephalosporin-resistant *Escherichia coli* in feral birds in Switzerland. International Journal of Antimicrobial Agents 41, 296−297.

Zurfluh, K., Hächler, H., Nüesch-Inderbinen, M., Stephan, R., 2013b. Characteristics of extended-spectrum β-lactamase- and carbapenemase-producing *Enterobacteriaceae* isolates from rivers and lakes in Switzerland. Applied and Environmental Microbiology 79, 3021−3026.

Zurfluh, K., Glier, M., Hächler, H., Stephan, R., 2015. Replicon typing of plasmids carrying *bla*_{CTX-M-15} among *Enterobacteriaceae* isolated at the environment, livestock and human interface. The Science of the Total Environment 521−522, 75−78.

Chapter 15

Escherichia coli

Chapter outline

Theodor Escherich (1885) first isolated *Escherichia coli* from the faeces of human infants (Shulman et al., 2007). *E. coli* is considered as a complex bacterial species consisting of both commensal and pathogenic strains. Pathogenic *E. coli* are associated with traveller's diarrhoea, bacillary dysentery, haemolytic uraemic syndrome (HUS), haemorrhagic colitis, thrombocytopenic purpura, urinary tract infections (UTIs) in human and edema disease (pigs), colisepticaemia and haemorrhagic colitis (calves), postweaning diarrhoea (pigs), coliform mastitis (cattle), cystitis and pyometra (dogs) and avian colibacillosis (poultry) in livestock and birds.

Evolution of antimicrobial-resistant *E. coli* or other bacteria is dependent on several factors such as contaminated environment, congested and unhygienic living conditions, poor quality of drinking water, rearing of livestock and poultry with indiscriminate use of antibiotics, consumption of antibiotics without medical supervision, lack of proper drug control and monitoring system and, moreover, lack of financial resources and political support to solve the issue precisely. Extended-spectrum β-lactamase (ESBL)−producing and ampC-β-lactamase-producing *E. coli* is considered as major resistant bugs since its global emergence during 1990 (Pitout and Laupland, 2008).

Properties

Morphology: *E. coli* are Gram-negative, short rods, 0.5 μm × 1−3 μm varying from coccoid shape to long filamentous forms. They occur singly, in pair or in short chain. They are nonspore forming and mostly motile by peritrichous flagella. However, the motility may not be observed in some strains because of absence of flagella. The strains adopted outside the intestine are encapsulated producing mucoid type of colonies in the solid media. The capsules are polysaccharide in nature and important virulence determinants, which enable the pathogenic bacteria to evade or counteract the unspecific host defense during the early phase of the infection.

Classification: The genus *Escherichia* is classified under the family *Enterobacteriaceae* that belongs to the order *Enterobacteriales*. There are total six species under the genus *Escherichia*, namely, *E. coli, E. albertii, E. blattae, E. fergusonii, E. hermannii* and *E. vulneris*. Recently, *Escherichia marmotae* sp. *nov.* was proposed isolated from faecal samples of Himalayan marmot (*Marmota himalayana*) in China (Liu et al., 2015). Pathogenic strains of *E. coli* are broadly classified into intestinal (Shiga toxin–producing *E. coli* (STEC), ETEC, EHEC, EPEC, EIEC, enteroaggregative *E. coli* (EAEC), avian pathogenic *E. coli* (APEC)) and extraintestinal pathotypes (UPEC, mastitic *E. coli*, septicaemic *E. coli*) (Table 15.1). Moreover, the *E. coli* strains are further assigned under four phylogenetic groups designated as A, B1, B2 and D (Escobar-Páramo et al., 2004). Distribution of virulence genes, ecological niches and types of *E. coli* infection varies according to the phylogenetic groups. Extraintestinal pathotypes of *E. coli* mostly belonged to group B2 (except some

TABLE 15.1 Major toxins and virulence factors produced by different *Escherichia coli* pathotypes.

E. coli pathotype	Toxins produced	Virulence factors possessed

Avian pathogenic *E. coli* (APEC)	(a) Heat-labile enterotoxin (LT)
	(b) Homolog of the heat-stable enterotoxin
	(c) Enterohaemolysin
	(d) Cytotoxic necrotising factor 1 (CNF 1)
	(e) Cytolethal distending toxin
	(f) Cytotoxin designated as VT2y
	(g) Vacuolating autotransporter toxin (encoded by VAT-PAI pathogenicity island)
		(A) Fimbriae:
		    (i) Mannose-binding type I fimbriae (F1)
		    (ii) Pap/Prs fimbriae
		    (iii) Avian *E. coli* 1 (AC/1) fimbriae
		    (iv) type IV pili
		(B) Adhesins:
		    (i) afa-8 gene cluster
		    (ii) Curli (coiled surface structure)
		    (iii) Temperature-sensitive haemagglutinin (Tsh)
		(C) Invasin:
		    (i) ibeA gene cluster
		    (ii) Homologue of the 25 kDa 'Tia' protein
		(D) Iron acquisition systems:
		    (i) Aerobactin system
		    (ii) Salmochelin siderophore system (encoded by the *iro*BCDEN locus).
		    (iii) *sit*ABC iron transport systems
		    (iv) Putative iron transport system novel to APEC (*eit*)
		(E) Outer membrane proteins encoded by *traT* and *iss* genes present in ColV plasmid

Shiga toxin–producing *E. coli* (STEC)	(a) Shiga toxins (stx_1 and stx_2); these toxins are encoded by stx_1 and stx_2 genes (b) Enterohaemolysin (encoded by *hlyA*)	(a) Non-LEE-encoded effectors (Nles): 32 molecules are distributed among 20 families encoded by prophages. Examples are NleA, NleB, NleC, NleD, NleE, NleF and NleG. (b) F18 fimbriae
Enterotoxigenic *E. coli* (ETEC)	(a) Heat-labile enterotoxin (LT) (b) Heat-stable enterotoxin (ST)	(a) K99/F5 fimbriae (b) 987P/F6 fimbriae (c) K88/F4 fimbriae (d) F18 fimbriae
Enteroinvasive *E. coli* (EIEC)		Inv plasmid
Enteropathogenic *E. coli* (EPEC)		'Intimin' encoded by *eae* gene present in the locus for enterocyte effacement (LEE)
Enterohaemorrhagic *E. coli* (EHEC)	Shiga toxins like STEC	'Intimin' encoded by *eae* gene present in the locus for enterocyte effacement (LEE)
Enteroaggregative *E. coli* (EAEC)	Heat-stable toxin-1 (EAST-1) (encoded by high molecular weight virulence plasmid)	Aggregative adherence Fimbriae I and II (AAF/I and AAF/II)
	Plasmid-encoded toxin (Pet) (encoded by high molecular weight virulence plasmid)	

Continued

TABLE 15.1 Major toxins and virulence factors produced by different *Escherichia coli* pathotypes.—cont'd

E. coli pathotype	Toxins produced	Virulence factors possessed
Diffusely adherent *E. coli* (DAEC)		Afa/Dr adhesins (produced by Afa/Dr DAEC)
		Adhesin involved in diffuse adherence (AIDA-I). It is produced along with EspA, EspB and EspD protein homologues.

Uropathogenic *E. coli* (UPEC) [O1, O2, O4, O6,O7, O8, O16, O18, O25 and O75]	α-Haemolysin	**(A)** Fimbriae:
		  (i) Type I (encoded by *fim*)
		  (ii) P (*Pap*)
		  (iii) S (*sfa*)
		  (iv) F1C (*foc*)

	Vacuolating autotransporter toxin (VAT)/Secreated auto transporter toxin (SAT)	**(B)** Iron acquisition system:
		  (i) Enterobactin siderophore (*ent*)
		  (ii) Salmochelin siderophore (*chu*) (hemin uptake system) (*iro*)
		  (iii) Iron/manganese transport (*Sit*)
		  (iv) Aerobactin siderophore (*iutA*)
		  (v) Yersiniabactin siderophore (*fyuA*)

	CNF 1	—
Mastitic *E. coli*	Endotoxin (LPS)	Capsule, serum resistance
Septicaemic *E. coli* (O1, O2, O78:K80)	Endotoxin (LPS)	Serum resistance
		Iron acquisition system
Necrotoxigenic *E. coli* (NTEC)	CNF1, CNF2	

strains of diffusely adherent *E. coli* and enteropathogenic *E. coli*) and D (Picard et al., 1999). The phylogenetic group B2 is further subdivided into nine subgroups (Le Gall et al., 2007).

The clonal lineage ST131 (sequence type 131 belonged to B2-ST complex) is considered as a predominant extraintestinal pathotype throughout the world, which was originated during 2003. The lineage ST131 is associated with UTIs such as cystitis and pyelonephritis, bacteremia, meningitis, osteoarticular infection, myositis, orchitis and septic shock in human patients. Virulence genes such as *malX* (pathogenicity island marker), *iha* (adhesion siderophore receptor), *kpsM*II (group 2 capsule synthesis), *usp* (uropathogen-specific protein), *sat* (secreted autotransporter toxin), *fimH* (type 1 fimbriae), *fyuA* (yersiniabactin receptor), *ompT* (outer membrane receptor), *iucD* (aerobactin), *iutA* (aerobactin receptor) and *tratT* (serum resistance associated) are commonly observed in ST131 strains (Nicolas-Chanoine et al., 2014). Resistance to higher generation cephalosporins (associated with CTX-M-15) and fluoroquinolones is observed in ST131 strains (Coque et al., 2008). Plasmids belonged to different incompatibility groups, especially IncF, were isolated and characterized from ST131 strains.

Another clinically 'successful' phylogenetic lineage is STC95 which also belonged to B2-ST complex. STC95 mostly causes septicaemia in poultry and human (Ewers et al., 2007). The pandemicity of STC95 is not well-established like ST131 strains.

Susceptibility to disinfectants: *E. coli* survive for months in dust, water, faeces of animals and poultry houses. They are susceptible to drying and common disinfectants such as phenol, cresol, etc.

Natural habitat: Intestine of all vertebrates including human is the most common natural habitat of *E. coli*. The sterile intestine after birth is gradually inhabited by the bacteria from mother/dam or the environment. Throughout the life, it remains as major flora of the gastrointestinal tract. They are excreted through the faeces of animal and human and act as a major contaminant of the environment.

Genome

E. coli has a larger genome of 4.6 Mb in size containing approximately 4288 genes. Several DNA binding proteins (HU, H1) are found in their genome like eukaryotes. The HU protein condenses DNA and helps in its replication. Apart from genomic DNA, *E. coli* also has a variety of plasmids associated with virulence (incompatibility family type Inc) encoding antimicrobial resistance, toxins, adhesins, colonization factors, etc. The linkage between antimicrobial resistance and virulence genes in *E. coli* is not always established. In a study with cefotaxime-susceptible and cefotaxime-resistant *E. coli* isolates from poultry, no major virulence genes such as *stx*s, *eae*, *ehxA*, *cdt*, heat-stable enterotoxin (ST) and heat-labile enterotoxin (LT) were detected. Few minor virulence genes detected in the *E. coli* isolates did not correlate with antimicrobial resistance (Baron et al., 2016).

IncF plasmids (50—200 bp) are not only self-replicating but also they can encode addiction system to control their copy number and inheritance during cell division. These types of plasmids can carry resistance determinants against all major classes of antimicrobials such as β-lactams, aminoglycosides, tetracyclines, chloramphenicol and quinolones (Liu et al., 2013). Several replicon types of IncF plasmids exist, and among them, IncFII plasmids were considered as a complex one with combinations of the replicons FIA, FIB and FII (Marcade et al., 2009). Association of IncFII plasmids possessing different resistance genes ($bla_{CTX-M-15}$, bla_{TEM-1}, bla_{OXA}, aminoglycoside or fluoroquinolone resistance) with *E. coli* epidemic clone (ST 131) was reported (Coque et al., 2008). Other large plasmids detected in *E. coli* ST 131 clones carrying virulence genes (*iss*, *eitA/eitB*, *cvaB/cvaC*, *ompT*, *hlyF*) generally do not possess resistance determinants such as β-lactamase genes (Ewers et al., 2010).

IncX plasmids are another group of self-transmissible plasmid which can encode several resistance determinants including ESBL and carbapenemase. The IncX plasmid has five subtypes designated as IncX1 to IncX5 (Lo et al., 2014). Recently, IncX4 plasmids carrying colistin resistance genes were detected in *E. coli* isolated from livestock, food and human in different geographical locations (Li et al., 2016). Similarity in nucleotide sequences of all IncX4 plasmids carrying colistin resistance genes isolated from different locations suggests their role in transmission of colistin resistance throughout the world (Fernandes et al., 2016).

Antigenic characteristics

E. coli can be classified into several serotypes on the basis of three major antigens, i.e., somatic (O-antigen), capsular (K-antigen) and flagellar (H-antigen). Approximately, 173 O, 80 K and 56 H antigens have been identified and numbered accordingly. Antigenically distinct groups can be formed by each of the antigen (O, H, K), known as 'serogroup' (e.g., O-serogroup), whereas an antigenically distinct entity formed by all the major antigens is known as 'serotype', e.g., O140: K 56:H7.

O-antigen is the extracellular whisker-like part of the Gram-negative bacterial lipopolysaccharide (LPS). It is polysaccharide in nature and heat-stable (destroyed at >100°C). The sequence variability in the repeat structure of the O-antigen is the basis of the O-serogroup formation. K-antigen is heat-labile capsular polysaccharide produced by some *E. coli* strains. Presence of K-antigen hinders the O-antigen agglutination with its homologous serum. In some cases, capsules are poorly immunogenic in vivo because of the structural relationship with host cellular polysaccharides. The strains with such capsules (K1, K5) are highly virulent. H-antigens are flagellar antigens present in motile *E. coli*. It is protein in nature. It acts as virulence marker for some strains. For example, *E. coli* O157: *H7* is a virulent strain causing HUS in human. Another pathogenic strain (ST 131) mostly belongs to O25: *H4* serotype, although nontypeable or O16: *H5* serotype have also documented in Asia (Japan, Pakistan), Australia and Europe (Denmark) (Nicolas-Chanoine et al., 2014).

In addition to these major antigens, the strains of *E. coli* also possess fimbrial antigen like other members of *Enterobacteriaceae* family. It helps in adhesion of bacteria with the host cells (K88/F4 and K99/F5). These antigens are not type or group-specific.

Many members of the *Enterobacteriaceae* family including *E. coli* O14, O56, O124, O144 and *Salmonella*, *Shigella* share a common heat-stable antigen known as 'enterobacterial common antigen (ECA)' or 'Kunin antigen'. The family specificity of ECA can be used for taxonomic and diagnostic purposes. ECA is located in the outer leaflet of the outer membrane. It is a glycophospholipid built up by an amino sugar heteropolymer linked to an L-glycerophosphatidyl residue. The genetical determination of ECA is closely related to that of LPS. For biosynthesis of ECA and LPS, partly the same sugar precursors and the same carrier lipid is used.

Toxins and virulence factors produced

(a) Enterotoxins: Two classes of enterotoxins are produced by *E. coli*. They are heat-labile enterotoxin (LT) and heat-stable enterotoxin (ST). Both of them are responsible for diarrhoea production in different ways.

Heat-labile enterotoxin (LT): It is a large protein molecule (88 KDa) having structural similarity with cholera toxin. Each molecule of toxin has one 'A' and 5 'B' subunits. This 'B' subunit helps in adherence of the toxin with enterocytes having ganglioside (GM1) receptors or intestinal brush borders having glycoprotein receptors. The active site of 'A' subunit (A_1), after adherence with the host cell, activates adenylate cyclase system located near the basal membrane region of the cell. This system converts adenosine triphosphate into cyclic adenosine monophosphate (cAMP) by the enzyme adenylate cyclase. A_1 toxin is adenosine diphosphate ribosyltransferase that causes ADP ribosylation of the regulatory protein of this adenylate cyclase system. The system is active when it is complexed with guanosine triphosphate (GTP) and regulatory protein. It becomes inactive when the GTP is converted into guanosine diphosphate by GTPase. Ribosylation of regulatory protein inhibits this GTPase. So, the system remains in permanently active form. Activation of this system results in elevated level of cAMP. In turn, it increases the efflux of the ions (Na^+ and Cl^-) which enhances the osmotic pressure of the intestinal lumen. This enhanced osmotic pressure removes more amount of water from intestinal cells into the lumen. It results in increased volume of the contents causing diarrhoea.

Heat-stable enterotoxin (ST): These are heat-stable low molecular weight toxins having two major types STa (STI) and STb (STII).

STa (STI): The toxin is resistant to acidic pH and protease enzyme. The receptor of the toxin is glycoprotein in nature and is present in the enterocytes. Receptors in younger and weaned pigs are more active in toxin binding than adults and unweaned pigs. The toxin activates guanylate cyclase in the intestinal cells. The guanylate cyclase itself can act as receptor also. This enzyme enhances the cGMP activity and produces diacylglycerol, inositol 1,4,5-triphosphate and C-kinase from phosphatidylinositol present in the intestinal villi border. These three products are responsible for Ca^{++} mobilization from intracellular compartments into the villi and this Ca^{++} impairs the absorption of Na^+ and Cl^- from the villi as well as stimulates the secretion of Cl^- from crypts. Thus the toxin acts as antiabsorptive and more amount of fluid is accumulated into the intestinal lumen causing diarrhoea.

STb (ST II): The gene encoding this toxin resides in the plasmid. It stimulates the production of prostaglandin (PGE2) in the intestinal mucosal cells causing diarrhoea.

(b) Verotoxin/Shiga-like toxin/Shiga toxin: It is a heat-labile toxin and protein in nature. It produces cytopathic effect in Vero cell culture, so previously it was known as verotoxin. It has structural and functional similarity with the toxin produced by *Shigella dysenteriae*. So, it is designated as 'Shiga-like toxin' or 'Shiga toxin'. Strains of *E. coli* producing this toxin are known as STEC. Like LT, it is a heterohexamer, in which one 'A' subunit (32 kDa) is noncovalently associated with a pentamer of 'B' subunits (7.7 kDa each) (A1B5). The 'B' subunit helps in adherence of the toxin with the cell membrane ceramide receptor. Activated A_1 enters the cell and acts as N-glycosidase on 28S rRNA. It prevents the binding of amino acyl t-RNA with the ribosome and thus protein synthesis of the cell is hampered. These toxins are subdivided into two major groups, Shiga toxin 1 (stx1) and Shiga toxin 2 (stx2). Stx1 is a rather homologous group in which three variants (stx1, stx1c and stx1d) have been described. The stx2 group is more heterogeneous and is comprised of several subtypes (stx2, stx2c, stx2d, stx2e, stx2f, stx2g and activatable stx2d).

(c) Haemolysin: Mainly three types of haemolysins are produced by different strains of *E. coli*: α-haemolysin, enterohaemolysin and contact haemolysin.

(d) Cytolethal distending toxin (CDT): CDT is a bacterial toxin produced by some strains of *E. coli* and other bacteria such as *Salmonella, Shigella, Campylobacter*, etc. It causes eukaryotic cell cycle block at the G2 stage before mitosis. The functional toxin is composed of three proteins: CdtA, CdtB and CdtC. The CdtA and CdtC function as dimeric subunits, which help to deliver CdtB into the mammalian cell interior. The CdtB enters the nucleus and exhibits a DNase I-like activity that results in DNA double-strand breaks, cell cycle arrest, cellular distension and ultimately cell death.

(e) Cytotoxic necrotizing factor (CNF): The toxin has two types, i.e., CNF1 and CNF2 (previously known as 'Vir' toxin). They are 115 and 110 KDa proteins, respectively, and immunologically related. Both of them cause multinucleation of cells in the culture and skin necrosis in rabbits.

Table 15.1 describes the toxins and virulence factors produced by different *E. coli* pathotypes.

Transmission

Ruminants (cattle, sheep, goat), other farm animals (pigs, horses, rabbits), companion animals (dogs, cats) and poultry act as major reservoir of *E. coli*. In an animal or poultry farm, *E. coli* is mainly transmitted through feed, drinking water, aerosols, fomites and carriers. The stress conditions such as transport, dietary change and extreme climate also help to establish the infection. The studies showed that the cattle fed with diets rich in energy but low in fiber content (grass silage or maize silage) excretes more STEC than others (Franz and van Bruggen, 2008). In piglets, the dietary change during weaning with increased protein and less fiber causes more multiplication of ETEC/STEC. Young animals or birds are more susceptible to the infection as their immune system is underdeveloped and some receptors for *E. coli* adhesins are only expressed in young animals. Neonatal infection of chicks can occur horizontally from the environment or vertically from the hen. A laying hen suffering with *E. coli*—induced oophoritis (inflammation of ovaries) or salpingitis (inflammation of oviducts) may infect the internal egg before shell formation (vertical transmission). Faecal contamination of the eggshell is possible during the passage of the egg through the cloaca and also after laying (horizontal transmission).

In human, *E. coli* pathotypes (e.g., STEC, enterohaemorrhagic *E. coli*) are considered as major foodborne pathogens. Raw or undercooked foods and food products (meat or milk-based), fruits and vegetables (spinach, hazelnuts, coleslaw, sprouts, Spanish onions, watercress, salad) and contaminated drinking water act as source of human infection (Alegbeleye et al., 2018). Other than food-originated infection, *E. coli* can also be transmitted into human through direct contact with infected animals (farmers, animal attendants, veterinarians, visitors of farms or animal fares), environment contaminated with infected manure, recreational water (swimming pool) and aquaculture (Petersen et al., 2002). Few reports documented high ESBL-producing *E. coli* colonization in human having direct contact with poultry (Dierikx et al., 2013) and companion animals (Meyer et al., 2012). However, influences of climate (flood, draught), stress, drinking water sources, housing, bedding choice and birthing pens are considered as datagaps in livestock sector acting as reservoir of resistant *E. coli* (Horigan et al., 2016). Our studies documented contaminated environment as a possible source of ESBL/β-lactamase-producing *E. coli* in backyard pigs and Kuroiler birds in India (Samanta et al., 2015; Ghosh et al., 2017).

Foodborne *E. coli* infection becomes more complicated with the transmission of antimicrobial-resistant *E. coli* (whole bacterium transmission) or transfer of antimicrobial resistance genes into gut commensal including *E. coli*. Horizontal transfer of antimicrobial resistance genes (plasmid or mobile genetic elements mediated) is possible in all kinds of food matrices with more probabilities in fermented, minimally processed (undercooked) or raw foods (Rossi et al., 2014). Transfer of ampicillin resistance genes from *Salmonella typhimurium* to *E. coli* was documented in certain food matrices such as milk and ground beef (Walsh et al., 2008). A United States—based study detected the occurrence of resistant *E. coli* in beef production chain with highest occurrence in hides followed by a decreasing order of contamination level along the production chain (Schmidt et al., 2015). Processing of meat during generation of meat-based products can reduce the contamination level of resistant bacterial population (Noyes et al., 2016). In comparison to porcine rectal swabs, occurrence of resistant *Enterobacteriaceae* was detected in significantly lower proportion in minced pork products originated from the same pigs (Sabia et al., 2017). Furthermore, proper cooking of meat, milk or eggs or their products reduces the possibility of transmission to the consumers, but not eliminating the risk, as the transmission may occur before cooking. Moreover, human intestine also acts as a suitable place for transfer or exchange of antimicrobial resistance genes between the same or different kinds of bacteria. In vitro transfer of ESBL genes was documented from donor to recipient *E. coli* (Smet et al., 2011). A whole genome—based study with cephalosporin-resistant *E. coli* isolates failed to reveal the evidence for direct transmission into human from chicken meat and pork. The authors suggested the role of plasmids in transmission (de Been et al., 2014). Whole bacterium transmission of expanded-spectrum cephalosporin-resistant *E. coli* from food items such as chicken meat was appropriately documented in the Netherlands, which used representative samples from different corners of the country and authentic molecular typing techniques (Overdevest et al., 2011; Kluytmans et al., 2012). Considerable proportion of ESBL-producing *E. coli* (up to 39%) isolated from human was found similar with the isolates from chicken meat (Leverstein-van Hall et al., 2011). A recent study conducted in Japan identified imported chicken meat as a source of CTX-M-8-producing *E. coli* in handlers through acquisition of either whole bacterium or its $bla_{\text{CTX-M-8}}$/IncI1 plasmids (Norizuki et al., 2017). However, the German study conducted in Hamburg did not reveal chicken meat as a major source of ESBL-producing *Enterobacteriaceae* for the consumers (Campos et al., 2014). The studies conducted in the countries such as Spain, North America, United Kingdom and Taiwan documented mobile genetic elements mediated transmission of expanded-spectrum cephalosporin-resistant *E. coli* from food animals, birds or meats (Yan et al., 2004; Mulvey et al., 2009; Paterson et al., 2010; Stokes et al., 2012).

Sometimes, foods procured from the livestock treated with antimicrobials may act as a niche for generation of resistant bacteria during storage. In a study in the United Kingdom with waste milk (unsuitable for human consumption), samples derived from the milch animals treated with β-lactams revealed the presence of penicillins and cephalosporins (Randall et al., 2014). Occurrence of resistant *E. coli* or any other bacteria in cefquinome-containing milk was 20 times higher than the milk samples without traces of antibiotics. Removal of waste milk from the ration can reduce the level of resistant *E. coli* in calves (Hordijk et al., 2013).

Diffusion of antimicrobial-resistant *E. coli* is a dynamic process which can flow from human to animals also. Transmission of human clinical isolates of antimicrobial-resistant *E. coli* (ESBL-producing ST131 lineage) to susceptible animals such as cattle, pigs, wildlife, companion animals and poultry was documented (Ewers et al., 2010; Mora et al., 2010; Platell et al., 2011). During this reverse transmission from human to animals, human clinical ST131 strains have gained new resistance genes (ESBL) linked to various plasmids (Rogers et al., 2011). Acquisition of new resistance genes generally causes retarded bacterial growth ('fitness cost') by compensatory mutations which was absent in clinical ST131 strains (Andersson and Hughes, 2010).

Person to person transmission of *E. coli* occurs through faecal—oral route (WHO, 2018). Human to human transmission of ESBL-producing *E. coli* can occur through direct contact also (Wu et al., 2013). A few studies using case—control approach pointed out the risk factors for colonization of ESBL-producing *E. coli* in human. Residing with a UTI patient acted as a risk factor for transmission of ESBL-producing *E. coli* in human, especially among those who preferred to take the meals at home than outside. It suggested a possibility of cross-transmission within the home (Rodríguez-Bano et al., 2008). Another hospital-based study in the United States revealed that vegetarians were more prone to colonization with resistant *E. coli* than the nonvegetarians (poultry meat consumers) (Sannes et al., 2008).

Diagnosis

Human clinical samples include stool, urine, blood, sputum, bile, endotracheal aspirate and bronchoalveolar lavage. Clinical samples from suspected animals and birds include fresh faeces/rectal or cloacal swabs, urine, milk, vaginal exudates, cardiac blood and affected tissues such as the liver, spleen, pericardium or bone marrow after postmortem. Specimens should be collected from fresh carcasses as the organisms readily invade the tissues after death. Cold chain should be maintained during transport without direct contact to the ice or coolants to prevent freezing of the collected samples. The samples should be processed within 24—48 h (holding period) in the laboratory.

Laboratory examinations

Direct examination

A smear can be prepared from centrifuged deposit of collected milk and urine or exudate samples or tissues and stained by Gram's Method. *E. coli* appears as Gram-negative small rod arranged singly, in a pair or short chain (Fig. 15.1).

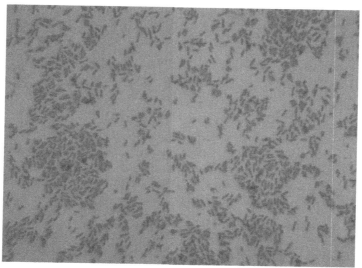

FIGURE 15.1   Gram-stained smear of *Escherichia coli* isolated from pigs (100X). *Courtesy: Arindam Samanta, Department of Veterinary Microbiology, West Bengal University of Animal and Fishery Sciences, Kolkata, India.*

Isolation of Escherichia coli

Blood agar and MacConkey's agar are the primary media for isolation of *E. coli*. The selective and differential medium 'sorbitol MacConkey agar (SMA)' is used to isolate EHEC serotype O157:H7. The plates are generally incubated at 37°C for 24 h. *E. coli* can grow at the temperature range between 15 and 45°C. In blood agar, *E. coli* colonies are smooth or rough, 2–3 mm in diameter, convex, moist, shiny and entire. Haemolysis depends on the strains. In MacConkey's agar, the colonies are pink in colour. The bacteria ferment the lactose sugar, present in the medium and make the medium acidic. Now neutral red, present in the media as a pH indicator, produces pink colour in this acidic pH. Bile salts of the medium prevent the growth of the Gram-positive bacteria. Lactose nonfermenters (*Salmonella, Proteus, Shigella*) produce pale or colourless colonies in MacConkey's agar because of production of basic pH by peptide digestion. In eosine methylene blue (EMB) agar, *E. coli* produces characteristic 'metallic sheen' that appears on the surface of the bacterial colonies. The lactose present in the media is fermented by the bacteria and at an acidic pH both the dyes (eosin methylene blue) combine to form a greenish metallic precipitate. Certain species of *Citrobacter* and *Enterobacter* also produce similar kind of metallic sheen in EMB agar. In SMA, colourless colonies are produced as O157 cannot ferment the sorbitol.

Pathogenicity of the *E. coli* isolates from clinical samples should be confirmed as they are present as normal bacterial flora within the body. Pathogenicity can be ascertained by ligated loop assay, cell culture cytotoxicity assay, typing of the isolates and detection of toxin by serological or DNA-based methods.

Ligated loop assay: LT/STb, CNF-2 toxins can be assayed in rabbit/weaned pig ligated ileal loop. In this assay, six-inch segments of small intestine without any feed are cut off by ligatures of silk and are inoculated with the suspected bacteria with the help of a 22-gauge needle. A part of the same intestine is ligated in similar way with tryptic soy broth inoculation (control). After 24 h, in positive case, distension of the inoculated portion with fluid is found. The fluid in the loop is turbid, sanguineous and usually contains clots of precipitated mucus. Occasionally there is oedema of the associated mesentery. Fluid weight per gut length of the loop can be calculated to measure the potency of toxin. The control shows no distension with fluid.

Cell culture cytotoxicity assay: Profound cytotoxicity of Vero (or HeLa) cells by Shiga toxins is the 'gold standard' method for detection of STEC/EHEC. The test involves treatment of vero monolayer with sterile extract of the test bacteria and examining cells for cytopathic effect after 48–72 h of incubation. The specificity of the assay can be improved by the addition of Shiga toxin–specific antisera. *E. coli* such as EAEC/DAEC/NTEC can be detected by Hep-2 or HeLa cell line adherence test.

Serological tests

Latex agglutination test and ELISA have been developed for detection of APEC whole bacterial antigen (O2, O78) or fimbrial antigen. For detection of STEC/EHEC antigens (stx antigen), sandwich ELISA with immune sera, affinity purified polyclonal antibodies, immobilized monoclonal antibody or Gb3 receptor as a capture system has been developed. Shiga toxin antigens can be detected in culture supernatant, bacterial extract or directly in the faecal samples or saliva. Reverse passive latex agglutination test and colony blot have also been developed for detection of STEC/EHEC.

Histopathology

Histopathological slide of the intestine (ileum) showing characteristic attaching effacing (AE) lesion helps in diagnosis of attaching and effacing E. coli (AEEC).

Typing methods

Typing and subtyping of strains is a valuable aid to identify outbreaks. Serotyping can be performed with specific antisera against *E. coli* O, H and K antigens in tube or plate agglutination tests. However, it cannot be used for all *E. coli* pathotypes. EAEC strains autoagglutinate because of 'aggregative phenotype' and are often described as 'untypeable (UT)' or 'rough' in serotyping report. Modern methods of typing include pulsed field gel electrophoresis, multiple-locus variable number tandem repeat analysis, plasmid replicon typing, multiple locus sequence typing, etc.

Molecular biology

DNA-based assay for STEC detection involves either colony hybridization with polynucleotide probe or polymerase chain reaction (PCR). In PCR-based detection, crude lysate or DNA extract from single colony, mixed broth cultures, colony sweeps, direct extract of faeces or food can be used as template. The troubleshooting may arise during use of PCR with faecal sample as it contains PCR inhibitory substances producing false negative results. Sometimes false positive result is found by detection of 'cryptic gene' (free *stx* encoding phages or presence of defective *stx* gene in bacteria). For detection of other pathotypes such as EAEC, multiplex PCR targeting the genes such as antiaggregation protein transporter, EAST and a chromosomal gene present in the pheU pathogenicity island was described.

Characteristics of antimicrobial resistance

Certain antibiotics are considered critically important in human medicine based on either nonavailability of alternative drugs or for treatment of infections caused by resistant organisms (WHO, 2007). Cephalosporins (third- and fourth-generation), quinolones and aminoglycosides are considered as critically important for treatment of *E. coli* infection in human.

Cephalosporin resistance

Higher generation cephalosporin resistance is offered by ESBLs that can lyse cephalosporins (ceftazidime, cefotaxime, ceftriaxone), monobactams (aztreonam) and penicillin. Since the late 1990s, ESBL-producing *E. coli* have emerged globally. Among the three major types of ESBLs (TEM, SHV, CTX-M) prevalent in human, occurrence of TEM and SHV is mostly replaced with CTX-M. Several cephalosporins such as first-generation (cefadroxil, cefapirin, cephalexin), third-generation (cefovecin, cefpodoxime, ceftiofur) and fourth-generation cephalosporins (cefquinome) are recommended for treatment of livestock and companion animals in different parts of the globe (Ewers et al., 2012). Livestock, poultry and companion animals are considered as potential reservoir of ESBL-producing *E. coli* throughout the world. Isolation of SHV-12-producing *E. coli* from a dog with UTI and CMY-2, CTX-M-14, SHV-12-producing *E. coli* from healthy chickens in Spain are the earliest reports of ESBL *E. coli* from animal sources (Teshager et al., 2000; Brinas et al., 2003). Prevalence of ESBL-producing *E. coli* in livestock and poultry varied between 0.6% and 44.7% in European countries and 1.7% and 11.8% in Asian countries (Ewers et al., 2012).

CTX-M (CTX-M-1, 2, 9, 14, 15, 32, 55) was detected as most prevalent among the ESBL-producing *E. coli* isolates followed by TEM (TEM-52) and SHV (SHV-12) in livestock, poultry and companion animals. Higher prevalence of CTX-M-1 in European *E. coli* isolates from animals (companion animals: 28%, poultry: 28%, cattle and pigs: 72%; carried by IncN, IncFII, IncFIB and IncI1 plasmids), CTX-M-9 and CTX-M-55 in Asian pigs and aquatic environment and CTX-M-14 (IncFII/FIB and IncK plasmids) in companion animals and poultry in Asia (30%−33%) was documented (Ewers et al., 2012; Seiffert et al., 2013). In human, CTX-M-15 was detected in *E. coli* isolates irrespective of geographical regions (Canton et al., 2008). SHV-12 (IncFIB, IncN, IncI1 plasmids) and TEM-52 (IncI1 plasmids) were predominantly documented in *E. coli* strains isolated from poultry in European countries (Seiffert et al., 2013). Distribution of ESBL/ampC genes in *E. coli* strains isolated from the livestock and companion animals in different parts of the world is described in Table 15.2.

In addition to ESBL, chromosome or plasmid-mediated ampC β-lactamases encoded by bla_{AmpC} or bla_{CMY-2} confer resistance against higher generation cephalosporins and β-lactam/β-lactamase inhibitor combinations (amoxicillin/clavulanate) (EFSA Panel on Biological Hazards, 2011). The chromosomal bla_{AmpC} of *E. coli* is repressed or weakly expressed, although mutation in the promoter region may cause constitutive overexpression. The CMY-2 gene belongs to a small family of plasmid-mediated ampC-like enzymes (LAT-1, LAT-2, BIL-1, CMY-2 and 2b, CMY-3, CMY-4, CMY-5), which share homology with the chromosomal *ampC* from *Citrobacter freundii* (Winokur et al., 2001). In addition to cephamycins, third-generation cephalosporins and aztreonam, CMY-2-β-lactamase of *E. coli* also conferred resistance to carbapenems (Poirel et al., 2004). CMY-2-β-lactamase encoding gene (bla_{CMY-2}) resides on a plasmid (incompatibility group IncI1-Iγ, IncA/C, IncF, IncK) (Carattoli, 2009). Higher prevalence of CMY-2-producing *E. coli* was detected in livestock of North America and Asia and in poultry of European countries (38%−78%) (Smet et al., 2010; Seiffert et al., 2013). The plasmids such as IncI1-Iγ and IncK were identified as vehicles of bla_{CMY-2} gene, associated with transmission of *E. coli* strains in human from broilers and chicken meat in the Netherlands and Sweden (Dierikx et al., 2013; Börjesson et al., 2013). Recent study in Denmark although found partial similarity between the plasmids carrying CMY-2 gene in *E. coli* strains isolated from dogs, poultry and human (Hansen et al., 2016). Discontinuation of higher generation cephalosporins in hatcheries (poultry) reduced occurrence of CMY-2-producing *E. coli* in chicken meat in Denmark (Baron et al., 2014).

TABLE 15.2 Worldwide distribution and molecular characteristics of extended-spectrum cephalosporin-resistant *Escherichia coli* in animals and birds.

Country	Prevalence of ESBL-producing *E. coli*	Prevalence of AmpC-producing *E. coli*	Livestock/Poultry
China	6%–10% (CTX-M-14, 22, 65)	1%–4% (CMY-2)	Pigs
	6% (CTX-M-14, 55)	—	Cattle
	12%–25% (CTX-M-14, 55, 65)	—	Poultry
HongKong	64% (CTX-M-3,14)	—	Pigs
	33% (CTX-M-14, 55)	—	Cattle
	33% (CTX-M-14, 55)	—	Poultry
	7.7%–13.9% (CTX-M-1, 9)	—	Brown rats (*Rattus norvegicus*), black rats (*Rattus rattus*)
Japan	—	1% (CMY-2)	Pigs
	3% (CTX-M-2)	1%–3% (CMY-2)	Cattle
	8%–60% (CTX-M-2, 25; SHV-12)	5%–13% (CMY-2)	Poultry
Indonesia	8.6% (CTX-M-1, 9)	—	Cattle
Korea	1% (CTX-M-14)	—	Cattle
India	6.3% (CTX-M, SHV, TEM)	—	Poultry (broilers)
	23.3% (CTX-M, SHV, TEM)	—	Poultry (Kuroilers)
	0%	—	Poultry (backyard layers)
	6% (CTX-M-9, SHV-12, TEM-1)	—	Pigs
Czech Republic	6% (CTX-M-1)	—	Pigs
	1%–39% (CTX-M-1)	—	Cattle
Denmark	CTX-M-1,2,9	—	Poultry
	11% (CTX-M-1, 14)	—	Pigs
France	1%–5% (CTX-M-1,9, 14,15; SHV-12; TEM-71; OXA-1)	0%–2%	Cattle
Germany	44% (CTX-M-1, SHV-12)	—	Poultry
	1% (CTX-M-1, 15; TEM-52)	—	Cattle
	4% (CTX-M-15)	—	Pigs cattle, turkey, poultry and their respective meats
Holland (the Netherland)	94% (CTX-M-1; TEM-52; SHV-12)	83% (ESBL + AmpC) (CMY-2)	Poultry
Poland	33% (ESBL + AmpC) (CTX-M-1)	33% (ESBL + AmpC) (CMY-2)	Pigs
	55% (ESBL + AmpC) (CTX-M-1)	55% (ESBL + AmpC) (CMY-2)	Poultry
Spain	13%–30% (CTX-M-1,9,14; SHV-12)	0%–4%	Pigs
	CTX-M-gr-9	CMY-2	Poultry
Italy	CTX-M-1, 32; SHV-12	—	Poultry
Portugal	25% (CTX-M-1)	—	Pigs
	7% (CTX-M-1, 32)	—	Sheep

Continued

TABLE 15.2 Worldwide distribution and molecular characteristics of extended-spectrum cephalosporin-resistant *Escherichia coli* in animals and birds.—cont'd

Country	Prevalence of ESBL-producing *E. coli*	Prevalence of AmpC-producing *E. coli*	Livestock/Poultry
Switzerland	4%–14% (CTX-M-1,14,15)	0%	Cattle
	25%–63% (CTX-M-1; SHV-12)	2% (CMY-2)	Poultry
	3%–15% (CTX-M-1,3,14)	0%–13% (CMY-2)	Pigs
United Kingdom	1%–42% (CTX-M-1,14,15; OXA-1)	–	Cattle
	54.5% (CTX-M-1,15)	–	Poultry
	6.3%–53.4% (CTX-M, TEM, SHV)	–	Horses
Czech Republic, France, Germany, Italy, Poland, Serbia, Spain and Switzerland	14% (CTX-M-1, 14, 15, 24, 25, 28, 55; SHV-12)	–	Rooks (*Corvus frugilegus*)
United States	–	CMY-2	Pigs
	CTX-M-1/-14/-15, TEM	CMY-2	Cattle
South Africa (Eastern Cape)	CTX-M, TEM	AmpC, CMY	Cattle

Quinolone resistance

Quinolone derivatives are broad spectrum in nature and are commonly used for treatment of various infections in animals and human. Emergence of resistance caused legal restrictions of fluroquinolone use in livestock and poultry in the United States and Denmark. Food and drug administration (FDA) of the United States banned the use of sarafloxacin and enrofloxacin in poultry since 2005 (Hammerum and Heuer, 2009). Resistance to quinolones is associated with mutation in topoisomerase enzyme (GyrA, GyrB, ParC, ParE), decreased expression of porin, overexpression of efflux pumps (qepA) to expel the drug molecule from the bacterial cell (Hopkins et al., 2005). Fluroquinolone resistance genes (*qnrA, qnrB, qnrC, qnrD, qnrS*), which can protect the bacterial genome from quinolones, are mostly transferred through the plasmids. Presence of *qnr* (*qnrB, qnrS*) was documented in *E. coli* isolates from poultry and pigs in China (Yue et al., 2008). Other quinolone resistance determinants such as *aac(6′)-Ib-cr* can act as aminoglycoside-acetyl-transferase. In ESBL-producing *E. coli* strains isolated from human, occurrences of *qnr* and *aac(6′)-Ib-cr* were estimated as 10% and 15%–50%, respectively, with an increasing trend specially in pandemic strain of ST131 lineage (Pitout et al., 2008; Karah et al., 2010). High phenotypical resistance to ciprofloxacin (84.2%) and levofloxacin (78.9%) was also detected in ESBL-producing *E. coli* isolated from Mongolian hospitals. Characterization of CTX-M-producing *E. coli* strains from Mongolian hospitals revealed the occurrence of *aac(6′)-lb-cr* and *oqxAB* along with *bla*CTX-M-15, no other determinants such as *qnrA, qnrB, qnrC, qnrD, qnrS, qnrVC* and *qepA* (Kao et al., 2016). Absence of quinolone resistance gene (*qnrA*) in *E. coli* strains isolated from backyard poultry in India was found to be correlated with lack of ESBL genes (Samanta et al., 2014). Moreover, ESBL/β-lactamase-producing *E. coli* were isolated with significantly more frequency from backyard pigs than the organized farm pigs along with significantly more phenotypical resistance against enrofloxacin (Samanta et al., 2015). Linkage of ESBL and quinolone resistance determinants (*qnrB*) was also detected in *E. coli* isolated from poultry in India (Kar et al., 2015). Fluoroquinolone-resistant *E. coli* strains isolated from livestock (cattle, goats, sheep) and companion animals (cats and dogs) in Turkey revealed the occurrence of *qnrA, qnrS, oqxB, aac(6′)lb-cr, acrB* and *soxS* determinants (Şahintürk et al., 2016).

Aminoglycoside resistance

Resistance to aminoglycosides in *E. coli* is primarily associated with production of three classes of enzymes (acetyltransferase, nucleotidyltransferase, phosphor transferase), which can lyse the drug molecule. Enzymatic methylation of nucleotides present in the A-site of 16S rRNA is another way of aminoglycoside resistance as it prevents the binding of the drug with 30S ribosomal subunits. The 16S rRNA methylases (ArmA, RmtA, RmtB, RmtC, RmtD, NpmA) are transferable between different species through the plasmids (Wachino et al., 2007). In human, association of *rmtB* with ESBL genes in *E. coli* was detected with growing trend in China (Yu et al., 2010). In animals (pigs), plasmid-mediated 16S rRNA methylase genes, i.e., *rmtB* and *armA*, was documented in *E. coli* isolates from China and Spain, respectively (Gonzalez-Zorn et al., 2005; Chen et al., 2007). Apramycin (aminoglycoside analogue used in animals) resistance was detected to be associated with *aac(3)-IV* gene, which also produced cross-resistance against gentamicin (Chaslus-Dancla et al., 1991). Increased consumption of apramycin with feed was linked with occurrence of *aac(3)-IV*-producing *E. coli* in healthy and infected pigs (Jensen et al., 2006).

Sulfonamide resistance

Sulfonamide resistance genes can encode modified target molecule of the drug (dihydropteroate synthase) in the folic acid synthesis pathway. All the sulfonamide resistance genes (*sul1, sul2, sul3*) were detected as prevalent in animal and human *E. coli* isolates in different countries (Grape et al., 2003; Hammerum et al., 2006; Kar et al., 2015).

Nitrofurantoin resistance

Nitrofurantoin resistance in *E. coli* is associated with a plasmid-encoded efflux pump (*OqxAB*) or mutation of chromosomal nitroreductase genes (*nfsA* and *nfsB*) (Breeze and Obaseiki-Ebor, 1983). Multidrug-resistant (including nitrofurantoin) *E. coli* possessing *OqxAB* was detected in pigs fed with olaquindox as feed additive in Denmark (Sørensen et al., 2003). In a recent study conducted with *E. coli* isolates from human UTI patients and food animals (chicken, pigs, cattle) in Hong Kong revealed the strong association of *oqxAB* genes of *E. coli* with nitrofurantoin resistance. The gene (*oqxAB*) was carried by plasmids of varied replicon types (Ho et al., 2016).

Tetracycline resistance

Tetracycline resistance is associated with *tet* gene causing efflux pump activation, ribosomal protection and enzymatic inactivation of the drug. Among the different *tet* genes (approximately 40), *tet*(A), *tet*(B), *tet*(C), *tet*(D) and *tet*(G) were found to be associated with *E. coli* strains (Chopra and Roberts, 2001). High prevalence of tetracycline-resistant *E. coli* possessing *tet*(A) (46.5%), *tet*(B) (45.1%) and *tet*(C) (5.8%) genes was documented from beef cattle in South Korea (Shin et al., 2015). Different Gram-negative organisms including *E. coli* isolated from milk samples of cattle suffering with subclinical mastitis possessed *tet (A)* (10%) and *tet(B)* (16%) genes in India (Das et al., 2017). *E. coli* isolated from backyard poultry in India showing phenotypical resistance to oxytetracycline was detected to possess a specific RAPD profile and was associated with a precise agro-climatic zone (Samanta et al., 2014). Enterotoxigenic *E. coli* and necrotoxigenic *E. coli* isolated from water buffaloes, STEC strains isolated from goats and raw yak milk or milk products in India were also detected to possess phenotypical resistance to tetracycline (Bandyopadhyayet al., 2012; Mahanti et al., 2014, 2015). Association of ESBL and ampC genes with *tet* genes was also documented (Endimiani et al., 2012).

Colistin resistance

Colistin was considered as a last-resort antibiotic for the treatment of infectious diseases. Emergence of colistin resistance is associated with the enzyme phosphatidylethanolamine transferase (encoded by 'mobilized colistin resistance' gene or *mcr-1*), which alters the 'lipid A' structure of the bacterial LPS, present in outer membrane of Gram-negative bacteria. Bacterial LPS is the major target for colistin and because of its structural modification, the colistin cannot bind with it. The plasmid-mediated *mcr-1* was first documented in China in 2013 (Liu et al., 2016). Since its first report, *mcr-1*-producing *E. coli* strains have been described in food animals, poultry, meat and meat products and human throughout the world (Table 15.3). Chromosomal *mcr-1* of *E. coli* isolated from veal calves in the Netherlands was also documented. Presence of insertion sequence (ISApl1) in the upstream of *mcr-1* facilitated its chromosomal translocation (Veldman et al., 2016). Additional colistin-resistance genes such as *mcr-2*, *mcr-3* and their variants were recently documented (Qiao et al., 2018).

TABLE 15.3 Worldwide occurrence of *mcr-1*-producing *Escherichia coli* in food animals, foods, environment and human.

Source	Country	Year	Numbers of isolates/occurrence rate of *mcr-1*-producing *E. coli*
Chicken	China	1980–2014	104
Chicken	Brazil	2003–2015	5%
Veal calves	France	2005–2014	106
Pigs	Japan	2008–2010	2
Ground beef	Canada	2010	2
Pigs	Germany	2010–2011	3
Food items	Portugal	2011	1
Chicken meat, pork	China	2011	5%–6%
Gastronomy tube	Canada	2011	1
Septicaemia in human	The Netherlands	2011	0.08%
Chicken meat, pork	China	2013	23%–25%
Chicken meat	China	2014	28%
Chicken meat	Denmark	2012–2014	5
Pigs	Brazil	2012–2014	1.8%
Retail meat (chicken, turkey)	The Netherlands	2009–2016	2%
River water	Switzerland	2012	1
Chickens, veal calves, turkeys	The Netherlands	2010–2015	<1%
Pigs	France	2011	0.5%
Pigs, veal calves	Belgium	2011–2012	6–7
Human stool	Thailand	2012	2
Human stool	Laos	2012	6
Pigs	Laos	2012	3
Human stool	Cambodia	2012	1
Cattle	Japan	2012–2013	4
Water	Malaysia	2013	1
Chicken, pigs	Malaysia	2013	1–3
Chickens, pigs	France	2013–2014	1%–2%
Turkey	Italy	2014	1
Pigs	Vietnam	2014–2015	38%
Pigs	China	2014	21%
Vegetables	Switzerland	2014	2
Wound in feet (human)	Germany	2014	1
Human patients	China	2014	1%
Turkey	France	2014	5.9%
Chickens	Tunisia	2015	67%
Chickens	Algeria	2015	1
Poultry meat	United Kingdom	2012–2015	2

Continued

TABLE 15.3 Worldwide occurrence of *mcr-1*-producing *Escherichia coli* in food animals, foods, environment and human.—cont'd

Source	Country	Year	Numbers of isolates/occurrence rate of *mcr-1*-producing *E. coli*
Human urinary tract infection	Switzerland	2015	1
Chicken meat	Denmark	2015	5
Chicken, pigs	South Korea	2016	0.1%
Chicken meat	Brazil	2017	19.5%

Characteristics of antimicrobial resistance in *E. coli* isolates observed in different livestock, poultry, wildlife, fishes and in human are discussed in the following section.

Livestock (cattle/buffalo/goat/yak)

In Europe, annual surveillance and reporting of antimicrobial-resistant *E. coli* and other commensal bacteria from livestock is mandatory since 2014. All the member countries of the European Union (EU) followed a standard protocol for detection of resistance in the commensal bacteria developed by European Food Safety Authority (EFSA). In a kind of report from Belgium based on data collected between 2011 and 2014, high occurrence (>50%) of ampicillin, tetracycline and sulfamethoxazole-resistant *E. coli* was detected in veal calves. Although multidrug resistance (at least against three drugs) of *E. coli* showed a decreasing trend in beef cattle and veal calves associated with decreased antibiotic consumption, better animal husbandry practices in comparison to broiler chickens. A greater occurrence of resistant *E. coli* was detected in calves (81.5%) compared to adult beef cattle (39.2%) reflecting the greater exposure of calves with antimicrobials (Hanon et al., 2015). Reliable data are lacking on the occurrence of AMR *E. coli* in cull dairy cattle at slaughter, although lower prevalence is expected because of lesser antimicrobial usage in beef cattle in comparison to the dairy cattle (Call et al., 2008). The decreasing trend of antimicrobial resistance in *E. coli* isolates of livestock (veal calves and chicken) from Belgium continued, although with a slow pace during 2015. Emergence of multidrug-resistant *E. coli* isolate became low but resistance against diversity of antimicrobials increased. Chloramphenicol resistance gene was still detected in the isolates, although with a decreasing trend, albeit the drug was banned for veterinary use since 1997 in Europe. Chloramphenicol resistance of *E. coli* was not because of cross-resistance with other phenicol antibiotics (florfenicol), licensed for veterinary use. Intensity of these 'ancient' resistance genes of chloramphenicol might have been further influenced by co-selection of other antimicrobial resistance genes, if their usage in livestock was not regulated properly (Callens et al., 2018). Reduced sales of antimicrobials for veterinary use was correlated with lower occurrence of resistance determinants in *E. coli* in veal calves, pigs and chicken in the Netherlands also (Dorado-Garcia et al., 2016).

In a similar kind of antimicrobial resistance (AMR) surveillance program conducted in Germany (GERM-Vet monitoring program), 6849 *E. coli* strains isolated from infected cattle, pigs and poultry during 2008—14 were screened for ESBL production. In total, 6.1% of *E. coli* strains including 11.2% isolates from cattle, 4.8% from pigs and 0.8% from poultry were confirmed as ESBL producers. Among the ESBL genes, $bla_{CTX-M-1}$ was the most prevalent among all the studied species and $bla_{CTX-M-2}$, $bla_{CTX-M-3}$ and $bla_{CTX-M-14}$ were confirmed in cattle only. Mostly the bovine isolates belonged to phylogroup 'A' and 'D'. Co-resistance study against non-β-lactam antibiotics revealed maximum resistance against sulfamethoxazole and minimum against amikacin, banned in livestock in Germany. Higher occurrence of ESBL-producing *E. coli* was detected in calves than adult cattle probably because of differences in sampling pattern. Faeces or intestinal contents were collected from calves and milk were the preferred samples from the adult cattle. Horizontal transfer of ESBL gene is consistently low in bovine udder because of lack of commensal present in the udder (Michael et al., 2017). In another study, *E. coli* isolated from mastitic milk samples of cattle during 2009—13 were studied for detection of ESBL production in Germany. ESBL genes such as $bla_{CTX-M-1}$, $bla_{CTX-M-2}$, $bla_{CTX-M-14}$ and $bla_{CTX-M-15}$ were confirmed on conjugative plasmids of different incompatibility groups (IncF, IncI1). ESBL gene possessing plasmids also harboured the resistance genes for sulphonamides, tetracycline, trimethoprim and chloramphenicol/florfenicol, which indicate about occurrence of ESBL genes even in absence of β-lactam antibiotics. Nine of the ESBL-producing isolates showed a multidrug resistance phenotype against at least three classes of antimicrobial agents (Freitag et al., 2017).

In Africa, *E. coli* isolated from livestock showed highest resistance against tetracycline, penicillin and sulphonamide with an increasing trend for quinolone resistance and ESBL production. CTX-M-1 was the predominant ESBL detected in African countries, and within the CTX-M-1 group, $bla_{CTX-M-15}$-producing *E. coli* was most prevalent in animals and human. Certain *E. coli* clonal types possessing bla_{CTX-M} (ST131/B2 or ST405/D) or plasmids such as IncI1/ST3 possessing $bla_{CTX-M-1}$(Tunisia), IncY possessing *qnrS1* and $bla_{CTX-M-15}$(Tanzania), IncF possessing $bla_{CTX-M-15}$ circulate between human and different animals (Alonso et al., 2017). *E. coli* isolated from faecal samples of healthy cattle, chicken and pigs in Nigeria during 2012−13 revealed highest resistance to tetracycline, trimethoprim/sulfamethoxazole and ampicillin. Approximately 40% of the isolates were susceptible to amikacin, cefepime, ceftazidime, ertapenem, meropenem and tigecycline (Adenipekun et al., 2015). Implementation of antimicrobial resistance surveillance programme is required to explore more data in Africa.

In India, synergistic intramammary infection of ESBL-producing *E. coli*, methicillin-resistant *Staphylococcus epidermidis* and methicillin-resistant *Staphylococcus aureus* was detected in Holstein Friesian crossbred cows with subclinical mastitis and nondescript cow with clinical mastitis (Bandyopadhyay et al., 2015a,b). STEC strains isolated from water buffaloes in India were detected as phenotypically resistant to several common antibiotics such as erythromycin, cephalothin, amikacin, kanamycin and gentamicin, although no ESBL producing and quinolone resistance genes were detected (Mahanti et al., 2013). STEC and enteropathogenic *E. coli* isolated from raw yak milk and milk products ('churpi') exhibited phenotypical resistance against erythromycin, amikacin, azithromycin, amoxicillin, ampicillin−cloxacillin, cephalothin, furazolidone, gentamicin, kanamycin, streptomycin and tetracycline (Bandyopadhyay et al., 2012). Multidrug-resistant diarrhoeagenic *E. coli* was reported from healthy goats and free-range yaks in India (Mahanti et al., 2015). In a retrospective study conducted in Kashmir valley (India), *E. coli* isolated from calves with diarrhoea exhibited resistance against several common antibiotics such as oxytetracycline, nalidixic acid and co-trimoxazole (Kawoosa et al., 2007).

Poultry

Higher occurrence of cephalosporin-resistant *E. coli* was detected in broiler chickens in Belgium during 2011−12 because of off-label use of ceftiofur sprayed on day old chicks or use of imported chicks from the countries where use of cephalosporins are common in hatcheries. Since 2010, use of cephalosporins was banned in European Union countries (Hanon et al., 2015). National antimicrobial resistance monitoring programme conducted in European countries (Denmark, France, Italy, Finland, Belgium, the Netherlands, Germany, Norway, Sweden) during 2005−11 revealed higher occurrence of nalidixic acid−resistant *E. coli* in broilers in almost all the studied countries except Finland, Denmark and Norway. Increasing trend in prevalence of ciprofloxacin-resistant *E. coli* was documented during 2005−11 in the Netherlands (50.8%−56.2%), Denmark (5.7%−9%) and France (19%−40.1%) (Garcia-Migura et al., 2014). In France, *E. coli* strains isolated from hens and broilers showed resistance to flumequine (97%), ceftiofur (97%), amoxicillin (98%), gentamicin (96%), enrofloxacin (97%), tetracycline (98%) and trimethoprim/sulphonamides (97%) (McNulty et al., 2016). In a Norwegian broiler farm, occurrence of extended-spectrum cephalosporin-resistant *E. coli* was detected in spite of rare usage of antibiotics because of strict implementation of restrictive policies. In addition to lack of antibiotic use, strict implementation of biosecurity policies such as restricted human entry into the farm, regular cleaning and disinfection were identified as additional factors to prevent the emergence of superbugs (Mo et al., 2016). A study conducted in Romania revealed high occurrence rate (69%) of ESBL and AmpC-producing *E. coli* in chickens. Genotyping of the *E. coli* isolates detected $bla_{CTX-M-15}$ and bla_{CMY-2} with highest frequency. Pulsed-field gel electrophoresis (PFGE) and multi locus sequence typing (MLST)-based comparison between human and chicken *E. coli* isolates in Romania did not find any clonal similarity (Maciuca et al., 2015).

Cefotaxime-resistant *E. coli* isolates were recovered (35%) from poultry faecal samples in Tunisia belonging to three phylogenetic groups (B1, A and D) and different clonal lineages such as ST542-B1, ST212-B1, ST58-B1, ST155-B1, ST349-D, ST405-D, ST1056-B1, ST117-D, ST2197-A and ST155-B1. ESBL and ACBL genes such as $bla_{CTX-M-1}$, $bla_{CTX-M-15}$, $bla_{CTX-M-14}$ and bla_{CMY-2} were prevalent among the studied *E. coli* isolates. The authors speculated use of antibiotics as growth promoter in poultry (although banned but not enforced) as the root cause of emerging cefotaxime-resistant *E. coli* infection in Tunisia (Maamar et al., 2016). IncI1 and IncF were the most common plasmid replicon types detected in cefotaxime-resistant *E. coli* strains from poultry in Tunisia and other parts of the world (Carattoli, 2009; Ben Sallem et al., 2014; Maamar et al., 2016).

In a comparative study between broiler and layer farms in India with substantial amount of faecal samples, higher occurrence of ESBL producing (87% in broilers compared to 42% in layers) and other antibiotic-resistant *E. coli* isolates were detected in broiler farms than layer farms. The authors could not establish a definite linkage between the use of antibiotics in farm and emergence of resistant bacteria as they could not rule out the role of contaminated environment (Brower et al., 2017). In another study conducted in India, multidrug-resistant ESBL-producing *E. coli* isolated from poultry and cattle were characterized. The isolates possessed class I integron (*int1*), sulphonamide resistance (*sul1*) and quinolone resistance genes (*qnrB*) along with *bla*$_{SHV}$, *bla*$_{CTXM}$, *bla*$_{TEM}$ and *bla*$_{ampC}$ (Kar et al., 2015). In a retrospective study in Kashmir valley (India), *E. coli* isolated from chicken with diarrhoea exhibited resistance against several common antibiotics such as penicillin, tetracycline, nitrofurantoin and sulfamethazine (Wani et al., 2004).

Pigs

National antimicrobial resistance monitoring programme conducted in European countries (Denmark, France, Italy, Finland, Belgium, the Netherlands, Germany, Norway, Sweden) during 2005–11 revealed negligible occurrence of ciprofloxacin-resistant *E. coli* in pigs and cattle. Prevalence of aminopenicillin (amoxicillin and ampicillin) resistant *E. coli* in swine industry was detected in highest proportion in the Netherlands, Denmark and Switzerland in comparison to Sweden and Norway where the occurrence was low (Garcia-Migura et al., 2014).

However, annual resistance monitoring programme based on the protocols developed by the European Committee of Antimicrobial Susceptibility Testing (EUCAST) revealed gradual increase in occurrence of multidrug-resistant *E. coli* in pigs in Sweden during the period 2008–14 (14%–42%) (SVARM, 2014). A few number of studies revealed the variable prevalence of ESBL-producing *E. coli* in pigs in different European countries such as 5.7% in Portugal, 15.3% in Switzerland, 18.2% in Denmark, 36.5% in Spain and 43.8% in Germany (Blanc et al., 2006; Jørgensen et al., 2007; Machado et al., 2008; Geser et al., 2012; Friese et al., 2013). A cross-sectional study of German fattening pig farms documented the occurrence of cefotaxime-resistant *E. coli* in faeces (61%), boot swabs (54%) and dust samples (11%). At least one sample from majority of the farms (85%) was found as positive for the target bacterium. Separate pen for infected pigs was identified as a risk factor for occurrence of cefotaxime-resistant *E. coli* in pig fattening farms (Hering et al., 2014). VIM-1-carbapenemase-*E. coli* was also detected in faecal samples of a German pig farm (Fischer et al., 2012). Manures and dust samples collected from pig farms in Germany also showed the presence of ESBL-producing *E. coli* (18.8%, García-Cobos et al., 2015).

Horses

E. coli isolated from horses showed resistance to different common groups of antibiotics such as penicillins, fluoroquinolones, cephalosporins, tetracyclines, aminoglycosides and sulphonamides (Anzai et al., 1987; Lavoie et al., 1991; Bucknell et al., 1997). Occurrence of antimicrobial-resistant *E. coli* was detected more in hospitalized equines than the nonhospitalized ones (Ahmed et al., 2010; Johns et al., 2012). Multidrug-resistant ESBL-producing *E. coli* was associated with soft tissue and wound infections in horses (Damborg et al., 2012). CTX-M-15-producing *E. coli* belonged to ST131 clonal lineage was also detected in horses (Ewers et al., 2010).

Companion animals

In Portugal, ESBL-producing *E. coli* was confirmed to be associated with chronic UTI in a dog. The isolate belonged to ST131 lineage and possessed an IncFII plasmid containing *bla*$_{CTX-M-15}$, *aac(60)-Ib-cr* and quinolone resistance (*qnrB2*) genes (Pomba et al., 2009). Multidrug-resistant *E. coli* belonged to ST131 lineage and possessing ST131-associated virulence genes were detected in a dog with chronic asymptomatic bacteriuria in the United States (Johnson et al., 2009). Majority (90%) of the ST131 strains detected in Europe belonged to canine population as observed in a prevalence study conducted with the samples from dogs, cats, cattle, guinea pigs, rabbit, pig and bird (Ewers et al., 2010). In Australia, quinolone-resistant *E. coli* belonging to ST131 lineage were isolated from urine and postoperative wounds in dogs (Platell et al., 2010).

Wildlife

Multidrug-resistant *E. coli* (ampicillin, doxycycline, streptomycin, tetracycline, trimethoprim/sulfamethoxazole) were isolated (13.3%) from wild animals in Botswana (Africa). Occurrence was significantly higher in carnivores, water animals and the animals inhabiting surrounding the urban residential area or peridomestic animals such as baboon, banded mongoose and warthog. Similarity in resistance pattern between the isolates from wild animals, human clinical samples and environment was noted suggesting a cross-transmission cycle (Jobbins and Alexander, 2015). Another study with land iguana as a model animal also showed that minimum exposure to antibiotics and anthropogenic activities was correlated with absence of antibiotic resistance determinants in the commensal bacteria in wild animals (Thaller et al., 2010). Similarly, microbiome study of sharks from tourist beach in Brazil having frequent contact with human also revealed the presence of *Enterobacteriaceae* with resistance against penicillin, cephalosporin, tetracycline, gentamicin, ciprofloxacin and chloramphenicol (Interaminense et al., 2010). Furthermore, study with wild deer and small mammals revealed the existence of antimicrobial-resistant *E. coli* in faeces, although the prevalence was substantially low (Alonso et al., 2016). ESBL-producing *E. coli* belonged to phylogroup D and sequence types ST117, ST115, ST2001 and ST69 with diverse combination of ESBL genes were detected in different wild animals (Iberian wolf (*Canis lupus signatus*), gilt-head seabream (*Sparusaurata*), Iberian lynx (*Lynx pardinus*), wild boars (*Sus scrofa scrofa*), red fox (*Vulpes vulpes*)) in Portugal and Spain (Cristovao et al., 2017).

Food animal products

Prevalence of ESBL-producing *E. coli* in different meat samples varied between geographical locations such as 60% in chicken meat in Germany (Campos et al., 2014), 20% in beef in Austria (Petternel et al., 2014), 1.2% in pork in Denmark (Agersø et al., 2011), 73.3% in chicken meat and 2% in beef in Switzerland (Vogt et al., 2014), 1.6% of indigenously generated chicken meat and 37% of imported chicken meat in United Kingdom (Warren et al., 2008). The later finding in the United Kingdom was also supported by other study (Randall et al., 2017). Maximum prevalence of ESBL/AmpC-producing *E. coli* was reported in South American chicken meat (95%) (McNulty et al., 2016). In beef cattle production system, prevalence of cephalosporin-resistant *E. coli* (100%) in hides was correlated with carcass contamination before evisceration (Schmidt et al., 2015).

Human

The retrospective study revealed increasing trend of resistance against ampicillin, sulfonamide and tetracycline in human *E. coli* isolates collected during 1950—2002. Prevalence of multidrug-resistant *E. coli* was also increased from 7% to 63% during the period 1950—2002 (Tadesse et al., 2012).

ESBL-producing extraintestinal *E. coli* infection in human was mostly associated with ST131 clonal lineage throughout the world and the strains possessed $bla_{CTX-M-15}$ with fluoroquinolone (100% resistance to ciprofloxacin) and other antibiotic resistance genes (70%—80% resistance to aminoglycosides) (Platell et al., 2011). In a few European countries (Spain, Russia, Italy, Germany, Poland, France, Hungary and Austria), ST131 *E. coli* strains were detected without CTX-M-15 production (Cagnacci et al., 2008). In South American countries, mostly $bla_{CTX-M-2}$ and in a few cases, $bla_{CTX-M-1}$, $bla_{CTX-M-9}$ and $bla_{CTX-M-8}$-producing *E. coli* strains were reported from human earlier 2010. A shift from CTX-M-2 producers to CTX-M-15 was detected later in Bolivia, Brazil and Argentina (Sennatiet al., 2012). Fluoroquinolone resistance among human clinical *E. coli* isolates was detected as another major issue in South American countries.

Environment

Discharge of antibiotics after human or livestock use is a considerable factor for generation of antibiotic-resistant bacteria in the environment. China is a leading producer and consumer of antibiotics with 48% consumption by human and 52% by livestock and poultry. Majority of the used antibiotics were discharged into the river through sewage system, followed by soil through manure treatment (Zhang et al., 2015). Human hospitals act as another major contributor in environmental generation of resistant microbes. China Antimicrobial Resistance Surveillance System (CARSS) revealed the greater occurrence of cefotaxime and fluroquinolone-resistant *E. coli* in clinical establishment environment (Qiao et al., 2018). Food contact surfaces such as wet poultry market, air of the livestock farm, farm building floors in contact with animal faeces were also detected as a source of ESBL-producing *E. coli* to the environment (Cortes et al., 2010; Aliyu et al., 2016; Navajas-Benito et al., 2017).

References

Adenipekun, E.O., Jackson, C.R., Oluwadun, A., Iwalokun, B.A., Frye, J.G., Barrett, J.B., Hiott, L.M., Woodley, T.A., 2015. Prevalence and antimicrobial resistance in *Escherichia coli* from food animals in Lagos, Nigeria. Microbial Drug Resistance 21 (3), 358—365.

Agersø, Y., Aarestrup, F.M., Pedersen, K., Seyfarth, A.M., Struve, T., Hasman, H., 2011. Prevalence of extended-spectrum cephalosporinase (ESC)-producing *Escherichia coli* in Danish slaughter pigs and retail meat identified by selective enrichment and association with cephalosporin usage. Journal of Antimicrobial Chemotherapy 67 (3), 582—588.

Ahmed, M., Clegg, P., Williams, N., Baptiste, K., Bennett, M., 2010. Antimicrobial resistance in equine faecal *Escherichia coli* isolates from North West England. Annals of Clinical Microbiology and Antimicrobials 9, 12.

Alegbeleye, O.O., Singleton, I., Sant'Ana, A.S., 2018. Sources and contamination routes of microbial pathogens to fresh produce during field cultivation: a review. Food Microbiology 73, 177–208.

Aliyu, A.B., Saleha, A.A., Jalila, A., Zunita, Z., 2016. Risk factors and spatial distribution of extended spectrum β-lactamase-producing-*Escherichia coli* at retail poultry meat markets in Malaysia: a cross-sectional study. BMC Public Health 16 (1), 699.

Alonso, C.A., González-Barrio, D., Tenorio, C., Ruiz-Fons, F., Torres, C., 2016. Antimicrobial resistance in faecal *Escherichia coli* isolates from farmed red deer and wild small mammals. Detection of a multiresistant *E. coli* producing extended-spectrum beta-lactamase. Comparative Immunology, Microbiology and Infectious Diseases 45, 34–39.

Alonso, C.A., Zarazaga, M., Ben Sallem, R., Jouini, A., Ben Slama, K., Torres, C., 2017. Antibiotic resistance in *Escherichia coli* in husbandry animals. The African Perspective. Letters in Applied Microbiology 64, 318–334.

Andersson, D.I., Hughes, D., 2010. Antibiotic resistance and its cost: is it possible to reverse resistance? Nature Reviews Microbiology 8, 260–271.

Anzai, T., Kamada, M., Ike, K., Kanemaru, T., Kumanomido, T., 1987. Drug susceptibility of *Escherichia coli* isolated from foals with diarrhea and mares with metritis. Bulletin of Equine Research Institute 24, 42–50.

Bandyopadhyay, S., Lodh, C., Rahaman, H., Bhattacharya, D., Bera, A.K., Ahmed, F.A., Mahanti, A., Samanta, I., Mondal, D.K., Sarkar, S., Dutta, T.K., 2012. Characterization of shiga toxin producing (STEC) and enteropathogenic *Escherichia coli* (EPEC) in raw yak (Poephagus grunniens) milk and milk products. Research in Veterinary Science 93 (2), 604–610.

Bandyopadhyay, S., Mahanti, A., Lodh, C., Samanta, I., Biswas, T.K., Dutta, T.K., Baruah, K.K., Bhattacharya, D., 2015a. The prevalence and drug resistance profile of Shiga-toxin producing (STEC), enteropathogenic (EPEC) and enterotoxigenic (ETEC) *Escherichia coli* in free ranging diarrheic and non-diarrheic yaks of West Kameng, Arunachal Pradesh, India. Veterinarski Arhiv 85 (5), 501–510.

Bandyopadhyay, S., Samanta, I., Bhattacharyya, D., Nanda, P.K., Kar, D., Chowdhury, J., Dandapat, P., Das, A.K., Batul, N., Mondal, B., Dutta, T.K., 2015b. Co-infection of methicillin-resistant Staphylococcus epidermidis, methicillin-resistant *Staphylococcus aureus* and extended spectrum β-lactamase producing *Escherichia coli* in bovine mastitis—three cases reported from India. Veterinary Quarterly 35 (1), 56–61.

Baron, S., Jouy, E., Larvor, E., Eono, F., Bougeard, S., Kempf, I., 2014. Impact of third-generation-cephalosporin administration in hatcheries on fecal *Escherichia coli* antimicrobial resistance in broilers and layers. Antimicrobial Agents and Chemotherapy 58, 5428–5434.

Baron, S., Delannoy, S., Bougeard, S., Larvor, E., Jouy, E., Balan, O., Fach, P., Kempf, I., 2016. Virulence genes in Expanded-spectrum-cephalosporin-resistant and-susceptible *Escherichia coli* isolates from treated and untreated Chickens. Antimicrobial Agents and Chemotherapy 60 (3), 1874–1877.

Ben Sallem, R., Ben Slama, K., Rojo-Bezares, B., Porres-Osante, N., Jouini, A., Klibi, N., Boudabous, A., Sáenz, Y., Torres, C., 2014. IncI1 plasmids carrying bla CTX-M-1 or bla CMY-2 genes in *Escherichia coli* from healthy humans and animals in Tunisia. Microbial Drug Resistance 20 (5), 495–500.

Blanc, V., Mesa, R., Saco, M., Lavilla, S., Prats, G., Miró, E., Navarro, F., Cortés, P., Llagostera, M., 2006. ESBL-and plasmidic class C β-lactamase-producing *E. coli* strains isolated from poultry, pig and rabbit farms. Veterinary Microbiology 118 (3–4), 299–304.

Börjesson, S., Jernberg, C., Brolund, A., Edquist, P., Finn, M., Landén, A., Olsson-Liljequist, B., Wisell, K.T., Bengtsson, B., Englund, S., 2013. Characterization of plasmid-mediated AmpC-producing *E. coli* from Swedish broilers and association with human clinical isolates. Clinical Microbiology and Infections 19, E309–E311.

Breeze, A.S., Obaseiki-Ebor, E.E., 1983. Transferable nitrofuran resistance conferred by R-plasmids in clinical isolates of *Escherichia coli*. Journal of Antimicrobial Chemotherapy 12 (5), 459–467.

Brinas, L., Moreno, M.A., Zarazaga, M., Porrero, C., Sáenz, Y., García, M., Dominguez, L., Torres, C., 2003. Detection of CMY-2, CTX-M-14, and SHV-12 β-lactamases in *Escherichia coli* fecal-sample isolates from healthy chickens. Antimicrobial Agents and Chemotherapy 47 (6), 2056–2058.

Brower, C.H., Mandal, S., Hayer, S., Sran, M., Zehra, A., Patel, S.J., Kaur, R., Chatterjee, L., Mishra, S., Das, B.R., Singh, P., 2017. The prevalence of extended-spectrum Beta-lactamase-producing multidrug-resistant *Escherichia coli* in poultry chickens and variation according to farming practices in Punjab, India. Environmental Health Perspectives 125 (7).

Bucknell, D.G., Gasser, R.B., Irving, A., Whithear, K., 1997. Antimicrobial resistance in *Salmonella* and *Escherichia coli* isolated from horses. Australian Veterinary Journal 75, 355–356.

Cagnacci, S., Gualco, L., Debbia, E., Schito, G.C., Marchese, A., 2008. European emergence of ciprofloxacin-resistant *Escherichia coli* clonal groups O25: H4-ST 131 and O15: K52: H1 causing community-acquired uncomplicated cystitis. Journal of Clinical Microbiology 46 (8), 2605–2612.

Call, D.R., Davis, M.A., Sawant, A.A., 2008. Antimicrobial resistance in beef and dairy cattle production. Animal Health Research Reviews 9 (2), 159–167.

Callens, B., Sarrazin, S., Cargnel, M., Welby, S., Dewulf, J., Hoet, B., Vermeersch, K., Wattiau, P., 2018. Associations between a decreased veterinary antimicrobial use and resistance in commensal *Escherichia coli* from Belgian livestock species (2011–2015). Preventive Veterinary Medicine 157, 50–58 (in press).

Campos, B.C., Fenner, I., Wiese, N., Lensing, C., Christner, M., Rohde, H., Aepfelbacher, M., Fenner, T., Hentschke, M., 2014. Prevalence and genotypes of extended spectrum beta-lactamases in *Enterobacteriaceae* isolated from human stool and chicken meat in Hamburg, Germany. International Journal of Medical Microbiology 304, 678–684.

Canton, R., Novais, A., Valverde, A., Machado, E., Peixe, L., Baquero, F., Coque, T.M., 2008. Prevalence and spread of extended-spectrum β-lactamase-producing Enterobacteriaceae in Europe. Clinical Microbiology and Infections 14 (s1), 144–153.

Carattoli, A., 2009. Resistance plasmid families in *Enterobacteriaceae*. Antimicrobial Agents and Chemotherapy 53, 2227–2238.

Chaslus-Dancla, E., Pohl, P., Meurisse, M., Marin, M., Lafont, J.P., 1991. High genetic homology between plasmids of human and animal origins conferring resistance to the aminoglycosides gentamicin and apramycin. Antimicrobial Agents and Chemotherapy 35, 590–593.

Chen, L., Chen, Z.L., Liu, J.H., Zeng, Z.L., Ma, J.Y., Jiang, H.X., 2007. Emergence of RmtB methylase-producing *Escherichia coli* and *Enterobacter cloacae* isolates from pigs in China. Journal of Antimicrobial Chemotherapy 59, 880–885.

Chopra, I., Roberts, M., 2001. Tetracycline antibiotics: mode of action, applications, molecular biology, and epidemiology of bacterial resistance. Microbiology and Molecular Biology Reviews 65 (2), 232–260.

Cortés, P., Blanc, V., Mora, A., Dahbi, G., Blanco, J.E., Blanco, M., López, C., Andreu, A., Navarro, F., Alonso, M.P., Bou, G., 2010. Isolation and characterization of potentially pathogenic antimicrobial-resistant *Escherichia coli* strains from chicken and pig farms in Spain. Applied and Environmental Microbiology 76 (9), 2799–2805.

Coque, T.M., Novais, A., Carattoli, A., Poirel, L., Pitout, J., Peixe, L., Baquero, F., Canton, R., Nordmann, P., 2008. Dissemination of clonally related *Escherichia coli* strains expressing extended-spectrum β-lactamase CTX-M-15. Emerging Infectious Diseases 14, 195–200.

Cristóvão, F., Alonso, C.A., Igrejas, G., Sousa, M., Silva, V., Pereira, J.E., Lozano, C., Cortés-Cortés, G., Torres, C., Poeta, P., 2017. Clonal diversity of extended-spectrum beta-lactamase producing *Escherichia coli* isolates in fecal samples of wild animals. FEMS Microbiology Letters 364 (5).

Damborg, P., Marskar, P., Baptiste, K.E., Guardabassi, L., 2012. Faecal shedding of CTX-M-producing *Escherichia coli* in horses receiving broad-spectrum antimicrobial prophylaxis after hospital admission. Veterinary Microbiology 154, 298–304.

Das, A., Guha, C., Biswas, U., Jana, P.S., Chatterjee, A., Samanta, I., 2017. Detection of emerging antibiotic resistance in bacteria isolated from sub-clinical mastitis in cattle in West Bengal. Veterinary World 10 (5), 517.

de Been, M., Lanza, V.F., de Toro, M., Scharringa, J., Dohmen, W., Du, Y., Hu, J., Lei, Y., Li, N., Tooming-Klunderud, A., Heederik, D.J., 2014. Dissemination of cephalosporin resistance genes between *Escherichia coli* strains from farm animals and humans by specific plasmid lineages. PLoS Genetics 10 (12), e1004776.

Dierikx, C., van der Goot, J., Fabri, T., van Essen-Zandbergen, A., Smith, H., Mevius, D., 2013. Extended-spectrum- β-lactamase- and AmpC- β -lactamase-producing *Escherichia coli* in Dutch broilers and broiler farmers. Journal of Antimicrobial Chemotherapy 68, 60–67.

Dorado-García, A., Mevius, D.J., Jacobs, J.J., Van Geijlswijk, I.M., Mouton, J.W., Wagenaar, J.A., Heederik, D.J., 2016. Quantitative assessment of antimicrobial resistance in livestock during the course of a nationwide antimicrobial use reduction in The Netherlands. Journal of Antimicrobial Chemotherapy 71 (12), 3607–3619.

EFSA Panel on Biological Hazards, 2011. Scientific Opinion on the public health risks of bacterial strains producing extended-spectrum β-lactamases and/or AmpC β-lactamases in food and food-producing animals. EFSA Journal 9, 2322.

Endimiani, A., Rossano, A., Kunz, D., Overesch, G., Perreten, V., 2012. First countrywide survey of third-generation cephalosporin-resistant *Escherichia coli* from broilers, swine, and cattle in Switzerland. Diagnostic Microbiology and Infectious Disease 73 (1), 31–38.

Escobar-Páramo, P., Sabbagh, A., Darlu, P., Pradillon, O., Vaury, C., Denamur, E., Lecointre, G., 2004. Decreasing the effects of horizontal gene transfer on bacterial phylogeny: the *Escherichia coli* case study. Molecular Phylogenetics and Evolution 30 (1), 243–250.

Ewers, C., Bethe, A., Semmler, T., Guenther, S., Wieler, L.H., 2012. Extended-spectrum β-lactamase-producing and AmpC-producing *Escherichia coli* from livestock and companion animals, and their putative impact on public health: a global perspective. Clinical Microbiology and Infections 18 (7), 646–655.

Ewers, C., Grobbel, M., Stamm, I., Kopp, P.A., Diehl, I., Semmler, T., Fruth, A., Beutlich, J., Guerra, B., Wieler, L.H., Guenther, S., 2010. Emergence of human pandemic O25:H4-ST131 CTX-M-15 extended-spectrumbeta-lactamase-producing *Escherichia coli* among companion animals. Journal of Antimicrobial Chemotherapy 65, 651–660.

Ewers, C., Li, G., Wilking, H., Kießling, S., Alt, K., Antáo, E.M., Laturnus, C., Diehl, I., Glodde, S., Homeier, T., Böhnke, U., 2007. Avian pathogenic, uropathogenic, and newborn meningitis-causing *Escherichia coli*: how closely related are they? International Journal of Medical Microbiology 297 (3), 163–176.

Fernandes, M.R., McCulloch, J.A., Vianello, M.A., Moura, Q., Pérez-Chaparro, P.J., Esposito, F., Sartori, L., Dropa, M., Matté, M.H., Lira, D.P., Mamizuka, E.M., 2016. First report of the globally disseminated IncX4 plasmid carrying the mcr-1 gene in a colistin-resistant *Escherichia coli* sequence type 101 isolate from a human infection in Brazil. Antimicrobial Agents and Chemotherapy 60 (10), 6415–6417.

Fischer, J., Rodríguez, I., Schmoger, S., Friese, A., Roesler, U., Helmuth, R., Guerra, B., 2012. *Escherichia coli* producing VIM-1 carbapenemase isolated on a pig farm. Journal of Antimicrobial Chemotherapy 67 (7), 1793–1795.

Franz, E., van Bruggen, A.H., 2008. Ecology of E. coli O157: H7 and *Salmonella enterica* in the primary vegetable production chain. Critical Reviews in Microbiology 34 (3e4), 143e161.

Freitag, C., Michael, G.B., Kadlec, K., Hassel, M., Schwarz, S., 2017. Detection of plasmid-borne extended-spectrum β-lactamase (ESBL) genes in *Escherichia coli* isolates from bovine mastitis. Veterinary Microbiology 200, 151–156.

Friese, A., Schulz, J., Laube, H., Hartung, J., Roesler, U., 2013. Faecal occurrence and emissions of livestock-associated methicillin-resistant *Staphylococcus aureus* (laMRSA) and ESbl/AmpC-producing E. coli from animal farms in Germany. Berliner und Münchener Tierärztliche Wochenschrift 126 (3–4), 175–180.

García-Cobos, S., Köck, R., Mellmann, A., Frenzel, J., Friedrich, A.W., Rossen, J.W., 2015. Molecular typing of Enterobacteriaceae from pig holdings in North-Western Germany reveals extended-spectrum and AmpC β-lactamases producing but no carbapenem resistant ones. PLoS One 10 (7), e0134533.

Garcia-Migura, L., Hendriksen, R.S., Fraile, L., Aarestrup, F.M., 2014. Antimicrobial resistance of zoonotic and commensal bacteria in Europe: the missing link between consumption and resistance in veterinary medicine. Veterinary Microbiology 170 (1–2), 1–9.

Geser, N., Stephan, R., Hächler, H., 2012. Occurrence and characteristics of extended-spectrum β-lactamase (ESBL) producing Enterobacteriaceae in food producing animals, minced meat and raw milk. BMC Veterinary Research 8 (1), 21.

Ghosh, P., Mahanti, A., Samanta, I., Joardar, S.N., Batabyal, K., Dey, S., Taraphder, S., Isore, D.P., 2017. Occurrence of extended-spectrum- cephalosporinase producing *Escherichia coli* in kuroiler birds. Veterinarski Arhiv 87 (6), 745–757.

Gonzalez-Zorn, B., Teshager, T., Casas, M., Porrero, M.C., Moreno, M.A., Courvalin, P., Dominguez, L., 2005. *armA* and aminoglycoside resistance in *Escherichia coli*. Emerging Infectious Diseases 11, 954–956.

Grape, M., Sundström, L., Kronvall, G., 2003. Sulphonamide resistance gene sul3 found in *Escherichia coli* isolates from human sources. Journal of Antimicrobial Chemotherapy 52 (6), 1022–1024.

Hammerum, A.E., Heuer, O.E., 2009. Human health hazards from antimicrobial-resistant *Escherichia coli* of animal origin. Clinical Infectious Diseases 48, 916–921.

Hammerum, A.M., Sandvang, D., Andersen, S.R., Seyfarth, A.M., Porsbo, L.J., Frimodt-Møller, N., Heuer, O.E., 2006. Detection of sul1, sul2 and sul3 in sulphonamide resistant *Escherichia coli* isolates obtained from healthy humans, pork and pigs in Denmark. International Journal of Food Microbiology 106 (2), 235–237.

Hanon, J.B., Jaspers, S., Butaye, P., Wattiau, P., Méroc, E., Aerts, M., Imberechts, H., Vermeersch, K., Van der Stede, Y., 2015. A trend analysis of antimicrobial resistance in commensal *Escherichia coli* from several livestock species in Belgium (2011–2014). Preventive Veterinary Medicine 122 (4), 443–452.

Hansen, K.H., Bortolaia, V., Nielsen, C.A., Nielsen, J.B., Schønning, K., Agersø, Y., Guardabassi, L., 2016. Host-specific patterns of genetic diversity among IncI1-Iγ and IncK plasmids encoding CMY-2 β-lactamase in *Escherichia coli* isolates from humans, poultry meat, poultry, and dogs in Denmark. Applied and Environmental Microbiology 82 (15), 4705–4714.

Hering, J., Hille, K., Frömke, C., von Münchhausen, C., Hartmann, M., Schneider, B., Friese, A., Roesler, U., Merle, R., Kreienbrock, L., 2014. Prevalence and potential risk factors for the occurrence of cefotaxime resistant *Escherichia coli* in German fattening pig farms-a cross-sectional study. Preventive Veterinary Medicine 116 (1–2), 129–137.

Ho, P.L., Ng, K.Y., Lo, W.U., Law, P.Y., Lai, E.L.Y., Wang, Y., Chow, K.H., 2016. Plasmid-mediated OqxAB is an important mechanism for nitrofurantoin resistance in *Escherichia coli*. Antimicrobial Agents and Chemotherapy 60 (1), 537–543.

Hopkins, K.L., Davies, R.H., Threlfall, J., 2005. Mechanisms of quinolone resistance in *Escherichia coli* and *Salmonella*: recent developments. International Journal of Antimicrobial Agents 25, 358–373.

Hordijk, J., Mevius, D.J., Kant, A., Bos, M.E.H., Graveland, H., Bosman, A.B., et al., 2013. Within-farm dynamics of ESBL/AmpC-producing *Escherichia coli* in veal calves: a longitudinal approach. Journal of Antimicrobial Chemotherapy 68, 2468e2476.

Horigan, V., Kosmider, R.D., Horton, R.A., Randall, L., Simons, R.R.L., 2016. An assessment of evidence data gaps in the investigation of possible transmission routes of extended spectrum β-lactamase producing *Escherichia coli* from livestock to humans in the UK. Preventive Veterinary Medicine 124, 1–8.

Interaminense, J.A., Nascimento, D.C.O., Ventura, R.F., Batista, J.E.C., Souza, M.M.C., Hazin, F.H.V., Pontes-Filho, N.T., Lima-Filho, J.V., 2010. Recovery and screening for antibiotic susceptibility of potential bacterial pathogens from the oral cavity of shark species involved in attacks on humans in Recife, Brazil. Journal of Medical Microbiology 59 (8), 941–947.

Jensen, V.F., Jakobsen, L., Emborg, H.D., Seyfarth, A.M., Hammerum, A.M., 2006. Correlation between apramycin and gentamicin use in pigs and an increasing reservoir of gentamicin-resistant *Escherichia coli*. Journal of Antimicrobial Chemotherapy 58 (1), 101–107.

Jobbins, S.E., Alexander, K.A., 2015. From whence they came-antibiotic-resistant *Escherichia coli* in African wildlife. Journal of Wildlife Diseases 51 (4), 811–820.

Johns, I., Verheyen, K., Good, L., Rycroft, A., 2012. Antimicrobial resistance in faecal *Escherichia coli* isolates from horses treated with antimicrobials: a longitudinal study in hospitalised and non-hospitalised horses. Veterinary Microbiology 159, 381–389.

Johnson, J.R., Miller, S., Johnston, B., Clabots, C., DebRoy, C., 2009. Sharing of *Escherichia coli* sequence type ST131 and other multidrug-resistant and urovirulent *E. coli* strains among dogs and cats within a household. Journal of Clinical Microbiology 47 (11), 3721–3725.

Jørgensen, C.J., Cavaco, L.M., Hasman, H., Emborg, H.D., Guardabassi, L., 2007. Occurrence of CTX-M-1-producing *Escherichia coli* in pigs treated with ceftiofur. Journal of Antimicrobial Chemotherapy 59 (5), 1040–1042.

Kao, C.Y., Udval, U., Wu, H.M., Bolormaa, E., Yan, J.J., Khosbayar, T., Wu, J.J., 2016. First characterization of fluoroquinolone resistance mechanisms in CTX-M-producing *Escherichia coli* from Mongolia. Infection, Genetics and Evolution 38, 79.

Kar, D., Bandyopadhyay, S., Bhattacharyya, D., Samanta, I., Mahanti, A., Nanda, P.K., Mondal, B., Dandapat, P., Das, A.K., Dutta, T.K., Bandyopadhyay, S., 2015. Molecular and phylogenetic characterization of multidrug resistant extended spectrum beta-lactamase producing *Escherichia coli* isolated from poultry and cattle in Odisha, India. Infection, Genetics and Evolution 29, 82–90.

Karah, N., Poirel, L., Bengtsson, S., Sundqvist, M., Kahlmeter, G., Nordmann, P., Sundsfjord, A., Samuelsen, O., 2010. Plasmid-mediated quinolone resistance determinants qnr and aac(6-)-Ib-cr in *Escherichia coli* and *Klebsiella* spp. from Norway and Sweden. Diagnostic Microbiology and Infectious Disease 66, 425–431.

Kawoosa, S.S., Samanta, I., Wani, S.A., 2007. In vitro drug sensitivity profile of stx and eaeA positive *Escherichia coli* from diarrhoeic calves in Kashmir valley. Indian Journal of Animal Sciences 77 (7), 573–575.

Kluytmans, J.A., Overdevest, I.T., Willemsen, I., Kluytmans-Van Den Bergh, M.F., Van Der Zwaluw, K., Heck, M., Rijnsburger, M., Vandenbroucke-Grauls, C.M., Savelkoul, P.H., Johnston, B.D., Gordon, D., 2012. Extended-Spectrum β-lactamase—producing *Escherichia coli* from retail chicken meat and humans: comparison of strains, plasmids, resistance genes, and virulence factors. Clinical Infectious Diseases 56 (4), 478–487.

Lavoie, J.P., Couture, L., Higgins, R., Laverty, S., 1991. Aerobic bacterial isolates in horses in a university hospital, 1986–1988. Canadian Veterinary Journal 32, 292–294.

Le Gall, T., Clermont, O., Gouriou, S., Picard, B., Nassif, X., Denamur, E., Tenaillon, O., 2007. Extraintestinal virulence is a coincidental by-product of commensalism in B2 phylogenetic group *Escherichia coli* strains. Molecular Biology and Evolution 24, 2373–2384.

Leverstein-van Hall, M.A., Dierikx, C.M., Cohen Stuart, J., Voets, G.M., van den Munckhof, M.P., van Essen-Zandbergen, A., Platteel, T., Fluit, A.C., van de Sande-Bruinsma, N., Scharinga, J., Bonten, M.J., Mevius, D.J., 2011. Dutch patients, retail chicken meat and poultry share the same ESBL genes, plasmids and strains. Clinical Microbiology and Infections 17, 873–880.

Li, A., Yang, Y., Miao, M., Chavda, K.D., Mediavilla, J.R., Xie, X., Feng, P., Tang, Y.W., Kreiswirth, B.N., Chen, L., Du, H., 2016. Complete sequences of *mcr-1*-harboring plasmids from extended spectrum β-lactamase- and carbapenemase-producing *Enterobacteriaceae*. Antimicrobial Agents and Chemotherapy 60 (7), 4351–4354.

Liu, B.T., Yang, Q.E., Li, L., Sun, J., Liao, X.P., Fang, L.X., Yang, S.S., Deng, H., Liu, Y.H., 2013. Dissemination and characterization of plasmids carrying *oqxAB-bla*CTX−M genes in *Escherichia coli* isolates from food-producing animals. PLoS One 8, e73947.

Liu, S., Jin, D., Lan, R., Wang, Y., Meng, Q., Dai, H., Lu, S., Hu, S., Xu, J., 2015. Escherichia marmotae sp. nov., isolated from faeces of Marmota himalayana. International Journal of Systematic and Evolutionary Microbiology 65 (7), 2130–2134.

Liu, Y.Y., Wang, Y., Walsh, T.R., Yi, L.X., Zhang, R., Spencer, J., Doi, Y., Tian, G., Dong, B., Huang, X., Yu, L.F., 2016. Emergence of plasmid-mediated colistin resistance mechanism MCR-1 in animals and human beings in China: a microbiological and molecular biological study. The Lancet Infectious Diseases 16 (2), 161–168.

Lo, W.U., Chow, K.H., Law, P.Y., Ng, K.Y., Cheung, Y.Y., Lai, E.L., Ho, P.L., 2014. Highly conjugative IncX4 plasmids carrying *bla*CTX-M in *Escherichia coli* from humans and food animals. Journal of Medical Microbiology 63, 835–840.

Machado, E., Coque, T.M., Canton, R., Sousa, J.C., Peixe, L., 2008. Antibiotic resistance integrons and extended-spectrum β-lactamases among Enterobacteriaceae isolates recovered from chickens and swine in Portugal. Journal of Antimicrobial Chemotherapy 62 (2), 296–302.

Maciuca, I.E., Williams, N.J., Tuchilus, C., Dorneanu, O., Guguianu, E., Carp-Carare, C., Rimbu, C., Timofte, D., 2015. High prevalence of *Escherichia coli*-producing CTX-M-15 extended-spectrum beta-lactamases in poultry and human clinical isolates in Romania. Microbial Drug Resistance 21 (6), 651–662.

Mahanti, A., Samanta, I., Bandopaddhay, S., Joardar, S.N., Dutta, T.K., Batabyal, S., Sar, T.K., Isore, D.P., 2013. Isolation, molecular characterization and antibiotic resistance of Shiga Toxin–Producing *Escherichia coli* (STEC) from buffalo in India. Letters in Applied Microbiology 56 (4), 291–298.

Mahanti, A., Samanta, I., Bandyopadhyay, S., Joardar, S.N., 2015. Molecular characterization and antibiotic susceptibility pattern of caprine Shiga toxin producing-*Escherichia coli* (STEC) isolates from India. Iranian Journal of Veterinary Research 16 (1), 31.

Mahanti, A., Samanta, I., Bandyopadhyay, S., Joardar, S.N., Dutta, T.K., Sar, T.K., 2014. Isolation, molecular characterization and antibiotic resistance of Enterotoxigenic *E. coli* (ETEC) and Necrotoxigenic *E. coli* (NTEC) from healthy water buffalo. Veterinarski Arhiv 84 (3), 241–250.

Maamar, E., Hammami, S., Alonso, C.A., Dakhli, N., Abbassi, M.S., Ferjani, S., Hamzaoui, Z., Saidani, M., Torres, C., Boubaker, I.B.B., 2016. High prevalence of extended-spectrum and plasmidic AmpC beta-lactamase-producing *Escherichia coli* from poultry in Tunisia. International Journal of Food Microbiology 231, 69–75.

Marcade, G., Deschamps, C., Boyd, A., Gautier, V., Picard, B., Branger, C., Denamur, E., Arlet, G., 2009. Replicon typing of plasmids in *Escherichia coli* producing extended-spectrum beta-lactamases. Journal of Antimicrobial Chemotherapy 63, 67–71.

Mc Nulty, K., Soon, J.M., Wallace, C.A., Nastasijevic, I., 2016. Antimicrobial resistance monitoring and surveillance in the meat chain: a report from five countries in the European Union and European Economic Area. Trends in Food Science and Technology 58, 1–13.

Meyer, E., Gastmeier, P., Kola, A., Schwab, F., 2012. Pet animals and foreign travel are risk factors for colonisation with extended-spectrum β-lactamase-producing *Escherichia coli*. Infection 40, 685–687.

Michael, G.B., Kaspar, H., Siqueira, A.K., de Freitas Costa, E., Corbellini, L.G., Kadlec, K., Schwarz, S., 2017. Extended-spectrum β-lactamase (ESBL)-producing *Escherichia coli* isolates collected from diseased food-producing animals in the GERM-Vet monitoring program 2008–2014. Veterinary Microbiology 200, 142–150.

Mo, S.S., Kristoffersen, A.B., Sunde, M., Nødtvedt, A., Norström, M., 2016. Risk factors for occurrence of cephalosporin-resistant *Escherichia coli* in Norwegian broiler flocks. Preventive Veterinary Medicine 130, 112–118.

Mora, A., Herrera, A., Mamani, R., López, C., Alonso, M.P., Blanco, J.E., Blanco, M., Dahbi, G., García-Garrote, F., Pita, J.M., Coira, A., 2010. Recent emergence of clonal group O25b: K1: H4-B2-ST131 ibeA strains among *Escherichia coli* poultry isolates, including CTX-M-9-producing strains, and comparison with clinical human isolates. Applied and Environmental Microbiology 76 (21), 6991–6997.

Mulvey, M.R., Susky, E., McCracken, M., Morck, D.W., Read, R.R., 2009. Similar cefoxitin-resistance plasmids circulating in *Escherichia coli* from human and animal sources. Veterinary Microbiology 134, 279–287.

Navajas-Benito, E.V., Alonso, C.A., Sanz, S., Olarte, C., Martínez-Olarte, R., Hidalgo-Sanz, S., Somalo, S., Torres, C., 2017. Molecular characterization of antibiotic resistance in *Escherichia coli* strains from a dairy cattle farm and its surroundings. Journal of the Science of Food and Agriculture 97 (1), 362–365.

Nicolas-Chanoine, M.H., Bertrand, X., Madec, J.Y., 2014. *Escherichia coli* ST131, an intriguing clonal group. Clinical Microbiology Reviews 27 (3), 543–574.

Norizuki, C., Wachino, J.-I., Suzuki, M., Kawamura, K., Nagano, N., Kimura, K., Arakawa, Y., 2017. Specific *bla*CTX-M-8/IncI1 plasmid transfer among genetically diverse *Escherichia coli* isolates between humans and chickens. Antimicrobial Agents and Chemotherapy 61 e00663-17.

Noyes, N.R., Yang, X., Linke, L.M., Magnuson, R.J., Dettenwanger, A., Cook, S., Geornaras, I., Woerner, D.E., Gow, S.P., McAllister, T.A., Yang, H., 2016. Resistome diversity in cattle and the environment decreases during beef production. Elife 5.

Overdevest, I., Willemsen, I., Rijnsburger, M., Eustace, A., Xu, L., Hawkey, P., Heck, M., Savelkoul, P., Vandenbroucke-Grauls, C., van der Zwaluw, K., Huijsdens, X., 2011. Extended-spectrum β-lactamase genes of *Escherichia coli* in chicken meat and humans, the Netherlands. Emerging Infectious Diseases 17 (7), 1216.

Paterson, D.L., Egea, P., Pascual, A., López-Cerero, L., Navarro, M.D., Adams-Haduch, J.M., Qureshi, Z.A., Sidjabat, H.E., Rodríguez-Baño, J., 2010. Extended-spectrum and CMY-type β-lactamase-producing *Escherichia coli* in clinical samples and retail meat from Pittsburgh, USA and Seville, Spain. Clinical Microbiology and Infections 16 (1), 33–38.

Petersen, A., Andersen, J.S., Kaewmak, T., Somsiri, T., Dalsgaard, A., 2002. Impact of integrated fish farming on antimicrobial resistance in a pond environment. Applied and Environmental Microbiology 68 (12), 6036–6042.

Petternel, C., Galler, H., Zarfel, G., Luxner, J., Haas, D., Grisold, A.J., Reinthaler, F.F., Feierl, G., 2014. Isolation and characterization of multidrug-resistant bacteria from minced meat in Austria. Food Microbiology 44, 41–46.

Picard, B., Garcia, J.S., Gouriou, S., Duriez, P., Brahimi, N., Bingen, E., Elion, J., Denamur, E., 1999. The link between phylogeny and virulence in *Escherichia coli* extraintestinal infection. Infection and Immunity 67 (2), 546–553.

Pitout, J.D., Laupland, K.B., 2008. Extended-spectrum beta-lactamase-producing *Enterobacteriaceae*: an emerging public-health concern. The Lancet Infectious Diseases 8, 159–166.

Pitout, J.D., Wei, Y., Church, D.L., Gregson, D.B., 2008. Surveillance for plasmid-mediated quinolone resistance determinants in Enterobacteriaceae within the Calgary Health Region, Canada: the emergence of aac (6')-Ib-cr. Journal of Antimicrobial Chemotherapy 61 (5), 999–1002.

Platell, J.L., Cobbold, R.N., Johnson, J.R., Trott, D.J., 2010. Clonal group distribution of fluoroquinolone-resistant *Escherichia coli* among humans and companion animals in Australia. Journal of Antimicrobial Chemotherapy 65 (9), 1936–1938.

Platell, J.L., Johnson, J.R., Cobbold, R.N., Trott, D.J., 2011. Multidrug-resistant extraintestinal pathogenic *Escherichia coli* of sequence type ST131 in animals and foods. Veterinary Microbiology 153 (1–2), 99–108.

Poirel, L., Héritier, C., Spicq, C., Nordmann, P., 2004. In vivo acquisition of high-level resistance to imipenem in *Escherichia coli*. Journal of Clinical Microbiology 42, 3831–3833.

Pomba, C., da Fonseca, J.D., Baptista, B.C., Correia, J.D., Martínez-Martínez, L., 2009. Detection of the pandemic O25-ST131 human virulent *Escherichia coli* CTX-M-15-producing clone harboring the qnrB2 and aac (6')-Ib-cr genes in a dog. Antimicrobial Agents and Chemotherapy 53 (1), 327–328.

Qiao, M., Ying, G.G., Singer, A.C., Zhu, Y.G., 2018. Review of antibiotic resistance in China and its environment. Environment International 110, 160–172.

Randall, L., Heinrich, K., Horton, R., Brunton, L., Sharman, M., Bailey-Horne, V., Sharma, M., McLaren, I., Coldham, N., Teale, C., Jones, J., 2014. Detection of antibiotic residues and association of cefquinome residues with the occurrence of Extended-Spectrum β-Lactamase (ESBL)-producing bacteria in waste milk samples from dairy farms in England and Wales in 2011. Research in Veterinary Science 96 (1), 15–24.

Randall, L.P., Lodge, M.P., Elviss, N.C., Lemma, F.L., Hopkins, K.L., Teale, C.J., Woodford, N., 2017. Evaluation of meat, fruit and vegetables from retail stores in five United Kingdom regions as sources of extended-spectrum beta-lactamase (ESBL)-producing and carbapenem-resistant *Escherichia coli*. International Journal of Food Microbiology 241, 283–290.

Rodríguez-Bano, J., López-Cerero, L., Navarro, M.D., Díaz de Alba, P., Pascual, A., 2008. Faecal carriage of extended-spectrum β-lactamase-producing *Escherichia coli*: prevalence, risk factors and molecular epidemiology. Journal of Antimicrobial Chemotherapy 62, 1142e1149.

Rogers, B.A., Sidjabat, H.E., Paterson, D.L., 2011. *Escherichia coli* O25b-ST131: a pandemic, multiresistant, community-associated strain. Journal of Antimicrobial Chemotherapy 66, 1–14.

Rossi, F., Rizzotti, L., Felis, G.E., Torriani, S., 2014. Horizontal gene transfer among microorganisms in food: current knowledge and future perspectives. Food Microbiology 42, 232–243.

Sabia, C., Stefani, S., Messi, P., de Niederhäusern, S., Bondi, M., Condò, C., Iseppi, R., Anacarso, I., 2017. Extended-spectrum B-lactamase and plasmid-mediated AMPC genes in swine and ground pork. Journal of Food Safety 37 (1).

Şahintürk, P., Arslan, E., Büyükcangaz, E., Sonal, S., Sen, A., Ersoy, F., Webber, M.A., Piddock, L.J., Cengiz, M., 2016. High level fluoroquinolone resistance in *Escherichia coli* isolated from animals in Turkey is due to multiple mechanisms. Turkish Journal of Veterinary and Animal Sciences 40 (2), 214–218.

Samanta, I., Joardar, S.N., Das, P.K., Das, P., Sar, T.K., Dutta, T.K., Bandyopadhyay, S., Batabyal, S., Isore, D.P., 2014. Virulence repertoire, characterization, and antibiotic resistance pattern analysis of *Escherichia coli* isolated from backyard layers and their environment in India. Avian Diseases 58 (1), 39–45.

Samanta, I., Joardar, S.N., Mahanti, A., Bandyopadhyay, S., Sar, T.K., Dutta, T.K., 2015. Approaches to characterize extended spectrum beta-lactamase/beta-lactamase producing *Escherichia coli* in healthy organized vis-à-vis backyard farmed pigs in India. Infection, Genetics and Evolution 36, 224–230.

Sannes, M.R., Belongia, E.A., Kieke, B., Smith, K., Kieke, A., Vandermause, M., Bender, J., Clabots, C., Winokur, P., Johnson, J.R., 2008. Predictors of antimicrobial-resistant *Escherichia coli* in the feces of vegetarians and newly hospitalized adults in Minnesota and Wisconsin. The Journal of Infectious Diseases 197 (3), 430–434.

Schmidt, J.W., Agga, G.E., Bosilevac, J.M., Brichta-Harhay, D.M., Shackelford, S.D., Wang, R., Wheeler, T.L., Arthur, T.M., 2015. Occurrence of antimicrobial-resistant *Escherichia coli* and *Salmonella enterica* in the beef cattle production and processing continuum. Applied and Environmental Microbiology 81 (2), 713–725.

Seiffert, S.N., Hilty, M., Perreten, V., Endimiani, A., 2013. Extended-spectrum cephalosporin-resistant Gram-negative organisms in livestock: an emerging problem for human health? Drug Resistance Updates 16 (1–2), 22–45.

Sennati, S., Santella, G., Di Conza, J., Pallecchi, L., Pino, M., Ghiglione, B., Rossolini, G.M., Radice, M., Gutkind, G., 2012. Changing epidemiology of extended-spectrum β-lactamases in Argentina: emergence of CTX-M-15. Antimicrobial Agents and Chemotherapy 56 (11), 6003–6005.

Shin, S.W., Shin, M.K., Jung, M., Belaynehe, K.M., Yoo, H.S., 2015. Prevalence of antimicrobial resistance and transfer of tetracycline resistance genes in *Escherichia coli* isolated from beef cattle. Applied and Environmental Microbiology. https://doi.org/10.1128/AEM.01511-15.

Shulman, S.T., Friedmann, H.C., Sims, R.H., 2007. Theodor Escherich: the first pediatric infectious diseases physician? Clinical infectious diseases 45 (8), 1025–1029.

Smet, A., Martel, A., Persoons, D., Dewulf, J., Heyndrickx, M., Herman, L., Haesebrouck, F., Butaye, P., 2010. Broad-spectrum β-lactamases among Enterobacteriaceae of animal origin: molecular aspects, mobility and impact on public health. FEMS Microbiology Reviews 34 (3), 295–316.

Smet, A., Rasschaert, G., Martel, A., Persoons, D., Dewulf, J., Butaye, P., Catry, B., Haesebrouck, F., Herman, L., Heyndrickx, M., 2011. In situ ESBL conjugation from avian to human *Escherichia coli* during cefotaxime administration. Journal of Applied Microbiology 110 (2), 541–549.

Sørensen, A.H., Hansen, L.H., Johannesen, E., Sørensen, S.J., 2003. Conjugative plasmid conferring resistance to olaquindox. Antimicrobial Agents and Chemotherapy 47 (2), 798–799.

Stokes, M.O., Cottell, J.L., Piddock, L.J.V., Wu, G., Wootton, M., Mevius, D.J., Randall, L.P., Teale, C.J., Fielder, M.D., Coldham, N.G., 2012. Detection and characterization of pCT-like plasmid vectors for bla CTX-M-14 in *Escherichia coli* isolates from humans, turkeys and cattle in England and Wales. Journal of Antimicrobial Chemotherapy 67 (7), 1639–1644.

SVARM, 2014. Consumption of Antibiotics and Occurrence of Antibiotic Resistance in Sweden. http://www.sva.se/globalassets/redesign2011/pdf/om_sva/publikationer/swedres_svarm2014.pdf.

Tadesse, D.A., Zhao, S., Tong, E., Ayers, S., Singh, A., Bartholomew, M.J., McDermott, P.F., 2012. Antimicrobial drug resistance in *Escherichia coli* from humans and food animals, United States, 1950–2002. Emerging Infectious Diseases 18 (5), 741.

Teshager, T., Domınguez, L., Moreno, M.A., Saénz, Y., Torres, C., Cardeñosa, S., 2000. Isolation of an SHV-12 β-lactamase-producing *Escherichia coli* strain from a dog with recurrent urinary tract infections. Antimicrobial Agents and Chemotherapy 44 (12), 3483–3484.

Thaller, M.C., Migliore, L., Marquez, C., Tapia, W., Cedeño, V., Rossolini, G.M., Gentile, G., 2010. Tracking acquired antibiotic resistance in commensal bacteria of Galapagos land iguanas: no man, no resistance. PLoS One 5 (2), e8989.

Veldman, K., van Essen-Zandbergen, A., Rapallini, M., Wit, B., Heymans, R., van Pelt, W., Mevius, D., 2016. Location of colistin resistance gene mcr-1 in Enterobacteriaceae from livestock and meat. Journal of Antimicrobial Chemotherapy 71 (8), 2340–2342.

Vogt, D., Overesch, G., Endimiani, A., Collaud, A., Thomann, A., Perreten, V., 2014. Occurrence and genetic characteristics of third-generation cephalosporin-resistant *Escherichia coli* in Swiss retail meat. Microbial Drug Resistance 20 (5), 485–494.

Wachino, J., Shibayama, K., Kurokawa, H., Kimura, K., Yamane, K., Suzuki, S., Shibata, N., Ike, Y., Arakawa, Y., 2007. Novel plasmid-mediated 16S rRNA m1A1408 methyl transferase, *NpmA*, found in a clinically isolated *Escherichia coli* strain resistant to structurally diverse aminoglycosides. Antimicrobial Agents and Chemotherapy 51, 4401–4409.

Walsh, C., Duffy, G., Nally, P., O'Mahony, R., McDowell, D.A., Fanning, S., 2008. Transfer of ampicillin resistance from *Salmonella* Typhimurium DT104 to *Escherichia coli* K12 in food. Letters in Applied Microbiology 46 (2), 210–215.

Wani, S.A., Bhat, M.A., Samanta, I., Buchh, A.S., 2004. In vitro drug sensitivity profile and characterization of *Escherichia coli* isolated from diarrhoeic chicken in Kashmir valley. Indian Journal of Animal Sciences 74 (8), 818–821.

Warren, R.E., Ensor, V.M., O'neill, P., Butler, V., Taylor, J., Nye, K., Harvey, M., Livermore, D.M., Woodford, N., Hawkey, P.M., 2008. Imported chicken meat as a potential source of quinolone-resistant *Escherichia coli* producing extended-spectrum β-lactamases in the UK. Journal of Antimicrobial Chemotherapy 61 (3), 504–508.

WHO, 2007. Critically Important Antimicrobials for Human Medicine: Categorization for the Development of Risk Management Strategies to Contain Antimicrobial Resistance Due to Non-Human Antimicrobial Use: Report of the Second WHO Expert Meeting, Copenhagen, 29–31 May 2007.

WHO, 2018. http://www.who.int/mediacentre/factsheets/fs125/en/.

Winokur, P.L., Vonstein, D.L., Hoffman, L.J., Uhlenhopp, E.K., Doern, G.V., 2001. Evidence for transfer of CMY-2 AmpC β-lactamase plasmids between *Escherichia coli* and Salmonella isolates from food animals and humans. Antimicrobial Agents and Chemotherapy 45, 2716–2722.

Wu, G., Day, M.J., Mafura, M.T., Nunez-Garcia, J., Fenner, J.J., Sharma, M., van Essen-Zandbergen, A., Rodríguez, I., Dierikx, C., Kadlec, K., Schink, A.-K., Wain, J., Helmuth, R., Guerra, B., Schwarz, S., Threlfall, J., Woodward, M.J., Woodford, N., Coldham, N., Mevius, D., 2013. Comparative analysis of ESBL-positive *Escherichia coli* isolates from animals and humans from the UK, The Netherlands and Germany. PLoS One 8, e75392.

Yan, J.J., Hong, C.Y., Ko, W.C., Chen, Y.J., Tsai, S.H., Chuang, C.L., Wu, J.J., 2004. Dissemination of blaCMY-2 among *Escherichia coli* isolates from food animals, retail ground meats, and humans in southern Taiwan. Antimicrobial Agents and Chemotherapy 48 (4), 1353–1356.

Yu, F.Y., Yao, D., Pan, J.Y., Chen, C., Qin, Z.Q., Parsons, C., Yang, L.H., Li, Q.Q., Zhang, X.Q., Qu, D., Wang, L.X., 2010. High prevalence of plasmid-mediated 16S rRNA methylase gene *rmtB* among *Escherichia coli* clinical isolates from a Chinese teaching hospital. BMC Infectious Diseases 10, p184.

Yue, L., Jiang, H.X., Liao, X.P., Liu, J.H., Li, S.J., Chen, X.Y., Chen, C.X., Lü, D.H., Liu, Y.H., 2008. Prevalence of plasmid-mediated quinolone resistance qnr genes in poultry and swine clinical isolates of *Escherichia coli*. Veterinary Microbiology 132 (3–4), 414–420.

Zhang, Q.Q., Ying, G.G., Pan, C.G., Liu, Y.S., Zhao, J.L., 2015. Comprehensive evaluation of antibiotics emission and fate in the river basins of China: source analysis, multimedia modeling, and linkage to bacterial resistance. Environmental Science and Technology 49 (11), 6772–6782.

Chapter 16

Staphylococcus

Chapter outline

Sir Alexander Ogston, a physician from Scotland, first elucidated the precise role of *Micrococcus* in formation of pus (Ogston, 1880). He proposed the name '*Staphylococcus*' (Greek 'staphyle' means bunch of grapes and 'kokkos' means berry). Anton J. Rosenbach isolated two different species of *Staphylococcus* and named them according to the pigmented appearance of colonies i.e., *S. aureus* (Latin 'aurum' means gold) and *S. albus* (Latin 'albus' means white) (Rosenbach, 1884). Experiments of Bumm (1885) established the relationship of *Staphylococcus* with human infections. Nocard (1887) and Guillebeau (1890) isolated *Staphylococcus* from mastitis in sheep and cattle, respectively and established its pathogenic role in animals (Jonsson and Wadstorm, 1993).

Staphylococcus aureus is a commensal as well as a human or animal pathogen. Approximately 30% of the human population is colonized with *S. aureus* specially in skin, nose and mucous membrane (Wertheim et al., 2005). In human, *S. aureus* is associated with folliculitis, furuncles, carbuncles, impetigo, wound infections, scalded skin syndrome, pneumonia, endocarditis, bone and joint infections, toxic shock syndrome, mastitis, food poisoning and rarely urinary tract infection (0.5%–1%). In livestock, *S. aureus* is the key etiology of mastitis in cattle, buffalo, sheep, goat and other ruminants, lethal systemic infections in rabbits, and bumble foot (ulcerative pododermatitis) in poultry.

Emergence of antibiotic resistant *Staphylococcus* (penicillin resistant) began in human patients during mid-1940s after the introduction of penicillin (Kirby, 1944). Penicillin-resistant *Staphylococcus* became pandemic during 1950–60 with the spread of a specific *Staphylococcus* clone (phage-type 80/81) (Blair and Carr, 1960). Since then, 90%–95% of *S. aureus* strains are detected as penicillin resistant with the production of penicillinase throughout the world. Introduction of methicillin (penicillinase resistant) although cleared the phage type 80/81from the population, methicillin resistant

Antimicrobial Resistance in Agriculture. https://doi.org/10.1016/B978-0-12-815770-1.00016-X

S. aureus (MRSA) appeared in 1961 (Barber, 1961). The earliest MRSA strain (COL) was reported from three human patients in Colindale, United Kingdom (Jevons, 1961). MRSA infection was restricted among hospitalized and immunocompromised patients till 1980. In late 1980s and 1990s, the ancient COL-MRSA strains disappeared from the European population and descendent strains (Iberian, Rome clones) appeared causing endemic infections in Europe and United States (Peacock et al., 1980; Mato et al., 2004).Currently, community associated-MRSA infection is a major concern in United States, Asia, Canada, South America, Australia and Europe. It is estimated that 53 million people globally may be colonized with MRSA (Grundmann et al., 2006). In United States and European Union, MRSA caused infection of about 80,000 and 150,000 persons annually, respectively (Köck et al., 2010; Dantes et al., 2013). First report of MRSA infection in animals was obtained from Belgium describing the association of MRSA with clinical mastitis in dairy cattle (Devriese et al., 1972). An emerging MRSA clone (ST398) was detected in pigs and farmers in contact in the Netherlands and other European countries (Fluit, 2012).

Properties

Morphology: Staphylococci are gram positive cocci, capsulated, non-sporing and non-motile. Each coccus cell is 1 μm in diameter. They are arranged in a group or grape like cluster as cell division occurs in more than one plane. During preparation of smear and staining the cluster is sometimes broken and cocci are seen in pair or single (Fig. 16.1). Staphylococcal capsule is polysaccharide in nature. The capsule can inhibit phagocytosis and helps in virulence. Staphylococcal cell wall contains three major components i.e., peptidoglycan (PG), teichoic acid (TA) and surface proteins.

(a) Peptidoglycan (PG): PG is a polymer of glucosamine and muramic acid cross linked by pentaglycine (L-glycine) bridge. This bridge is sequentially synthesized by Fem ABX non-ribosomal peptide transferases. In other gram positive bacteria these glucosamine and muramic acids are N-acetylated. In *Staphylococcus* they are O-acetylated making them resistant to lysozyme.
(b) Teichoic acids (TA): They are found in the cell wall of Staphylococci like other gram positive bacteria. TA is either peptidoglycan associated or sometimes present outside the cell. TA contains ribitol in *S. aureus* cell wall whereas glycerol in *S. epidermidis* and *S. intermedius*.
(c) Surface proteins: The surface proteins are known as 'microbial surface components recognizing adhesive matrix molecules'(MSCRAMMs) that mediate attachment of the bacteria to the host tissues and initiate colonization prior to an infection. This protein group includes fibronectin binding protein, clumping factors, collagen binding proteins etc. A kind of immunoglobulin binding protein is found in the surface of *S. aureus* known as 'Protein-A'. Carotenoid pigments present in the bacterial cell membrane produce golden colored colonies of *S. aureus* in agar plates.

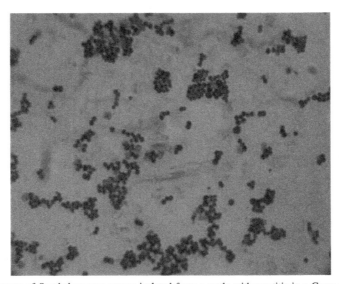

FIGURE 16.1   Appearance of *Staphylococcus aureus* isolated from a cattle with mastitis in a Gram –stained smear (100X).

Classification: *Staphylococcus* belongs to *Micrococcaceae* family and the genus contains 32 recognized species among them 13 are restricted to human and rest to the animals. Major pathogenic species are *Staphylococcus aureus*, *S. intermedius*, *S. pseudintermedius*, *S. hyicus*, *S. epidermidis*, *S. schleiferi* subsp. *coagulans*, *s. haemolyticus*, *S. delphini*.

S. aureus strains are further classified into several clonal complexes based on multilocus sequence typing (MLST) of housekeeping genes. The strains having identical sequences at all loci of the studied housekeeping genes are considered as a clone and designated with a unique sequence type (ST). The sequence types which vary in sequences at more than three loci are grouped into clonal complexes (CC). Assignment of ST/CC of the sequences can be done by eBURST algorithm (http://eburst.mlst.net).

Most of the methicillin sensitive *S. aureus* strains (88%) isolated worldwide belonged to 11 clonal complexes (CC1, CC5, CC8, CC9, CC12, CC15, CC22, CC25, CC30, CC45, CC51/121) (Enright et al., 2002). The first well characterized penicillin resistant *S. aureus* pandemic strain (phage type 80/81), originally isolated in Australia, belonged to CC30 group (Robinson et al., 2005). Preliminary methicillin resistant *S. aureus* (MRSA) strains (COL) belonged to CC8 (ST 250) which circulated in European population during 1970-80. Major human originated MRSA clones are CC1, CC5, CC8, CC22, CC30 and CC45 which were prevalent throughout the world even before the emergence of methicillin resistance (Gomes et al., 2006). Seventeen epidemic strains of human methicillin resistant *S. aureus* (EMRSA1-17) were described with frequent detection of EMRSA-15 and EMRSA-16 associated with clinical infection (Hardy et al., 2004). The hospital associated ST36 (EMRSA-16) clone in Australia and United Kingdom, and southwest pacific clone of community associated-MRSA (CA-MRSA) in Australia are considered as current descendant of CC30 (Johnson et al., 2001; Robinson et al., 2005). In United States and European countries, EMRSA-16 was detected as predominant strain associated with human clinical MRSA infection (Holden et al., 2004). The EMRSA-16 lineage was originated from sub-saharan Africa and was detected to cause hospital and community acquired infections in Algeria (Abdulgader et al., 2014).

The evolution of CA-MRSA strains are geographical location specific. For example, prevalent CA-MRSA clones in Europe, United Kingdom, Taiwan and Australia are ST 80, EMRSA-15 (ST 22) and EMRSA-16 (ST 36), ST 59 and ST 30, respectively (Chambers and DeLeo, 2009). African epidemic *S. aureus* (CA-MRSA) strains belonged to ST88-IV, ST5-IV and ST239-III (Breurec et al., 2011).

S. aureus clonal complexes present in livestock and poultry is still not well characterized. The most widely prevalent livestock associated MRSA (LA MRSA), belonged to CC 398 lineage, was described in pigs and other food animals in different parts of the world (Feßler et al., 2012). The LA MRSA was originated as methicillin sensitive *S. aureus* strains in human which acquired the methicillin and tetracycline resistance attributes from pigs and transferred back to human as MRSA (Price et al., 2012). In South-East Asia, ST 9 clonal complex is widely prevalent among farmed pigs (Yan et al., 2014).

Susceptibility to disinfectants: *Staphylococcus* can withstand drying for several weeks specially within pus or within the medium containing 7.5% salt concentration. Common disinfectants like phenol, mercuric chloride and several antimicrobials can destroy them. They are also sensitive to bacteriostatic dye like crystal violet (1: 500,000 concentration) and bile salts.

Natural habitat: Staphylococci are ubiquitously present in the environment such as in soil, water and air. The bacteria have the inherent ability to form biofilms on biotic and abiotic surfaces. All warm blooded animals and human can act as the reservoir. The bacteria reside in the external nares, nasal passage, saliva, skin, perineum, external genitalia, respiratory and intestinal tract of human and animals. Bovine udder is another important site of bacterial residence.

Genome

S. aureus genome is circular in shape and is 2.8−2.9 Mb in size with 33 mol% GC content. The genome is composed of core genome, accessory component and foreign genes, acquired by intra-species gene transfer. The core genome occupies 75% of the genome and is responsible for metabolism and housekeeping. Rest 25% of the genome consists of mobile genetic elements such as transposons and staphylococcal cassette chromosome (SCC). The genome also contains several genomic islands (GI) harbouring the foreign genes, and the genes associated with virulence (toxic shock syndrome toxin and enterotoxin) and antibiotic resistance. *S. aureus* GIs are composed of integrated prophage, *oriC* environ, *v*Sa (*v* = island). The *v*Sa has two classes i.e., *v*Sa*n* ('*n*' denotes location of the attachment site in the chromosome) and *v*Saα-*v*Saε. The *v*Sa*n* is associated with pathogenicity and resistance genes whereas, *v*Saα-*v*Saε contains genes encoding staphylococcal superantigens, exfoliative toxin, virulence gene regulators (T and U) (Hiramatsu et al., 2013). The plasmids of *S. aureus* belong to three classes. Class I plasmids are 1−5 kb and occur in high copy numbers (15−50 per cell). They usually encode a single antibiotic resistance determinant. Class II plasmids are of intermediate size and occur in intermediate copy numbers, and they usually encode for β-lactamase only. Class III consists of large conjugative plasmids (40−60 kb). It can carry multiple resistance determinants against trimethoprim, gentamycin and ethidium bromide.

Staphylococcal cassette chromosome *mec* (SCCmec), present in MRSA isolates confers resistance against methicillin. It is composed of *mecA* gene complex (encoding penicillin-binding protein 2a or PBP2a), regulation genes *mecR1* (signal transducer protein MecR1) and *mecI* (repressor protein MecI) and insertion sequences such as site-specific recombinase or cassette chromosome recombinase (ccrAB and/or ccrC) (Ito et al., 2001). J-regions (junkyard/joining region) containing pseudogenes and truncated copies of transposons and insertion sequences are also detected in SCC mec which encodes resistance against other antibiotics and heavy metals (IWG-SCC, 2009). The *mec* gene complex is further subdivided into five classes (A-E). Among the five classes, class A is considered as prototype which contains *mecA*, *mecR1* and *mecI* upstream of *mecA*, and the hypervariable region and insertion sequence (IS431) downstream of *mecA*. Animal originated (dairy cattle) *mecC* possessing *S. aureus* isolates belonged to different clonal types was prevalent in human and other animals (Cuny et al., 2010). SCCmec is so far classified into 11 types (I-XI) with numerous subtypes. Characteristics of major SCCmec types and their association with different kinds of MRSA infections are described in Table 16.1. Insertion sequences present in SCCmec were found responsible for resistance against non-β-lactam antibiotics such as macrolides and fluroquinolones (Gorwitz, 2008).

Antigenic characteristics

Serotyping of the Staphylococcal isolates is possible using the capsular antigen. The capsule is polysaccharide in nature. It can be subdivided into 12 types. Most animal (mastitic) and human clinical isolates of *S. aureus* produce thin microcapsule of five or eight type.

TABLE 16.1 Characteristics of SCCmec types.

Scc mec types	Size (Kb)	mec	ccr	Numbers of insertion sequences (IS431)	Numbers of transposons (Tn554)	Resistance to other antibiotics/chemicals	Type of infection
Type I	34	B	A1B1	1	0	None	Healthcare associated-MRSA infection
Type II	53	A	A2B2	2	1	Erythromycin, tobramycin	Healthcare associated-MRSA infection
Type III	67	A	A3B3	4	2	Erythromycin, tetracycline	Healthcare associated-MRSA infection
Type IV	21-24	B	A2B2	1	0	None	Community associated-MRSA/MRSE infection
Type V	28	C2	C	2	0	None	Community associated-MRSA/MRSH infection
Type VI	24	B	A4B4	1	0	None	-
Type VII	49	C1/C2	C2, C8	1	0	None	-
Type VIII	32	A	A4B4	1	1	Erythromycin	-
Type IX	-	C2	A1B1	1	-	Heavy metal	-
Type X	-	C1	A1B6	1	-	Heavy metal	-
Type XI	-	C	-	-	-	-	-

MRSE, Methicillin resistant *S. epidermidis*; *MRSH*, Methicillin resistant *S. haemolyticus.*

Toxins and virulence factors produced

(a) Alpha-toxin (α-haemolysin): This is the best characterized exotoxin produced by animal and human strains of Staphylococci. Specially, 20%−50% strains causing bovine mastitis produce α-toxin. It is encoded by *hla* gene. It causes lysis of red blood cells collected from several species such as rabbit, sheep and ox at 37°C by formation of pores in the cellular membrane. Through the pores cellular contents come out causing osmotic cytolysis. The toxin causes local tissue damage by interfering the macrophage function. It can act as a dermonecrotic toxin after injection into the skin of the rabbit and lethal to the rabbit if injected intravenously. It also causes lysis of leukocytes (leukocidal).

(b) Beta-toxin (β-haemolysin): It is a type of sphingomyelinase (phopholipase C) causing lysis of cellular membrane having higher content of sphingomyelin. It is encoded by *hlb* gene. It is produced by animal strains of Staphylococci specially those associated with bovine mastitis (75%−100% mastitis causing strains). This toxin enhances bacterial growth in the udder. It is also known as *hot cold lysin*. It produces a zone of incomplete haemolysis at 37°C in a blood agar plate prepared with red blood cells of cattle, sheep and goat. This haemolysis becomes clear and complete at 4°C. This type of haemolytic activity is referred as *hot cold lysis*. The toxin has no lethal, dermonecrotising and leukocidal activities.

(c) Gamma-toxin (γ-haemolysin): It can act on rabbit, sheep and human red blood cells but not on horse RBC. It is a bi-compartmental toxin and the 'protease' part helps in unmasking the second part. The second compartment is associated with cell membrane binding. It is encoded by *hlgA,B,C* gene.

(d) Delta-toxin (δ-haemolysin): It produces narrow zone of complete haemolysis with red blood cells of different species. It has a detergent like cell damaging activity. It is encoded by *hld* gene. Serum and skin lipids can neutralize the toxin.

(e) Leukocidin (Panton-Valentine Leukocidin): Methicillin resistant *S. aureus* (MRSA) strains, specially community acquired (CA-MRSA) strains, produce leukocidin responsible for lysis of leukocytes (human, cattle, rabbit) by formation of a pore in cellular membrane. The toxin is associated with severe skin infections. The toxin has two components known as F (fast) and S (slow). This nomenclature is based on their electrophoretic mobility. This is encoded by *lukF,M* gene. This is the first bacterial leukocidin observed.

(f) Toxic shock syndrome toxin (TSST-1): This toxin is 22 Kda protein and also known as superantigen. It can form a trimolecular complex with MHC class II present in the surface of antigen presenting cells and T-cell receptor (V_β domain). The complex can stimulate T-cell proliferation in antigen independent way (mitogenic stimulation) to produce excessive cytokines such as tumour necrosis factor (TNF), interleukin (IL-1). It causes capillary leak, epithelial damage, hypotension and cardiovascular shock. The cells to which the toxin binds are also destroyed by cytotoxic T cells. This toxin lowers the cellular and humoral immunity level to allow the bacteria to propagate. It is encoded by *tst* gene. This toxin is resistant to heat and protease enzyme.

(g) Enterotoxin: It is a heat stable protein and like TSST-1 acts as mitogen to stimulate lymphocytes to produce more amount of IL-1 (superantigen). It is the most potent protein mitogen. It is resistant to pepsin and trypsin. There are 10 antigenic types described till date (A, B, C1, C2, C3, D, E, G, H, I). The toxin is produced by 30% of *S.aureus* strains and *S. intermedius* strains associated with food poisoning in human. When the preformed toxin is ingested along with the food it causes nausea, vomition and diarrhoea in human. The symptoms appear within 1−6 h of ingestion. Animals are found resistant to this toxin (except kitten and monkeys). The toxins are encoded by *SE (s)* gene.

(h) Exfoliative toxin (epidermolytic toxin): This is a 30Kda protein and like TSST-1 acts as superantigen. It is produced by some strains of *S. aureus* and *S. hyicus*. It has two types ETA (encoded by chromosomal gene *eta*) and ETB (encoded by plasmid gene *etb*). It causes separation of cells from one another in stratum granulosum and blisters in infants or adults. In infants the condition is known as 'Staphylococcal scalded skin syndrome'. In animals, it is associated with 'exudative dermatitis' in pigs.

Virulence factors

In addition to the exotoxins, Staphylococci produce several virulence factors like exoenzymes, cell surface structures, adhesins encoded by more than 50 virulence associated genes (virulons).

Exoenzymes

(i) Coagulase: The production of heat stable coagulase enzyme can sub divide Staphylococci into two major groups i.e., coagulase positive Staphylococci and coagulase negative Staphylococci (CNS). *S. aureus, S. intermedius, S. schleiferi* subsp. *coagulans* are coagulase positive. Whereas *S. lugdunensis, S. epidermidis, S. hyicus, S. haemolyticus* are example of CNS. Coagulase positive Staphylococci can produce two major types of coagulase i.e., cell bound coagulase and extracellular free coagulase. This free coagulase can convert fibrinogen into fibrin that forms a layer surrounding the bacterial cells in vivo and protects the bacteria from phagocytosis. It coagulates plasma in vitro. However its role in pathogenesis is uncertain as few strains of CNS are found equally pathogenic like coagulase producers. Currently *S. lugdunensis* displays an unusual rate of virulence in human close to *S. aureus* (Douiri et al., 2016).

  (ii) Lipid degrading enzymes: *S. aureus* can produce lipases, esterases and fatty acid modifying enzymes (FAME). First two enzymes degrade skin lipids and help in bacterial multiplication. Lipid degradation can generate antibacterial fatty acids, modified by 'FAME'. So the skin abscess producing strains of *S. aureus* can generate FAME to neutralize the antibacterial effects of the fatty acids.

 (iii) Catalase: All Staphylococci produce catalase enzyme to survive in presence of oxygen. As the oxygen can produce superoxide radicals that generate hydrogen peroxide in a sequential chemical reaction. Catalase can neutralize this hydrogen peroxide which is otherwise toxic to the bacterial cell.

 (iv) Proteases: *S. aureus* produces a variety of proteases like hyaluronidase, nuclease, staphylokinase, serine proteases, cysteine proteases, zinc metalloproteinase (aureolysin). They are encoded by *hysA, nuc, sak,htrA, sspBC, aur* genes, respectively. Hyaluronidase acts as 'spreading factor' and helps in tissue invasion of the bacteria and diffusion of the toxins produced. Hyaluronidase along with nuclease can degrade the pus materials to generate nutrients for the growing bacteria within a lesion.

Table 16.2 describes the toxins and virulence factors produced by Staphylococci.

Transmission

S. aureus is mostly transmitted in human and animals by direct contact with contaminated living or non-living objects and indirectly through ingestion. The bacteria are common resident of bovine udder and external nares, nasal passage, skin, perineum, external genitalia, respiratory and intestinal tract of human and animals. Loss of skin barrier, presence of immunocompromising diseases such as diabetes and HIV, defects in neutrophil function are predisposing factors. Most of the animal infection is endogenous in nature.

TABLE 16.2 Major virulence factors produced by Staphylococci.

Virulence factors	Function
Capsule	Antiphagocytic as it prevents opsonization.
Peptidoglycan	PG can stimulate the production of endogenous pyrogen and act as chemoattractant for the leukocytes. So more amount of PG is found in the local infections such as skin abscess and joint infections.
Teichoic acid	Extracellular TA can prevent opsonization by reducing the availability of complement components to the bacteria and helps in bacterial virulence.
Protein A (It is found in 98% surface of *S. aureus* animal and human strains. It is encoded by *spa* gene.)	**(a)** It can bind with Fc portion of IgG1, IgG2 and IgG4 subclasses and mask the Fc portion to prevent opsonization & phagocytosis. **(b)** It can also bind with 'Von Willebrand factor', a protein found in the endothelium. Thus 'protein-A' helps in attachment of the bacteria to cause endovascular diseases. **(c)** It helps in biofilm formation of MRSA strains (*ica* independent pathway)
'SecA' secretion system	Precursor proteins of the bacteria are transported into their destinations through this secretion system which also changes the protein structure to make it active.

'Microbial surface components recognizing adhesive matrix molecules' (MSCRAMMs)
They are cell wall anchored proteins produced by 'Sec A' secretion system. There are total 21 proteins identified till date. Important ones are discussed below.

Continued

TABLE 16.2 Major virulence factors produced by Staphylococci.—cont'd

Virulence factors	Function
(a) Fibronectin binding protein (FnbpA and FnbpB). It is encoded by *fnbA,B* gene.	It helps in attachment of bacterial cells to an extra-cellular matrix component, fibronectin. Its binding with fibronectin interacts with the host cell integrin. Integrins initiate a signaling pathway causing rearrangement of the host cell actin filaments and helps in bacterial uptake (staphylococci can survive within certain kind of cells like fibroblasts, osteoblasts, keratinocytes and endothelial cells). Binding of *S. aureus* FnBPA to human fibronectin is a primary step in pathogenesis of prosthetic device infections.
(b) Collagen binding protein (Cna). It is encoded by *cna* gene.	It is necessary for adherence of *S. aureus* to collagenous tissues and cartilages.
(c) Clumping factor A and B (ClfA and ClfB), encoded by *clfA,B* gene.	They can mediate clumping and adherence of bacterial cells to fibrinogen in the presence of fibronectin. ClfB is also found to help in adherence with nasal epithelium (it specifically binds cytokeratin-10 ligand).
(d) Plasma-sensitive surface protein (PLs)	It participates in binding of the bacteria to both the fibrinogen and fibronectin
(e) Polysaccharide intercellular adhesin (PIA/ica)	It helps in 'biofilm' production after attachment of staphylococci with the surface of biomaterials. 'Biofilm' is a shelter for pathogenic bacteria making them inaccessible to host defence and antibiotics. Biofilms are commonly seen in intramammary devices, milking machine, catheters for urinary bladder etc. Biofilms are made of complex bacterial populations within a polysaccharide matrix, composed of poly-*N*-acetylglucosamine (PNAG). This PNAG production is induced by *ica* locus composed of *icaR* (regulatory) and *icaADBC* (biosynthetic) genes.
(f) staphylococcal Respiratory response regulator (SrrAB)	The *ica* locus is upregulated during anaerobic condition, suitable for biofilm production. SrrAB helps in PIA induction under anaerobic conditions through binding with a DNA sequence present at the upstream of icaADBC operon.
Rbf, Spx (global regulator of stress response), *arlRS* two-component system, staphylococcal accessory regulator (sarA), sigB operon	Regulator of biofilm formation
Biofilm-associated protein (Bap)	Formation of biofilm (*ica* independent pathway)
cidA protein	Cell lysis and DNA release which helps in biofilm formation
Accessory gene regulator (agr) quorum sensing system (RNA II, RNA III and AIP)	RNA II helps in Agr-sensing mechanism transcribed by genes *agrA, agrC, agrD* and *agrB*. RNA III acts as intracellular effector molecule which upregulates transcription of extracellular protein genes and downregulates surface protein Genes. AIP (autoinducer protein) regulates exotoxin production and biofilm dispersal.
Ribosomal protein L2 (RAP)	Alternative 'agr' activator during early growth phase
Autolysin (Atl)	It helps in cell wall turnover, cell division, cell separation, lysis of bacteria required during biofilm formation
SERAMs (Secreatable Expanded Repertoire adhesive molecules)	After secreation from the bacterial cell they can bind fibrinogen, fibronectin, prothrombin, vitronectin. Then they rebind to *S. aureus* and mediate adhesion by acting as a bridge between bacteria and the host cells.

Contaminated food items are considered as potent source of antimicrobial resistant *S. aureus* in human (Wegener, 2012). Infant milk and contaminated food items was identified as a source of MRSA associated human outbreaks in United States and Netherlands (Parks et al., 1987; Kluytmans et al., 1995; Jones et al., 2002). Biofilm formation in surfaces of food processing plants by both methicillin resistant and sensitive *S. aureus* isolates was associated with food borne outbreaks due to consumption of fresh or processed foods worldwide (Oulahal et al., 2008). MRSA was detected in all the major steps of food processing plant starting from pig farm, slaughter house to food production units (EFSA, 2009).

Other than ingestion, direct contact is alternative route of MRSA whole bacterium transmission. Occupational exposure to contaminated animals was detected as a greater source of MRSA (LA MRSA) than handling raw meat in human (de Jonge et al., 2010; Van Cleef et al., 2010). In human hospitals, droplets, stools and skin cells of infected patients, medical instruments, beddings, clothing, furniture, toiletries and the atmosphere act as the source of MRSA infection (Dancer, 2008). Similarly, environment of small animal and equine hospitals also act as a source of MRSA (Loeffler et al., 2005). Airborne MRSA transmission through dust particles originated from pig farms was detected among the farm workers in The Netherlands (Van Den Broek et al., 2009). Statistical analysis revealed a positive correlation between airborne transmission of MRSA and working at the pig stables containing sows and finishing pigs.

In addition to whole bacterium transmission, spread of antibiotic resistance determinants can take place horizontally through plasmids, transposons and insertion sequences. Horizontal spread of SCCmec occurs between competent bacterial cells or by experimental transduction in the laboratory (Stewart and Rosenblum, 1980). Acquisition of SCCmec is detected in few *S. aureus* lineages belonged to CC1, CC5, CC8, CC22, CC30, and CC45 (Enright et al., 2002). Other resistance genes such as *vanA* (resistance to vancomycin) located on a Tn*1546*-containing plasmid, *tetL* (resistance to tetracycline), *dfrK* (resistance to trimethoprim), *lsa(E)* (resistance to streptograminA) and *cfr* (resistance to muti-drugs) were transmitted into *S. aureus* strains from enterococci (López et al., 2012; Wendlandt et al., 2012).

Diagnosis

Clinical samples from human include swabs from nose and skin lesions. Animal clinical samples are mastitic milk, pus and exudate from lesion, skin scrapings, urine and affected tissues. Cold chain should be maintained during transport without direct contact to the ice or coolants to prevent freezing of the collected samples.

Laboratory examinations

Direct examination

A smear can be prepared from clinical samples or tissues and stained by Gram's method. Staphylococci appear as gram positive cocci arranged in classical grape like bunch. Although the smear from the colony reveals gram positive cocci randomly distributed over the field.

Isolation of staphylococcus

Staphylococci can be isolated in routinely used bacteriological media like nutrient agar, blood agar or specific media like mannitol salt agar (MSA), lipovitellin salt mannitol agar (LSM), Vogel-Johnson agar (VJ), Baird Parker agar, potassium thiocyanate-actidione-sodium azide-egg yolk-pyruvate agar (KRANEP), *Staphylococcus* medium number 110. The bacteria can tolerate 5%−10% sodium chloride. This property is used in the selective medium to inhibit the growth of other bacteria (MSA, LSM). Potassium tellurite and lithium chloride are also used as selective agents to inhibit the growth of contaminants as found in Vogel-Johnson and Baird Parker agar. Fermentation of mannitol will shift pH of the medium which is detected by phenol red indicator.

If the bacteria are present in low number in the samples, initially they are inoculated into enrichment broths like tryptone soya broth with sodium chloride and pyruvate, Giolitti and Cantoni Broth and liquid Baird−Parker medium. All enrichment broths or media plates are incubated at 37°C. Sometimes reduced oxygen tension with increased CO_2 concentration favours the growth. It has a wide pH range for growth but the optimum is 7.2. Colony characteristics of *S. aureus* in different isolation media are described in Table 16.3.

Small colony variants (SCV): Small colony variants of *S. aureus* are a type of slow growing subpopulation producing non-pigmented, tiny colonies in the agar. They may persist within lung, udder for a long time and cause chronic fibrosed lungs in human and persistent mastitis in cattle, respectively. They exhibit reduced rate of metabolism and are less virulent, but due to their slow growth and reduced cell wall synthesis, they are more tolerant of β-lactam antibiotics than their wild-type parents. In lungs with chronic fibrosis, synergistic interaction between *Pseudomonas aeruginosa* and *S. aureus*

TABLE 16.3 Colony characteristics of *S. aureus* or antibiotic resistant *S. aureus* in different isolation media.

Media	Colony characteristics
Nutrient agar	Round, smooth, convex, glistening with entire edge. *S. aureus* from cattle, human and other domestic animals produces golden yellow coloured colonies in nutrient agar. The canine *S. aureus* isolates, *S. intermedius* and *S. hyicus* produce non-pigmented colonies
Blood agar	Haemolytic
Mannitol salt agar	Colonies are surrounded by bright yellow zone. Phenol red indicator produces yellow colour in acidic pH due to fermentation of mannitol
Lipovitellin salt mannitol agar	Colonies are found with opaque zone against yellow background
Vogel-Johnson agar	Black, convex and shiny surrounded by yellow zone
Baird Parker agar	Black, shiny and convex with narrow white entire margin and surrounded by a clear zone
Potassium thiocyanate-actidione-sodium azide-egg yolk-pyruvate agar (KRANEP)	*S. aureus* produces golden yellow colonies with a precipitation zone of egg yolk after 48 h of incubation. The medium remains opaque
Oxacillin resistant Screening Agar base (ORSAB)	MRSA produce intense blue coloured colonies
CHROM agar	MRSA produce rose to mauve coloured colonies
MRSA ID	Green coloured colonies

(SCV) was detected. Quorum sensing molecule (2-heptyl-4-hydroxyquinoline N-oxide) secreted by *P. aeruginosa* activates alternative sigma factor B in *S. aureus* which is a pre-requisite for SCV induction. SCV induction acts as a protective mechanism for survival of *S. aureus* during competition with *P. aeruginosa* (Hoffman et al., 2006). Vancomycin-intermediate *S. aureus* (VISA) and heterogenous vancomycin-intermediate *S. aureus* (hVISA) produce 'mixed' type of colonies (large and small variants) with different pigmentation (Marlowe et al., 2001).

Serological tests

(a) Latex agglutination test
(b) An agar diffusion method using micro titer plates is used to detect antibodies to the DNases produced by *S. aureus*.
(c) Enzyme-linked immunosorbent assay (ELISA)

Tests for pathogenicity

(a) Coagulase test: Detection of coagulase enzyme produced by *S. aureus* either in bound or free form is used as pathogenicity test although now a day coagulase is not considered as exclusive virulence marker of *S. aureus*. The bound coagulase is detected by the slide test and the free coagulase is detected by the tube test.
  (i) In slide coagulase test, a loop full staphylococcal culture is placed over a drop of normal saline in a slide. Equal amount of rabbit plasma is added and mixed gently. In positive case clumping will be visible under naked eye. Fibrinogen of the plasma is converted into fibrin by coagulase and clumping is produced.
  (ii) In tube coagulase test, 1:5 diluted rabbit plasma is placed into two sugar tubes. Now five drops of overnight grown culture is poured into one tube. Another will act as control. Both the tubes are incubated at 37°C. In positive cases clot will be produced within 1−3 h or longer. In the control tube no clot will be detected.
(b) PCR can be used to detect the genes for major virulence factors

Typing of S. aureus *isolates*

(a) Capsular serotyping of the isolates is performed by the use of direct cell agglutination and immuno-precipitation of cell extracts with antisera specific for 12 capsular types.
(b) Phage typing: It is carried out with the help of different bacteriophages capable of lysing *Staphylococcus*.

(c) Molecular techniques such as pulsed-field gel electrophoresis (PFGE), multilocus sequence typing (MLST) and DNA sequencing of the X region present in the protein A gene (spa typing) are used for *S. aureus* typing. The same *S. aureus* isolate can be designated by different nomenclature systems depending on the test used for typing. *S. aureus* isolates are named as CMRSA1, ST followed by a number and 't' followed by a number in PFGE, MLST and spa typing, respectively.

Molecular Biology: PCR assay is developed with the oligonucleotide primers for the detection of *Staphylococcus* specific 16S ribosomal RNA and the *nuc* gene (*S. aureus*− specific). Other than detection of virulence associated genes, whole genome sequencing is currently used for prediction of antimicrobial resistance genes in *S. aureus* genome (Gordon et al., 2014).

Detection of antimicrobial resistant S. aureus

For isolation of MRSA, enrichment media containing indicators, inhibitory agents and antibiotics (oxacillin or cefoxitin) can be used (Table 16.3). Other than isolation in specific media, detection of antibiotic sensitivity with oxacillin and/or cefoxitin, and minimum inhibitory concentration of *S. aureus* isolates can identify MRSA. Cefoxitin disc diffusion is the most sensitive method for detecting MRSA isolates showing negative and positive predictive values of 100% and 98%, respectively. Oxacillin/cefoxitin are preferred for detection of MRSA instead of methicillin itself due to unavailability of methicillin, better detection of heterogenous strains by oxacillin, and greater induction of *mecA* by cefoxitin. Conventional PCR for *mecA*, SCCmec typing, PFGE or MLST based typing in combination with phenotypic methods can confirm MRSA isolates (CDC, 2017).

Detection of antibiotic sensitivity in Mueller-Hinton agar with teicoplanin (5 µg/mL) and minimum inhibitory concentration of *S. aureus* isolates by modified E-test can identify VRSA/VISA/hVISA. The brain-heart infusion agar is a better choice than Mueller−Hinton agar for detection of vancomycin resistance. For confirmation of hVISA strains in the laboratory, population analysis profile (PAP) is the method of choice. Test culture grown in tryptone soya broth is inoculated into brain heart infusion agar with vancomycin (0, 0.5, 1, 2, 2.5, 4 µg per ml) and the plates are incubated for 48 h. The area under the concentration-time (AUC) is calculated with software and if AUC ratio is $\geq$ 0.9 and vancomycin MIC is $\leq$ 2 µg per ml, the isolate is considered as hVISA (Howden et al., 2010).

Characteristics of antimicrobial resistance

Penicillin resistance

Within few years after introduction, penicillin resistant *S. aureus* appeared in hospitals and community during 1942 (Rammelkamp and Maxon, 1942). The penicillin resistant *S. aureus* strains was first observed in 1944 (Kirby, 1944) and the precise role of penicillinase was discovered subsequently (Bondi and Dietz, 1945). In diversified clinical establishments, more than 90% of staphylococcal infections are penicillin resistant (Lowy, 2003).

Penicillin resistance of *S. aureus* is mediated by a serine β-lactamase (*blaZ*) which lyses the β-lactam ring present in the antibiotic structure. The blaZ protein is located at outer face of the cytoplasmic membrane of bacterial cell wall and the soluble part is released into the surrounding medium. The gene (*blaZ*) is carried by transposon (Tn*552*), located in large plasmid or integrated within the chromosome (Jensen and Lyon, 2009). Activation of *blaZ* occurs during exposure to penicillin and cleavage of BlaR1, a transmembrane sensor-transducer. The cleaved BlaR1 protein acts as protease and lyses the repressor protein (BlaI) to activate *blaZ* (Zhang et al., 2001).

Methicillin resistance

Methicillin (a type of penicillin) was introduced to combat penicillinase enzyme produced by penicillin resistant *S. aureus*. Soon after the introduction, methicillin resistant *S. aureus* (MRSA) appeared in 1961 (Barber, 1961). Methicillin can block the penicillin binding proteins (PBPs) of the bacteria required for cell wall synthesis i.e., both transglycosylation and transpeptidation. N-acetyl-glucosamine and N-acetyl-muramic acid disaccharides are attached with the growing peptidoglycan chain by transglycosylation. The newly incorporated repeating unit is cross-linked to an already synthesized peptidoglycan strand by transpeptidation. The cross linking takes place between 4 D-alanine and 3 L-lysine of two adjacent peptidoglycan strands in *S. aureus* (Giesbrecht et al., 1998). Precisely methicillin or other β-lactams inhibit the transpeptidation by formation of an acyl-enzyme complex with PBPs. Dissociation of this acyl-enzyme complex is inhibited due to accumulation of active site of the enzyme with the β-lactam ring structure. The cell wall cross-linking is progressively lost during subsequent bacterial cell division which causes defective cell wall formation followed by leakage of bacterial cytoplasm and cell death (Giesbrecht et al., 1998). MRSA can synthesize a new form of PBP known as PBP2a (MRSA-PBP) which has reduced affinity for β-lactam antibiotics. The active-site serine of PBP2a which binds with β-lactams is present within a narrow cleft and remains inaccessible to the antibiotics (Lim and Strynadka, 2002).

This PBP2a is encoded by *mecA* gene (earlier described as *mecr*), found on an extra/foreign portion of bacterial chromosome (SCCmec), absent in methicillin susceptible strains (Stewart and Rosenblum, 1980). The *mecA* was originated from animal associated Staphylococci such as *S. sciuri* and *S. fleuretti* which was transferred horizontally to *S. aureus* (Tsubakishita et al., 2010). Other than *mecA*/SCCmec, *fem* (factors essential for methicillin resistance), *aux* (auxiliary factors), *hmt* (high methicillin resistance) are also associated with lowered cell-wall biosynthesis in the presence of methicillin or other β-lactams and resistance to the antibiotics (De Lencastre et al., 1999). Modified *S. aureus* (MODSA) strains, possessing point mutations in PBP2 are another example of *mecA* independent methicillin resistance, associated with few clinical infections (Ba et al., 2013). Borderline oxacillin-resistant *S. aureus* (BORSA) strains produce low level of resistance against oxacillin and are rarely associated with clinical infections (1.2%) (Maalej et al., 2012).

Most of the MRSA isolates show heterogenous methicillin resistance, even cultured from a single colony. Majority of the cells produce lowered resistance to methicillin and only 0.01%—0.1% cells display higher levels of resistance. Heterogenous MRSA cells are converted into homogenous population through alterations in gene expression in the presence of β-lactams (Finan et al., 2002).

MRSA is not only resistant to methicillin but also to all β-lactam antibiotics, including synthetic penicillins, cephalosporins and carbapenems as well as other group of antibiotics like aminoglycosides, macrolides, lincosamides, streptogramins, tetracyclines.

Vancomycin resistance

Kornfield (1950), an organic chemist at Eli Lilly, first isolated a bacterium namely *Amycolatopsis orientalis* (*Streptomyces orientalis* or *Nocardia orientalis*) from mud collected by a missionary from forests of Borneo island. A compound ('Mississippi mud' or compound 05,865) was extracted from the isolated bacteria and it was approved by FDA as vancomycin drug after clinical trials (Levine, 2006). MRSA was successfully treated with vancomycin for several years since its introduction (1958). In 1997, reduced susceptibility of *S. aureus* clinical isolates to vancomycin was reported from Japan (strain Mu50, vancomycin-intermediate *S. aureus* or VISA) (Hiramatsu et al., 1997). Vancomycin-resistant *S. aureus* (VRSA, MIC ≥16 μg/mL) was reported from Michigan and Pennsylvania in 2002 and New York in 2004 due to acquisition of *vanA* from enterococci (CDC, 2002; Sievert et al., 2008). Isolation of VRSA from human was further reported from United States, India and Iran (Sievert et al., 2008; Aligholi et al., 2008; Saha et al., 2008). Most of the VRSA strains isolated from United States possessed Tn*1546* and belonged to CC5. The VISA (or hVISA) phenotype have been reported from human in many countries such as Japan, United States, Mexico, Australia, United Kingdom, Germany, Belgium, France, Scotland, Brazil, Oman, South Korea, Hong Kong, South Africa, Thailand, Israel, Jordan, China, Bangladesh (Bierbaum et al., 1999; Elhag et al., 2000; Denis et al., 2002; Bataineh, 2006; Delgado et al., 2007; Howden et al., 2010; Melo-Cristino et al., 2013; Paul et al., 2014; Shang et al., 2016). In contrast, there is paucity of documents on the occurrence of VRSA in animals possibly due to the fact that glycopeptides (vancomycin) are not regularly used in veterinary practices. The reports of livestock associated VRSA is coming in current years as observed from South Africa (Adegoke and Okoh, 2014). Our group recently documented occurrence of VRSA (MIC ≥ 16 μg/mL) and VISA (MIC ≥ 8 μg/mL) in milk samples of cattle and goats suffering with mastitis in India (West Bengal). All the isolates were resistant to cefoxitin and oxacillin and possessed *mecA* gene, none of them carried vancomycin resistance gene (*vanA*/*vanB*). Occurrence of VRSA and VISA could probably be due to intensive use of vancomycin in human healthcare which might have led to the development of glycopeptide-resistant strains and further dissemination into the environment (Bhattacharyya et al., 2016).

The cell wall of *S. aureus* is typically composed of peptidoglycan like other gram-positive bacteria. The peptidoglycan consists of glycan chains (*N*-acetyl-glucosamine and *N*-acetyl-muramic acid) with cross-linkage. The degree of peptidoglycan cross-linkage in the *S. aureus* cell wall is high (80%—90%) (Dmitriev et al., 2004). One of the key components in the synthesis of peptidoglycan is lipid II. Vancomycin has high affinity for D-alanyl-D-alanine (D-ala-D-ala) residue of lipid II and thus blocks the transglycosylation and transpeptidation reactions of cell wall synthesis. In VRSA isolates, alteration of D-ala-D-ala to D-alanyl-D-lactate (D-ala-D-lac) causes reduced affinity for vancomycin (Arthur and Courvalin, 1993).

VISA strains (MIC: 4—8 μg/mL) are emerging concern now a days in patients with MRSA infections undergoing vancomycin therapy for a prolonged period (Howden et al., 2010). Heterogenous VISA (hVISA) is the precursor of VISA strains which consists of cell subpopulations with various degrees of vancomycin resistance (Hiramatsu et al., 1997). Current definition of VRSA or VISA is based on their mechanism of vancomycin resistance. Horizontal acquisition of *vanA* and accumulation of mutations in regulator genes (sensor kinase gene *vraUTSR*, sensor histidine kinase *walK*, cognate response regulator *walR*, response regulator gene *graR*, and non-regulator gene *rpoB*) are considered as major mechanisms of vancomycin resistance in VRSA and VISA isolates, respectively. Mutations in *rpoB*, *walRK* and *vraUTSR* are the first-step towards conversion of VSSA into VISA. Other than vancomycin, use of non-glycopeptide antibiotics such as rifampicin, daptomycin and β-lactams (imipenem, cefmetazole, flomoxef) also acts as selection pressure for generation of hVISA/VISA (Watanabe et al., 2011). Under electron microscopy, VISA cells are observed with thick cell wall. Two different strategies for vancomycin resistance are observed in VISA cells. Peptidoglycan layer of VISA cells absorbs huge quantity of vancomycin molecules. Bound vancomycin molecules cause destruction of the layer and prevent further diffusion of vancomycin from exterior ('clogging effect'). Second strategy depends on thickness of cell wall in VISA cells. Vancomycin cannot completely inhibit peptidoglycan synthesis even in higher dosage (Hiramatsu et al., 2014). Another phenotype of VISA/hVISA is described as slow VISA which grows usually after 3 days of incubation at 37°C. The slow VISA is probably generated due to *rpoB* mutation and they can resist greater concentration of vancomycin. The hVISA may temporarily switch over into slow VISA form during vancomycin therapy and revert back to hVISA when the therapy is discontinued (Hiramatsu et al., 2014).

Telavancin resistance

Telavancin is a semisynthetic lipoglycopeptide, approved by United States Food and Drug Administration (FDA) for treatment of skin and skin structure infections, hospital-acquired bacterial pneumonia, and ventilator-associated pneumonia. Telavancin increases bacterial membrane permeability causing depolarization and inhibits peptidoglycan synthesis (Higgins et al., 2005). It was found active against MRSA and VISA/hVISA except one report of in vivo development of resistance against hVISA in a heart transplanted patient undergoing telavancin therapy (Swartz et al., 2013). Recent study indicated sustained potency of telavancin against clinical isolates of MSSA, MRSA and coagulase-negative staphylococci in United States (Pfaller et al., 2017).

Quinolone resistance

Quinolones were initially introduced to treat gram-negative bacterial infection. Due to their broad spectrum activity they were started to use against Staphylococcal infection and quinolone resistance emerged specially among the MRSA isolates. Sometimes, when the quinolones are used to treat other bacterial infection, *S. aureus* present on the skin or mucosa are exposed to sub-therapeutic concentration of the drug and become resistant (Hooper, 2002). Quinolone antibiotics act on DNA gyrase (gram-negative) or topoisomerase IV (gram-positive), relieve DNA supercoiling and inhibit bacterial DNA replication. Mutation in GrlA subunit of topoisomerase IV in *S. aureus* reduces affinity of enzyme-DNA complex for quinolones and generates resistance (Ng et al., 1996). Increased expression of NorA multidrug resistance efflux pump is also associated with quinolone resistance (Ng et al., 1994).

Aminoglycoside resistance

Aminoglycosides (neomycin, gentamicin) were introduced for topical or systemic use against *S. aureus* infection. Emergence of aminoglycoside resistant *S. aureus* strains occurred due to acquisition of aminoglycoside modifying enzymes encoded by mobile genetic elements. Examples of such enzymes conferring resistance against gentamicin and neomycin are acetyl transferase-phosphotransferase (*aacA-aphD*) carried by Tn*4001*, phosphotransferase (*aphA*) carried by Tn*5405*, adenyl transferase (*aadD*) carried by plasmid pUB110. The modified aminoglycoside drug is unable to bind ribosomes (Jensen and Lyon, 2009).

Sulfonamide resistance

Sulfonamides inhibit dihydropteroate synthase (DHPS) which condenses pteroate and p-aminobenzoic acid (pABA) to form dihydropteroate from which folic acid is generated. The folic acid is an essential enzyme for bacteria which can synthesize it. The sulfonamide competes with pABA at the active site of the enzyme to act as an alternative substrate and produce pteroate-sulfonamide complex from which the bacteria cannot generate folic acid. Resistance to sulfonamide is associated with amino acid substitutions in DHPS enzyme which prevents the drug binding. The sulfonamide resistant

S. aureus strains have chromosomally encoded genes producing amino acid substitutions in DHPS enzyme (Hampele et al., 1997).

Tetracycline/tigecycline resistance

Tetracyclines bind to the 30S ribosomal subunit of bacteria, disrupt amino acyl tRNA binding and inhibit protein synthesis. Tigecycline is a third generation derivative of tetracycline which was approved for treatment of MRSA infection. Due to substitutions on 'D' ring of Tet nucleus, the tigecycline binds with 30S subunit with $10-100$-fold higher affinity. Tetracycline resistance is associated with *tet* gene causing efflux pump activation, ribosomal protection, and enzymatic inactivation of the drug. Among different Tet proteins, TetK is associated with efflux pump activation, encoded by plasmid pT181 and is detected in SCCmecIII of MRSA strains (Jensen and Lyon, 2009). The TetO/M, encoded by chromosomally located transposons (Tn*916* and Tn*1545*) can bind with the EF-G binding site on the bacterial ribosome and dislodges the bound drug molecule from the ribosome. Tigecycline is not affected by these 'tet' proteins (TetK, TetO/M) due to bulky substitutions on ring D (Chopra and Roberts, 2001). Experimentally, resistance to tigecycline in *S. aureus* strains was found to be associated with increased transcription of TetM, MepA (multidrug and toxin extrusion family transporter) and mutations in *rpsJ* that encodes ribosomal protein S10 (McAleese et al., 2005; Beabout et al., 2015). The conformational changes in tigecycline binding site causes reduced binding of the drug and resistance.

Macrolide resistance

Currently macrolide (erythromycin) is not recommended to treat MRSA infection. The semisynthetic macrolides (clarithromycin, azithromycin, telithromycin) are still used to treat infection other than *S. aureus*. There is a possibility that the commensal *S. aureus* present in skin and mucosa are exposed to semisynthetic macrolides and become resistant. Specific methylation of 23S rRNA in *S. aureus* possessing *ermA* was associated with resistance to macrolides (Lai et al., 1973). Transfer of erythromycin resistance from one *S. aureus* strain to another was found experimentally possible (Noble et al., 1992).

Chloramphenicol/florfenciol resistance

Chloramphenicol is currently recommended only for topical use in conjunctivitis. Florfenicol [*d*-threo-3-fluoro-2-dichloroacetamido-1-(4-methylsulfonylphenyl)-1-propanol], fluorinated derivative of thiamphenicol is exclusively used in veterinary medicine. Since 1995, florfenicol is approved to treat respiratory tract infections in cattle in European Union, and to treat infectious pododermatitis in cattle and other bacterial infections in fishes in non-European countries. Chloramphenicol and florfenicol interfere with the peptidyl transferase action and inhibit protein synthesis (Schwarz et al., 2016). The genes (*cfr*, *fexA*) detected in *S. aureus* isolates were found to be associated with florfenicol resistance. The *cfr* gene was originally transferred from *S. sciuri* and it encodes an rRNA methylase. The gene product causes methylation of 23S rRNA at position A2503 and induces resistance against florfenicol, chloramphenicol and clindamycin (Kehrenberg et al., 2005). The *fexA* gene was transferred from *S. lentus* and it encodes a novel efflux protein associated with florfenicol and chloramphenicol resistance (Kehrenberg and Schwarz, 2004).

Linezolid/tidezolid resistance

Linezolid, an oxazolidinone derivative, was approved in 2000 to treat chronic nosocomial MRSA infection. It interferes with amino acyl moiety of aatRNA, inhibits peptidyl transferase and bacterial protein synthesis. Tedizolid (second generation oxazolidinone), having enhanced potency than linezolid, was recommended to treat skin and soft tissues infections in 2014. It also binds with amino acyl moiety of aatRNA but with increased affinity due to more contact sites. Resistance to linezolid in clinical isolates of *S. aureus* is associated with mutations in 23S rRNA genes (G2576U mutation) which can modify the bases present at linezolid binding site. Alternate mechanisms include modified expression of housekeeping enzymes causing rRNA alteration (pseudouridylation of U2504), loss of activity of RlmN methyl transferase and amino acid substitutions in ribosomal proteins (L3, L4) (Long and Vester, 2012). Tidezolid is effective against linezolid resistant strains with mutated genes encoding 23S rRNA and ribosomal proteins. Resistance to *both* linezolid and tidezolid in enterococci, coagulase-negative staphylococci (not in *S. aureus*) is associated with *o*xazolidinine and *p*henicol *t*ransferable *r*esistance determinant (OptrA). The OptrA causes resistance by displacing the drug molecule and protecting the target (Sharkey et al., 2016).

Streptogramin resistance

Streptogramin A and B antibiotic groups (quinupristin and dalfopristin, collectively called QDA) act synergistically on the bacterial 50S ribosomal subunit and inhibit protein synthesis. They are recommended to treat MRSA infection since 1999. Virginiamycin and pristinamycin belongs to the same antibiotic group and is widely used for treatment of *S. aureus* infection. Virginiamycin is also used as animal growth promoter in poultry, cattle and swine except in European countries. In *S. aureus*, resistance to streptogramin A (not B) can confer resistance against both the compounds (QDA). Resistance to streptogramin A is associated with the genes *vat* (virginiamycin acetyl transferase, Allignet et al., 1998), *vga* (virginiamycin A lyases, Schwendener and Perreten, 2011), *lsa* (lincosamide, streptogramin A, Wendlandt et al., 2012, and *cfr* (methyl transferase, Long et al., 2006). The virginiamycin acetyl transferase (Vat) acetylates the hydroxyl group at position O8 of streptogramin A molecules and inactivates the molecule. Lsa belongs to ABC-F (ATP binding cassette domain) group of resistance determinant which can protect the ribosome either by removing the attached dug molecules or by preventing the binding of drug molecule with the ribosome (Sharkey et al., 2016). The *lsa(E)* gene is detected in *S. aureus* isolates belonged to multilocus sequence types ST 398, ST 125 and ST 9 of human (Wendlandt et al., 2014), pig (Li et al., 2013), dairy cow (Silva et al., 2014) and poultry (Wendlandt et al., 2014).

Daptomycin resistance

Daptomycin (Dap) is a cyclic peptide antibiotic with a decanoyl fatty acid side chain and is approved to treat MRSA infections. Daptomycin forms a complex with calcium and the Ca-Dap complex acts as cationic peptide. The complex after binding with negatively charged phosphatidylglycerol enters bacterial cytoplasmic membrane and causes leakage of ions (K+) followed by cell death. Daptomycin resistance is associated with mutational changes in multiple peptide resistance factor (*mrpF*) gene. The mutations in *mrpF* add positively charged lysine residue to phosphatidylglycerol and generates lysyl-phosphatidylglycerol. Consequently, overall charge of cytoplasmic membrane becomes positive and Ca-Dap complex is repelled. Changes to the fluidity of the membrane and increased rigidity also cause reduced binding with Ca-Dap complex (Bayer et al., 2013). Persistent infections caused by daptomycin resistant MRSA isolates can be treated successfully with daptomycin and β-lactams ('see-saw' effect). The daptomycin resistant isolates paradoxically become sensitive to β-lactams due to increased expression of lipoprotein chaperone (PrsA) on the outer face of bacterial cytoplasmic membrane associated with generation of lysyl-phosphatidylglycerol. PrsA is needed for localization of PBP2a and absence of PBP2a in spite of its normal expression is the cause behind β-lactam sensitivity (Renzoni et al., 2017). Generation of VISA phenotype is also observed in daptomycin resistant *S. aureus* isolates due to similarity in resistance mechanism such as increase in cell wall thickness and positive charges of the cytoplasmic membrane (Allington and Rivey, 2001).

Fusidic acid resistance

Fusidic acid has topical use against *S. aureus* associated skin disorders. Chronic MRSA infection can also be treated with fusidic acid-rifampicin combination. Fusidic acid binds with elongation factor-G (EF-G) and inhibits bacterial protein synthesis. Resistance to fusidic acid in *S. aureus* is associated with plasmid encoded *fusB* and chromosomal *fusC* genes (SCCfus/SCCmec). Fus mediated resistance is based on either inhibition of drug binding with EF-G or release of the drug molecule from EF-G due to conformational changes (Fernandes, 2016; Tomlinson et al., 2016).

Mupirocin resistance

Mupirocin is used topically to treat skin infections and to reduce nasal carriage of MRSA. Mupirocin acts on isoleucyl-tRNA synthetase and inhibits bacterial protein synthesis. Resistance to mupirocin in *S. aureus* isolates is associated with plasmid encoded *MupA* which prevents the binding of drug molecule with the target (Thomas et al., 2010).

Rifampicin resistance

Rifampicin is used as adjunct therapy with β-lactam or glycopeptides to treat bacteraemia and endocarditis caused by *S. aureus*. Target of rifampicin is bacterial RNA polymerase. The drug binds with B subunit of the enzyme and prevents transcription. Mutation results conformational changes of the drug binding site in rifampicin resistant isolates (Wichelhaus et al., 1999).

Characteristics of antimicrobial resistance in *Staphylococcus* isolates observed in different livestock, poultry, wildlife as well as in human are discussed in the following section.

Livestock

MRSA belonged to ST398 lineage was reported from livestock such as pigs, sheep, and goats in European countries (Denmark, The Netherlands, Belgium, Ireland), United States, Canada and Asia (Fluit, 2012; Stefani et al., 2012; Hartley et al., 2014). In China, CC9 was detected as major clonal lineage of MRSA prevalent in pigs and pig farmers (Ho et al., 2012). Transmission of livestock associated MRSA (LA-MRSA) from human to animals (humanosis) or the reverse particularly in individuals with frequent animal contact was documented (Paterson et al., 2012). The LA-MRSA ST 398 strain was originated from a human MSSA strain which was transferred to pigs (Price et al., 2012).

Poultry

In European countries such as in The Netherlands and Denmark highest prevalence of MRSA was detected in poultry (Rodríguez-Lázaro et al., 2015). In The Netherlands, another study with broilers at slaughterhouse revealed the presence of MRSA in birds (6.9%). The birds were originated from Dutch flocks of which 35% was positive. Most of the MRSA isolates belonged to ST398/ST9 and *spa* type t1430 (Mulders et al., 2010). In Belgium, occurrence of MRSA was confirmed in broilers, not in layers due to restricted use of antimicrobials in laying birds. All the MRSA isolates belonged to *spa* type t1456 (Persoons et al., 2009). The retrospective study with *S. aureus* strains isolated between 1970 and 2006 in Belgium, methicillin resistance was mostly detected in recent isolates and the isolates belonged to MLST type 398 and *spa* types t011 and t567 (Nemati et al., 2008).

Horses

MRSA was isolated from a postoperative wound infection in a horse (Hartmann et al., 1997). Other than ST 398, ST 1, ST eight and ST 254 were reported from healthy or diseased horses reared in different countries (Cuny et al., 2008; Loeffler et al., 2009; Carfora et al., 2016; Guérin et al., 2017). Transmission of MRSA to veterinary personnel despite short-term contact with a foal infected with CA-MRSA was observed. The isolates from the foal and human belonged to MRSA-5 (SCC*mec*IV) and were indistinguishable by PFGE (Weese et al., 2005). Similar kind of PFGE based similarity was detected in MRSA strains isolated from nasal swabs of healthy horses and human in close contact in Italy (De Martino et al., 2010).

Companion animals

Among companion animals, MRSA infection is more associated with dogs (Morgan, 2008). In a study in United Kingdom, MRSA was detected in companion animals (1.5%) associated with skin and soft tissue infections or post-operative infections after surgery (Rich and Roberts, 2004). Canine-associated MRSA mostly belonged to ST 22 and ST 36 lineages in UK (Loeffler et al., 2009). The studies have documented transmission of MRSA from pet (*spa* type t037) or hospitalized dogs (ST 22) to owners or hospital staffs (Baptiste et al., 2005; Rutland et al., 2009). Transmission of MRSA from infected owner to her asymptomatic family members and healthy pet cat (humanosis) was also documented (Sing et al., 2008).

Wildlife

Occurrence of MRSA was documented in lesser yellow migratory shore bird, wild rat, wood mice, red deer, Spanish wild goat, vulture, wild boar (Wardyn et al., 2012; Porrero et al., 2013; Himsworth et al., 2014; Gómez et al., 2014). Most common lineage of MRSA associated with wildlife belonged to CC 130 and ST 425.

Food animal products

Meat (pork, mutton, beef, chicken, turkey, rabbit), milk, cheese and pancake was identified as sources of MRSA infection. Comparing the literature available worldwide it seems that pork from United States and Canada (Weese et al., 2010) and chicken from the Netherlands and Denmark (Rodríguez-Lázaro et al., 2015) acts as major sources of MRSA. Overall prevalence of MRSA in meat in European countries is 37% with predominance of ST 398, originated from livestock (Feßler et al., 2011). The studies conducted between 1999 and 2006 in few European countries (Spain, Hungary, France, Germany), Japan, Korea revealed lower prevalence (0%−1.3%) of MRSA in different food items (Doulgeraki et al., 2017). The studies with milk samples from Pakistan (10.4%), meat samples or meat products from Egypt (24%−52%),

United States (5%) and The Netherlands (2.5%−11.9%) revealed higher occurrence of MRSA (Farzana and Hameed, 2006; Van Loo et al., 2007; De Boer et al., 2009; Pu et al., 2009; Karmi, 2013). Fluoroquinolone-resistant *S. aureus* isolates were detected in chicken products collected from United states, although the drug was used in United States broiler industry during 1995−2005 (Waters et al., 2011). Other than ST 398, human associated lineages (ST five and ST 125) possessing SCCmec III and IV was also reported from food items (Lozano et al., 2009).

Human

Healthcare associated/hospital associated MRSA (HA-MRSA) infection in human depends on colonization of bacteria within the body. Anterior nares is the usual site for MRSA colonization, although other anatomical sites such as hands, perineal region, skin wounds, throat, genitourinary tract and the digestive tract may also be colonized. The colonization takes place from infected patients and contaminated objects. HA-MRSA causes dermatitis, septicaemia, cardiac and pulomanry infections specially in immunocompromised patients. Higher occurrence rate of HA-MRSA (>50%) was detected in United States, Asia (South Korea, Vietnam, Taiwan, Honng Kong) and Malta, and intermediate rate (25%−50%) of occurrence was detected in Africa, China and Europe (Mejía et al., 2010; Stefani et al., 2012). The common lineage detected as HA-MRSA in different countries was ST 239 (CC 8) (Harris et al., 2010).

References

Abdulgader, S.M.A., Shittu, A., Nicol, M.P., Kaba, M., 2014. Molecular epidemiology of methicillin-resistant *Staphylococcus aureus* in Africa: a systematic review of the published literature. International Journal of Infectious Diseases 21, 107.

Adegoke, A.A., Okoh, A.I., 2014. Species diversity and antibiotic resistance properties of *Staphylococcus* of farm animal origin in Nkonkobe municipality, South Africa. Folia Microbiologica 59 (2), 133−140.

Aligholi, M., Emaneini, M., Jabalameli, F., Shahsavan, S., Dabiri, H., Sedaght, H., 2008. Emergence of high-level vancomycin-resistant *Staphylococcus aureus* in the Imam Khomeini hospital in Tehran. Medical Principles and Practice 17 (5), 432−434.

Allignet, J., Liassine, N., El Solh, N., 1998. Characterization of a staphylococcal plasmid related to pUB110 and carrying two novel genes, vatC andvgbB, encoding resistance to streptogramins A and B and similar antibiotics. Antimicrobial Agents and Chemotherapy 42 (7), 1794−1798.

Allington, D.R., Rivey, M.P., 2001. Quinupristin/dalfopristin: a therapeutic review. Clinical Therapeutics 23 (1), 24−44.

Arthur, M., Courvalin, P., 1993. Genetics and mechanisms of glycopeptide resistance in enterococci. Antimicrobial Agents and Chemotherapy 37 (8), 1563.

Ba, X., Harrison, E.M., Edwards, G.F., Holden, M.T., Larsen, A.R., Petersen, A., Skov, R.L., Peacock, S.J., Parkhill, J., Paterson, G.K., Holmes, M.A., 2013. Novel mutations in penicillin-binding protein genes in clinical *Staphylococcus aureus* isolates that are methicillin resistant on susceptibility testing, but lack the mec gene. Journal of Antimicrobial Chemotherapy 69 (3), 594−597.

Baptiste, K.E., Williams, K., Willams, N.J., Wattret, A., Clegg, P.D., Dawson, S., Corkill, J.E., O'Neill, T., Hart, C.A., 2005. Methicillin-resistant staphylococci in companion animals. Emerging Infectious Diseases 11 (12), 1942.

Barber, M., 1961. Methicillin-resistant staphylococci. Journal of Clinical Pathology 14, 385−393.

Bataineh, H.A., 2006. Resistance of *Staphylococcus aureus* to vancomycin in Zarqa, Jordan. Pakistan Journal of Medical Sciences 22 (2), 144.

Bayer, A.S., Schneider, T., Sahl, H.G., 2013. Mechanisms of daptomycin resistance in *Staphylococcus aureus*: role of the cell membrane and cell wall. Annals of the New York Academy of Sciences 1277 (1), 139−158.

Beabout, K., Hammerstrom, T.G., Perez, A.M., Magalhães, B.F., Prater, A.G., Clements, T.P., Arias, C.A., Saxer, G., Shamoo, Y., 2015. The ribosomal S10 protein is a general target for decreased tigecycline susceptibility. Antimicrobial Agents and Chemotherapy 59 (9), 5561−5566.

Bhattacharyya, D., Banerjee, J., Bandyopadhyay, S., Mondal, B., Nanda, P.K., Samanta, I., Mahanti, A., Das, A.K., Das, G., Dandapat, P., Bandyopadhyay, S., 2016. First report on vancomycin-resistant *Staphylococcus aureus* in bovine and caprine milk. Microbial Drug Resistance 22 (8), 675−681.

Bierbaum, G., Fuchs, K., Lenz, W., Szekat, C., Sahl, H.G., 1999. Presence of *Staphylococcus aureus* with reduced susceptibility to vancomycin in Germany. European Journal of Clinical Microbiology & Infectious Diseases 18 (10), 691−696.

Blair, J.E., Carr, M., 1960. Distribution of phage groups of *Staphylococcus aureus* in the years 1927 through 1947. Science 132, 1247−1248.

Bondi, J.A., Dietz, C.C., 1945. Penicillin resistant staphylococci. Proceedings of the Society for Experimental Biology and Medicine 60, 55−58.

Breurec, S., Zriouil, S.B., Fall, C., Boisier, P., Brisse, S., Djibo, S., Etienne, J., Fonkoua, M.C., Perrier-Gros-Claude, J.D., Pouillot, R., Ramarokoto, C.E., 2011. Epidemiology of methicillin-resistant *Staphylococcus aureus* lineages in five major African towns: emergence and spread of atypical clones. Clinical Microbiology and Infections 17 (2), 160−165.

Bumm, E., 1885. Der Mikroorganismus der Gonoirhoischen Scheimhaut Erkrankungen "Gonococcus Neisser," Wiesbaden.

Carfora, V., Caprioli, A., Grossi, I., Pepe, M., Alba, P., Lorenzetti, S., Amoruso, R., Sorbara, L., Franco, A., Battisti, A., 2016. A methicillin-resistant *Staphylococcus aureus* (MRSA) sequence type 8, spa type t11469 causing infection and colonizing horses in Italy. Pathogens and Disease 74 (4).

Centers for Disease Control and Prevention (CDC), 2002. *Staphylococcus aureus* resistant to vancomycin−United States, 2002. MMWR. Morbidity and Mortality Weekly Report 51 (26), 565.

Centres for Disease Control and Prevention (CDC), 2017. Available at: https://www.cdc.gov/mrsa/lab/index.html.

Chambers, H.F., DeLeo, F.R., 2009. Waves of resistance: *Staphylococcus aureus* in the antibiotic era. Nature Reviews Microbiology 7 (9), 629.

Chopra, I., Roberts, M., 2001. Tetracycline antibiotics: mode of action, applications, molecular biology, and epidemiology of bacterial resistance. Microbiology and Molecular Biology Reviews 65 (2), 232–260.

Cuny, C., Friedrich, A., Kozytska, S., Layer, F., Nübel, U., Ohlsen, K., Strommenger, B., Walther, B., Wieler, L., Witte, W., 2010. Emergence of methicillin-resistant *Staphylococcus aureus* (MRSA) in different animal species. International Journal of Medical Microbiology 300 (2–3), 109–117.

Cuny, C., Strommenger, B., Witte, W., Stanek, C., 2008. Clusters of infections in horses with MRSA ST1, ST254, and ST398 in a veterinary hospital. Microbial Drug Resistance 14 (4), 307–310.

Dancer, S.J., 2008. Importance of the environment in meticillin-resistant *Staphylococcus aureus* acquisition: the case for hospital cleaning. The Lancet Infectious Diseases 8 (2), 101–113.

Dantes, R., Mu, Y., Belflower, R., Aragon, D., Dumyati, G., Harrison, L.H., Lessa, F.C., Lynfield, R., Nadle, J., Petit, S., Ray, S.M., 2013. National burden of invasive methicillin-resistant *Staphylococcus aureus* infections, United States, 2011. JAMA Internal Medicine 173 (21), 1970–1978.

De Boer, E., Zwartkruis-Nahuis, J.T.M., Wit, B., Huijsdens, X.W., De Neeling, A.J., Bosch, T., Van Oosterom, R.A.A., Vila, A., Heuvelink, A.E., 2009. Prevalence of methicillin-resistant *Staphylococcus aureus* in meat. International Journal of Food Microbiology 134 (1–2), 52–56.

de Jonge, R., Verdier, J.E., Havelaar, A., 2010. Prevalence of meticillin-resistant *Staphylococcus aureus* amongst professional meat handlers in The Netherlands, March-July 2008. Euro Surveillance 15 (46).

De Lencastre, H., Wu, S.W., Pinho, M.G., Ludovice, A.M., Filipe, S., Gardete, S., Sobral, R., Gill, S., Chung, M., Tomasz, A., 1999. Antibiotic resistance as a stress response: complete sequencing of a large number of chromosomal loci in *Staphylococcus aureus* strain COL that impact on the expression of resistance to methicillin. Microbial Drug Resistance 5 (3), 163–175.

De Martino, L., Lucido, M., Mallardo, K., Facello, B., Mallardo, M., Iovane, G., Pagnini, U., Tufano, M.A., Catalanotti, P., 2010. Methicillin-resistant staphylococci isolated from healthy horses and horse personnel in Italy. Journal of Veterinary Diagnostic Investigation 22 (1), 77–82.

Delgado, A., Riordan, J.T., Lamichhane-Khadka, R., Winnett, D.C., Jimenez, J., Robinson, K., O'Brien, F.G., Cantore, S.A., Gustafson, J.E., 2007. Hetero-vancomycin-intermediate methicillin-resistant *Staphylococcus aureus* isolate from a medical center in Las Cruces, New Mexico. Journal of Clinical Microbiology 45 (4), 1325–1329.

Denis, O., Nonhoff, C., Byl, B., Knoop, C., Bobin-Dubreux, S., Struelens, M.J., 2002. Emergence of vancomycin-intermediate *Staphylococcus aureus* in a Belgian hospital: microbiological and clinical features. Journal of Antimicrobial Chemotherapy 50 (3), 383–391.

Devriese, L.A., Damme, L.V., Fameree, L., 1972. Methicillin (cloxacillin)-resistant *Staphylococcus aureus* strains isolated from bovine mastitis cases. Zoonoses and Public Health 19 (7), 598–605.

Dmitriev, B.A., Toukach, F.V., Holst, O., Rietschel, E.T., Ehlers, S., 2004. Tertiary structure of *Staphylococcus aureus* cell wall murein. Journal of Bacteriology 186 (21), 7141–7148.

Douiri, N., Hansmann, Y., Lefebvre, N., Riegel, P., Martin, M., Baldeyrou, M., Christmann, D., Prevost, G., Argemi, X., 2016. *Staphylococcus lugdunensis*: a virulent pathogen causing bone and joint infections. Clinical Microbiology and Infections 22 (8), 747–748.

Doulgeraki, A.I., Di Ciccio, P., Ianieri, A., Nychas, G.J.E., 2017. Methicillin-resistant food-related *Staphylococcus aureus*: a review of current knowledge and biofilm formation for future studies and applications. Research in Microbiology 168 (1), 1–15.

Elhag, K.M., Al Jardani, A.K., Al Yaqubi, F.M., Mohsin, N., 2000. The first glycopeptide-intermediate *Staphylococcus aureus* in Oman. Clinical Microbiology and Infections 6 (3), 173–174.

Enright, M.C., Robinson, D.A., Randle, G., Feil, E.J., Grundmann, H., Spratt, B.G., 2002. The evolutionary history of methicillin-resistant *Staphylococcus aureus* (MRSA). Proceedings of the National Academy of Sciences 99 (11), 7687–7692.

European Food Safety Authority (EFSA), 2009. Assessment of the public health significance of meticillin resistant *Staphylococcus aureus* (MRSA) in animals and foods. EFSA Journal 993, 20–73.

Farzana, K., Hameed, A., 2006. Resistance pattern of clinical isolates of *Staphylococcus aureus* against five groups of antibiotics. Journal of Research Science 17, 19–26.

Fernandes, P., 2016. Fusidic acid: a bacterial elongation factor inhibitor for the oral treatment of acute and chronic staphylococcal infections. Cold Spring Harbor Perspectives in Medicine 6 (1), a025437.

Feßler, A.T., Kadlec, K., Hassel, M., Hauschild, T., Eidam, C., Ehricht, R., Monecke, S., Schwarz, S., 2011. Characterization of methicillin-resistant *Staphylococcus aureus* isolates from food and food products of poultry origin in Germany. Applied and Environmental Microbiology 77 (20), 7151–7157.

Feßler, A.T., Riekerink, R.G.O., Rothkamp, A., Kadlec, K., Sampimon, O.C., Lam, T.J., Schwarz, S., 2012. Characterization of methicillin-resistant *Staphylococcus aureus* CC398 obtained from humans and animals on dairy farms. Veterinary Microbiology 160 (1–2), 77–84.

Finan, J.E., Rosato, A.E., Dickinson, T.M., Ko, D., Archer, G.L., 2002. Conversion of oxacillin-resistant staphylococci from heterotypic to homotypic resistance expression. Antimicrobial Agents and Chemotherapy 46 (1), 24–30.

Fluit, A.C., 2012. Livestock-associated *Staphylococcus aureus*. Clinical Microbiology and Infections 18 (8), 735–744.

Giesbrecht, P., Kersten, T., Maidhof, H., Wecke, J., 1998. Staphylococcal cell wall: morphogenesis and fatal variations in the presence of penicillin. Microbiology and Molecular Biology Reviews 62 (4), 1371–1414.

Gomes, A.R., Westh, H., De Lencastre, H., 2006. Origins and evolution of methicillin-resistant *Staphylococcus aureus* clonal lineages. Antimicrobial Agents and Chemotherapy 50 (10), 3237–3244.

Gómez, P., González-Barrio, D., Benito, D., García, J.T., Viñuela, J., Zarazaga, M., Ruiz-Fons, F., Torres, C., 2014. Detection of methicillin-resistant *Staphylococcus aureus* (MRSA) carrying the *mecC* gene in wild small mammals in Spain. Journal of Antimicrobial Chemotherapy 69 (8), 2061–2064.

Gordon, N.C., Price, J.R., Cole, K., Everitt, R., Morgan, M., Finney, J., Kearns, A.M., Pichon, B., Young, B., Wilson, D.J., Llewelyn, M.J., 2014. Prediction of Staphylococcus aureus antimicrobial resistance by whole-genome sequencing. Journal of Clinical Microbiology 52 (4), 1182−1191.

Gorwitz, R.J., 2008. A review of community-associated methicillin resistant Staphylococcus aureus and soft tissue infections. The Pediatric Infectious Disease Journal 27, 1e5.

Grundmann, H., Aires-de-Sousa, M., Boyce, J., Tiemersma, E., 2006. Emergence and resurgence of meticillin-resistant Staphylococcus aureus as a public-health threat. The Lancet 368 (9538), 874−885.

Guérin, F., Fines-Guyon, M., Meignen, P., Delente, G., Fondrinier, C., Bourdon, N., Cattoir, V., Léon, A., 2017. Nationwide molecular epidemiology of methicillin-resistant Staphylococcus aureus responsible for horse infections in France. BMC Microbiology 17 (1), 104.

Hampele, I.C., D'Arcy, A., Dale, G.E., Kostrewa, D., Nielsen, J., Oefner, C., Page, M.G., Schönfeld, H.J., Stüber, D., Then, R.L., 1997. Structure and function of the dihydropteroate synthase from Staphylococcus aureus. Journal of Molecular Biology 268, 21−30.

Hardy, K.J., Hawkey, P.M., Gao, F., Oppenheim, B.A., 2004. Methicillin resistant Staphylococcus aureus in the critically ill. British Journal of Anaesthesia 92 (1), 121−130.

Harris, S.R., Feil, E.J., Holden, M.T., Quail, M.A., Nickerson, E.K., Chantratita, N., Gardete, S., Tavares, A., Day, N., Lindsay, J.A., Edgeworth, J.D., 2010. Evolution of MRSA during hospital transmission and intercontinental spread. Science 327 (5964), 469−474.

Hartley, H., Watson, C., Nugent, P., Beggs, N., Dickson, E., Kearns, A., 2014. Confirmation of LA-MRSA in pigs in the UK. The Veterinary Record 175 (3), 74−75.

Hartmann, F.A., Trostle, S.S., Klohnen, A.A., 1997. Isolation of methicillin-resistant Staphylococcus aureus from a postoperative wound infection in a horse. Journal of the American Veterinary Medical Association 211 (5), 590−592.

Higgins, D.L., Chang, R., Debabov, D.V., Leung, J., Wu, T., Krause, K.M., Sandvik, E., Hubbard, J.M., Kaniga, K., Schmidt, D.E., Gao, Q., 2005. Telavancin, a multifunctional lipoglycopeptide, disrupts both cell wall synthesis and cell membrane integrity in methicillin-resistant Staphylococcus aureus. Antimicrobial Agents and Chemotherapy 49 (3), 1127−1134.

Himsworth, C.G., Miller, R.R., Montoya, V., Hoang, L., Romney, M.G., Al-Rawahi, G.N., Kerr, T., Jardine, C.M., Patrick, D.M., Tang, P., Weese, J.S., 2014. Carriage of methicillin-resistant Staphylococcus aureus by wild urban Norway rats (Rattus norvegicus). PLoS One 9 (2), e87983.

Hiramatsu, K., Aritaka, N., Hanaki, H., Kawasaki, S., Hosoda, Y., Hori, S., Fukuchi, Y., Kobayashi, I., 1997. Dissemination in Japanese hospitals of strains of Staphylococcus aureus heterogeneously resistant to vancomycin. The Lancet 350 (9092), 1670−1673.

Hiramatsu, K., Ito, T., Tsubakishita, S., Sasaki, T., Takeuchi, F., Morimoto, Y., Katayama, Y., Matsuo, M., Kuwahara-Arai, K., Hishinuma, T., Baba, T., 2013. Genomic basis for methicillin resistance in Staphylococcus aureus. Infection and Chemotherapy 45 (2), 117−136.

Hiramatsu, K., Kayayama, Y., Matsuo, M., Aiba, Y., Saito, M., Hishinuma, T., Iwamoto, A., 2014. Vancomycin-intermediate resistance in Staphylococcus aureus. Journal of Global Antimicrobial Resistance 2 (4), 213−224.

Ho, P.L., Chow, K.H., Lai, E.L., Law, P.Y., Chan, P.Y., Ho, A.Y., Ng, T.K., Yam, W.C., 2012. Clonality and antimicrobial susceptibility of Staphylococcus aureus and methicillin-resistant S. aureus isolates from food animals and other animals. Journal of Clinical Microbiology 50 (11), 3735−3737.

Hoffman, L.R., Déziel, E., D'Argenio, D.A., Lépine, F., Emerson, J., McNamara, S., Gibson, R.L., Ramsey, B.W., Miller, S.I., 2006. Selection for Staphylococcus aureus small-colony variants due to growth in the presence of Pseudomonas aeruginosa. Proceedings of the National Academy of Sciences 103 (52), 19890−19895.

Holden, M.T., Feil, E.J., Lindsay, J.A., Peacock, S.J., Day, N.P., Enright, M.C., Foster, T.J., Moore, C.E., Hurst, L., Atkin, R., Barron, A., 2004. Complete genomes of two clinical Staphylococcus aureus strains: evidence for the rapid evolution of virulence and drug resistance. Proceedings of the National Academy of Sciences of the United States of America 101 (26), 9786−9791.

Hooper, D.C., 2002. Fluoroquinolone resistance among Gram-positive cocci. The Lancet Infectious Diseases 2 (9), 530−538.

Howden, B.P., Davies, J.K., Johnson, P.D., Stinear, T.P., Grayson, M.L., 2010. Reduced vancomycin susceptibility in Staphylococcus aureus, including vancomycin-intermediate and heterogeneous vancomycin-intermediate strains: resistance mechanisms, laboratory detection, and clinical implications. Clinical Microbiology Reviews 23 (1), 99−139.

International Working Group on the Classification of Staphylococcal Cassette Chromosome Elements (IWG-SCC), 2009. Classification of staphylococcal cassette chromosome mec (SCCmec): guidelines for reporting novel SCCmec elements. Antimicrobial Agents and Chemotherapy 53 (12), 4961−4967.

Ito, T., Katayama, Y., Asada, K., Mori, N., Tsutsumimoto, K., Tiensasitorn, C., Hiramatsu, K., 2001. Structural comparison of three types of staphylococcal cassette chromosome mec integrated in the chromosome in methicillin-resistant Staphylococcus aureus. Antimicrobial Agents and Chemotherapy 45 (5), 1323−1336.

Jensen, S.O., Lyon, B.R., 2009. Genetics of antimicrobial resistance in Staphylococcus aureus. Future Microbiology 4 (5), 565−582.

Jevons, M., 1961. "Celbenin"-resistant staphylococci. British Medical Journal 1, 124−125.

Johnson, A.P., Aucken, H.M., Cavendish, S., Ganner, M., Wale, M.C., Warner, M., Livermore, D.M., Cookson, B.D., UK EARSS participants, T., 2001. Dominance of EMRSA-15 and-16 among MRSA causing nosocomial bacteraemia in the UK: analysis of isolates from the European antimicrobial resistance surveillance system (EARSS). Journal of Antimicrobial Chemotherapy 48 (1), 143−144.

Jones, T.F., Kellum, M.E., Porter, S.S., Bell, M., Schaffner, W., 2002. An outbreak of community-acquired foodborne illness caused by methicillin-resistant Staphylococcus aureus. Emerging Infectious Diseases 8 (1), 82.

Jonsson, P., Wadstrom, T., 1993. Staphylococcus. In: Gyles, C.L., Thoen, C.O. (Eds.), Pathogenesis of Bacterial Infections in Animals. The Iowa State University Press, USA, pp. 21−43.

Karmi, M., 2013. Prevalence of methicillin-resistant Staphylococcus aureus in poultry meat in Qena, Egypt. Veterinary World 6 (10).

Kehrenberg, C., Schwarz, S., 2004. fexA, a novel *Staphylococcus lentus* gene encoding resistance to florfenicol and chloramphenicol. Antimicrobial Agents and Chemotherapy 48 (2), 615—618.

Kehrenberg, C., Schwarz, S., Jacobsen, L., Hansen, L.H., Vester, B., 2005. A new mechanism for chloramphenicol, florfenicol and clindamycin resistance: methylation of 23S ribosomal RNA at A2503. Molecular Microbiology 57 (4), 1064—1073.

Kirby, W., 1944. Extraction of a highly potene penicillin inactivator from penicillin resistant Staphylococci. Science 99, 452—453.

Kluytmans, J., Van Leeuwen, W., Goessens, W., Hollis, R., Messer, S., Herwaldt, L., Bruining, H., Heck, M., Rost, J., Van Leeuwen, N., 1995. Food-initiated outbreak of methicillin-resistant *Staphylococcus aureus* analyzed by pheno-and genotyping. Journal of Clinical Microbiology 33 (5), 1121—1128.

Köck, R., Becker, K., Cookson, B., van Gemert-Pijnen, J.E., Harbarth, S., Kluytmans, J.A.J.W., Mielke, M., Peters, G., Skov, R.L., Struelens, M.J., Tacconelli, E., 2010. Methicillin-resistant *Staphylococcus aureus* (MRSA): burden of disease and control challenges in Europe. Euro Surveillance 15 (41), 19688.

Lai, C.J., Dahlberg, J.E., Weisblum, B., 1973. Structure of an inducibly methylatable nucleotide sequence in 23S ribosomal ribonucleic acid from erythromycin-resistant *Staphylococcus aureus*. Biochemistry 12 (3), 457—460.

Levine, D.P., 2006. Vancomycin: a history. Clinical Infectious Diseases 42 (Suppl. 1), S5—S12.

Li, B., Wendlandt, S., Yao, J., Liu, Y., Zhang, Q., Shi, Z., Wei, J., Shao, D., Schwarz, S., Wang, S., Ma, Z., 2013. Detection and new genetic environment of the pleuromutilin—lincosamide—streptogramin A resistance gene lsa (E) in methicillin-resistant *Staphylococcus aureus* of swine origin. Journal of Antimicrobial Chemotherapy 68 (6), 1251—1255.

Lim, D., Strynadka, N.C., 2002. Structural basis for the β lactam resistance of PBP2a from methicillin-resistant *Staphylococcus aureus*. Nature Structural & Molecular Biology 9 (11), 870.

Loeffler, A., Boag, A.K., Sung, J., Lindsay, J.A., Guardabassi, L., Dalsgaard, A., Smith, H., Stevens, K.B., Lloyd, D.H., 2005. Prevalence of methicillin-resistant *Staphylococcus aureus* among staff and pets in a small animal referral hospital in the UK. Journal of Antimicrobial Chemotherapy 56 (4), 692—697.

Loeffler, A., Kearns, A.M., Ellington, M.J., Smith, L.J., Unt, V.E., Lindsay, J.A., Pfeiffer, D.U., Lloyd, D.H., 2009. First isolation of MRSA ST398 from UK animals: a new challenge for infection control teams? Journal of Hospital Infection 72 (3), 269—271.

Long, K.S., Vester, B., 2012. Resistance to linezolid caused by modifications at its binding site on the ribosome. Antimicrobial Agents and Chemotherapy 56 (2), 603—612.

Long, K.S., Poehlsgaard, J., Kehrenberg, C., Schwarz, S., Vester, B., 2006. The Cfr rRNA methyltransferase confers resistance to phenicols, lincosamides, oxazolidinones, pleuromutilins, and streptogramin A antibiotics. Antimicrobial Agents and Chemotherapy 50 (7), 2500—2505.

López, M., Kadlec, K., Schwarz, S., Torres, C., 2012. First detection of the staphylococcal trimethoprim resistance gene dfrK and the dfrK-carrying transposon Tn 559 in enterococci. Microbial Drug Resistance 18 (1), 13—18.

Lowy, F.D., 2003. Antimicrobial resistance: the example of *Staphylococcus aureus*. Journal of Clinical Investigation 111 (9), 1265—1273.

Lozano, C., López, M., Gómez-Sanz, E., Ruiz-Larrea, F., Torres, C., Zarazaga, M., 2009. Detection of methicillin-resistant *Staphylococcus aureus* ST398 in food samples of animal origin in Spain. Journal of Antimicrobial Chemotherapy 64 (6), 1325—1326.

Maalej, S.M, Rhimi, F.M., Fines, M., Mnif, B., Leclercq, R., Hammami, A., 2012. Analysis of borderline oxacillin-resistant Staphylococcus aureus (BORSA) strains isolated in Tunisia. Journal of Clinical Microbiology 50 (10), 3345—3348.

Marlowe, E.M., Cohen, M.D., Hindler, J.F., Ward, K.W., Bruckner, D.A., 2001. Practical strategies for detecting and confirming vancomycin-intermediate *Staphylococcus aureus*: a tertiary-care hospital laboratory's experience. Journal of Clinical Microbiology 39 (7), 2637—2639.

Mato, R., Campanile, F., Stefani, S., Crisostomo, M.I., Santagati, M., Sanches, S.I., De Lencastre, H., 2004. Clonal types and multidrug resistance patterns of methicillin-resistant *Staphylococcus aureus* (MRSA) recovered in Italy during the 1990s. Microbial Drug Resistance 10 (2), 106—113.

McAleese, F., Petersen, P., Ruzin, A., Dunman, P.M., Murphy, E., Projan, S.J., Bradford, P.A., 2005. A novel MATE family efflux pump contributes to the reduced susceptibility of laboratory-derived *Staphylococcus aureus* mutants to tigecycline. Antimicrobial Agents and Chemotherapy 49 (5), 1865—1871.

Mejía, C., Zurita, J., Guzmán-Blanco, M., 2010. Epidemiology and surveillance of methicillin-resistant *Staphylococcus aureus* in Latin America. Brazilian Journal of Infectious Diseases 14, 79—86.

Melo-Cristino, J., Resina, C., Manuel, V., Lito, L., Ramirez, M., 2013. First case of infection with vancomycin-resistant *Staphylococcus aureus* in Europe. The Lancet 382 (9888), 205.

Morgan, M., 2008. Methicillin-resistant *Staphylococcus aureus* and animals: zoonosis or humanosis? Journal of Antimicrobial Chemotherapy 62 (6), 1181—1187.

Mulders, M.N., Haenen, A.P.J., Geenen, P.L., Vesseur, P.C., Poldervaart, E.S., Bosch, T., Huijsdens, X.W., Hengeveld, P.D., Dam-Deisz, W.D.C., Graat, E.A.M., Mevius, D., 2010. Prevalence of livestock-associated MRSA in broiler flocks and risk factors for slaughterhouse personnel in The Netherlands. Epidemiology and Infection 138 (5), 743—755.

Nemati, M., Hermans, K., Lipinska, U., Denis, O., Deplano, A., Struelens, M., Devriese, L.A., Pasmans, F., Haesebrouck, F., 2008. Antimicrobial resistance of old and recent *Staphylococcus aureus* isolates from poultry: first detection of livestock-associated methicillin-resistant strain ST398. Antimicrobial Agents and Chemotherapy 52 (10), 3817—3819.

Ng, E.Y., Trucksis, M., Hooper, D.C., 1994. Quinolone resistance mediated by norA: physiologic characterization and relationship to flqB, a quinolone resistance locus on the *Staphylococcus aureus* chromosome. Antimicrobial Agents and Chemotherapy 38 (6), 1345—1355.

Ng, E.Y., Trucksis, M., Hooper, D.C., 1996. Quinolone resistance mutations in topoisomerase IV: relationship to the flqA locus and genetic evidence that topoisomerase IV is the primary target and DNA gyrase is the secondary target of fluoroquinolones in *Staphylococcus aureus*. Antimicrobial Agents and Chemotherapy 40 (8), 1881–1888.

Noble, W.C., Virani, Z., Cree, R.G., 1992. Co-transfer of vancomycin and other resistance genes from *Enterococcus faecalis* NCTC 12201 to *Staphylococcus aureus*. FEMS Microbiology Letters 93 (2), 195–198.

Ogston, A., 1880. Ueber Abscesse. Archiv fuer Klinische Chirurgie 25, 588–600.

Oulahal, N., Brice, W., Martial, A., Degraeve, P., 2008. Quantitative analysis of survival of *Staphylococcus aureus* or *Listeria innocua* on two types of surfaces: polypropylene and stainless steel in contact with three different dairy products. Food Control 19 (2), 178–185.

Parks, Y.A., Noy, M.F., Aukett, M.A., Webb, C.A., 1987. Methicillin resistant *Staphylococcus aureus* in milk. Archives of Disease in Childhood 62, 82–88.

Paterson, G.K., Larsen, A.R., Robb, A., Edwards, G.E., Pennycott, T.W., Foster, G., Mot, D., Hermans, K., Baert, K., Peacock, S.J., Parkhill, J., 2012. The newly described mecA homologue, mecA LGA251, is present in methicillin-resistant *Staphylococcus aureus* isolates from a diverse range of host species. Journal of Antimicrobial Chemotherapy 67 (12), 2809–2813.

Paul, S.K., Ghosh, S., Kawaguchiya, M., Urushibara, N., Hossain, M.A., Ahmed, S., Mahmud, C., Jilani, M.S.A., Haq, J.A., Ahmed, A.A., Kobayashi, N., 2014. Detection and genetic characterization of PVL-positive ST8-MRSA-IVa and exfoliative toxin D-positive European CA-MRSA-Like ST1931 (CC80) MRSA-IVa strains in Bangladesh. Microbial Drug Resistance 20 (4), 325–336.

Peacock, J.E., Marsik, F.J., Wenzel, R.P., 1980. Methicillin-resistant *Staphylococcus aureus*: introduction and spread within a hospital. Annals of Internal Medicine 93 (4), 526–532.

Persoons, D., Van Hoorebeke, S., Hermans, K., Butaye, P., De Kruif, A., Haesebrouck, F., Dewulf, J., 2009. Methicillin-resistant *Staphylococcus aureus* in poultry. Emerging Infectious Diseases 15 (3), 452.

Pfaller, M.A., Sader, H.S., Flamm, R.K., Castanheira, M., Smart, J.I., Mendes, R.E., 2017. In vitro activity of telavancin against clinically important gram-positive pathogens from 69 US medical centers (2015): potency analysis by US census divisions. Microbial Drug Resistance 23 (6), 718–726.

Porrero, M.C., Mentaberre, G., Sánchez, S., Fernández-Llario, P., Gómez-Barrero, S., Navarro-Gonzalez, N., Serrano, E., Casas-Díaz, E., Marco, I., Fernández-Garayzabal, J.F., Mateos, A., 2013. Methicillin resistant *Staphylococcus aureus* (MRSA) carriage in different free-living wild animal species in Spain. The Veterinary Journal 198 (1), 127–130.

Price, L.B., Stegger, M., Hasman, H., Aziz, M., Larsen, J., Andersen, P.S., Pearson, T., Waters, A.E., Foster, J.T., Schupp, J., Gillece, J., 2012. *Staphylococcus aureus* CC398: host adaptation and emergence of methicillin resistance in livestock. mBio 3 (1), e00305–e00311.

Pu, S., Han, F., Ge, B., 2009. Isolation and characterization of methicillin-resistant *Staphylococcus aureus* strains from Louisiana retail meats. Applied and Environmental Microbiology 75 (1), 265–267.

Rammelkamp, C.H., Maxon, T., 1942. Resistance of *Staphylococcus aureus* to the action of penicillin. Proceedings of the Society for Experimental Biology and Medicine 51 (3), 386–389.

Renzoni, A., Kelley, W.L., Rosato, R.R., Martinez, M.P., Roch, M., Fatouraei, M., Haeusser, D.P., Margolin, W., Fenn, S., Turner, R.D., Foster, S.J., 2017. Molecular bases determining daptomycin resistance-mediated resensitization to β-lactams (seesaw effect) in methicillin-resistant *Staphylococcus aureus*. Antimicrobial Agents and Chemotherapy 61 (1) e01634-16.

Rich, M., Roberts, L., 2004. Methicillin-resistant *Staphylococcus aureus* isolates from companion animals. The Veterinary Record 154 (10), 310.

Robinson, D.A., Kearns, A.M., Holmes, A., Morrison, D., Grundmann, H., Edwards, G., O'Brien, F.G., Tenover, F.C., McDougal, L.K., Monk, A.B., Enright, M.C., 2005. Re-emergence of early pandemic *Staphylococcus aureus* as a community-acquired meticillin-resistant clone. The Lancet 365 (9466), 1256–1258.

Rodríguez-Lázaro, D., Ariza-Miguel, J., Diez-Valcarce, M., Fernández-Natal, I., Hernández, M., Rovira, J., 2015. Foods confiscated from non-EU flights as a neglected route of potential methicillin-resistant *Staphylococcus aureus* transmission. International Journal of Food Microbiology 209, 29–33.

Rosenbach, A.J.F., 1884. Mikro-organismen bei den Wund-infections-krankheiten des Menschen. JF Bergmann.

Rutland, B.E., Weese, J.S., Bolin, C., Au, J., Malani, A.N., 2009. Human-to-dog transmission of methicillin-resistant *Staphylococcus aureus*. Emerging Infectious Diseases 15 (8), 1328.

Saha, B., Singh, A.K., Ghosh, A., Bal, M., 2008. Identification and characterization of a vancomycin-resistant *Staphylococcus aureus* isolated from Kolkata (South Asia). Journal of Medical Microbiology 57 (1), 72–79.

Schwarz, S., Shen, J., Kadlec, K., Wang, Y., Michael, G.B., Feßler, A.T., Vester, B., 2016. Lincosamides, streptogramins, phenicols, and pleuromutilins: mode of action and mechanisms of resistance. Cold Spring Harbor Perspectives in Medicine 6 (11), a027037.

Schwendener, S., Perreten, V., 2011. New transposon Tn6133 in methicillin-resistant *Staphylococcus aureus* ST398 contains vga (E), a novel streptogramin A, pleuromutilin, and lincosamide resistance gene. Antimicrobial Agents and Chemotherapy 55 (10), 4900–4904.

Shang, W., Hu, Q., Yuan, W., Cheng, H., Yang, J., Hu, Z., Yuan, J., Zhang, X., Peng, H., Yang, Y., Hu, X., 2016. Comparative fitness and determinants for the characteristic drug resistance of ST239-MRSA-III-t030 and ST239-MRSA-III-t037 strains isolated in China. Microbial Drug Resistance 22 (3), 185–192.

Sharkey, L.K., Edwards, T.A., O'Neill, A.J., 2016. ABC-F proteins mediate antibiotic resistance through ribosomal protection. mBio 7 (2) e01975-15.

Sievert, D.M., Rudrik, J.T., Patel, J.B., McDonald, L.C., Wilkins, M.J., Hageman, J.C., 2008. Vancomycin-resistant *Staphylococcus aureus* in the United States, 2002–2006. Clinical Infectious Diseases 46 (5), 668–674.

Silva, N.C.C., Guimarães, F.F., Manzi, M.P., Júnior, A.F., Gómez-Sanz, E., Gómez, P., Langoni, H., Rall, V.L.M., Torres, C., 2014. Methicillin-resistant *Staphylococcus aureus* of lineage ST398 as cause of mastitis in cows. Letters in Applied Microbiology 59 (6), 665–669.

Sing, A., Tuschak, C., Hörmansdorfer, S., 2008. Methicillin-resistant *Staphylococcus aureus* in a family and its pet cat. New England Journal of Medicine 358 (11), 1200−1201.

Stefani, S., Chung, D.R., Lindsay, J.A., Friedrich, A.W., Kearns, A.M., Westh, H., MacKenzie, F.M., 2012. Meticillin-resistant *Staphylococcus aureus* (MRSA): global epidemiology and harmonisation of typing methods. International Journal of Antimicrobial Agents 39 (4), 273−282.

Stewart, G.C., Rosenblum, E.D., 1980. Genetic behavior of the methicillin resistance determinant in *Staphylococcus aureus*. Journal of Bacteriology 144 (3), 1200−1202.

Swartz, T.H., Huprikar, S., Labombardi, V., Pinney, S., Anyanwu, A., Lee, M., Patel, G., 2013. Heart transplantation in a patient with heteroresistant vancomycin-intermediate *Staphylococcus aureus* ventricular assist device mediastinitis and bacteremia. Transplant Infectious Disease 15 (5).

Thomas, C.M., Hothersall, J., Willis, C.L., Simpson, T.J., 2010. Resistance to and synthesis of the antibiotic mupirocin. Nature Reviews Microbiology 8 (4), 281.

Tomlinson, J.H., Thompson, G.S., Kalverda, A.P., Zhuravleva, A., O'Neill, A.J., 2016. A target-protection mechanism of antibiotic resistance at atomic resolution: insights into FusB-type fusidic acid resistance. Scientific Reports 6, 19524.

Tsubakishita, S., Kuwahara-Arai, K., Sasaki, T., Hiramatsu, K., 2010. Origin and molecular evolution of the determinant of methicillin resistance in staphylococci. Antimicrobial Agents and Chemotherapy 54 (10), 4352−4359.

Van Cleef, B.A.G.L., Broens, E.M., Voss, A., Huijsdens, X.W., Züchner, L., Van Benthem, B.H.B., Kluytmans, J.A.J.W., Mulders, M.N., Van De Giessen, A.W., 2010. High prevalence of nasal MRSA carriage in slaughterhouse workers in contact with live pigs in The Netherlands. Epidemiology and Infection 138 (5), 756−763.

Van Den Broek, I.V.F., Van Cleef, B.A.G.L., Haenen, A., Broens, E.M., Van Der Wolf, P.J., Van Den Broek, M.J.M., Huijsdens, X.W., Kluytmans, J.A.J.W., Van De Giessen, A.W., Tiemersma, E.W., 2009. Methicillin-resistant *Staphylococcus aureus* in people living and working in pig farms. Epidemiology and Infection 137 (5), 700−708.

Van Loo, I.H., Diederen, B.M., Savelkoul, P.H., Woudenberg, J.H., Roosendaal, R., Van Belkum, A., Lemmens-den Toom, N., Verhulst, C., Van Keulen, P.H., Kluytmans, J.A., 2007. Methicillin-resistant *Staphylococcus aureus* in meat products, The Netherlands. Emerging Infectious Diseases 13 (11), 1753.

Wardyn, S.E., Kauffman, L.K., Smith, T.C., 2012. Methicillin-resistant *Staphylococcus aureus* in central Iowa wildlife. Journal of Wildlife Diseases 48 (4), 1069−1073.

Watanabe, Y., Cui, L., Katayama, Y., Kozue, K., Hiramatsu, K., 2011. Impact of rpoB mutations on reduced vancomycin susceptibility in *Staphylococcus aureus*. Journal of Clinical Microbiology 49 (7), 2680−2684.

Waters, A.E., Contente-Cuomo, T., Buchhagen, J., Liu, C.M., Watson, L., Pearce, K., Foster, J.T., Bowers, J., Driebe, E.M., Engelthaler, D.M., Keim, P.S., 2011. Multidrug-resistant *Staphylococcus aureus* in US meat and poultry. Clinical Infectious Diseases 52 (10), 1227−1230.

Weese, J.S., Reid-Smith, R., Rousseau, J., Avery, B., 2010. Methicillin-resistant *Staphylococcus aureus* (MRSA) contamination of retail pork. The Canadian Veterinary Journal 51 (7), 749.

Weese, J.S., Rousseau, J., Traub-Dargatz, J.L., Willey, B.M., McGeer, A.J., Low, D.E., 2005. Community-associated methicillin-resistant *Staphylococcus aureus* in horses and humans who work with horses. Journal of the American Veterinary Medical Association 226 (4), 580−583.

Wegener, H.C., 2012. A15 Antibiotic resistance—linking human and animal health. In: Institute of Medicine (US). Improving Food Safety Through a One Health Approach: Workshop Summary. National Academies Press, Washington, DC, USA.

Wendlandt, S., Li, J., Ho, J., Porta, M.A., Feßler, A.T., Wang, Y., Kadlec, K., Monecke, S., Ehricht, R., Boost, M., Schwarz, S., 2014. Enterococcal multiresistance gene cluster in methicillin-resistant *Staphylococcus aureus* from various origins and geographical locations. Journal of Antimicrobial Chemotherapy 69 (9), 2573−2575.

Wendlandt, S., Lozano, C., Kadlec, K., Gómez-Sanz, E., Zarazaga, M., Torres, C., Schwarz, S., 2012. The enterococcal ABC transporter gene lsa (E) confers combined resistance to lincosamides, pleuromutilins and streptogramin A antibiotics in methicillin-susceptible and methicillin-resistant *Staphylococcus aureus*. Journal of Antimicrobial Chemotherapy 68 (2), 473−475.

Wertheim, H.F., Melles, D.C., Vos, M.C., van Leeuwen, W., van Belkum, A., Verbrugh, H.A., Nouwen, J.L., 2005. The role of nasal carriage in *Staphylococcus aureus* infections. The Lancet Infectious Diseases 5 (12), 751−762.

Wichelhaus, T.A., Schäfer, V., Brade, V., Böddinghaus, B., 1999. Molecular characterization of rpoB mutations conferring cross-resistance to rifamycins on methicillin-resistant *Staphylococcus aureus*. Antimicrobial Agents and Chemotherapy 43 (11), 2813−2816.

Yan, X., Yu, X., Tao, X., Zhang, J., Zhang, B., Dong, R., Xue, C., Grundmann, H., Zhang, J., 2014. *Staphylococcus aureus* ST398 from slaughter pigs in northeast China. International Journal of Medical Microbiology 304 (3−4), 379−383.

Zhang, H.Z., Hackbarth, C.J., Chansky, K.M., Chambers, H.F., 2001. A proteolytic transmembrane signaling pathway and resistance to β-lactams in staphylococci. Science 291 (5510), 1962−1965.

Chapter 17

Streptococcus

Chapter outline

Rivolta (1873) first described the chain forming cocci in pus collected from the equine infection (Todd, 1910). Later Rosenbach established the genus as 'Streptococcus' (Rosenbach, 1884). Nocard and Mollereau (1887) first observed the relationship between the bovine mastitis and *Streptococcus agalactiae*. Lancefield classified beta-haemolytic streptococci on the basis of group specific-carbohydrate antigens (Lancefield, 1933).

Community acquired pneumonia (CAP) and invasive pneumococcal pneumonia (IPD), major clinical and economic disease burden throughout the world is mostly associated with *S. pneumoniae* (pneumococcus) (File and Marrie, 2010). The global study estimated more than 860,000 deaths annually due to *S. pneumoniae* infection in children worldwide (O'Brien et al., 2009). World health organization (WHO) also identified pneumonia as the single cause for 15% of child death under 5 years age group throughout the world (WHO, 2016).In Europe and United States, incidence rate of IPD was 11 and 49 cases per 100,000 populations, respectively before the introduction of vaccine (Blasi et al., 2012; Drijkoningen and Rohde, 2014). A Dutch study estimated the economic burden of CAP as €10,284 per episode of infection for 50−64 year olds admitted to the hospital (Rozenbaum et al., 2015).

Development of antibiotic (penicillin) resistance during 1980−90s in clinical pneumococcal isolates shifted the treatment to macrolides. Due to high selection pressure, pneumococcal isolates soon started to develop macrolide resistance and currently, <10% to >90% *S. pneumoniae* isolates show macrolide resistance worldwide (Pan et al., 2015). *S. suis* besides causing encephalitis, arthritis, endocarditis and meningitis in pigs is currently considered as a major zoonotic pathogen associated with human meningitis specially in Asian countries.

Antimicrobial Resistance in Agriculture. https://doi.org/10.1016/B978-0-12-815770-1.00017-1

Properties of genus

Morphology

Streptococci are gram positive cocci, capsulated, non-sporing and non-motile. Each coccus cell is 1 μm in diameter. They are arranged in a pair or chain of cells as the cell division occurs in one plane. The chain formation and the chain length are variable. *Streptococcus equi* ssp. *equi* is a constant chain producer, other species are not. Young cultures are gram positive whereas bacteria present in the pus and older cultures in the laboratory are often stained as gram negative.

Streptococcal capsule is polysaccharide in nature. The capsules of *S. equi, S. pyogenes* are made of nonantigenic hyaluronic acids containing repeating units of glucuronic acid and *N*-acetyl-glucosamine. Synthesis of the polymer involves the products of three genes, *hasA*, *hasB*, and *hasC*, which are all in the same operon.

In group A Streptococci, underneath the capsule, the cell wall is present. This cell wall has three layers. Outer most layer contains three major surface proteins: M, T and R. Among them M-protein is antiphagocytic and the major virulence factor. It is encoded by *emm* gene. The M-protein structure consists of A, B, C, and D repeat regions followed by the protein anchor and pepsin cleavage site. The anchor region contains the LPXTGX motif required to anchor gram-positive proteins in the host cell membrane. Middle layer of the cell wall consists of group specific carbohydrate antigen (C-substances). Inner layer of the cell wall consists of peptidoglycan. Peptidoglycan can stimulate the production of endogenous pyrogen and act as chemoattractant for leukocytes. Teichoic acids are found in the cell wall of streptococci like other gram positive bacteria.

Classification

Streptococcus belongs to *Micrococcaceae* family and the genus *Streptococcus* consists of 104 recognized species, both commensal and pathogenic. Major pathogenic species for human and animals are *S. pneumoniae* (middle ear infections, meningitis and pneumonia in children and pneumonia with sepsis in adults or immunocompromised persons), *S. pyogenes* (scarlet fever, rheumatic fever), *S. agalactiae* (neonatal pneumonia in human, mastitis in animals), *S. dysagalactiae* ssp. *dysagalactiae* (mastitis), *S. equi* ssp. *equi* (strangles in horses), *S. equi* ssp. *zooepidermicus* (joint ill, mastitis in animals), *S. gordonii* (infective endocarditis in human), *S. parasanguinis* (infective endocarditis in human), *S. sanguinis* (infective endocarditis in human), *S. mutans* (dental caries). The species such as *S. dysgalactiae* subsp. *dysgalactiae*, *S. iniae*, *S. agalactiae* and *S. parauberis* are considered as fish pathogens. 16S rRNA based phylogenetic typing identified five clusters namely *S. mitis*, *S. mutans*, *S. salivarius* (viridians streptococci), *S. agalactiae* and *S. pyogenes* (pyogenic group) which correlated with earlier clustering based on ecological niche and pathogenicity.

Susceptibility to disinfectants

Streptococci are lysed by 6.5% salt, 40% bile (except *S. agalactiae*), 0.1% methylene blue and common disinfectants. They are resistant to 0.02% sodium azide which can be added into media to isolate streptococci (azide blood agar).

Natural habitat

Streptococci are ubiquitously present in the nature specially in the soil, water and air. All warm blooded animals and human can act as their reservoir. Bacteria reside in the mucous membranes of upper respiratory, lower genital and alimentary tract, skin, nose, mouth and throat of human and animals. For example, *S. pneumoniae* is carried by young children (40%−60%), older children (12%), adolescents (6%−10%) and adults (3%−4%) in their nasopharynx (Cardozo et al., 2008). Pneumococcal serotypes with low immunogenicity (6, 14, 19, 23) are colonized in the nasopharynx for prolonged period. Colonization is also influenced by overcrowding, winter season, passive smoke, viral respiratory infection and maternal pneumococcal carriage. Use of antibiotics does not alter the carriage rate but can act as selection pressure to produce carriage of resistant pneumococci specially among the low immunogenic serotypes (Sulikowska et al., 2004). Oral streptococci (20% of total oral bacteria) can colonize and produce biofilm on the surface of teeth. The oral bacteria compete with each other for binding with the teeth surface by producing bacteriocins as observed in dental caries produced by *S. mutans* (Kreth et al., 2008).

Genome: *S. agalactiae* genome is circular and 2 Mb in size. The genome (G + C) content is low. It contains approximately 2100 protein coding sequences as well as structural and regulatory RNAs. The genome also contains certain regions that share some properties with pathogenicity islands (PAI). These islands contain genes for surface proteins and putative virulence factors. The islands are also related to mobile genetic elements such as prophages, plasmids, and conjugative transposons, suggesting that they have been laterally transferred from other sources.

Pneumococci are naturally transformable and they take up and incorporate exogenous DNA by homologous recombination. The rate of recombination varies between pneumococcal strains which can be estimated as the rate at which nucleotide polymorphisms accumulate through recombination compared with mutation (r/m). Micro and macro types of recombination are observed producing replacement of a single/short DNA fragment or uptake of long DNA fragment causing major phenotypic changes (Mostowy et al., 2014).Uncapsulated Pneumococcal lineages showed more tendencies to uptake exogenous DNA and more probabilities to develop antimicrobial resistance (Hanage et al., 2009). Horizontal gene transfer frequently takes place between pneumococci and other streptococci (*S. mitis*, *S. infantis*, *S. oralis*) or any other genera inhabiting the nasopharynx or oral cavity (Donati et al., 2010).

Antigenic characteristics

On the basis of group specific carbohydrate antigen (C-substances) pathogenic streptococci can be sub divided into 21 serogroups. They are designated by letters of the alphabets (A to V, except 'I' and 'J'). This is known as 'Lancefield classification' as per the name of its first proposer, Rebecca Lancefield. The antigen can be extracted by hot hydrochloric acid, formamide or enzymes. The distribution of Lancefield group, streptococcal species and major virulence factors are described in Table 17.1. Some species such as *S. pneumoniae*, *S. uberis,* and *S. parauberis* and are non-groupable.

Differentiation of streptococcal species into serotypes is based on 'type specific' antigen. Group-A Streptococci (*S. pyogenes*) has more than 70 serotypes based on M-protein. Variability of the amino terminal region of M-protein is the basis of this typing. Instead of the serotyping, currently *emm*-typing (M-protein encoding) is also used based on the variation of the hyper variable sequences of the *emm* gene. *Streptococcus suis* is classified into 35 serotypes based on capsular antigens. Among them, serotype 2 is most frequently associated with swine infections (Wisselink et al., 2000). The serotype 2 was also reported as zoonotic agent causing human infections in southeast and east Asia, Europe, North and South America, Australia and New Zealand (Hughes et al., 2009; Gottschalk et al., 2010).

Variations in capsular structure substantiated with molecular analysis differentiate pneumococci into 97 serotypes (Geno et al., 2015). Certain pneumococcal serotypes such as 6A, 6B, 9V, 14, 19A, 19 and 23F are associated with children and the serotype 3 was detected in adults with pneumococcal infection (Cilloniz et al., 2016). The serotypes 1, 5, 6A/6B, and 14 are the predominant strains causing invasive pneumococcal disease (IPD) throughout the world (Johnson et al., 2010). Among these pathogenic serotypes, serotype 1 in Nepal, serotype 14 in Bangladesh and India and serotype 19F in Sri Lanka and Pakistan are commonly detected (Jaiswal et al., 2014). Certain pneumococcal strains are non-typeable (NTPn) due to down-regulated or defective capsule genes (Hathaway et al., 2004). The NTPn are common in carrier people but are sometimes associated with mucosal and eye infections, and rarely with invasive infection (Scott et al., 2012). Introduction of pneumococcal vaccine in children recently changed the distribution of pneumococcal serotypes in the circulation ('serotype replacement'). For example, recent emergence of 19A serotype replacing 19F serotype was associated with 'capsular switching' (Wyres et al., 2012). Capsular switching is the substitution of a particular capsule type gene with another one. The newly emerged serotype can *escape* the vaccine and is associated with multiple antibiotic resistances probably due to high rate of recombination across the genome (Croucher et al., 2013).

Toxins and virulence factors produced

Toxins

(a) Streptolysin-O (SLO): It is an oxygen labile haemolysin at room temperature. It is produced by Lancefield group A, C, G of streptococci. It can lyse the red blood cells, leukocytes, platelets, myocardial cells. It is lethal for mice, guinea pig and rabbit.

(b) Streptolysin-S (SLS): It is an oxygen stable haemolysin at room temperature. It is associated with β—haemolytic streptococci.

(c) Streptokinase: It is a type of fibrinolysin that helps in dissolving the fibrin clot. It is produced by Lancefield group A, C, G of streptococci.

(d) Erythrogenic toxin: It is only produced by Group A streptococci, responsible for erythema production in scarlet fever of human. It is used as antigen in 'Dick test' for diagnosis of scarlet fever.

TABLE 17.1 Distribution of Lancefield group, and major virulence factors of pathogenic streptococcal species.

Bacteria	Lancefield group	Virulence factors	Role of virulence factors
S. agalactiae	B	Capsule (capsular polysaccharide)	Human strains produce it to inhibit complement activation, C3 deposition and thus prevent opsonization and phagocytosis. However, bovine strains do not produce or produce fewer amounts
		CAMP factor	Ceramide binding protein and lethal for mice. It potentiates the activity of haemolysin and it's cytotoxic to mammary tissues.
		R- protein [R28, member of alpha like protein (ALP) family]	Enhances colonization of the human strains to the epithelium, but its role in udder pathogenesis is not known
		Streptococcal C5a peptidase (scpA and scpB): Surface-localized Serine protease	(a) It inactivates human C5a, a neutrophil chemoattractant produced during complement activation. This streptococcal enzyme contributes to virulence by interfering the neutrophil recruitment and results poor inflammatory response in the infected tissues. (b) It can also bind fibronectin and promotes bacterial invasion of epithelial cells
		Neuraminidase Haemolysin Lipoteichoic acid	Exact role in pathogenesis in udder is un-established
		BibA	Immunogenic adhesin with antiphagocytic activity
S. dysgalactiae ssp. *dysgalactiae*	C	Hyaluronidase	Acts as 'spreading factor', enhances the tissue permeability of the bacteria by dissolving the hyaluronic acid
		Streptokinase	As discussed above
		Fibronectin binding protein	It helps in attachment of bacterial cells to an extra-cellular matrix component, fibronectin.
		Serum opacity factor [SOF]	SOF detected in fish isolates. The SOF binds to HDL and then disrupts its structure, which may contribute to the virulence of streptococci
Streptococcus dysgalactiae subsp. *equisimilis*	C, G, A (rare)	M Protein	It can bind fibrinogen and complement control factor 'H'. These interactions mask C3b binding sites on the bacterial surface and inhibit the alternative C3 and classical C5 convertases. It prevents the accumulation of complements on the surface and opsonization
		C5a peptidase (scpA)	It inactivates human C5a, a neutrophil chemoattractant produced during complement activation. This streptococcal enzyme contributes to virulence by interfering the neutrophil recruitment

TABLE 17.1 Distribution of Lancefield group, and major virulence factors of pathogenic streptococcal species.—cont'd

Bacteria	Lancefield group	Virulence factors	Role of virulence factors
S. equi ssp. *equi*	C	Capsule (non antigenic hyaluronic acid make)	Hyaluronic acid capsule enhances negative charge and hydrophilicity of the bacterial surface. So it can maintain the reducing environment adjacent to the bacteria to protect the oxygen labile toxins and enzymes released by it
		M-protein (58 KDa): No antigenic variations is found in the M-protein of this streptococcal species	Antiphagocytic because it can bind fibrinogen and complement control factor 'H'. These interactions mask C3b binding sites on the bacterial surface and inhibit the alternative C3 and classical C5 convertases. Thus it prevents the accumulation of complements on the surface and opsonization.
		Streptokinase	a) It helps in dissemination of the bacteria within the tissue b) It activates complement and produces low molecular weight nitrogenous substrates for bacterial growth
		Streptolysin-O	As discussed above
		IgG binding protein	It binds Fc region of Ig-G. Probably it masks the Fc portion to prevent opsonization & phagocytosis.
		Leukocidin	It can destroy leukocytes
		Bacterial peptidoglycan	(a) It activates alternative complement pathway and produces C3a, C5a that acts as chemoattractant for neutrophils. It has major pathological consequences in the disease production. (b) It acts as pyrogen by release of cytokines like IL-6, TNF from leukocytes and is responsible for fever in the course of the infection.
S. equi ssp. *zooepidemicus*	C	M-protein/Szp, haemolysin, streptokinase	As discussed for *S. equi* ssp *equi*
S. canis	G	M-protein, Streptolysin-O	As discussed above
S. suis	D, R, S, T	Capsule	Antiphagocytic. However, reduced capsule expression or absence of capsule is associated with attachment to epithelial/endothelial cells and formation of biofilms. Substantial amount of S. suis (34%) isolated from infective endocarditis are unencapsulated
		100 KDa and 136 KDa soluble proteins	Exact mechanism of action is not known, but they are required for full expression of virulence
		Suilysin	Suilysin is toxic for different cells, lyses complement, increases blood brain barrier and blood-CSF barrier permeability and induces an inflammatory reaction
		Galα1-4Gal binding adhesin	Adhesion with host cells

Continued

TABLE 17.1 Distribution of Lancefield group, and major virulence factors of pathogenic streptococcal species.—cont'd

Bacteria	Lancefield group	Virulence factors	Role of virulence factors
S. porcinus	E, P, U, V	Capsule, streptokinase, M -protein	As discussed above
S. pneumoniae	Ungroupable	Capsule	Antiphagocytic
		Pilli	Pilli help in adhesion process, associated with pilus Cpa protein/collagen I binding protein. Pilli also help in bacterial cell aggregation in liquid culture/saliva, formation of biofilms
		Pneumococcal surface protein K (PspK)	PspK, present in non-encapsulated subtypes of pneumococci helps in adhesion of the bacteria with respiratory epithelium of the host. PspK also neutralizes secretory IgA on mucosal surfaces
		Pneumolysin	A toxin which is similar to the streptolysin- O, has cell membrane damaging effects and slows the ciliar beat to reduce bacterial clearance
		Neuraminidase	It removes N-acetyl neuraminic acid from the oligosaccharides present in the mucosal cells, alters its structure and thus exposes receptors for bacterial attachment.
		Ig-A protease	It can destroy Ig-A antibody present in the secreation
		PbIB (platelet-binding protein)	It binds to galactose containing residues on lung epithelium and promotes nasopharyngeal colonization
		GH20C (β-hexosamidase)	Involved in nutrient acquisition by processing hexosaminide sugars from host glycans and promotes growth and persistence
		Spbhp-37 (hemoglobin binding protein)	Associated with iron acquisition, growth and infectivity of the bacteria
		Bg1A3 (β-glucosidase)	Converts phosphorylated substrates to monosaccharides, used by the bacteria as nutrient
		DiiA (cell wall protein)	It binds to collagen and lactoferrin and promotes nasopharyngeal colonization and dissemination
		Elongation factor Tu (Tuf)	Binds inactivators of the complement systems (factor H and complement factor H-related protein 1) preventing complement-mediated lysis of the bacteria
		Polyamine transporter (potABCD)	It helps in uptake of polyamines which protect against acid and reactive oxygen species and promotes biofilm formation

TABLE 17.1 Distribution of Lancefield group, and major virulence factors of pathogenic streptococcal species.—cont'd

Bacteria	Lancefield group	Virulence factors	Role of virulence factors
		L-Ascorbate-6-phosphate lactonase	Metallo-β-lactamase activity and produce resistance against β-lactam antibiotics
		Fibronectin binding protein (F1/SfbI, F2)	Invasion of eukaryotic cells
		Serum opacity factor (SfbII)	It promotes adhesion of bacteria with human pharyngeal epithelial cells
		pneumococcal Adhesion and virulence factor (PavA)	It has fibronectin binding activity and it is critical for invasive diseases such as sepsis and meningitis
		Laminin binding protein	It helps in adhesion to basement membrane components and helps in bacterial colonization of damaged epithelium and invasion of bacteria into the bloodstream
		Choline binding proteins (CBP)	CBPs bind to the phosphorylcholine of cell wall noncovalently through a choline binding domain. It binds secretory IgA and complement factor H. It acts as an 'adhesin' and it promotes invasion of epithelial cells and biofilm formation
S. uberis	Ungroupable	Capsule, hyaluronidase	As discussed above
		65 kDa protein (R-like protein, trypsin resistant)	Antiphagocytic
		uberis factor	Analogous to the CAMP factor
		Plasmin binding protein	It binds with plasmin and helps in invasion of the bacteria
		Streptococcus uberis adhesion molecule (*SUAM*)	It can adhere to bovine mammary epithelial cells

Virulence factors

Table 17.1 describes the virulence factors produced by different groups of streptococci.

Transmission

Streptococci are transmitted by ingestion, inhalation, congenital routes and coitus in animals and human. Pneumococci are transmitted from person-to-person by direct contact with respiratory secreations, saliva or mucus (CDC, 2017). Transmission of *S. pyogenes* occurs by inhalation, ingestion of contaminated and untreated foods (salads, milk, eggs), direct contact with nasal discharges and skin lesions of infected persons, and direct contact with skin, vagina, anus and pharynx of carrier peoples (Bessen, 2009). *S. equi* subsp. *zooepidemicus* resides on the tonsil, upper respiratory tract, skin and urogenital tract of horses. Transmission of *S. equi* subsp. *zooepidemicus* to human occurs by inhalation, ingestion or through skin contact. Transmission of *S. suis* and *S. canis* from infected pigs and dogs, respectively to human can take place through direct contact. Fish associated streptococci (*S. iniae*) are transmitted through abraded skin during handling of live or freshly killed fishes.

Diagnosis

Broncho alveolar lavage, broncho aspirate, blood and sputum can be collected from pneumonia patients. Ideal sputum sample for detection of etiological bacteria should contain less than 10 epithelial cells and more than 25 lymphocyte cells and it should be collected before initiation of antimicrobial therapy. The clinical samples from animals include mastitic milk, pus and exudate from lesion, skin scrapings, cerebrospinal fluid, urine and affected tissues. All the samples should be carried into the laboratory in transport medium maintaining the cold chain as streptococci are highly susceptible to drying.

Laboratory examinations

Direct examination

A smear can be prepared from centrifuged deposit of collected broncho alveolar lavage, broncho aspirate, sputum, milk, urine, pus or exudate samples or tissues and stained by Gram's Method. Streptococci appear as gram positive cocci arranged in a pair or chain of spherical cells. The chains are specially observed either in clinical samples or in the liquid medium (broth) culture. All species of streptococci are not always chain producers (except *S. equi* ssp *equi*). *S. pneumoniae* is found as pair of cocci.

Isolation of *Streptococcus* spp.: Isolation of pneumococci from blood samples is a major diagnostic approach for confirmation of community-acquired pneumonia. Role of blood culture in confirmation of ventilator-associated pneumonia and hospital-acquired pneumonia is although limited (Chastre and Fagon, 2002). Streptococci cannot be isolated in ordinary bacteriological media. They are fastidious and auxotrophic for a number of amino acids. Presence of salt (6.5%), bile (40%), bacitracin and higher pH (9.6) can inhibit the streptococcal growth. Blood agar with sodium azide, Columbia blood agar, Edwards medium can be used for isolation. Group D Streptococci can be isolated in Bile-aesculin media, eosine methylene blue agar, citrate-azide-tween-carbonate-agar (CATC), kanamycin-aesculin-azide-agar (KAA). Fish associated strains of *Streptococcus dysgalactiae* subsp. *dysgalactiae* (GCSD) are isolated in Todd-Hewitt agar containing congo red and oxolinic acid. Majority of them do no grow in MacConkey agar. Incubation temperature is 37°C, however thermophilic strains prefer higher temperature like 42°C.

After overnight incubation, translucent, convex 1−2 mm diameter colonies are produced. Varieties of haemolysis as described below are observed in blood agar.

(a) Beta haemolysis (β-haemolysis): A zone of complete haemolysis surrounding the colony is found. It is found in *S. pyogenes, S. agalactiae, S. equi* ssp. *equi* etc.

(b) Alpha haemolysis (α-haemolysis): a narrow zone of greenish partial haemolysis is observed adjacent to the colony which is surrounded by clear zone of complete haemolysis. It is produced by *S.equinus, S. uberis, S. suis* etc. Streptococcal strains isolated from fish initially produce α-hemolysis on cattle and sheep blood agar which is converted into β-hemolysis after prolonged incubation at 37°C or 4°C.

(c) α′-haemolysis (alpha prime): A hazy zone of partial haemolysis adjacent to the colony which is less well demarcated from the rest of the medium.

(d) Gamma haemolysis (γ-haemolysis): Non-haemolytic and mostly non-pathogenic strains are described as γ-haemolytic.

In a liquid medium, growth after incubation is characterized by either evenly dispersed turbidity or as sediment with clear supernatant. GCSD is excellent congo red binder and produces orange coloured colonies in Todd-Hewitt agar containing congo red and oxolinic acid. The oxolinic acid is inhibitory for contaminant staphylococci and Gram-negative bacteria.

Immunological tests: An antigen capture-ELISA for detection of pneumolysin in urine of children is developed (del Mar García-Suárez et al., 2007).

Serological tests: Serological tests are not useful for detection of pneumococci in patients who require immediate treatment. For detection of persistent infections in carrier people, ELISA is developed against pneumococcal surface adhesin A (PsaA) or capsular polysachharide (Jado et al., 2001).

Molecular biology: PCR targeting *ply* (pneumolysin) or *lytA* gene can confirm pneumococcal infection in suspected patients (Murdoch, 2004; Carvalho et al., 2007).

Characteristics of antimicrobial resistance

A moderate proportion of pneumococci (20%—30%) associated with CAP are increasingly detected as multi-drug resistant (MDR) against several classes of antibiotics such as penicillins, cephalosporins, macrolides and fluoroquinolones throughout the world (Draghi et al., 2006). In South Asian countries, resistance of clinical pneumococci against co-trimoxazole varied between 56% and 74%, whereas in Sri Lanka, resistance to penicillin (90%), erythromycin (60%), cefotaxime (50%), and chloramphenicol (26%) was detected (Jaiswal et al., 2014). Vaccination against pneumococci followed by 'serotype replacement' was also detected as a contributing factor for generation of MDR strains other than horizontal transfer of mobile genetic elements. Serotype replacement was associated with change in antibiotic selection pressure causing 'soft selective sweep' of the strains mediated by multiple adaptive alleles across the population at the same time (Croucher et al., 2014). Moreover, capsulated pneumococcal strains sometimes became non-encapsulated to escape vaccine and remained in a higher transformation stage with more efficiency to accept virulence and antibiotic resistance genes (Chewapreecha et al., 2014a, 2014b).

Penicillin and β-lactam resistance

Currently, Pneumococcal isolates having MIC of 2 mg/L for penicillin are considered as penicillin resistant during treatment of human meningitis. For parenteral treatment of pneumococcal pneumonia, MIC of 8 mg/L or more is considered as resistant (Cillóniz et al., 2016). Penicillin resistant (MIC: 0.6 mg/L) pneumococci was first reported from Australia in 1967 (Hansman and Bullen, 1967). In 1977, pneumococci (serotypes 6 and 19A) with much higher resistance to penicillin (MIC: 0.12—4 mg/L) and other antibiotics was detected in hospitalized children in South Africa (Jacobs et al., 1978). In Spain, penicillin resistant pneumococci (MIC: 0.5—2 mg/L) was detected from adult patients (Liñares et al., 1983). Subsequently penicillin resistant pneumococci (serotypes 6A, 6B, 9V, 14, 15A, 19A, 19F, 23F) spread throughout the countries in Europe, North America, South America and Asia (Low, 2005). A comprehensive study with published data of penicillin sensitivity among the pneumococcal isolates in Asia during 1993—2013 revealed a decreasing trend of the sensitivity in certain countries such as Malaysia, Singapore, Taiwan, Hong Kong and Nepal (Mamishi et al., 2014). Although pneumococcal isolates with high penicillin sensitivity were reported from few Asian countries for example Japan, India, Iran and Bangladesh (Fahimzad et al., 2006; Sonavane et al., 2008; Saha et al., 2009; Hishiki et al., 2011).

Three phases of peptidoglycan synthesis were described in streptococci (pneumococci). Sidewall growth (primary step) is followed by septal growth and final septation. The septal growth occurs across the middle plane of the bacterial cell and it produces a distinct ring shaped structure on the surface (annulus) made of peptidoglycan. The annulus helps in final septation (Wheeler et al., 2011). Six classes of penicillin binding proteins (PBPs) are engaged in peptidoglycan synthesis of pneumococci. Three of the PBPs (PBP1a, PBP1b, PBP2a) are class 'A' PBPs having both transglycosylase and transpeptidase activities. Two of them (PBP2b and PBP2x) belong to class 'B' and act as transpeptidase. The PBP3 is a class 'C' carboxypeptidase. The PBP2b acts as a component of 'elongation complex' and helps in peptidoglycan elongation (annulus formation) and PBP2x acts as a member of 'divisome complex' synthesizing the septum peptidoglycan (Philippe et al., 2014). Mutations in PBP1a, PBP2b and PBP2x are associated with resistance against penicillin and other β-lactams in pneumococci (Zapun et al., 2008). Pneumococci can select the PBP to produce resistance against β-lactams according to the potentiality of PBPs. For example, to generate resistance against piperacillin (a kind of penicillin), pneumococci preferred to produce mutations in PBP2b although having greater affinity for PBP2x ('piperacillin paradox'). Mutation in PBP2b can arrest bacterial growth due to erroneous elongation of peptidoglycan, whereas, mutation in PBP2x can hamper the septation process but cannot arrest the bacterial growth (Kocaoglu et al., 2015). Cephalosporins have affinity for PBP2x and the resistant strains of pneumococci generate mutations in PBP2x. The resistance is associated with loss of hydrogen bond in PBP2x, used for recognition of the cephalosporins (Gordon et al., 2000).

The genome-wide association study identified single nucleotide polymorphism in the genes other than PBPs associated with β-lactam resistance in pneumococci such as genes for peptidoglycan synthesis (*mraW*, *mraY*) and cell-division pathway (*ftsL*, *gpsB*), genes encoding chaperones (*clpL*, *clpX*), gene in the recombination pathway (*recU*) (Chewapreecha et al., 2014a, 2014b). The genes associated with penicillin resistance and other β-lactam resistance is not always similar. The single point mutation in PBP2x conferred resistance against cefotaxime, not against penicillins

(Kocaoglu et al., 2015). Other resistance mechanism of pneumococci involves possession of murMN operon encoding transferase enzyme that add L-Ala-L-Ala (or L-Ser-LAla) cross-bridge extension to the L-Lysine residue of the peptidoglycan. The cross bridge can increase PBP2b-dependent transpeptidation and generate β-lactam resistance (Berg et al., 2013).

Macrolide resistance

Macrolides bind reversibly to the 23S rRNA at a site near the peptidyl transferase center of the bacterial ribosomal (50S). The 14/15 membered smaller macrolides block the formation of nascent peptide chain and the >16 membered larger macrolides cause ribosomal dissociation and inhibit bacterial protein synthesis. Macrolide resistance in pneumococci or other streptococci is mediated by common mechanisms used by other gram-positive bacteria.

Macrolide efflux is the most common mechanism of resistance, encoded by the *mef* (E)/*mel* operon possessed by pneumococci (M-phenotype) isolated from North America, United Kingdom, Canada, Germany and other countries (Chancey et al., 2012). The *mef* (E)/*mel* is carried by macrolide efflux genetic assembly (Mega) element which is inducible with erythromycin, clarithromycin, and azithromycin during nasopharyngeal colonization of pneumococci (Chancey et al., 2015). The *mef* (E) is common throughout the world, whereas the homolog *mef* (A) is detected in pneumococci in Germany, Denmark and Australia and another homolog, *mef* (I) is relatively rare in occurrence (Cochetti et al., 2005). The *mef* (E) encodes a protein of major facilitator superfamily which utilizes proton motive force-driven efflux pump to expel the drug from bacterial cells (Tait-Kamradt et al., 1997). The Mef(E) acts synergistically with Mel as a two-compartment efflux pump to generate macrolide resistance. The *mel* encodes an ATP-binding cassette (ABC) transporter protein which helps in displacement of macrolide from the ribosome and transfer to Mef(E) for effective efflux (Nunez-Samudio and Chesneau, 2013).

Ribosomal binding of macrolides can be prevented by methylation of 23SrRNA. Adenine specific N-methyl transferases, encoded by erythromycin ribosomal methylase (*erm*) causes the methylation of rRNA. This mechanism is associated with higher level macrolide resistance in pneumococci and is more prevalent in Europian countries such as Belgium, France, Poland, Italy, and Spain (Cillóniz et al., 2016). Pneumococci commonly possess *erm* (B) and rarely *erm*(A) and *erm*(TR), associated with resistance against lincosamides and streptograminB in addition to macrolides (Johnston et al., 1998). Usually expression of *erm* [except *erm* (B)] is repressed in absence of inducible macrolides through a mechanism known as 'translational attenuation'. Expression of *erm* (B) is both inducible and constitutive in the cost of bacterial 'fitness' (Min et al., 2008; Gupta et al., 2013). *S. pneumoniae* possessing both *erm* (B) and *mef* (E)/*mel* (dual macrolide resistance genotype) is increasingly reported throughout the globe since 1990s specially in Asian countries, Russia, South Africa, and United States (Farrell et al., 2008).

Mutation of ribosomal proteins (L4 and L22) was seldom found associated with macrolide resistance in pneumococci (Franceschi et al., 2004). In *S. pyogenes*, macrolide resistance was associated with ATP-binding cassette proteins [*msr* (D)] which protect the bacterial ribosome by displacement of macrolides attached (Sharkey et al., 2016).

Quinolone resistance

Point mutations in quinolone resistance-determining regions of DNA topoisomerase IV (ParC2ParE2) and DNA gyrase (GyrA2GyrB2) were associated with quinolone resistance in pneumococci. Intraspecies or interspecies recombination (with mitis group of streptococci) contributes also in emergence of quinlone resistance in pneumococci (de la Campa, 2004).

Chloramphenicol resistance

Resistant strains of pneumococci produce chloramphenicol acetyltransferase enzyme (encoded by *cat*) which can break down the drug and make it incapable to bind with bacterial ribosome (Dang-Van et al., 1978). The *cat* gene is carried by a transposon (Tn*5253*) present in clinical isolates of pneumococci. The Tn*5253* is a composite transposon consisting of the tetracycline resistance transposon Tn*5251* and Tn*5252*, a 47-kb transposon carrying the chloramphenicol resistance determinant (Ayoubi et al., 1991).

Tetracycline resistance

The drug prevents bacterial protein synthesis by binding with either the acceptor site (A-site) or the peptidyl-donor site (P-site) of the 30S ribosomal subunit. Ribosomal protection mediated by *tet*(M) and *tet*(O) is the resistance mechanism detected in pneumococci against tetracycline (Martin et al., 1986). The Tet(M) helps in release of tetracycline from the ribosome by a GTP mediated process and it modifies tRNA in such a manner that tRNA binding with ribosome is not affected by the drug (Burdett, 1993; Dantley et al., 1998). The resistance determinant *tet*(M) is transferred through the transposons Tn*1545*, Tn*525* and Tn*916* from diverse sources (Ayoubi et al., 1991; Cochetti et al., 2007). The Tn*916* also carries other resistance genes [*erm*(B)] in addition to *tet*(M) and is highly conserved. The conserved nature of Tn*916* may be attributed to the persistence of antibiotic resistance in pneumococci throughout the era (Wyres et al., 2013).

Trimethoprim-sulfamethoxazole resistance

Trimethoprim resistance in clinical isolates of pneumococci was associated with single amino acid substitution (isoleucine replaced with leucine) in the chromosomal-encoded dihydrofolate reductase and disruption of its function (Adrian and Klugman, 1997). Pneumococcal resistance to sulfamethoxazole was correlated with duplicaton (position 66 and 67, Ser-61, Arg-58, Pro-59) or insertion of amino acids (insertion of arginine between Gly-60 and Ser-61) in chromosomal-encoded dihydropteroate synthase (Lopez et al., 1987; Padayachee and Klugman, 1999).

Glycopeptide resistance

Vancomycin-resistant pneumococci did not appear in the circulation so far. Clinically important enterococci (*E. faecalis* and *E. faecium*) associated with meningitis, urinary tract infections, intra-abdominal and intra-pelvic abscesses and bacteraemia are increasingly found resistant to vancomycin due to possession of *vanA* gene (Sood et al., 2008).

Spectinomycin resistance

It is an aminocyclitol antibiotic and is used therapeutically in farm animals in combination with lincomycin. Spectinomycin resistance in *S. suis* isolates was correlated with *spw* and *spw_like* determinants causing mutation in the 30S ribosomal protein s5. A mobile genetic element carrying *spw_like-aadE-lnu*(B)-*lsa*(E) multidrug resistance cluster was also identified in *S. suis* isolates (Huang et al., 2016).

Cationic antimicrobial peptide (CAMP) resistance

The cationic antimicrobial peptides (cathelicidins, defensins) are produced by circulating neutrophils, macrophages and epithelial cells to encounter the invading pathogens including streptococci. CAMPs can produce bactericidal effect after getting attracted to the negative charge of the bacterial membrane. Resistance to CAMP is associated with increased charge of bacterial membrane which can repel the CAMPs. The *dlt* operon of pathogenic streptococci can produce D-alanylation of teichoic acids, an acidic polymer present on the cell wall. The highly cationic side chain of alanine increases cell surface charge and repeal CAMPs in group A and B streptococci, pneumococci, *S. suis* and *S. mutans* (Saar-Dover et al., 2012). Group A streptococci possessing N-acetylglucosamine side-chain in Lancefield group-specific carbohydrate was detected to produce CAMP resistance (van Sorge et al., 2014). The LytA protein of pneumococci can mask the bacterial surface with highly charged choline and thus repeal CAMPs (Swiatlo et al., 2002).

Characteristics of antimicrobial resistance of streptococcal isolates observed in different livestock, horses, birds, wildlife, marine animals as well as in human are discussed in the following section.

Livestock (cattle, buffalo)

An antimicrobial resistance study in European countries (Poland) with the antibiotics commonly used in the country and substantial numbers of streptococcal isolates (*S. uberis*, *S. dysgalactiae*, *S. agalactiae*) from clinical bovine mastitis revealed the resistance against gentamicin, kanamycin, and tetracycline and susceptibility for penicillin, enrofloxacin, and marbofloxacin. In most of the isolates tetracycline resistance gene [*tet*(M), *tet*(K), *tet*(L)] was detected but no correlation between possession of resistance gene and phenotypical resistance was observed (Kaczorek et al., 2017). In Asian countries such as in China, streptococcal isolates from bovine mastitis showed resistance against penicillin-tetracycline-erythromycin-clindamycin and majority of the isolates possessed *pbp2b, tetL, tetM*, and *ermB* genes (Ding et al., 2016). *S. suis* associated with diverse clinical conditions in calves showed multi drug resistance (trimethoprim-sulfamethoxazole, sulfadimethoxine, oxytetracycline, chlortetracycline, gentamicin, florfenicol, neomycin, tilmicosin, clindamycin, enrofloxacin, spectinomycin) in majority (67%) of the isolates in United States (Okwumabua et al., 2017). Another United States (Wisconsin) based study exhibited phenotypic susceptibility of all *Streptococcus* spp. (isolated from bovine mastitis) to ceftiofur, cephalothin, and oxacillin (Ruegg et al., 2015). In New Zealand, *S. dysgalactiae* and *S. uberis* isolated from bovine milk showed resistance against trimethoprim/sulfamethoxazole (McDougall et al., 2014). Whole-genome sequence-based study of *S. uberis* and *S. dysgalactiae* strains isolated from dairy cows in Canada revealed the presence of unique resistance gene sequences (8.1/genome) such as *TEM, Linb, Lnub, Ermb, Ermc,* and *TetS*. Significant correlation between possession of *tetM* (P = .015) and *tetS* (P = .064) genes and phenotypic resistance to tetracyclines was detected in *S. uberis* isolates (Vélez et al., 2017). Vancomycin resistant *Streptococcus gallolyticus* subsp. *gallolyticus* was isolated from a calf. The isolate possessed Tn*1546*-like element, integrated into the bacterial chromosome, and showed excess chromosomal rearrangement, deletion or insertion of gene (Romero-Hernández et al., 2015). β-lactam resistant streptococci were isolated from mastitic milk of buffaloes in India (Preethirani et al., 2015).

Livestock (pigs)

Antibiotic resistance pattern of *S. suis* isolated from pigs with or without clinical infections in United Kingdom over a period of 2009—14 was studied. The isolates from healthy animals were more resistant than the isolates from infected animals to cephalosporins, sulphonamides and tetracyclines. Clinical *S. suis* isolates showed increased resistance against aminoglycosides, cephalosporins, fluoroquinolones, sulphonamides and tetracyclines in recent times (2013—14) than earlier (2009—11) (Hernandez-Garcia et al., 2017). Antibiotic resistance of *S. suis*, isolated from different organs of pigs after post-mortem with wider variation (0.1%—78%) was observed against penicillin, ampicillin, ceftiofur, clindamycin, tetracycline, florfenicol, enrofloxacin and trimethoprim/sulfamethoxazole (van Hout et al., 2016). Serotype 9 of *S. suis* was detected as endemic in swine population of certain European countries such as Spain. Most of the serotype 9 strains isolated from pigs in Spain and Canada were found resistant to tetracycline, lincosamides and macrolides (Zheng et al., 2018). In China, ST7 sequence type of *S. suis* was most prevalent and the sequence type was associated with *ermB, mefA, tet*(O) genes (Huang et al., 2015).

Horses

Streptococcus zooepidemicus was isolated from sick horses during 2000—14 in Japan and 32.3% isolated strains possessed one of the tetracycline resistance genes i.e., *tet*(M), *tet*(O), or *tet*(W). Presence of *tet*(O) was associated with phenotypical resistance and high MIC against minocycline, commonly used in racing horses in Japan (Kinoshita et al., 2018). A retrospective study with streptococcal isolates (*S. zooepidemicus*) from equine clinical samples collected during 1999—2012 revealed increased resistance over time against tetracycline (Johns and Adams, 2015).

Ducks

Streptococcus gallolyticus subsp. *pasteurianus* is an under-studied and opportunistic pathogen for human. *S. gallolyticus* subsp. *pasteurianus* isolated from dead ducklings in China during 2010—13 showed high macrolide resistance (MIC ≥ 1024 mg/L for erythromycin and 512 mg/L for clarithromycin) associated with possession of *ermB* and *ermT* genes in Tn*916* and IS*1216*, respectively (Li et al., 2016).

Wildlife

β-hemolytic streptococci isolated from captive mink (*Neovison vison*) showed high levels of resistance to tetracycline and erythromycin in Denmark. The antibiotics such as aminopenicillins, tetracyclines and macrolides were prescribed for the studied mink (off-label use) (Nikolaisen et al., 2017).

Marine animals

The complete genome sequence of multiple-drug-resistant *S. parauberis* was reported, isolated from a diseased olive flounder (Japanese halibut) in South Korea. The bacterium possessed a circular chromosome (2,128,740 bp) and a plasmid (23,538 bp) harboring 2123 and 24 genes, respectively (Lee et al., 2018).

Human

Global study (Alexander Project) revealed increased prevalence of penicillin resistant pneumococci in human during 2001 in comparison to 1992 in different countries, such as, in United States (5.6%—20.4%), Spain (24.9%—30.2%),

France (7.7%—35.8%), Italy, Germany and United Kingdom (below 5%). Macrolide resistance of pneumococci was detected as 16.5%—21.9% in 1996—97 which increased up to 24.6% in 1998—2000 (Felmingham et al., 2005). Afterward study (PROTEKT-US) in United States detected a decreasing trend in occurrence of penicillin resistant pneumococci from 26.3% (2000—01) to 16.5% (2003—04). The PROTEKT study also detected penicillin-non-susceptibility (resistance and intermediate sensitivity) in pneumococci isolated from human in South Africa (74%), the Far East (63%), and the Middle East (54%). Overall prevalence rate of macrolide resistant pneumococci in human was 31.0% in 1999—2000 which increased up to 37.2% in 2003—04 (Jenkins et al., 2008). In Mediterranean region, Algeria (44%) and Lebanon (40%) were reported to possess majority of the penicillin non-susceptible pneumococci in human (Borg et al., 2009). European Antimicrobial Resistance Surveillance System (EARSS) reported low prevalence (5%) of penicillin non-susceptible pneumococci in northern European countries and higher prevalence (25%) in southern and eastern European countries (EARSS, 2008).

References

Adrian, P.V., Klugman, K.P., 1997. Mutations in the dihydrofolate reductase gene of trimethoprim-resistant isolates of *Streptococcus pneumoniae*. Antimicrobial Agents and Chemotherapy 41 (11), 2406—2413.

Ayoubi, P., Kilic, A.O., Vijayakumar, M.N., 1991. Tn*5253*, the pneumococcal omega (*cat tet*) BM6001 element, is a composite structure of two conjugative transposons, Tn5251 and Tn5252. Journal of Bacteriology 173 (5), 1617—1622.

Berg, K.H., Stamsås, G.A., Straume, D., Håvarstein, L.S., 2013. Effects of low PBP2b levels on cell morphology and peptidoglycan composition in *Streptococcus pneumoniae* R6. Journal of Bacteriology 195 (19), 4342—4354.

Bessen, D.E., 2009. Population biology of the human restricted pathogen, *Streptococcus pyogenes*. Infection, Genetics and Evolution 9 (4), 581—593.

Blasi, F., Mantero, M., Santus, P., Tarsia, P., 2012. Understanding the burden of pneumococcal disease in adults. Clinical Microbiology and Infections 18, 7—14.

Borg, M.A., Tiemersma, E., Scicluna, E., Van De Sande-Bruinsma, N., De Kraker, M., Monen, J., Grundmann, H., ARMed Project members and collaborators, 2009. Prevalence of penicillin and erythromycin resistance among invasive *Streptococcus pneumoniae* isolates reported by laboratories in the southern and eastern Mediterranean region. Clinical Microbiology and Infections 15 (3), 232—237.

Burdett, V., 1993. tRNA modification activity is necessary for Tet (M)-mediated tetracycline resistance. Journal of Bacteriology 175 (22), 7209—7215.

Cardozo, D.M., Nascimento-Carvalho, C.M., Andrade, A.L.S., Silvany-Neto, A.M., Daltro, C.H., Brandao, M.A.S., Brandao, A.P., Brandileone, M.C.C., 2008. Prevalence and risk factors for nasopharyngeal carriage of *Streptococcus pneumoniae* among adolescents. Journal of Medical Microbiology 57 (2), 185—189.

Carvalho, M.D.G., Tondella, M.L., McCaustland, K., Weidlich, L., McGee, L., Mayer, L.W., Steigerwalt, A., Whaley, M., Facklam, R.R., Fields, B., Carlone, G., Ades, E.W., Dagan, R., Sampson 469, J.S., 2007. Evaluation and improvement of real-time PCR assays targeting *lytA*, *ply*, and *psaA* 470 genes for detection of pneumococcal DNA. Journal of Clinical Microbiology 45, 2460—2466.

CDC, 2017. Available at: https://www.cdc.gov/pneumococcal/about/risk-transmission.html.

Chancey, S.T., Bai, X., Kumar, N., Drabek, E.F., Daugherty, S.C., Colon, T., Ott, S., Sengamalay, N., Sadzewicz, L., Tallon, L.J., Fraser, C.M., 2015. Transcriptional attenuation controls macrolide inducible efflux and resistance in *Streptococcus pneumoniae* and in other gram-positive bacteria containing *mef/mel* [*msr* (D)] elements. PLoS One 10 (2), e0116254.

Chancey, S.T., Zähner, D., Stephens, D.S., 2012. Acquired inducible antimicrobial resistance in gram-positive bacteria. Future Microbiology 7 (8), 959—978.

Chastre, J., Fagon, J.Y., 2002. Ventilator-associated pneumonia. American Journal of Respiratory and Critical Care Medicine 165 (7), 867—903.

Chewapreecha, C., Harris, S.R., Croucher, N.J., Turner, C., Marttinen, P., Cheng, L., Pessia, A., Aanensen, D.M., Mather, A.E., Page, A.J., Salter, S.J., 2014a. Dense genomic sampling identifies highways of pneumococcal recombination. Nature Genetics 46 (3), 305.

Chewapreecha, C., Marttinen, P., Croucher, N.J., Salter, S.J., Harris, S.R., Mather, A.E., Hanage, W.P., Goldblatt, D., Nosten, F.H., Turner, C., Turner, P., 2014b. Comprehensive identification of single nucleotide polymorphisms associated with beta-lactam resistance within pneumococcal mosaic genes. PLoS Genetics 10 (8), e1004547.

Cillóniz, C., Ardanuy, C., Vila, J., Torres, A., 2016. What is the clinical relevance of drug-resistant pneumococcus? Current Opinion in Pulmonary Medicine 22 (3), 227—234.

Cilloniz, C., Martin-Loeches, I., Garcia-Vidal, C., San Jose, A., Torres, A., 2016. Microbial etiology of pneumonia: epidemiology, diagnosis and resistance patterns. International Journal of Molecular Sciences 17 (12), 2120.

Cochetti, I., Tili, E., Vecchi, M., Manzin, A., Mingoia, M., Varaldo, P.E., Montanari, M.P., 2007. New Tn*916*-related elements causing *erm*(B)-mediated erythromycin resistance in tetracycline-susceptible pneumococci. Journal of Antimicrobial Chemotherapy 60 (1), 127—131.

Cochetti, I., Vecchi, M., Mingoia, M., Tili, E., Catania, M.R., Manzin, A., Varaldo, P.E., Montanari, M.P., 2005. Molecular characterization of pneumococci with efflux-mediated erythromycin resistance and identification of a novel mef gene subclass, mef (I). Antimicrobial Agents and Chemotherapy 49 (12), 4999—5006.

Croucher, N.J., Chewapreecha, C., Hanage, W.P., Harris, S.R., McGee, L., van der Linden, M., Song, J.H., Ko, K.S., de Lencastre, H., Turner, C., Yang, F., 2014. Evidence for soft selective sweeps in the evolution of pneumococcal multidrug resistance and vaccine escape. Genome Biology and Evolution 6 (7), 1589—1602.

Croucher, N.J., Finkelstein, J.A., Pelton, S.I., Mitchell, P.K., Lee, G.M., Parkhill, J., Bentley, S.D., Hanage, W.P., Lipsitch, M., 2013. Population genomics of post-vaccine changes in pneumococcal epidemiology. Nature Genetics 45 (6), 656.

Dang-Van, A., Tiraby, G., Acar, J.F., Shaw, W.V., Bouanchaud, D.H., 1978. Chloramphenicol resistance in Streptococcus pneumoniae: enzymatic acetylation and possible plasmid linkage. Antimicrobial Agents and Chemotherapy 13 (4), 577–583.

Dantley, K.A., Dannelly, H.K., Burdett, V., 1998. Binding interaction between Tet (M) and the ribosome: requirements for binding. Journal of Bacteriology 180 (16), 4089–4092.

de la Campa, A.G., balsalobre, L., Ardanuy, C., Fenoll, A., Pérez-Trallero, E., Liñares, J., 2004. Spanish pneumococcal infection study network G03/103. Fluoroquinolone resistance in penicillin-resistant Streptococcus pneumoniae clones, Spain. Emerging Infectious Diseases 10 (10), 1751–1759.

del Mar García-Suárez, M., Cima-Cabal, M.D., Villaverde, R., Espinosa, E., Falguera, M., Juan, R., Vázquez, F., Méndez, F.J., 2007. Performance of a pneumolysin enzyme-linked immunosorbent assay for diagnosis of pneumococcal infections. Journal of Clinical Microbiology 45 (11), 3549–3554.

Ding, Y., Zhao, J., He, X., Li, M., Guan, H., Zhang, Z., Li, P., 2016. Antimicrobial resistance and virulence-related genes of Streptococcus obtained from dairy cows with mastitis in Inner Mongolia, China. Pharmaceutical Biology 54 (1), 162–167.

Donati, C., Hiller, N.L., Tettelin, H., Muzzi, A., Croucher, N.J., Angiuoli, S.V., Oggioni, M., Hotopp, J.C.D., Hu, F.Z., Riley, D.R., Covacci, A., 2010. Structure and dynamics of the pan-genome of Streptococcus pneumoniae and closely related species. Genome Biology 11 (10), R107.

Draghi, D.C., Jones, M.E., Sahm, D.F., Tillotson, G.S., 2006. Geographically-based evaluation of multidrug resistance trends among Streptococcus pneumoniae in the USA: findings of the FAST surveillance initiative (2003–2004). International Journal of Antimicrobial Agents 28 (6), 525–531.

Drijkoningen, J.J.C., Rohde, G.G.U., 2014. Pneumococcal infection in adults: burden of disease. Clinical Microbiology and Infections 20, 45–51.

European Antimicrobial Resistance Surveillance System (EARSS), 2008. Available at: http://www.rivm.nl/earss/Images/EARSS%202008_final_tcm61-65020.pdf.

Fahimzad, A.R., Mamaishi, S., Noorbakhsh, S., Siadati, A., Hashemi, F.B., Tabatabaei, S.R., Pourakbari, B., Aligholi, M., Abedini, M., 2006. Study of antibiotics resistance in pediatric acute bacterial meningitis with E-Test method. Iranian Journal of Pediatrics 16 (2), 149–156.

Farrell, D.J., Couturier, C., Hryniewicz, W., 2008. Distribution and antibacterial susceptibility of macrolide resistance genotypes in Streptococcus pneumoniae: PROTEKT year 5 (2003–2004). International Journal of Antimicrobial Agents 31 (3), 245–249.

Felmingham, D., White, A.R., Jacobs, M.R., Appelbaum, P.C., Poupard, J., Miller, L.A., Grüneberg, R.N., 2005. The Alexander project: the benefits from a decade of surveillance. Journal of Antimicrobial Chemotherapy 56 (Suppl. 1_2), ii3–ii21.

File Jr., T.M., Marrie, T.J., 2010. Burden of community-acquired pneumonia in North American adults. Postgraduate Medicine 122 (2), 130–141.

Franceschi, F., Kanyo, Z., Sherer, E.C., Sutcliffe, J., 2004. Macrolide resistance from the ribosome perspective. Current Drug Targets - Infectious Disorders 4 (3), 177–191.

Geno, K.A., Gilbert, G.L., Song, J.Y., Skovsted, I.C., Klugman, K.P., Jones, C., Konradsen, H.B., Nahm, M.H., 2015. Pneumococcal capsules and their types: past, present, and future. Clinical Microbiology Reviews 28 (3), 871–899.

Gordon, E., Mouz, N., Duee, E., Dideberg, O., 2000. The crystal structure of the penicillin-binding protein 2x from Streptococcus pneumoniae and its acyl-enzyme form: implication in drug resistance1. Journal of Molecular Biology 299 (2), 477–485.

Gottschalk, M., Xu, J., Calzas, C., Segura, M., 2010. Streptococcus suis: a new emerging or an old neglected zoonotic pathogen? Future Microbiology 5 (3), 371–391.

Gupta, P., Sothiselvam, S., Vázquez-Laslop, N., Mankin, A.S., 2013. Deregulation of translation due to post-transcriptional modification of rRNA explains why erm genes are inducible. Nature Communications 4, 1984.

Hanage, W.P., Fraser, C., Tang, J., Connor, T.R., Corander, J., 2009. Hyper-recombination, diversity, and antibiotic resistance in pneumococcus. Science 324 (5933), 1454–1457.

Hansman, D., Bullen, M.M., 1967. A resistant pneumococcus. Lancet 277, 264–265.

Hathaway, L.J., Meier, P.S., Bättig, P., Aebi, S., Mühlemann, K., 2004. A homologue of aliB is found in the capsule region of non-encapsulated Streptococcus pneumoniae. Journal of Bacteriology 186 (12), 3721–3729.

Hernandez-Garcia, J., Wang, J., Restif, O., Holmes, M.A., Mather, A.E., Weinert, L.A., Wileman, T.M., Thomson, J.R., Langford, P.R., Wren, B.W., Rycroft, A., 2017. Patterns of antimicrobial resistance in Streptococcus suis isolates from pigs with or without streptococcal disease in England between 2009 and 2014. Veterinary Microbiology 207, 117–124.

Hishiki, H., Ishiwada, N., Fukasawa, C., Abe, K., Hoshino, T., Aizawa, J., Ishikawa, N., Kohno, Y., 2011. Incidence of bacterial coinfection with respiratory syncytial virus bronchopulmonary infection in pediatric inpatients. Journal of Infection and Chemotherapy 17 (1), 87–90.

Huang, J., Shang, K., Kashif, J., Wang, L., 2015. Genetic diversity of Streptococcus suis isolated from three pig farms of China obtained by acquiring antibiotic resistance genes. Journal of the Science of Food and Agriculture 95 (7), 1454–1460.

Huang, K., Zhang, Q., Song, Y., Zhang, Z., Zhang, A., Xiao, J., Jin, M., 2016. Characterization of spectinomycin resistance in Streptococcus suis leads to two novel insights into drug resistance formation and dissemination mechanism. Antimicrobial Agents and Chemotherapy 60 (10), 6390–6392.

Hughes, J.M., Wilson, M.E., Wertheim, H.F., Nghia, H.D.T., Taylor, W., Schultsz, C., 2009. Streptococcus suis: an emerging human pathogen. Clinical Infectious Diseases 48 (5), 617–625.

Jacobs, M.R., Koornhof, H.J., Robins-Browne, R.M., Stevenson, C.M., Vermaak, Z.A., Freiman, I., Miller, G.B., Witcomb, M.A., Isaäcson, M., Ward, J.I., Austrian, R., 1978. Emergence of multiply resistant pneumococci. New England Journal of Medicine 299 (14), 735–740.

Jado, I., Fenoll, A., Casal, J., Pérez, A., 2001. Identification of the psaA gene, coding for pneumococcal surface adhesin A, in viridans group streptococci other than Streptococcus pneumoniae. Clinical and Diagnostic Laboratory Immunology 8 (5), 895–898.

Jaiswal, N., Singh, M., Das, R.R., Jindal, I., Agarwal, A., Thumburu, K.K., Kumar, A., Chauhan, A., 2014. Distribution of serotypes, vaccine coverage, and antimicrobial susceptibility pattern of *Streptococcus pneumoniae* in children living in SAARC countries: a systematic review. PLoS One 9 (9), e108617.

Jenkins, S.G., Brown, S.D., Farrell, D.J., 2008. Trends in antibacterial resistance among *Streptococcus pneumoniae* isolated in the USA: update from PROTEKT US years 1—4. Annals of Clinical Microbiology and Antimicrobials 7 (1), 1.

Johns, I.C., Adams, E.L., 2015. Trends in antimicrobial resistance in equine bacterial isolates: 1999—2012. The Veterinary Record 176, 334.

Johnson, H.L., Deloria-Knoll, M., Levine, O.S., Stoszek, S.K., Hance, L.F., Reithinger, R., Muenz, L.R., O'Brien, K.L., 2010. Systematic evaluation of serotypes causing invasive pneumococcal disease among children under five: the pneumococcal global serotype project. PLoS Medicine 7 (10) pii: e1000348.

Johnston, N.J., de Azavedo, J.C., Kellner, J.D., Low, D.E., 1998. Prevalence and characterization of the mechanisms of macrolide, lincosamide, and streptogramin resistance in isolates of *Streptococcus pneumoniae*. Antimicrobial Agents and Chemotherapy 42 (9), 2425—2426.

Kaczorek, E., Małaczewska, J., Wójcik, R., Rekawek, W., Siwicki, A.K., 2017. Phenotypic and genotypic antimicrobial susceptibility pattern of *Streptococcus spp.* isolated from cases of clinical mastitis in dairy cattle in Poland. Journal of Dairy Science 100 (8), 6442—6453.

Kinoshita, Y., Niwa, H., Katayama, Y., 2018. Minocycline resistance in *Streptococcus equi* subsp. *zooepidemicus* isolated from thoroughbred racehorses with respiratory disease in Japan. Journal of Equine Veterinary Science 63, 80—85.

Kocaoglu, O., Tsui, H.C.T., Winkler, M.E., Carlson, E.E., 2015. Profiling of β-lactam selectivity for penicillin-binding proteins in *Streptococcus pneumoniae* D39. Antimicrobial Agents and Chemotherapy 59 (6), 3548—3555.

Kreth, J., Zhang, Y., Herzberg, M.C., 2008. Streptococcal antagonism in oral biofilms: *Streptococcus sanguinis* and *Streptococcus gordonii* interference with *Streptococcus mutans*. Journal of Bacteriology 190 (13), 4632—4640.

Lancefield, R.C., 1933. A serological differentiation of human and other groups of hemolytic streptococci. Journal of Experimental Medicine 57 (4), 571—595.

Lee, Y., Nguyen, T.L., Kim, A., Kim, N., Roh, H.J., Han, H.J., Jung, S.H., Cho, M.Y., Kang, H.Y., Kim, D.H., 2018. Complete genome sequence of multiple-antibiotic-resistant *Streptococcus parauberis* strain SPOF3K, isolated from diseased olive flounder (*Paralichthys olivaceus*). Genome Announcements 6 (17) pii: e00248-18.

Li, M., Cai, C., Chen, J., Cheng, C., Cheng, G., Hu, X., Liu, C., 2016. Inducible expression of both ermB and ermT conferred high macrolide resistance in *Streptococcus gallolyticus* subsp. *pasteurianus* isolates in China. International Journal of Molecular Sciences 17 (10), 1599.

Liñares, J., Garau, J., Dominguez, C., Pérez, J.L., 1983. Antibiotic resistance and serotypes of *Streptococcus pneumoniae* from patients with community-acquired pneumococcal disease. Antimicrobial Agents and Chemotherapy 23 (4), 545—547.

Lopez, P., Espinosa, M., Greenberg, B., Lacks, S.T., 1987. Sulfonamide resistance in *Streptococcus pneumoniae*: DNA sequence of the gene encoding dihydropteroate synthase and characterization of the enzyme. Journal of Bacteriology 169 (9), 4320—4326.

Low, D.E., 2005. Changing trends in antimicrobial-resistant pneumococci: it's not all bad news. Clinical Infectious Diseases 41 (Suppl. 4), S228—S233.

Mamishi, S., Moradkhani, S., Mahmoudi, S., Hosseinpour-Sadeghi, R., Pourakbari, B., 2014. Penicillin-resistant trend of *Streptococcus pneumoniae* in Asia: a systematic review. Iranian Journal of Microbiology 6 (4), 198.

Martin, P., Trieu-Cuot, P., Courvalin, P., 1986. Nucleotide sequence of the tetM tetracycline resistance determinant of the streptococcal conjugative shuttle transposon Tn *1545*. Nucleic Acids Research 14 (17), 7047—7058.

McDougall, S., Hussein, H., Petrovski, K., 2014. Antimicrobial resistance in *Staphylococcus aureus*, *Streptococcus uberis* and *Streptococcus dysgalactiae* from dairy cows with mastitis. New Zealand Veterinary Journal 62 (2), 68—76.

Min, Y.H., Kwon, A.R., Yoon, E.J., Shim, M.J., Choi, E.C., 2008. Translational attenuation and mRNA stabilization as mechanisms of erm (B) induction by erythromycin. Antimicrobial Agents and Chemotherapy 52 (5), 1782—1789.

Mostowy, R., Croucher, N.J., Hanage, W.P., Harris, S.R., Bentley, S., Fraser, C., 2014. Heterogeneity in the frequency and characteristics of homologous recombination in pneumococcal evolution. PLoS Genetics 10 (5), e1004300.

Murdoch, D.R., 2004. Molecular genetic methods in the diagnosis of lower respiratory tract infections. Acta Pathologica Microbiologica et Immunologica Scandinavica 112 (11-12), 713—727.

Nikolaisen, N.K., Lassen, D.C.K., Chriél, M., Larsen, G., Jensen, V.F., Pedersen, K., 2017. Antimicrobial resistance among pathogenic bacteria from mink (*Neovison vison*) in Denmark. Acta Veterinaria Scandinavica 59 (1), 60.

Nocard, N., Mollereau, R., 1887. Sur une mammite contagieuse des vaches laitieres. Annales de l'Institut Pasteur 1, 109—126.

Nunez-Samudio, V., Chesneau, O., 2013. Functional interplay between the ATP binding cassette Msr (D) protein and the membrane facilitator superfamily Mef (E) transporter for macrolide resistance in *Escherichia coli*. Research in Microbiology 164 (3), 226—235.

O'Brien, K.L., Wolfson, L.J., Watt, J.P., Henkle, E., Deloria-Knoll, M., McCall, N., Lee, E., Mulholland, K., Levine, O.S., Cherian, T., 2009. Burden of disease caused by *Streptococcus pneumoniae* in children younger than 5 years: global estimates. The Lancet 374 (9693), 893—902.

Okwumabua, O., Peterson, H., Hsu, H.M., Bochsler, P., Behr, M., 2017. Isolation and partial characterization of *Streptococcus suis* from clinical cases in cattle. Journal of Veterinary Diagnostic Investigation 29 (2), 160—168.

Padayachee, T., Klugman, K.P., 1999. Novel expansions of the gene encoding dihydropteroate synthase in trimethoprim-sulfamethoxazole-resistant *Streptococcus pneumoniae*. Antimicrobial Agents and Chemotherapy 43 (9), 2225—2230.

Pan, F., Han, L., Huang, W., Tang, J., Xiao, S., Wang, C., Qin, H., Zhang, H., 2015. Serotype distribution, antimicrobial susceptibility, and molecular epidemiology of *Streptococcus pneumoniae* isolated from children in Shanghai, China. PLoS One 10 (11), e0142892.

Philippe, J., Vernet, T., Zapun, A., 2014. The elongation of ovococci. Microbial Drug Resistance 20 (3), 215—221.

Preethirani, P.L., Isloor, S., Sundareshan, S., Nuthanalakshmi, V., Deepthikiran, K., Sinha, A.Y., Rathnamma, D., Prabhu, K.N., Sharada, R., Mukkur, T.K., Hegde, N.R., 2015. Isolation, biochemical and molecular identification, and in-vitro antimicrobial resistance patterns of bacteria isolated from bubaline subclinical mastitis in south India. PLoS One 10 (11), e0142717.

Romero-Hernández, B., Tedim, A.P., Sánchez-Herrero, J.F., Librado, P., Rozas, J., Muñoz, G., Baquero, F., Cantón, R., del Campo, R., 2015. *Streptococcus gallolyticus subsp. gallolyticus* from human and animal origins: genetic diversity, antimicrobial susceptibility, and characterization of a vancomycin-resistant calf isolate carrying a vanA-Tn*1546*-like element. Antimicrobial Agents and Chemotherapy 59 (4), 2006−2015.

Rosenbach, F.J., 1884. Mikroorganismen bei den Wundinfektionskrankheiten des Menschen. J.F. Bergmann Verlag, Wiesbaden.

Rozenbaum, M.H., Mangen, M.J.J., Huijts, S.M., van der Werf, T.S., Postma, M.J., 2015. Incidence, direct costs and duration of hospitalization of patients hospitalized with community acquired pneumonia: a nationwide retrospective claims database analysis. Vaccine 33 (28), 3193−3199.

Ruegg, P.L., Oliveira, L., Jin, W., Okwumabua, O., 2015. Phenotypic antimicrobial susceptibility and occurrence of selected resistance genes in gram-positive mastitis pathogens isolated from Wisconsin dairy cows. Journal of Dairy Science 98 (7), 4521−4534.

Saar-Dover, R., Bitler, A., Nezer, R., Shmuel-Galia, L., Firon, A., Shimoni, E., Trieu-Cuot, P., Shai, Y., 2012. D-alanylation of lipoteichoic acids confers resistance to cationic peptides in group B *Streptococcus* by increasing the cell wall density. PLoS Pathogens 8 (9) e1002891.

Saha, S.K., Naheed, A., El Arifeen, S., Islam, M., Al-Emran, H., Amin, R., Fatima, K., Brooks, W.A., Breiman, R.F., Sack, D.A., Luby, S.P., 2009. Surveillance for invasive *Streptococcus pneumoniae* disease among hospitalized children in Bangladesh: antimicrobial susceptibility and serotype distribution. Clinical Infectious Diseases 48 (Suppl. 2), S75−S81.

Scott, J.R., Hinds, J., Gould, K.A., Millar, E.V., Reid, R., Santosham, M., O'brien, K.L., Hanage, W.P., 2012. Nontypeable pneumococcal isolates among Navajo and white mountain Apache communities: are these really a cause of invasive disease? The Journal of Infectious Diseases 206 (1), 73−80.

Sharkey, L.K., Edwards, T.A., O'Neill, A.J., 2016. ABC-F proteins mediate antibiotic resistance through ribosomal protection. mBio 7 (2) e01975-15.

Sonavane, A., Baradkar, V., Mathur, M., 2008. Pattern and antibiotic susceptibility of bacteria isolated in clinically suspected cases of meningitis in children. Journal of Pediatric Neurosciences 3 (2), 131.

Sood, S., Malhotra, M., Das, B.K., Kapil, A., 2008. Enterococcal infections and antimicrobial resistance. Indian Journal of Medical Research 128, 111−121.

Sulikowska, A., Grzesiowski, P., Sadowy, E., Fiett, J., Hryniewicz, W., 2004. Characteristics of *Streptococcus pneumoniae*, *Haemophilus influenzae*, and *Moraxella catarrhalis* isolated from the nasopharynges of asymptomatic children and molecular analysis of *S. pneumoniae* and *H. influenzae* strain replacement in the nasopharynx. Journal of Clinical Microbiology 42 (9), 3942−3949.

Swiatlo, E., Champlin, F.R., Holman, S.C., Wilson, W.W., Watt, J.M., 2002. Contribution of choline-binding proteins to cell surface properties of *Streptococcus pneumoniae*. Infection and Immunity 70 (1), 412−415.

Tait-Kamradt, A., Clancy, J., Cronan, M., Dib-Hajj, F., Wondrack, L., Yuan, W., Sutcliffe, J., 1997. Mef E is necessary for the erythromycin-resistant M phenotype in *Streptococcus pneumoniae*. Antimicrobial Agents and Chemotherapy 41 (10), 2251−2255.

Todd, A.G., 1910. Strangles. Journal of Comparative Pathology and Therapeutics 23, 212−229.

van Hout, J., Heuvelink, A., Gonggrijp, M., 2016. Monitoring of antimicrobial susceptibility of *Streptococcus suis* in The Netherlands, 2013−2015. Veterinary Microbiology 194, 5−10.

van Sorge, N.M., Cole, J.N., Kuipers, K., Henningham, A., Aziz, R.K., Kasirer-Friede, A., Lin, L., Berends, E.T., Davies, M.R., Dougan, G., Zhang, F., 2014. The classical lancefield antigen of group a *Streptococcus* is a virulence determinant with implications for vaccine design. Cell Host & Microbe 15 (6), 729−740.

Vélez, J.R., Cameron, M., Rodríguez-Lecompte, J.C., Xia, F., Heider, L.C., Saab, M., McClure, J., Sánchez, J., 2017. Whole-genome sequence analysis of antimicrobial resistance genes in *Streptococcus uberis* and *Streptococcus dysgalactiae* isolates from Canadian dairy herds. Frontiers in Veterinary Science 4, 63.

Wheeler, R., Mesnage, S., Boneca, I.G., Hobbs, J.K., Foster, S.J., 2011. Super-resolution microscopy reveals cell wall dynamics and peptidoglycan architecture in ovococcal bacteria. Molecular Microbiology 82 (5), 1096−1109.

Wisselink, H.J., Smith, H.E., Stockhofe-Zurwieden, N., Peperkamp, K., Vecht, U., 2000. Distribution of capsular types and production of muramidase-released protein (MRP) and extracellular factor (EF) of *Streptococcus suis* strains isolated from diseased pigs in seven European countries. Veterinary Microbiology 74 (3), 237−248.

World Health Organization (WHO), 2016. Pneumonia Fact Sheet; World Health Organization Report 2016. WHO, Geneva, Switzerland.

Wyres, K.L., Lambertsen, L.M., Croucher, N.J., McGee, L., von Gottberg, A., Liñares, J., Jacobs, M.R., Kristinsson, K.G., Beall, B.W., Klugman, K.P., Parkhill, J., 2012. Pneumococcal capsular switching: a historical perspective. The Journal of Infectious Diseases 207 (3), 439−449.

Wyres, K.L., van Tonder, A., Lambertsen, L.M., Hakenbeck, R., Parkhill, J., Bentley, S.D., Brueggemann, A.B., 2013. Evidence of antimicrobial resistance-conferring genetic elements among pneumococci isolated prior to 1974. BMC Genomics 14 (1), 500.

Zapun, A., Contreras-Martel, C., Vernet, T., 2008. PPBs and b-lactam resistance. FEMS Microbiology Reviews 32, 361−385.

Zheng, H., Du, P., Qiu, X., Kerdsin, A., Roy, D., Bai, X., Xu, J., Vela, A.I., Gottschalk, M., 2018. Genomic comparisons of *Streptococcus suis* serotype 9 strains recovered from diseased pigs in Spain and Canada. Veterinary Research 49 (1), 1.

Chapter 18

Actinobacillus

Chapter outline

Lignieres and Spitz (1902) first isolated *Actinobacillus*-like organism from infected cattle in Argentina. Brumpt named the bacterium as *Actinobacillus lignieresii* in memory of Lignieres (Brumpt, 1910). *Actinobacillus pleuropneumoniae*—like organism was first isolated from pigs in the United Kingdom in 1957 (Pattison et al., 1957). Shope (1964) described a similar kind of swine infection in Argentina as porcine contagious pleuropneumonia caused by *Haemophilus pleuropneumoniae*. Based on nucleotide sequence homology, *H. pleuropneumoniae* was transferred under the genus *Actinobacillus* (Pohl et al., 1983).

A. pleuropneumoniae is considered as a major aetiology of porcine respiratory disease complex having multifactorial reasons such as different pathogens, stress associated with management practices, environmental conditions and genetic predispositions. The disease complex causes significant economic losses in swine industry throughout the world, especially in Asia, Latin America, few European countries and sporadically in the United States and Canada (Gottschalk, 2012). The infection is characterized by exudative, fibrinous and hemorrhagic pneumonia and pleuritis (Bossé et al., 2014). Control strategy includes vaccination, proper husbandry practices and treatment with antibiotics which sometimes generate resistance (El Garch et al., 2016).

Aggregatibacter actinomycetemcomitans is associated with periodontitis and rarely with endocarditis in human.

Properties of genus

Morphology: *Actinobacillus* are Gram-negative small rods, occurring singly, in pairs or rarely in chains. In Gram-stained smear, the bacteria show both bacillus and coccus form together, known as 'morse code' appearances (dots and dashes appearance). The bacteria are nonmotile (both at room temperature and 37°C), nonsporing and nonacid fast. The pili and capsule are found in few strains of *A. pleuropneumoniae*. The slime layer is detected on the surface of other species such as *A. lignieresii*, *Actinobacillus suis* and *Actinobacillus equuli*. The slime layer is associated with stickiness of the bacterial colonies, enhanced resistance against chemical disinfectants, antibiotics and desiccation.

Classification: The family *Pasteurellaceae* contains several genera such as *Actinobacillus sensu stricto*, *Mannheimia*, *Pasteurella sensu stricto*, *Lonepinella*, *Phocoenobacter*, *Haemophilus sensu stricto*, *Gallibacterium*, *Histophilus* and *Volucribacter*. There are total 22 species or species-like taxa of *Actinobacillus* confirmed so far. Based on 16S rRNA phylogenetic analysis and DNA—DNA hybridizations studies, *A. sensu stricto* ('true' *Actinobacillus*) is restricted to include *A. lignieresii*, *A. pleuropneumoniae*, *A. equuli* subsp. *equuli*, *A. equuli* subsp. *haemolyticus* (taxon 11 of Bisgaard), *Actinobacillus hominis*, *A. suis*, *Actinobacillus ureae*, *Actinobacillus arthritidis* (sorbitol-positive taxon 9 of Bisgaard), *Actinobacillus* genomospecies 1 (*A. lignieresii* phenotype isolated from horses) and 2 (sorbitol-negative *A. arthritidis*), taxa 8 (guinea pig isolate) and taxa 26 (avian haemolytic *Actinobacillus*-like) of Bisgaard. Among the members of *A. sensu stricto*, only *A. pleuropneumoniae* is considered as a primary pathogen.

Antimicrobial Resistance in Agriculture. https://doi.org/10.1016/B978-0-12-815770-1.00018-3

Susceptibility to disinfectants: *Actinobacillus* are susceptible to common disinfectants such as phenol, cresol, etc. *A. pleuropneumoniae* contains resistance plasmids encoding the genes associated with resistance to sulfonamides, tetracycline and penicillin.

Natural habitat: Most of the *Actinobacillus* species are commensal in the mucous membrane of different carrier animals. *A. lignieresii* and *A. suis* are commonly found in the oropharynx of cattle and tonsil or upper respiratory tract of swine, respectively. Subclinically infected pigs (*Sus scrofa*) such as domestic and feral pigs and wild boars act as carrier of *A. pleuropneumoniae* in nasal cavities, tonsillar crypts and lungs (Tobias et al., 2014). The wild boars become carrier because of frequent contact with domestic pigs or boars of other countries.

Actinobacillus species do not survive in the environment for a prolonged period if not embedded in organic material. *A. pleuropneumoniae* can survive up to 30 days in water at 4°C (Assavacheep and Rycroft, 2013) and can produce biofilm for survival in drinking water at pig farms and during early or chronic stage of infection (Loera-Muro et al., 2013). Production of *A. pleuropneumoniae* biofilm during early or chronic stage of infection is associated with anaerobic condition, which upregulates the necessary genes (Li et al., 2014).

Genome: *A. equuli* subsp. *equuli* has a single circular chromosome (2,431,533 bp) with a GC content of 40.3%. The genome contains 2264 genes which can encode proteins (approximately 2182) and RNAs. Most of the predicted genes are assigned to 25 functional 'clusters of orthologous group' categories such as lipopolysaccharides (LPS), adhesins, fimbriae, filamentous haemagglutinin homologue, toxins and haemolysins (Huang et al., 2015).

Antigenic characteristics

A. lignieresii contains two major types of antigens, i.e., heat-stable (somatic) and heat-labile antigens. On the basis of somatic antigens, *A. lignieresii* has six serotypes, designated as type 1–6. Among these serotypes, type 1 is restricted to cattle, whereas types 2, 3 and 4 are found in sheep. In addition to the host, the serotype distribution is also influenced by different geographical locations. There is an antigenic relationship between *A. lignieresii*, *Burkholderia mallei* and *Burkholderia pseudomallei*.

On the basis of capsular polysaccharide and LPS O-chain *A. pleuropneumoniae* has 16 serotypes (Bossé et al., 2017a,b). Two of these serotypes (1, 5) have been further divided into subtypes (1a, 1b, 5a, 5b). The cross-reactivity between the serotypes 3, 6 and 8 are found due to similarities in structure of LPS. *A. pleuropneumoniae* is also classified into two biotypes known as biotype 1 (typical) and 2 (atypical), based on their nicotinamide adenine dinucleotide (NAD) requirements. Biotype 1 is NAD-dependent, whereas biotype 2 is independent (Ito, 2015). The serotypes 1–12 and 15 and 16 are classified under biotype 1, and the serotypes 13 and 14 belong to biotype 2 (Serrano-Rubio et al., 2008). In a few instances, variants of serotypes 2, 4, 7, 9 and 11 are identified as NAD-independent and occurrence of untypable serotypes is increasing throughout the world (Perry et al., 2012; Morioka et al., 2016). The global distribution of *A. pleuropneumoniae* serotypes is described in Table 18.1. The serotypes do not offer any cross-protection, and virulence of the serotypes differs between

TABLE 18.1 Global distribution of *Actinobacillus pleuropneumoniae* serotypes.

A. pleuropneumoniae serotype	Continent/country
1, 5, 7	America (North)
1, 4, 5, 6, 7	America (South)
2, 3, 4, 9, 11	Europe
2, 6, 7, 8, 12	England and Wales
2, 9, 11	Czech Republic
2, 4	Spain
2	Denmark, Norway, Sweden
2, 6, 15	Asia
1, 3, 4, 5, 7	China
1, 2, 5	South Korea
1, 5, 7, 12, 15	Australia

the geographical locations. European serotype 2 strains can produce Apx toxins and are highly virulent, while the serotype 2 isolated from North America cannot produce the toxin and are nonpathogenic (Gottschalk, 2015).

Toxins and virulence factors produced

Toxins

The cytotoxin belongs to 'RTX' (repeats-in-toxin structure) toxin family, a kind of pore-forming, cytolytic protein toxin found in Gram-negative bacteria. The RTX genes are present in *A. pleuropneumoniae, A. suis, A. lignieresii* and *A. equuli* subsp. *haemolyticus.* All of the RTX family members share a C-terminal calcium-binding domain consisting of glycine-rich nonapeptide repeats with a consensus sequence X-(L/I/F)-XG-G-X-G-(N/D)-D. The repeat varies between less than 10 to more than 40 in different toxins. After penetration, most of the RTX toxins make pores on the cellular membrane by an unknown mechanism. Two or more toxin molecules aggregate together before pore formation. The pores are cation-selective and short-lived (Benz et al., 1994).

In *A. pleuropneumoniae,* this cytotoxin has four types namely ApxI, ApxII, ApxIII and ApxIV. Among them, ApxI is strongly haemolytic and cytotoxic and is produced by serotypes 1, 5a, 5b, 9, 10, 11, 14 and 16, which are correlated with severe outbreaks. ApxII is weakly haemolytic and moderately cytotoxic and is detected in all serotypes except 10 and 14. ApxIII is nonhaemolytic, strongly cytotoxic and expressed by serotypes 2, 3, 4, 6, 8 and 15. ApxIII can lyse red blood cells, epithelial cells, T lymphocytes and macrophages by forming pore in their cell membrane. At low concentration, it can affect oxidative metabolism of phagocytic cells. ApxIV is produced by all serotypes and is widely used in diagnosis (Tegetmeyer et al., 2008).

In *A. suis,* proteins similar to ApxI and Apx II are detected.

In *A. lignieresii,* although RTX gene is detected, the expression of the toxin is yet not confirmed.

In *A. equuli* subsp. *haemolyticus*, this RTX toxin is known as 'Aqx'. Equine granulocytes are susceptible to this toxin.

Virulence factors

Most of the field isolates of *A. pleuropneumoniae* (5b, 11) produce biofilm which is chiefly composed of poly-N-acetyl-glucosamine (PGA). The protein is encoded by pgaABCD operon present in almost all serotypes (1−12) of *A. pleuropneumoniae* (Izano et al., 2007). Like other bacteria, biofilm-producing *A. pleuropneumoniae* is less sensitive to antibiotics such as ampicillin, florfenicol, tiamulin and tilmicosin, which are frequently used in pig farms (Archambault et al., 2012). Host immune response against biofilm-producing *A. pleuropneumoniae* is also reduced because of structural modification of bacterial LPS (Hathroubi et al., 2016).

Other virulence factors of *A. pleuropneumoniae* are described in Table 18.2.

TABLE 18.2 Major virulence factors of *Actinobacillus pleuropneumoniae*

Virulence factors	Function
Capsule	Antiphagocytic
Pili	It helps in adherence of the bacteria with the alveolar epithelium and cilia of terminal bronchioles.
Lipopolysaccharide (LPS)	(a) It can induce lesions in mice similar to whole cells, but less severe and without haemolysis. (b) LPS can mediate adhesion of *A. pleuropneumoniae* with tracheal epithelium.
Transferrin-binding protein (TBP), 'Afu-A' (*Actinobacillus* ferric uptake) protein, catecholamine	(a) TBP is an outer membrane protein, detected in *A. pleuropneumoniae*. It helps in acquisition of iron by binding porcine transferrin. Iron is required for metabolic electron transport chain of the bacteria. (b) 'Afu-A' protein is a periplasmic protein associated with iron transport. (c) Catecholamine binding to *A. pleuropneumoniae* Facilitates iron uptake.
Hyaluronidase	It helps in infiltration of the bacteria into the lungs.
Global anaerobic regulators (ArcA and HlyX), anaerobic enzymes (AspA, DmsA, FrdABCD)	Essential for *A. pleuropneumoniae* infection although the exact role is unexplored.

Transmission

A. pleuropneumoniae and *A. suis* are transmitted into susceptible pigs by direct contact or inhalation of the infected dust particles spread over short distances, except few experimental reports about airborne transmission of *A. pleuropneumoniae* over longer distances (Desrosiers and Moore, 1998). The droplets smaller in size (0.5—3 mm in diameter) showed highest infectivity which can penetrate deep into the lung (Nicolet and König, 1969). In a pig farm, high population density and poor ventilation are predisposing factors for transmission. Maternal antibodies from infected or vaccinated sow can protect the piglets up to 2—12 weeks of age (Chiers et al., 2002). Direct contact—based transmission from pigs to pigs is documented more from the pigs with less severe clinical infection (Tobias et al., 2013). A mathematical simulation study indicated about endogenous infection of *A. pleuropneumoniae* in pigs triggered by various factors (Klinkenberg et al., 2014).

A. lignieresii resides in the oropharynx, tonsil, tongue and rumen of cattle. Injury or trauma of buccal cavity or stomach helps in penetration of the bacteria into the underlying soft tissues. Continuous feeding with thorny vegetations and stemmy haylages may also produce such kind of buccal injuries and trigger endogenous infection.

Diagnosis

For detection of *A. pleuropneumoniae*, lung tissue after necropsy and oral fluids or bronchoalveolar lavage, nasal swabs and tonsillar scrapings can be collected from live pigs. *A. pleuropneumoniae* survives deep in the tonsillar crypts which make it difficult to detect the bacteria from tonsil (Costa et al., 2011). Pus exudates as antemortem samples, and lung tissues after necropsy can be collected for detection of *A. lignieresii*.

Laboratory examinations

Direct examination: For direct examination of *A. lignieresii* in pus samples, the grayish white granules present in the pus are washed with distilled water and are placed in one drop of 10% KOH in a glass slide. The granules are gently crushed with cover slip and observed under low power. In positive cases, 'club-shaped' bacterial colonies with Gram-negative rods at the centre are observed.

Isolation of *Actinobacillus* spp.:*Actinobacillus* spp. can be isolated in sheep blood agar. The plates are incubated at 37°C for 24 h with 5%—10% CO_2 tension. *A. pleuropneumoniae* requires 48 h incubation for optimal growth. Chocolate agar is suitable for isolation of *A. pleuropneumoniae,* as it requires factor 'V' (NAD) for its optimum growth (such as *Haemophilus*). Streaking of *Staphylococcus* in blood agar can also supply this factor 'V' for optimum growth of *A. pleuropneumoniae*. Haemolysis in blood agar is produced by *A. pleuropneumoniae*, *A. equuli* subsp. *haemolyticus* and *A. suis*. Colonies of *A. lignieresii* after primary culture and 24 h of growth are nonhaemolytic, translucent or grayish, 1—2 mm in diameter and very sticky or waxy.

Serological tests: ELISA can be used for detection of antibodies against *A. pleuropneumoniae* LPS, capsular polysaccharide and Apx toxins. LPS-based ELISA is serogroup-specific under both field and experimental conditions. Apx-IV-based ELISA is widely used although it cannot specify the virulence of the isolate and certain insertion sequence (ISApl1) can inhibit the expression of Apx-IV toxin (Tegetmeyer et al., 2008). Apx-II-based ELISA is not specific as cross-reaction with *A. suis* or *Actinobacillus porcitonsillarum* can take place. There is no universal rule to declare a pig herd free from *A. pleuropneumoniae*. In Denmark, serological testing of 20 animals is recommended once a month over a time period of 2—3 years. In Germany, seromonitoring of 15 samples four times in a year is preferred (Sassu et al., 2018). In piglet monitoring program, the sows are recommended to be tested for antibodies to evaluate the transmission risk, as maternal and acquired antibodies cannot be differentiated by routine serological tests (Vigre et al., 2002).

Molecular biology: Polymerase chain reaction (PCR)—based confirmation of *A. pleuropneumoniae* is described, which detects *omlA* or *ApxIVa* gene (Frey, 2003). Detection of *ApxIVa* gene permits direct identification of the bacteria from infected lung tissues and nasal fluids. The PCR-based serotyping of the *A. pleuropneumoniae* isolates is also carried out depending on the differences in *Apx* toxin gene or outer membrane lipoprotein (*omlA*) gene sequences (Angen et al., 2008). Healthy carrier pigs can be confirmed by parallel PCR testing of nasal, tonsillar and oropharyngeal swabs (Fablet et al., 2011).

Characteristics of antimicrobial resistance

Characteristics of antimicrobial resistance of *Actinobacillus* isolates observed in pigs, horses and human are discussed in the following section.

Pigs

Tetracycline and sulfamethoxazole/trimethoprim are recommended for treatment of porcine pleuropneumonia throughout the world (Burch et al., 2008). Resistance of *A. pleuropneumoniae* against tetracycline was detected to be associated with *tet*(H), *tet*(M)/*tet*(O) and *tet*(L) in Switzerland and Spain (Blanco et al., 2006; Matter et al., 2007); *tet*(B) or *tet*(H) in the United Kingdom (Bossé et al., 2017a,b); *tet*(B), *tet*(O), *tet*(H) and *tet*(C) in Canada (Archambault et al., 2012); *tet*(A), *tet*(H) and *tet*(M)/*tet*(O) in Japan (Morioka et al., 2008); *tet*(A), *tet*(H), *tet*(M)/*tet*(O) and *tet*(L) in South Korea (Kim et al., 2016) and *tet*(B) and *tet*(H) in Australia (Turni, 2014). Trimethoprim-resistant *A. pleuropneumoniae* strains isolated from porcine lung tissues in the United Kingdom showed the presence of *dfrA14* (Bossé et al., 2017a,b). The study with *A. pleuropneumoniae* strains isolated from pigs in Canada during 1980−84 revealed that majority (68%) of the isolates were resistant to tetracycline but were susceptible to trimethoprim, erythromycin and gentamicin (Nadeau et al., 1988). The studies conducted in recent times showed the changing scenario in the resistance and circulating serovar pattern of porcine *A. pleuropneumoniae* strains in Canada. Majority of the isolates became susceptible to most of the common antibiotics but resistance against chlortetracycline (88.4%) and oxytetracycline (90.7%) sustained high (Archambault et al., 2012).

β-Lactam group of antibiotics was shown to be effective against *A. pleuropneumoniae* isolates (Matter et al., 2007). Recent studies revealed the presence of β-lactam-resistant *A. pleuropneumoniae* isolates associated with *bla*$_{ROB-1}$ in Spain, Italy, United Kingdom and Australia (Gutiérrez-Martín et al., 2006; Vanni et al., 2012; Turni, 2014; Bossé et al., 2017a,b). However, *bla*$_{ROB-1}$-independent β-lactam−resistant *A. pleuropneumoniae* isolates were detected in pigs in South Korea (Kim et al., 2016).

Florfenicol (fluorinated chloramphenicol) is licenced in Europe since 2000 for the treatment of respiratory tract infections in pigs (Kehrenberg et al., 2004). Low resistance of *A. pleuropneumoniae* against florfenicol was observed in European (Germany, Spain and Switzerland) and Asian (Japan) countries (Gutiérrez-Martín et al., 2006; Morioka et al., 2008). In South Korea, high prevalence of florfenicol resistance (45%) was detected in *A. pleuropneumoniae* isolates (Yoo et al., 2014; Kim et al., 2016). The plasmids conferring resistance to florfenicol and chloramphenicol were detected in clinical isolates from Brazil and Greece (Bossé et al., 2015; da Silva et al., 2017).

Macrolide resistance in *A. pleuropneumoniae* strains isolated from pigs in Australia was associated with a mutation in the sequences of the bacterial 23S ribosomal subunit (Turni, 2014). In the United Kingdom, *A. pleuropneumoniae* isolated from the lung tissues of infected pigs showed resistance against erythromycin and tilmicosin without possession of macrolide resistance gene or any point mutation (Bossé et al., 2017a,b).

Horses

A comparative study with *Actinobacillus* spp. isolates (including *A. suis*) from diseased horses admitted to the equine hospital in Quebec (Canada) revealed increase in resistance to amikacin between 1996−98 and 2007−13; penicillin between 1986−88 and 1996−98; trimethoprim/sulfamethoxazole between 1986−88 and 1996−98. Decrease in resistance to penicillin, ampicillin and trimethoprim/sulfamethoxazole was observed between 1996−98 and 2007−13 (Malo et al., 2016).

Human

Resistance to tetracycline, penicillin G and metronidazole was detected in *A. actinomycetemcomitans* associated with refractory or recurrent periodontitis in the United States (Listgarten et al., 1993). Recent study revealed similar pattern of resistance in *A. actinomycetemcomitans* strains associated with chronic periodontitis against doxycycline, amoxicillin, metronidazole and clindamycin in the United States (Rams et al., 2014).

References

Angen, Ø., Ahrens, P., Jessing, S.G., 2008. Development of a multiplex PCR test for identification of *Actinobacillus pleuropneumoniae* serovars 1, 7, and 12. Veterinary Microbiology 132 (3−4), 312−318.

Archambault, M., Harel, J., Gouré, J., Tremblay, Y.D., Jacques, M., 2012. Antimicrobial susceptibilities and resistance genes of Canadian isolates of *Actinobacillus pleuropneumoniae*. Microbial Drug Resistance 18 (2), 198−206.

Assavacheep, P., Rycroft, A.N., 2013. Survival of *Actinobacillus pleuropneumoniae* outside the pig. Research in Veterinary Science 94 (1), 22−26.

Benz, R., Hardie, K.R., Hughes, C., 1994. Pore formation in artificial membranes by the secreted hemolysins of *Proteus vulgaris* and *Morganella morganii*. The FEBS Journal 220 (2), 339−347.

Blanco, M., Gutiérrez-Martin, C.B., Rodríguez-Ferri, E.F., Roberts, M.C., Navas, J., 2006. Distribution of tetracycline resistance genes in *Actinobacillus pleuropneumoniae* isolates from Spain. Antimicrobial Agents and Chemotherapy 50 (2), 702–708.

Bossé, J.T., Li, Y., Angen, Ø., Weinert, L.A., Chaudhuri, R.R., Holden, M.T., Williamson, S.M., Maskell, D.J., Tucker, A.W., Wren, B.W., Rycroft, A.N., 2014. Multiplex PCR assay for unequivocal differentiation of *Actinobacillus pleuropneumoniae* serovars 1 to 3, 5 to 8, 10, and 12. Journal of Clinical Microbiology 52 (7), 2380–2385.

Bossé, J.T., Li, Y., Atherton, T.G., Walker, S., Williamson, S.M., Rogers, J., Chaudhuri, R.R., Weinert, L.A., Holden, M.T., Maskell, D.J., Tucker, A.W., 2015. Characterization of a mobilisable plasmid conferring florfenicol and chloramphenicol resistance in *Actinobacillus pleuropneumoniae*. Veterinary Microbiology 178 (3–4), 279–282.

Bossé, J.T., Li, Y., Rogers, J., Fernandez Crespo, R., Li, Y., Chaudhuri, R.R., Holden, M.T., Maskell, D.J., Tucker, A.W., Wren, B.W., Rycroft, A.N., 2017a. Whole genome sequencing for surveillance of antimicrobial resistance in *Actinobacillus pleuropneumoniae*. Frontiers in Microbiology 8, 311.

Bossé, J.T., Li, Y., Sárközi, R., Gottschalk, M., Angen, Ø., Nedbalcova, K., Rycroft, A.N., Fodor, L., Langford, P.R., 2017b. A unique capsule locus in the newly designated *Actinobacillus pleuropneumoniae* serovar 16 and development of a diagnostic PCR assay. Journal of Clinical Microbiology 55 (3), 902–907.

Brumpt, F., 1910. Precis De Parasitologie. Masson Et Cie, Paris, p. 849.

Burch, D.G., Duran, C.O., Aarestrup, F.M., 2008. Guidelines for antimicrobial use in swine. In: Guide to Antimicrobial Use in Animals. Blackwell Publishing Oxford, UK, pp. 102–125.

Chiers, K., Donné, E., Van Overbeke, I., Ducatelle, R., Haesebrouck, F., 2002. *Actinobacillus pleuropneumoniae* infections in closed swine herds: infection patterns and serological profiles. Veterinary Microbiology 85 (4), 343–352.

Costa, G., Oliveira, S., Torrison, J., Dee, S., 2011. Evaluation of *Actinobacillus pleuropneumoniae* diagnostic tests using samples derived from experimentally infected pigs. Veterinary Microbiology 148 (2–4), 246–251.

da Silva, G.C., Rossi, C.C., Santana, M.F., Langford, P.R., Bossé, J.T., Bazzolli, D.M.S., 2017. p518, a small floR plasmid from a South American isolate of *Actinobacillus pleuropneumoniae*. Veterinary Microbiology 204, 129–132.

Desrosiers, R., Moore, C., 1998. Indirect transmission of *Actinobacillus pleuropneumoniae*. Journal of Swine Health and Production 6 (6), 263–265.

El Garch, F., de Jong, A., Simjee, S., Moyaert, H., Klein, U., Ludwig, C., Marion, H., Haag-Diergarten, S., Richard-Mazet, A., Thomas, V., Siegwart, E., 2016. Monitoring of antimicrobial susceptibility of respiratory tract pathogens isolated from diseased cattle and pigs across Europe, 2009–2012: VetPath results. Veterinary Microbiology 194, 11–22.

Fablet, C., Marois, C., Kuntz-Simon, G., Rose, N., Dorenlor, V., Eono, F., Eveno, E., Jolly, J.P., Le Devendec, L., Tocqueville, V., Quéguiner, S., 2011. Longitudinal study of respiratory infection patterns of breeding sows in five farrow-to-finish herds. Veterinary Microbiology 147 (3–4), 329–339.

Frey, J., 2003. Detection, identification, and subtyping of *Actinobacillus pleuropneumoniae*. In: PCR Detection of Microbial Pathogens. Humana Press, pp. 87–95.

Gottschalk, M., 2012. Actinobacillosis. In: Karriker, L., Ramirez, A., Schwartz, K., Stevenson, G., Zimmerman, J. (Eds.), Diseases of Swine, tenth ed. Wiley, Hoboken, NJ, pp. 653–669.

Gottschalk, M., 2015. The challenge of detecting herds sub-clinically infected with *Actinobacillus pleuropneumoniae*. The Veterinary Journal 206 (1), 30–38.

Gutiérrez-Martín, C.B., Del Blanco, N.G., Blanco, M., Navas, J., Rodríguez-Ferri, E.F., 2006. Changes in antimicrobial susceptibility of *Actinobacillus pleuropneumoniae* isolated from pigs in Spain during the last decade. Veterinary Microbiology 115 (1–3), 218–222.

Hathroubi, S., Beaudry, F., Provost, C., Martelet, L., Segura, M., Gagnon, C.A., Jacques, M., 2016. Impact of *Actinobacillus pleuropneumoniae* biofilm mode of growth on the lipid A structures and stimulation of immune cells. Innate Immunity 22 (5), 353–362.

Huang, B.F., Kropinski, A.M., Bujold, A.R., MacInnes, J.I., 2015. Complete genome sequence of *Actinobacillus equuli* subspecies *equuli* ATCC 19392 T. Standards in Genomic Sciences 10 (1), 32.

Ito, H., 2015. The genetic organization of the capsular polysaccharide biosynthesis region of *Actinobacillus pleuropneumoniae* serotype 14. Journal of Veterinary Medical Science 77 (5), 583–586.

Izano, E.A., Sadovskaya, I., Vinogradov, E., Mulks, M.H., Velliyagounder, K., Ragunath, C., Kher, W.B., Ramasubbu, N., Jabbouri, S., Perry, M.B., Kaplan, J.B., 2007. Poly-N-acetylglucosamine mediates biofilm formation and antibiotic resistance in *Actinobacillus pleuropneumoniae*. Microbial Pathogenesis 43 (1), 1–9.

Kehrenberg, C., Mumme, J., Wallmann, J., Verspohl, J., Tegeler, R., Kühn, T., Schwarz, S., 2004. Monitoring of florfenicol susceptibility among bovine and porcine respiratory tract pathogens collected in Germany during the years 2002 and 2003. Journal of Antimicrobial Chemotherapy 54 (2), 572–574.

Kim, B., Hur, J., Lee, J.Y., Choi, Y., Lee, J.H., 2016. Molecular serotyping and antimicrobial resistance profiles of *Actinobacillus pleuropneumoniae* isolated from pigs in South Korea. Veterinary Quarterly 36 (3), 137–144.

Klinkenberg, D., Tobias, T.J., Bouma, A., Van Leengoed, L.A.M.G., Stegeman, J.A., 2014. Simulation study of the mechanisms underlying outbreaks of clinical disease caused by *Actinobacillus pleuropneumoniae* in finishing pigs. The Veterinary Journal 202 (1), 99–105.

Li, L., Zhu, J., Yang, K., Xu, Z., Liu, Z., Zhou, R., 2014. Changes in gene expression of Actinobacillus pleuropneumoniae in response to anaerobic stress reveal induction of central metabolism and biofilm formation. Journal of Microbiology 52 (6), 473–481.

Lignieres, J., Spitz, G., 1902. Bulletin et Mémoires Société Centrale de Médecine Vétérinaire 20, 487.

Listgarten, M.A., Lai, C.H., Young, V., 1993. Microbial composition and pattern of antibiotic resistance in subgingival microbial samples from patients with refractory periodontitis. Journal of Periodontology 64 (3), 155–161.

Loera-Muro, V.M., Jacques, M., Tremblay, Y.D., Avelar-Gonzalez, F.J., Muro, A.L., Ramírez-López, E.M., Medina-Figueroa, A., Gonzalez-Reynaga, H.M., Guerrero-Barrera, A.L., 2013. Detection of *Actinobacillus pleuropneumoniae* in drinking water from pig farms. Microbiology 159 (3), 536−544.

Malo, A., Cluzel, C., Labrecque, O., Beauchamp, G., Lavoie, J.P., Leclere, M., 2016. Evolution of in vitro antimicrobial resistance in an equine hospital over 3 decades. The Canadian Veterinary Journal 57 (7), 747.

Matter, D., Rossano, A., Limat, S., Vorlet-Fawer, L., Brodard, I., Perreten, V., 2007. Antimicrobial resistance profile of *Actinobacillus pleuropneumoniae* and *Actinobacillus porcitonsillarum*. Veterinary Microbiology 122 (1−2), 146−156.

Morioka, A., Asai, T., Nitta, H., Yamamoto, K., Ogikubo, Y., Takahashi, T., Suzuki, S., 2008. Recent trends in antimicrobial susceptibility and the presence of the tetracycline resistance gene in *Actinobacillus pleuropneumoniae* isolates in Japan. Journal of Veterinary Medical Science 70 (11), 1261−1264.

Morioka, A., Shimazaki, Y., Uchiyama, M., Suzuki, S., 2016. Serotyping reanalysis of unserotypable *Actinobacillus pleuropneumoniae* isolates by agar gel diffusion test. Journal of Veterinary Medical Science 78 (4), 723−725.

Nadeau, M., Lariviere, S., Higgins, R., Martineau, G.P., 1988. Minimal inhibitory concentrations of antimicrobial agents against *Actinobacillus pleuropneumoniae*. Canadian Journal of Veterinary Research 52 (3), 315.

Nicolet, J., König, H., 1969. On haemophilus pleuropneumonia in swine. II. A contagious disease of scientific value. Schweizer Archiv fur Tierheilkunde 111 (3), 166−174.

Pattison, I.H., Howell, D.G., Elliot, J., 1957. A haemophilus-like organism isolated from pig lung and the associated pneumonic lesions. Journal of Comparative Pathology and Therapeutics 67. 320-IN37.

Perry, M.B., Angen, Ø., MacLean, L.L., Lacouture, S., Kokotovic, B., Gottschalk, M., 2012. An atypical biotype I *Actinobacillus pleuropneumoniae* serotype 13 is present in North America. Veterinary Microbiology 156 (3−4), 403−410.

Pohl, S., Bertschinger, H.U., Frederiksen, W., Mannheim, W., 1983. Transfer of *Haemophilus pleuropneumoniae* and the *Pasteurella haemolytica*-like organism causing porcine necrotic pleuropneumonia to the genus *Actinobacillus* (*Actinobacillus pleuropneumoniae* comb. nov.) on the basis of phenotypic and deoxyribonucleic acid relatedness. International Journal of Systematic and Evolutionary Microbiology 33 (3), 510−514.

Rams, T.E., Degener, J.E., van Winkelhoff, A.J., 2014. Antibiotic resistance in human chronic periodontitis microbiota. Journal of Periodontology 85 (1), 160−169.

Sassu, E.L., Bossé, J.T., Tobias, T.J., Gottschalk, M., Langford, P.R., Hennig-Pauka, I., 2018. Update on Actinobacillus pleuropneumoniae—knowledge, gaps and challenges. Transboundary and emerging diseases 65, 72−90.

Serrano-Rubio, L.E., Tenorio-Gutiérrez, V., Suárez-Güemes, F., Reyes-Cortés, R., Rodríguez-Mendiola, M., Arias-Castro, C., Godínez-Vargas, D., de la Garza, M., 2008. Identification of *Actinobacillus pleuropneumoniae* biovars 1 and 2 in pigs using a PCR assay. Molecular and Cellular Probes 22 (5−6), 305−312.

Shope, R.E., 1964. Porcine Contagious Pleuropneumonia: I. Experimental transmission, etiology, and pathology. Journal of Experimental Medicine 119 (3), 357−368.

Tegetmeyer, H.E., Jones, S.C., Langford, P.R., Baltes, N., 2008. ISApl1, a novel insertion element of *Actinobacillus pleuropneumoniae*, prevents ApxIV-based serological detection of serotype 7 strain AP76. Veterinary Microbiology 128 (3−4), 342−353.

Tobias, T.J., Bouma, A., Daemen, A.J., Wagenaar, J.A., Stegeman, A., Klinkenberg, D., 2013. Association between transmission rate and disease severity for *Actinobacillus pleuropneumoniae* infection in pigs. Veterinary Research 44 (1), 2.

Tobias, T.J., Bouma, A., Van Den Broek, J., Van Nes, A., Daemen, A.J.J.M., Wagenaar, J.A., Stegeman, J.A., Klinkenberg, D., 2014. Transmission of *Actinobacillus pleuropneumoniae* among weaned piglets on endemically infected farms. Preventive Veterinary Medicine 117 (1), 207−214.

Turni, C., 2014. Antibiotic Sensitivity of *Haemophilus parasuis* Plus *Actinobacillus pleuropneumoniae* and Other Respiratory Pathogens. Available at: https://pdfs.semanticscholar.org/a09a/43ae2e50f30356f67df57eecf5c1325cc198.pdf.

Vanni, M., Merenda, M., Barigazzi, G., Garbarino, C., Luppi, A., Tognetti, R., Intorre, L., 2012. Antimicrobial resistance of *Actinobacillus pleuropneumoniae* isolated from swine. Veterinary Microbiology 156 (1−2), 172−177.

Vigre, H., Angen, Ø., Barfod, K., Lavritsen, D.T., Sørensen, V., 2002. Transmission of *Actinobacillus pleuropneumoniae* in pigs under field-like conditions: emphasis on tonsillar colonization and passively acquired colostral antibodies. Veterinary Microbiology 89 (2−3), 151−159.

Yoo, A.N., Cha, S.B., Shin, M.K., Won, H.K., Kim, E.H., Choi, H.W., Yoo, H.S., 2014. Serotypes and antimicrobial resistance patterns of the recent Korean *Actinobacillus pleuropneumoniae* isolates. The Veterinary Record 174 (9), 223.

Chapter 19

Campylobacter

Chapter outline

In 1886, Escherich observed *Campylobacter*-like organisms in stool samples of children with diarrhoea (Vandamme, 2000). In 1913, McFaydean and Stockman first confirmed them as *Campylobacter* in foetal tissues of aborted sheep. Confirmatory tests were also carried out by Smith (1919) when similar organisms (*Vibrio foetus*) were isolated from aborted bovine foetus. Vandamme (2000) and Doyle (1944) isolated *Vibrio jejuni* and *Vibrio coli* from cattle and pigs, respectively, suffering with diarrhoea (Doyle, 1944; Vandamme, 2000). Sebald and Véron (1963) differentiated the bacteria from *Vibrionaceae* family, and the new genus *Campylobacter* ('curved rod') under *Campylobacteriaceae* family was proposed due to low DNA base composition, nonfermentative metabolism and microaerophilic growth requirements.

Campylobacter causes 400−500 million cases of infection in human each year throughout the world (García and Heredia, 2013). Campylobacteriosis is endemic among children in Asia, Africa and Middle East countries, and an increasing trend of occurrence was noticed in North America, Europe and Australia (Kaakoush et al., 2015). In the United States, prevalence of campylobacteriosis was detected as second highest after salmonellosis as foodborne infection, affecting 15% of the population, and was considered as a leading cause of hospitalization (Scallan et al., 2011; Crim et al., 2014). In European countries *Campylobacter* was considered as major pathogen associated with gastroenteritis with an incidence rate of 55.5 per 100,000 population (Gölz et al., 2014).

Human campylobacteriosis is characterized by acute diarrhoea, abdominal pain and fever, which are mostly self-limiting. Few complicated cases may yield severe bloody diarrhoea, inflammatory bowel diseases, esophageal complications (Barrett's oesophagus), periodontitis, cholecystitis, colon cancer and rarely Guillain−Barre syndrome (0.01%−0.03% cases), Miller Fisher syndrome and reactive arthritis (1%−5% cases). Bacteraemia, lung infections, meningitis and brain abscesses are also reported as extraintestinal complications (Man, 2011). Thermophilic *Campylobacter* (*Campylobacter coli*, *Campylobacter jejuni*) are mostly zoonotic and are transmitted through ingestion of raw or undercooked poultry meat, unpasteurized milk, contaminated drinking water and direct contact with animals.

Properties of genus

Morphology: *Campylobacter* are Gram-negative, comma-shaped rods especially in infected tissues and young cultures. When two bacterial cells are found together in a microscopic field, it appears like the alphabet 'S' or 'wing of gull'

Antimicrobial Resistance in Agriculture. https://doi.org/10.1016/B978-0-12-815770-1.00019-5

('flying seagull'). In older cultures, the chains of organisms appear as long spirals. They are motile by single unipolar/bipolar unsheathed flagella. Motility is darting or corkscrew type, best observed under dark-field microscope. Some species contain a surface layer (S-layer), a paracrystalline protein structure composed of S-layer proteins (SLPs) external to the outer membrane.

Classification: Campylobacteriaceae contains four genera namely *Campylobacter*, *Arcobacter*, *Sulfurospirillum* and *Thiovulum*. The genus *Campylobacter* currently consists of 26 species, 2 provisional species and 9 subspecies (Kaakoush et al., 2015). Major species with pathogenic significance in man and animals are *Campylobacter fetus* subsp. *venerealis*, *C. fetus* subsp. *fetus*, *C. jejuni* subsp. *jejuni*, *C. jejuni* subsp. *doyeli*, *C. coli*, *Campylobacter concisus*, *Campylobacter hyointestinalis*, *Campylobacter mucosalis*, *Campylobacter lari*, *Campylobacter upsaliensis*, *Campylobacter helveticus*, *Campylobacter insulaenigrae*, *Campylobacter rectus*, *Campylobacter sputorum* and *Campylobacter ureolyticus*. Among them, *C. jejuni* and *C. coli* are most frequently isolated from human gastroenteritis and poultry.

Susceptibility to disinfectants: *Campylobacter* are sensitive to common disinfectants such as phenol, cresol, etc.

Natural habitat: *Campylobacter* can be recovered from water, sewage, hay, manure and reservoir animals and birds. *C. jejuni* and *C. coli* can colonize the intestinal mucosa of food and companion animals, mucosal crypts of caeca and colon or to a lesser extent in small intestine, liver and organs of poultry (Hermans et al., 2012). In broilers *C. jejuni* is the predominant colonizer followed by *C. coli* in most of the countries except in Southeast Asian region where the reverse occurrence pattern was observed. In commercial turkeys and organic or free-range chicken, *C. coli* was reported as major species (Heuer et al., 2001). In birds, clinical symptoms are mild or absent in spite of extensive colonization of *Campylobacter* (10^9 colony-forming units/gram caecal contents) as the bacteria localize the intestinal crypts without invasion into the adjacent epithelial cells (Beery et al., 1988; Corry and Atabay, 2001). Experimental infections with *Campylobacter* developed diarrhoea and weight loss in birds (Humphrey et al., 2014). Occurrence of *Campylobacter* is uncommon in young birds aged less than 2—3 weeks because of the presence of maternal antibodies (Sahin et al., 2001). Probability of colonization is less in aged birds especially in layers having longer lifespan because of development of active immunity (Achen et al., 1998). *Campylobacter* are considered as a major source of poultry meat contamination and are responsible for 20%—40% foodborne infection in consumers. During processing of the poultry carcasses, the prevalence of *Campylobacter* increases after defeathering and evisceration and the rate decreases after scalding and chilling.

C. fetus is commonly found in genital and intestinal tract of domestic animals (cattle, sheep). *C. fetus* subsp. *venerealis* resides at the prepuce of the bull and the vagina of the cow. In cows, this carriage rate is generally reduced after two breeding seasons. *C. fetus* ssp. *fetus* commonly inhabits intestinal tract of healthy small ruminants (sheep). Natural habitat of *C. upsaliensis* is intestinal tract of healthy puppies and kittens.

Genome: The genome of *Campylobacter* is small in size (1.6—2 megabases) with GC content of 30.1—33.0 mol%. The genome contains several hypervariable regions harbouring genes required for biosynthesis or modification of capsule, lipooligosaccharide and flagellum (Parkhill et al., 2000). These hypervariable sequences consist of homopolymeric tracts and are heritable in nature. Variation in these sequences can produce phase variation, frameshift and point mutations, gene duplication or deletion which results in the generation of multiple serotypes in a single bird or a flock of birds (Parkhill et al., 2000; Linton et al., 2000). *C. jejuni* is naturally competent which can uptake plasmid or chromosomal DNA during colonization into the poultry. The natural transformation generates genome plasticity and helps in spread of antibiotic resistance genes even in absence of selection pressure (Boer et al., 2002). The natural transformation of *C. jejuni* is regulated by carbon dioxide and bacterial cell concentration and certain genes encoded by type II and type IV secretion systems. The complete sequencing of virulence plasmid (pVir) in *C. jejuni* revealed the presence of type IV secretion system, associated with cellular invasion and other roles in pathogenesis (Bacon et al., 2002). *C. jejuni* prefer to receive DNA from other strains of *C. jejuni* than any other bacterial species (Wilson et al., 2003).

Antigenic characteristics

Campylobacter is antigenically heterogeneous group of bacteria. *C. jejuni* has heat-stable (somatic) and heat-labile (flagellin) antigens. The flagella of *C. jejuni* are unsheathed and composed of flagellin protein having molecular weight of 57,000—66,000 Da. They can be divided into more than 600 Penner serotypes (heat-stable antigens) and more than 100 Lior serotypes (heat-labile antigens) (García and Heredia, 2013).

C. fetus has three major groups of antigens: somatic (O), flagellar (H) and SLPs. They have at least 50 heat-stable serotypes based on somatic and more than 36 heat-labile serotypes based on flagellar antigens. It has antigenic relationship with *Brucella abortus*.

Toxins and virulence factors produced

Toxins

Enterotoxin

The enterotoxin is produced by *C. jejuni, C. coli* and *C. lari*. It has structural and functional relationship with *Escherichia coli* heat-labile enterotoxin (LT) and cholera toxin (CT). *Campylobacter* enterotoxin is also heat-labile (inactivated at 56°C for 1 h or at 96°C for 10 min), trypsin and pH sensitive (pH two or 8) and has a molecular weight of 60–70 K Da. Like CT or LT, this toxin also attaches with ganglioside receptor of the host cell. It activates adenylate cyclase enzyme to increase the level of intracellular cAMP and disrupt the normal ion transport in the enterocytes, thus causing secreatory watery diarrhoea. Toxic activity of the crude toxin is progressively lost after storage for 1 month at 4°C or for 1 week at −20 or −70°C. The toxin can induce fluid accumulation in rabbit or rat ligated ileal loop assay.

Cytotoxin

It is produced by *C. jejuni, C. coli* and *C. lari*. It is trypsin-sensitive and toxic for HeLa, Vero cells in vitro. The toxin is destroyed at 70°C temperature for 30 min exposure.

Cytolethal distending toxin

It is heat-labile, trypsin-sensitive, nondialyzable cytotoxin with a molecular weight of 30 KDa and produced by *C. jejuni, C. coli* and *C. lari*. It is cytolethal to Chinese hamster ovary, Vero, HeLa, human epithelial carcinoma (Hep2) cell lines. The toxin cannot induce fluid accumulation in rabbit ligated ileal loop assay. The iron is required for expression of this toxin.

Virulence factors: Major virulence factors of *Campylobacter* are described in Table 19.1.

Transmission

C. jejuni is transmitted through faecal–oral route in poultry. After infection, caecum and colon are the major sites for bacterial multiplication followed by faecal shedding. The bacteria can contaminate the skin of the poultry carcass during slaughtering if an intestinal rupture takes place (Silva et al., 2011). Contaminated drinking water, old litter, farm animals such as cattle, sheep and pigs, wild animals, pets, house flies, insects (litter beetles), farm equipment, transport vehicles and farm workers act as potential source of infection (Sahin et al., 2015). Vertical route of transmission from breeder hen to chick is rare. Presence of *Campylobacter* was although detected in young hatchling (Chuma et al., 1997; Byrd et al., 2007), eggs laid by *Campylobacter* positive flocks (Doyle, 1984), reproductive tract of hens (Buhr et al., 2002) and semen of rooster (Cox et al., 2002).

Among the farm animals, prevalence of *Campylobacter* was highest in cattle (6%–90%), especially the feedlot cattle harboured *C. jejuni, C. coli, C. lari* and *Campylobacter lanienae* (Horrocks et al., 2009). Occurrence of *Campylobacter* in pigs, sheep and goats varies 32.8%–85.0% and 6.8%–17.5%, respectively. Companion animals such as 58% of healthy dogs and 97% of diarrhoeic dogs also harboured *Campylobacter* spp. (Kaakoush et al., 2015).

Human transmission of *C. jejuni* occurs because of extensive international travel, consumption of undercooked chicken or their products, unpasteurized milk, and contaminated water, direct contact with infected farm or companion animals (children) and environmental exposure (Kaakoush et al., 2015). Handling, processing and consumption of undercooked poultry meat or its products are responsible for 20%–30% of human cases (EFSA Panel on Biological Hazards, 2010).The poultry meat may contain high level of the bacteria at preharvest level, which is further contaminated during the time of slaughter and processing. Infective dose of *Campylobacter* in human is not determined but it was experimentally observed that 500 bacterial cells can cause the disease in human (Robinson, 1981). The susceptibility varies between individuals, foods carrying the organisms, and the children in general were found more susceptible than adults (Calva et al., 1988). Person to person transmission is reported at low frequency (Musher and Musher, 2004).

Use of certain antibiotics specially quinolones in animals and birds as therapeutic agent or growth promoter was associated with transmission of resistant *Campylobacter* strains from animals to human (Endtz et al., 1991).

TABLE 19.1 Major virulence factors of *Campylobacter*.

Virulence factors	Function
Motility and chemotaxis factors: Flagellin (FlaA, FlaB), hook basal body protein (FliF), flagellar motor proteins (FliM, FliY), P ring protein (FlgI), L-ring protein (FlgH), hook components (FlgE, FliK), chemotaxis proteins (Che A, Che B, Che R, Che V, Che W, Che Z), methyl-accepting chemotaxis proteins (MCPs), *Campylobacter* energy taxis system proteins CetA (Tlp9) and CetB (Aer2)	Motility is required for survival under the different chemotactic conditions in the gastrointestinal tract and for colonization of the small intestine. Chemotaxis is required for colonization into mucus-filled crypts of the ceca in avian gut.
Adhesins: (i) CadF (*Campylobacter ad*hesion to fibronectin [Fn])	It helps in binding of bacteria with fibronectin protein, found in extracellular matrix or regions of cell to cell contact. So it helps in bacterial adhesion with host tissues.
(ii) Periplasmic/membrane-associated protein (PEB1, PEB3)	Putative adhesin of *Campylobacter jejuni*.
(iii) CapA (*Campylobacter adhesion protein* A)	Acts as adhesin.
(iv) JlpA (*jejuni lipoprotein* A)	It helps in adherence of bacteria with human epithelial cells (Hep2).
(v) Cj1279c and Cj1349c protein	They act as fibronectin and fibrinogen-binding protein.
(vi) Type IV secretion system	Helps in adhesion of bacteria.
Invasion factors: (i) Flagellar proteins (FlhA, FlhB, FliO, FliP, FliQ, FliR)	Flagellar proteins also act as T3SS, an export apparatus required for invasion into the host.
(ii) FlaC protein	Colonization and invasion.
(iii) CiaB, CiaC, CiaI	Invasion and intracellular survival.
(iv) HtrA chaperone	Correct folding of adhesion proteins.
Capsule (capsular polysaccharide transport protein M, capsule biosynthesis proteins)	*C. jejuni* surface is covered with a capsule which helps in survival, adherence and evasion of the host immune system.
VirK protein	Protection against antimicrobial peptide.
Iron uptake system (i) Membrane ferric enterobactin (FeEnt) receptors (ii) CeuE lipoprotein (iron acquisition) (iii) Ferric uptake regulator (Fur) (iv) Outer membrane receptor for haemin and haemoglobin (ChuA)	Iron transport and regulation are required for survival of *Campylobacter*.
Major outer membrane protein (MOMP); encoded by *porA* gene	MOMP is known to allow passage of hydrophilic molecules across the outer membrane and provides structural stability to the outer membrane. It also helps in bacterial adhesion with host tissues.
Stress response factors [stringent control (spoT), catalase (katA), alkyl hydroperoxide reductase (AhpC), thiol peroxidase (Tpx), cytochrome *c* peroxidases, NADPH quinine reductase, heat shock protein]	These factors help in survival under oxidative stress such as starvation, heat, reduced pH occurred during food processing and storage. *Campylobacter* enter a viable but nonculturable state which is characterized by decreased metabolic activity, increased production of certain enzymes and cell shrinkage. This condition helps in survival of *Campylobacter* under unfavourable conditions.
Lipopolysaccharide (LPS)	LPS contains N-acetylneuraminic acid (NeuAc), responsible for serum resistance. 'NeuAc' is rarely found in prokaryotes although common in eukaryotic glycolipids.

Diagnosis

The infected poultry birds shed large numbers of organisms ($>10^6$ colony-forming units/g faeces). Clinical samples for isolation of *Campylobacter* are fresh faeces (without urine), caecal droppings or cloacal swabs and bile. Postmortem samples include caeca from poultry, intestinal content from cattle, sheep and pigs. The samples after collection should be carried in a transport media (Cary—Blair, Stuart, Amies, alkaline peptone water) into the laboratory to prevent the drying and oxygen exposure. The samples should be protected from light, freezing ($<0°C$) and high temperature ($>20°C$).

Laboratory examinations

Direct examination: A smear can be prepared from clinical samples and stained by dilute carbol fuchsin. *Campylobacter* appears as pink-coloured small curved rod arranged in a pair to produce characteristic 'S' or 'wing of gull' appearance. The bacteria can also be demonstrated by wet mounts of faeces by phase contrast or dark-field microscopy. *C. mucosalis* and *C. hyointestinalis* can be demonstrated by modified Ziehl—Neelsen stain. The organisms appear as pink-coloured, curved, intracellular rods.

Isolation of *Campylobacter* spp.: *Campylobacter* can be isolated from clinical samples without any enrichment. The samples are filtered through 0.65 or 0.45 µm filters before inoculation into the media. Selective media for *Campylobacter* isolation is broadly categorized into two types, i.e., charcoal based and blood based. Charcoal and blood components remove toxic derivatives of oxygen from the media. Examples of charcoal-based selective media are modified charcoal, cefoperazone, deoxycholate agar (mCCDA), Karmali agar or charcoal selective medium. The blood-based media are Preston agar, Skirrow agar, Butzler agar and Campy Cefex agar. Commonly used nonselective media for *Campylobacter* isolation are blood agar with or without 0.1% sodium thioglycolate (used to reduce oxygen tension of the media) and antibiotics. The antibiotics used in the media are cephalosporins, trimethoprim, bacitracin, actidione, amphotericin B, etc. Actidione and amphotericin B are used to prevent the growth of yeasts and moulds.

Campylobacter are microaerophilic in nature and require 3%—5% CO_2 with 3%—15% O_2 for growth. Optimum growth requires incubation at 37°C temperature for 2—5 days (24—48 h for *C. jejuni* and *C. coli*). *Campylobacter* spp. will not survive below a pH of 4.9 and above pH 9.0 and grow optimally at pH 6.5—7.5. Thermophilic *Campylobacter* (*C. jejuni*, *C. coli*) prefer to grow at 30—46°C in an atmosphere containing 10% CO_2 and 5% O_2.

C. jejuni is nonhaemolytic and produces finely granular, irregular margin, flat, greyish colonies in blood agar. On charcoal-based media, the colonies may produce 'metallic sheen'.

Serological tests: Fluorescence in situ hybridization, latex agglutination test and a physical enrichment method (filtration) can detect *Campylobacter* in the food matrix (Baggerman and Koster, 1992; Hazeleger et al., 1992; Lehtola et al., 2006).

Molecular biology: Multiplex polymerase chain reaction (PCR) is developed for detection of several *Campylobacter* species such as *C. jejuni* (23S RNA gene); *C. coli*, *C. lari* and *C. upsaliensis* (*glyA* gene) and *sapB2* gene from *C. fetus* subsp. *fetus* (Wang et al., 2002). PCR combined with immunomagnetic separation can detect *Campylobacter* present in low numbers in the samples (Waller and Ogata, 2000). Real-time PCR can confirm *Campylobacter* in very low copies (1 cfu) in less than 2 hours (Debretsion et al., 2007).

Characteristics of antimicrobial resistance

Erythromycin (macrolide) is the drug of choice for clinical campylobacteriosis, although fluoroquinolone, tetracyclines and gentamicin are also used for the treatment (Acheson and Allos, 2001). Increasing resistance of *Campylobacter* against common antibiotics is a public health concern. Intrinsic resistance in *C. jejuni* and *C. coli* was described against penicillins and cephalosporins, bacitracin, novobiocin, rifampin, streptogramin B and vancomycin (McNulty, 1987). The multidrug efflux pump (CmeABC) was detected to be associated with intrinsic resistance in *Campylobacter* (Lin et al., 2002).

Mutation of the essential genes and horizontal transfer of resistance determinants are two major pathways associated with generation of antimicrobial resistance in *Campylobacter*. Absence of DNA repair molecules such as methyl-directed mismatch repair (mutH and mutL), recombination repair (sbcB), repair of pyrimidine dimmers (phr), very short patch repair (vsr) and protecting protein from UV-induced mutagenesis (umuCD) and alkylating agents (ada) in *C. jejuni* isolates further promote the mutations (Parkhill et al., 2000).

Quinolone resistance

Use of fluoroquinolones in animal and poultry farms in the United States, Europe, Australia and Asia was correlated with generation of quinolone-resistant human *Campylobacter* isolates (Endtz et al., 1991; Nachamkin et al., 2002; Hart et al., 2004). Conversion of fluoroquinolone-susceptible *C. jejuni* into resistant population was observed after exposure to enrofloxacin (McDermott et al., 2002).

Amino acid substitution (Thr86Ile, Asp90Asn, Thr86Lys, Thr86Ala, Thr86Val, Asp90Tyr) in the quinolone resistance-determining region (QRDR) of topoisomerase enzyme is associated with quinolone resistance of *Campylobacter* spp. Mutation (C257T) in *gyrA* gene and subsequent Thr86Ile amino acid substitution was detected as most common mechanism of quinolone resistance in *Campylobacter* spp. (Payot et al., 2006). This substitution (Thr86Ile) produced high level of resistance in *C. jejuni* and *C. coli* isolates against ciprofloxacin (Ge et al., 2005). The frequencies of emergence of fluoroquinolone-resistant mutants range from approximately 10^{-6} to 10^{-8}/cell/generation (Yan et al., 2006). Strain to strain variation in emergence of mutant occurs as the mutation (C257T) might offer a 'fitness benefit' to one strain of *C. jejuni* but was 'costly' for a different strain (Luo et al., 2005).

The multidrug efflux pump (CmeABC) was also detected to be associated with quinolone resistance in *Campylobacter* spp. in synergy with *gyrA* mutations. CmeABC is encoded by three genes, i.e., *cmeA* (periplasmic fusion protein), *cmeB* (drug transporter) and *cmeC* (outer membrane protein). Blocking the efflux pump in *Campylobacter* reduced the MIC value against ciprofloxacin in spite of mutation in *gyrA* (Luo et al., 2003).

Mfd (mutant frequency decline), a transcription repair coupling factor associated with DNA repair, also develops quinolone-resistant *Campylobacter* strains (Han et al., 2008).

Tetracycline resistance

Resistance to tetracyclines in *Campylobacter* is associated with *tet(O)* gene, present in a self-transmissible plasmid (45–58 kb) and prevalent in both *C. jejuni* and *C. coli* strains (Connell et al., 2003a). *Campylobacter tet(O)* gene was acquired by horizontal gene transfer from *Streptomyces*, *Streptococcus* and *Enterococcus* spp. (Batchelor et al., 2004). The *tet(O)* gene encodes ribosomal protection proteins which can bind with open 'A' site on the bacterial ribosome and produces a conformational change of the ribosome in such a manner that all the bound tetracycline molecules are released(Connell et al., 2003b). The conformational change did not hamper the protein synthesis of the bacterial ribosome.

Macrolide resistance

Generation of macrolide resistance in *Campylobacter* is a stepwise process that requires exposure for a prolonged period. Exposure to quinolones although rapidly induces resistance in *Campylobacter* strains. Subtherapeutic exposure to tylosin, given continuously in feed, produced more macrolide resistance in *C. coli* isolates than therapeutic exposure (Schönberg-Norio et al., 2006; Ladely et al., 2007).

Resistance to macrolides in *Campylobacter* is associated with modification of the ribosomal target, ribosomal proteins and enzymatic inactivation of the drug. Mutation in 23S rRNA gene (A2074C, A2074G, A2075G) is the common way to generate erythromycin resistance (MIC > 128 mg/L) in *C. jejuni* and *C. coli* isolates (Jeon et al., 2008). Modifications (substitution, insertion, deletion) of the ribosomal proteins (L4, L22) were associated with generation of low-level macrolide resistance in *Campylobacter* isolates (Cagliero et al., 2006). The multidrug efflux pump (CmeABC) was also detected to be associated with macrolide resistance in *Campylobacter* spp. in synergy with 23S rRNA mutations and modifications of L4, L22 proteins (Corcoran et al., 2006; Cagliero et al., 2006).The frequency of emergence of macrolide-resistant mutants is lower than fluoroquinolone-resistant mutants (10^{-10}/cell/generation) (Lin et al., 2007).

Lower mutation rate, prolonged antibiotic exposure and required fitness cost are the probable explanations for the lower prevalence of macrolide resistance in *Campylobacter* isolates.

Aminoglycoside resistance

Aminoglycoside-modifying enzymes (aminoglycoside phosphor transferase types I, III, IV and VII, aminoglycoside adenyl transferase, 6-amino glycoside adenyl transferase) detected in *Campylobacter* spp. can decrease the affinity of aminoglycosides for the rRNA A-site (Llano-Sotelo et al., 2002). Kanamycin-resistance phosphotransferase [APH (3′) III and APH (3′) IV] was detected in a 14 Kbp plasmid present in *C. jejuni* isolates (Tenover et al., 1989). This plasmid can offer resistance against tetracyclines also and is transferred between *Campylobacter* strains (Gibreel et al., 2004).

β-Lactam antibiotic resistance

Majority of *Campylobacter* strains are inherently resistant to penicillins and narrow spectrum cephalosporins (except amoxicillin and ampicillin) because of production of β-lactamase enzyme or mediated through multidrug efflux pump (CmeABC) (Tajada et al., 1996; Lin et al., 2002). *C. jejuni/C. coli* strains were found susceptible to cefotaxime, ceftazidime, cefpirome and imipenem (Van der Auwera et al., 1985).

Chloramphenicol resistance

Plasmid-encoded chloramphenicol resistance gene (*cat*) was rarely detected in *Campylobacter* spp. (Wang and Taylor, 1990). The enzyme acetyltransferase, encoded by *cat* gene, modifies chloramphenicol in a way which prevents its binding with bacterial ribosomes. A recently explored mechanism suggested the synergistic role of efflux pump (CmeB) and radical S-adenosylmethionine enzyme in production of chloramphenicol resistance in *C. jejuni* strains (Li et al., 2017).

Sulphonamide resistance

Resistance to sulphonamides in *C. jejuni* strains was associated with mutational substitution of amino acids in dihydropteroate synthase enzyme resulting in reduced affinity for sulphonamides (Gibreel and Sköld, 1999).

Trimethoprim resistance

Resistance to trimethoprim in *Campylobacter* was associated with two dihydrofolate reductases (*dfr1* and *dfr9*) acquired from *Enterobacteriaceae* (Gibreel and Sköld, 2000).

Streptothricin resistance

The *sat4* gene present in *C. coli* was found to be associated with streptothricin resistance in animal and clinical isolates in Germany (Bischoff and Jacob, 1996).

Characteristics of antimicrobial resistance in *Campylobacter* isolates observed in poultry, pigs and human are discussed in the following section.

Poultry

Occurrence of *Campylobacter* in healthy poultry gut is high and use of antibiotics in poultry can induce the generation of antibiotic-resistant strains. The fluoroquinolones (sarafloxacin and enrofloxacin) were licenced by the FDA for therapeutic use in poultry during 1990 which generated quinolone-resistant *Campylobacter* in poultry in the United States (Gupta et al., 2004). National Antimicrobial Resistance Monitoring System (NARMS) in the United States revealed an increasing trend (20.3% in 2001 to 23.1% in 2010) of ciprofloxacin resistance in *C. jejuni* isolated from the chicken at slaughter (NARMS, 2010). Subsequently the licence for fluoroquinolone use in poultry was cancelled in the United States in 2005 after prolonged legal battle (Nelson et al., 2007). Higher occurrence of fluoroquinolone-resistant *Campylobacter* was observed in conventional poultry and associated retail meat than organic poultry in the United States (Cui et al., 2005; Luangtongkum et al., 2006). Throughout the world, prevalence of fluoroquinolone-resistant *Campylobacter* varied widely (0%−99%) in broilers. The prevalence was at lower side (0%−11%) in poultry in Australia, Denmark and Norway (Iovine, 2013) and higher occurrence was observed in Spain and Thailand (80%−99%) (Sáenz et al., 2000; Chokboonmongkol et al., 2013). Increasing trend in occurrence of quinolone-resistant *Campylobacter* strains was observed in poultry during 1994 (47%) to 2008 (90%) in Poland (Wozniak, 2011).

Macrolide resistance in poultry *C. jejuni* isolates was comparatively lower than *C. coli* in most of the countries (Gyles, 2008). The study in Portugal although revealed the higher rate of erythromycin resistance in *C. jejuni* (35%) isolates than *C. coli* (13%) in poultry (Fraqueza et al., 2014). Low erythromycin resistance (0%−10%, 2001−10) was observed in *C. jejuni* strains isolated from retail poultry meat in the United States (NARMS, 2010). Higher occurrence of macrolide-resistant *C. coli* (100%) than *C. jejuni* (9%−14%) was detected in poultry in China (Chen et al., 2010). In a systemic study in China, species shift from *C. jejuni* to *C. coli* was observed in poultry during 2008−14. Occurrence of macrolide-resistant *C. jejuni* strains reduced from 13.3% (2008−09) to 8.2% (2012−14), and subsequently, occurrence of resistant *C. coli* strains increased from 48.7% (2008−09) to 76.4% (2012−14). Excessive use of macrolides (tylosin, tilmicosin, erythromycin, kitasamycin, tulathromycin) in poultry and livestock industry in China was correlated with species shift of *Campylobacter* and increased macrolide resistance (Wang et al., 2015).

Pigs

Ciprofloxacin-resistant *C. coli* were detected in pigs in China with higher occurrence (96%—99% of the isolates) (Qin et al., 2011). Increased macrolide use in swine industry in China was also correlated with increased prevalence (44% during 2008—09 to 59% during 2012—14) of macrolide-resistant *C. coli* (Wang et al., 2015).

Human

Resistance to antibiotics (fluoroquinolone) was first detected in human *Campylobacter* isolates during late 1980s (Acheson and Allos, 2001). The resistance spreads rapidly throughout the world with introduction of fluoroquinolones in poultry and livestock industry. In the United States, fluoroquinolone resistance in human isolates raised from 1.3% in 1992 to 10.2% in 1998 (Nachamkin et al., 2002). Similar increasing trend of fluoroquinolone resistance in *Campylobacter* isolates was detected in Europe (Spain in 1993—2003, Germany in 1991—2002) (Luber et al., 2003; Ruiz et al., 2007) and Asia (India and Thailand, Hoge et al., 1998; Jain et al., 2005). In Denmark and Finland, a positive correlation between resistance to ciprofloxacin, nalidixic acid and tetracycline in human *Campylobacter* isolates and international travel (specially in Spain and Thailand) was detected (Hakanen et al., 2003; Skjøt-Rasmussen et al., 2009). In Australia, occurrence of resistant *Campylobacter* spp. in human was low because of restricted use of antibiotics both in human and food animals (Unicomb et al., 2003).

References

Achen, M., Morishita, T.Y., Ley, E.C., 1998. Shedding and colonization of *Campylobacter jejuni* in broilers from day-of-hatch to slaughter age. Avian Diseases 732—737.

Acheson, D., Allos, B.M., 2001. *Campylobacter jejuni* infections: update on emerging issues and trends. Clinical Infectious Diseases 32 (8), 1201—1206.

Bacon, D.J., Alm, R.A., Hu, L., Hickey, T.E., Ewing, C.P., Batchelor, R.A., Guerry, P., 2002. DNA sequence and mutational analyses of the pVir plasmid of *Campylobacter jejuni* 81—176. Infection and Immunity 70 (11), 6242—6250.

Baggerman, W.I., Koster, T., 1992. A comparison of enrichment and membrane filtration methods for the isolation of *Campylobacter* from fresh and frozen foods. Food Microbiology 9 (2), 87—94.

Batchelor, R.A., Pearson, B.M., Friis, L.M., Guerry, P., Wells, J.M., 2004. Nucleotide sequences and comparison of two large conjugative plasmids from different *Campylobacter* species. Microbiology 150 (10), 3507—3517.

Beery, J.T., Hugdahl, M.B., Doyle, M.P., 1988. Colonization of gastrointestinal tracts of chicks by *Campylobacter jejuni*. Applied and Environmental Microbiology 54 (10), 2365—2370.

Bischoff, K., Jacob, J., 1996. The *sat4* streptothricin acetyl transferase gene of *Campylobacter coli*: its distribution in the environment and use as epidemiological marker. Zentralblatt fur Hygiene und Umweltmedizin: International Journal of Hygiene and Environmental Medicine 198 (3), 241—257.

Boer, P.D., Wagenaar, J.A., Achterberg, R.P., van Putten, J.P., Schouls, L.M., Duim, B., 2002. Generation of *Campylobacter jejuni* genetic diversity *in vivo*. Molecular Microbiology 44 (2), 351—359.

Buhr, R.J., Cox, N.A., Stern, N.J., Musgrove, M.T., Wilson, J.L., Hiett, K.L., 2002. Recovery of *Campylobacter* from segments of the reproductive tract of broiler breeder hens. Avian Diseases 46 (4), 919—924.

Byrd, J., Bailey, R.H., Wills, R., Nisbet, D., 2007. Recovery of *Campylobacter* from commercial broiler hatchery trayliners. Poultry Science 86 (1), 26—29.

Cagliero, C., Mouline, C., Cloeckaert, A., Payot, S., 2006. Synergy between efflux pump CmeABC and modifications in ribosomal proteins L4 and L22 in conferring macrolide resistance in *Campylobacter jejuni* and *Campylobacter coli*. Antimicrobial Agents and Chemotherapy 50 (11), 3893—3896.

Calva, J., Lopez-Vidal, A., Ruiz-Palacios, G., Ramos, A., Bojalil, R., 1988. Cohort study of intestinal infection with *Campylobacter* in Mexican children. The Lancet 331 (8584), 503—506.

Chen, X., Naren, G.W., Wu, C.M., Wang, Y., Dai, L., Xia, L.N., Luo, P.J., Zhang, Q., Shen, J.Z., 2010. Prevalence and antimicrobial resistance of *Campylobacter* isolates in broilers from China. Veterinary Microbiology 144 (1—2), 133—139.

Chokboonmongkol, C., Patchanee, P., Gölz, G., Zessin, K.H., Alter, T., 2013. Prevalence, quantitative load, and antimicrobial resistance of *Campylobacter* spp. from broiler ceca and broiler skin samples in Thailand. Poultry Science 92 (2), 462—467.

Chuma, T., Yano, K., Omori, H., Okamoto, K., Yugi, H., 1997. Direct detection of *Campylobacter jejuni* in chicken cecal contents by PCR. Journal of Veterinary Medical Science 59 (1), 85—87.

Connell, S.R., Trieber, C.A., Dinos, G.P., Einfeldt, E., Taylor, D.E., Nierhaus, K.H., 2003a. Mechanism of Tet (O)-mediated tetracycline resistance. The EMBO Journal 22 (4), 945—953.

Connell, S.R., Tracz, D.M., Nierhaus, K.H., Taylor, D.E., 2003b. Ribosomal protection proteins and their mechanism of tetracycline resistance. Antimicrobial Agents and Chemotherapy 47 (12), 3675−3681.

Corcoran, D., Quinn, T., Cotter, L., Fanning, S., 2006. An investigation of the molecular mechanisms contributing to high-level erythromycin resistance in *Campylobacter*. International Journal of Antimicrobial Agents 27 (1), 40−45.

Corry, J.E.L., Atabay, H.I., 2001. Poultry as a source of *Campylobacter* and related organisms. Journal of Applied Microbiology 90 (S6).

Cox, N.A., Stern, N.J., Wilson, J.L., Musgrove, M.T., Buhr, R.J., Hiett, K.L., 2002. Isolation of *Campylobacter* spp. from semen samples of commercial broiler breeder roosters. Avian Diseases 46 (3), 717−720.

Crim, S.M., Iwamoto, M., Huang, J.Y., Griffin, P.M., Gilliss, D., Cronquist, A.B., Cartter, M., Tobin-D'Angelo, M., Blythe, D., Smith, K., Lathrop, S., 2014. Incidence and trends of infection with pathogens transmitted commonly through food—foodborne diseases active surveillance network, 10 US sites, 2006−2013. Morbidity and Mortality Weekly Report 63 (15), 328−332.

Cui, S., Ge, B., Zheng, J., Meng, J., 2005. Prevalence and antimicrobial resistance of *Campylobacter* spp. and *Salmonella* serovars in organic chickens from Maryland retail stores. Applied and Environmental Microbiology 71 (7), 4108−4111.

Debretsion, A., Habtemariam, T., Wilson, S., Nganwa, D., Yehualaeshet, T., 2007. Real-time PCR assay for rapid detection and quantification of *Campylobacter jejuni* on chicken rinses from poultry processing plant. Molecular and Cellular Probes 21 (3), 177−181.

Doyle, L.P., 1944. A vibrio associated with swine dysentery. American Journal of Veterinary Research 5 (3).

Doyle, M.P., 1984. Association of *Campylobacter jejuni* with laying hens and eggs. Applied and Environmental Microbiology 47 (3), 533−536.

EFSA Panel on Biological Hazards (BIOHAZ), 2010. Scientific opinion on quantification of the risk posed by broiler meat to human campylobacteriosis in the EU. European Food Safety Authority Journal 8 (1), 1437.

Endtz, H.P., Ruijs, G.J., van Klingeren, B., Jansen, W.H., van der Reyden, T., Mouton, R.P., 1991. Quinolone resistance in *Campylobacter* isolated from man and poultry following the introduction of fluoroquinolones in veterinary medicine. Journal of Antimicrobial Chemotherapy 27 (2), 199−208.

Fraqueza, M.J., Martins, A., Borges, A.C., Fernandes, M.H., Fernandes, M.J., Vaz, Y., Bessa, R.J.B., Barreto, A.S., 2014. Antimicrobial resistance among *Campylobacter* spp. strains isolated from different poultry production systems at slaughterhouse level. Poultry Science 93 (6), 1578−1586.

García, S., Heredia, N., 2013. Campylobacter. In: Labb_e, R.G., García, S. (Eds.), Guide to Foodborne Pathogens, second ed. Wiley Blackwell, Hoboken, NJ, p. 188e96.

Ge, B., McDermott, P.F., White, D.G., Meng, J., 2005. Role of efflux pumps and topoisomerase mutations in fluoroquinolone resistance in *Campylobacter jejuni* and *Campylobacter coli*. Antimicrobial Agents and Chemotherapy 49 (8), 3347−3354.

Gibreel, A., Sköld, O., 1999. Sulfonamide resistance in clinical isolates of *Campylobacter jejuni*: mutational changes in the chromosomal dihydropteroate synthase. Antimicrobial Agents and Chemotherapy 43 (9), 2156−2160.

Gibreel, A., Sköld, O., 2000. An integron cassette carrying dfr1 with 90-bp repeat sequences located on the chromosome of trimethoprim-resistant isolates of *Campylobacter jejuni*. Microbial Drug Resistance 6 (2), 91−98.

Gibreel, A., Tracz, D.M., Nonaka, L., Ngo, T.M., Connell, S.R., Taylor, D.E., 2004. Incidence of antibiotic resistance in *Campylobacter jejuni* isolated in Alberta, Canada, from 1999 to 2002, with special reference to *tet (O)*-mediated tetracycline resistance. Antimicrobial Agents and Chemotherapy 48 (9), 3442−3450.

Gölz, G., Rosner, B., Hofreuter, D., Josenhans, C., Kreienbrock, L., Löwenstein, A., Schielke, A., Stark, K., Suerbaum, S., Wieler, L.H., Alter, T., 2014. Relevance of *Campylobacter* to public health-the need for a One Health approach. International Journal of Medical Microbiology 304 (7), 817−823.

Gupta, A., Nelson, J.M., Barrett, T.J., Tauxe, R.V., Rossiter, S.P., Friedman, C.R., Joyce, K.W., Smith, K.E., Jones, T.F., Hawkins, M.A., Shiferaw, B., 2004. Antimicrobial resistance among campylobacter strains, United States, 1997−2001. Emerging Infectious Diseases 10 (6), 1102.

Gyles, C.L., 2008. Antimicrobial resistance in selected bacteria from poultry. Animal Health Research Reviews 9 (2), 149−158.

Hakanen, A., Jousimies-Somer, H., Siitonen, A., Huovinen, P., Kotilainen, P., 2003. Fluoroquinolone resistance in *Campylobacter jejuni* isolates in travelers returning to Finland: association of ciprofloxacin resistance to travel destination. Emerging Infectious Diseases 9 (2), 267.

Han, J., Sahin, O., Barton, Y.W., Zhang, Q., 2008. Key role of Mfd in the development of fluoroquinolone resistance in *Campylobacter jejuni*. PLoS Pathogens 4 (6), e1000083.

Hart, W.S., Heuzenroeder, M.W., Barton, M.D., 2004. Antimicrobial resistance in *Campylobacter* spp., *Escherichia coli* and enterococci associated with pigs in Australia. Journal of Veterinary Medicine − Series B 51 (5), 216−221.

Hazeleger, W.C., Beumer, R.R., Rombouts, F.M., 1992. The use of latex agglutination tests for determining *Campylobacter* species. Letters in Applied Microbiology 14 (4), 181−184.

Hermans, D., Pasmans, F., Messens, W., Martel, A., Van Immerseel, F., Rasschaert, G., Heyndrickx, M., Van Deun, K., Haesebrouck, F., 2012. Poultry as a host for the zoonotic pathogen *Campylobacter jejuni*. Vector Borne and Zoonotic Diseases 12 (2), 89−98.

Heuer, O.E., Pedersen, K., Andersen, J.S., Madsen, M., 2001. Prevalence and antimicrobial susceptibility of thermophilic *Campylobacter* in organic and conventional broiler flocks. Letters in Applied Microbiology 33 (4), 269−274.

Hoge, C.W., Gambel, J.M., Srijan, A., Pitarangsi, C., Echeverria, P., 1998. Trends in antibiotic resistance among diarrheal pathogens isolated in Thailand over 15 years. Clinical Infectious Diseases 26 (2), 341−345.

Horrocks, S.M., Anderson, R.C., Nisbet, D.J., Ricke, S.C., 2009. Incidence and ecology of *Campylobacter jejuni* and *coli* in animals. Anaerobe 15 (1−2), 18−25.

Humphrey, S., Chaloner, G., Kemmett, K., Davidson, N., Williams, N., Kipar, A., Humphrey, T., Wigley, P., 2014. *Campylobacter jejuni* is not merely a commensal in commercial broiler chickens and affects bird welfare. mBio 5 (4) e01364-14.

Iovine, N.M., 2013. Resistance mechanisms in *Campylobacter jejuni*. Virulence 4 (3), 230−240.

Jain, D., Sinha, S., Prasad, K.N., Pandey, C.M., 2005. *Campylobacter* species and drug resistance in a north Indian rural community. Transactions of the Royal Society of Tropical Medicine and Hygiene 99 (3), 207–214.

Jeon, B., Muraoka, W., Sahin, O., Zhang, Q., 2008. Role of Cj1211 in natural transformation and transfer of antibiotic resistance determinants in *Campylobacter jejuni*. Antimicrobial Agents and Chemotherapy 52 (8), 2699–2708.

Kaakoush, N.O., Castaño-Rodríguez, N., Mitchell, H.M., Man, S.M., 2015. Global epidemiology of *Campylobacter* infection. Clinical Microbiology Reviews 28 (3), 687–720.

Ladely, S.R., Harrison, M.A., Fedorka-Cray, P.J., Berrang, M.E., Englen, M.D., Meinersmann, R.J., 2007. Development of macrolide-resistant *Campylobacter* in broilers administered subtherapeutic or therapeutic concentrations of tylosin. Journal of Food Protection 70 (8), 1945–1951.

Lehtola, M.J., Pitkänen, T., Miebach, L., Miettinen, I.T., 2006. Survival of *Campylobacter jejuni* in potable water biofilms: a comparative study with different detection methods. Water Science and Technology 54 (3), 57–61.

Li, H., Wang, Y., Fu, Q., Wang, Y., Li, X., Wu, C., Shen, Z., Zhang, Q., Qin, P., Shen, J., Xia, X., 2017. Integrated genomic and proteomic analyses of high-level chloramphenicol resistance in *Campylobacter jejuni*. Scientific Reports 7 (1), 16973.

Lin, J., Michel, L.O., Zhang, Q., 2002. CmeABC functions as a multidrug efflux system in *Campylobacter jejuni*. Antimicrobial Agents and Chemotherapy 46 (7), 2124–2131.

Lin, J., Yan, M., Sahin, O., Pereira, S., Chang, Y.J., Zhang, Q., 2007. Effect of macrolide usage on emergence of erythromycin-resistant *Campylobacter* isolates in chickens. Antimicrobial Agents and Chemotherapy 51 (5), 1678–1686.

Linton, D., Gilbert, M., Hitchen, P.G., Dell, A., Morris, H.R., Wakarchuk, W.W., Gregson, N.A., Wren, B.W., 2000. Phase variation of a β-1, 3 galactosyltransferase involved in generation of the ganglioside GM1-like lipo-oligosaccharide of *Campylobacter jejuni*. Molecular Microbiology 37 (3), 501–514.

Llano-Sotelo, B., Azucena Jr., E.F., Kotra, L.P., Mobashery, S., Chow, C.S., 2002. Aminoglycosides modified by resistance enzymes display diminished binding to the bacterial ribosomal aminoacyl-tRNA site. Chemistry & Biology 9 (4), 455–463.

Luangtongkum, T., Morishita, T.Y., Ison, A.J., Huang, S., McDermott, P.F., Zhang, Q., 2006. Effect of conventional and organic production practices on the prevalence and antimicrobial resistance of *Campylobacter* spp. in poultry. Applied and Environmental Microbiology 72 (5), 3600–3607.

Luber, P., Wagner, J., Hahn, H., Bartelt, E., 2003. Antimicrobial resistance in *Campylobacter jejuni* and *Campylobacter coli* strains isolated in 1991 and 2001–2002 from poultry and humans in Berlin, Germany. Antimicrobial Agents and Chemotherapy 47 (12), 3825–3830.

Luo, N., Pereira, S., Sahin, O., Lin, J., Huang, S., Michel, L., Zhang, Q., 2005. Enhanced *in vivo* fitness of fluoroquinolone-resistant *Campylobacter jejuni* in the absence of antibiotic selection pressure. Proceedings of the National Academy of Sciences 102 (3), 541–546.

Luo, N., Sahin, O., Lin, J., Michel, L.O., Zhang, Q., 2003. In vivo selection of *Campylobacter* isolates with high levels of fluoroquinolone resistance associated with gyrA mutations and the function of the CmeABC efflux pump. Antimicrobial Agents and Chemotherapy 47 (1), 390–394.

Man, S.M., 2011. The clinical importance of emerging *Campylobacter* species. Nature Reviews Gastroenterology & Hepatology 8 (12), 669.

McDermott, P.F., Bodeis, S.M., English, L.L., White, D.G., Walker, R.D., Zhao, S., Simjee, S., Wagner, D.D., 2002. Ciprofloxacin resistance in *Campylobacter jejuni* evolves rapidly in chickens treated with fluoroquinolones. The Journal of Infectious Diseases 185 (6), 837–840.

McNulty, C.A., 1987. The treatment of *Campylobacter* infections in man. Journal of Antimicrobial Chemotherapy 19 (3), 281–284.

Musher, D.M., Musher, B.L., 2004. Contagious acute gastrointestinal infections. New England Journal of Medicine 351 (23), 2417–2427.

Nachamkin, I., Ung, H., Li, M., 2002. Increasing fluoroquinolone resistance in *Campylobacter jejuni*, Pennsylvania, USA, 1982–2001. Emerging Infectious Diseases 8 (12), 1501.

National Antimicrobial Resistance Monitoring System-Enteric Bacteria (NARMS), 2010. Executive Report. U.S. Department of Health and Human Services, Food and Drug Administration, Rockville, MD. Available at: https://www.fda.gov/downloads/animalveterinary/safetyhealth/antimicrobialresistance/nationalantimicrobialresistancemonitoringsystem/ucm312360.pdf.

Nelson, J.M., Chiller, T.M., Powers, J.H., Angulo, F.J., 2007. Fluoroquinolone-resistant *Campylobacter* species and the withdrawal of fluoroquinolones from use in poultry: a public health success story. Clinical Infectious Diseases 44 (7), 977–980.

Parkhill, J., Wren, B.W., Mungall, K., Ketley, J.M., Churcher, C., Basham, D., Chillingworth, T., Davies, R.M., Feltwell, T., Holroyd, S., Jagels, K., 2000. The genome sequence of the food-borne pathogen *Campylobacter jejuni* reveals hypervariable sequences. Nature 403 (6770), 665.

Payot, S., Bolla, J.M., Corcoran, D., Fanning, S., Mégraud, F., Zhang, Q., 2006. Mechanisms of fluoroquinolone and macrolide resistance in *Campylobacter* spp. Microbes and Infection 8 (7), 1967–1971.

Qin, S.S., Wu, C.M., Wang, Y., Jeon, B., Shen, Z.Q., Wang, Y., Zhang, Q., Shen, J.Z., 2011. Antimicrobial resistance in *Campylobacter coli* isolated from pigs in two provinces of China. International Journal of Food Microbiology 146 (1), 94–98.

Robinson, D.A., 1981. Infective dose of *Campylobacter jejuni* in milk. British Medical Journal(Clinical Research Edition) 282 (6276), 1584.

Ruiz, J., Marco, F., Oliveira, I., Vila, J., GascON, J., 2007. Trends in antimicrobial resistance in *Campylobacter* spp. causing traveler's diarrhea. Acta Pathologica Microbiologica et Immunologica Scandinavica 115 (3), 218–224.

Sáenz, Y., Zarazaga, M., Lantero, M., Gastañares, M.J., Baquero, F., Torres, C., 2000. Antibiotic resistance in *Campylobacter* strains isolated from animals, foods, and humans in Spain in 1997–1998. Antimicrobial Agents and Chemotherapy 44 (2), 267–271.

Sahin, O., Kassem, I.I., Shen, Z., Lin, J., Rajashekara, G., Zhang, Q., 2015. *Campylobacter* in poultry: ecology and potential interventions. Avian Diseases 59 (2), 185–200.

Sahin, O., Zhang, Q., Meitzler, J.C., Harr, B.S., Morishita, T.Y., Mohan, R., 2001. Prevalence, antigenic specificity, and bactericidal activity of poultry anti-*Campylobacter* maternal antibodies. Applied and Environmental Microbiology 67 (9), 3951–3957.

Scallan, E., Hoekstra, R.M., Angulo, F.J., Tauxe, R.V., Widdowson, M.A., Roy, S.L., Jones, J.L., Griffin, P.M., 2011. Foodborne illness acquired in the United States—major pathogens. Emerging Infectious Diseases 17 (1), 7.

Schönberg-Norio, D., Hänninen, M.L., Katila, M.L., Kaukoranta, S.S., Koskela, M., Eerola, E., Uksila, J., Pajarre, S., Rautelin, H., 2006. Activities of telithromycin, erythromycin, fluoroquinolones, and doxycycline against *Campylobacter* strains isolated from Finnish subjects. Antimicrobial Agents and Chemotherapy 50 (3), 1086—1088.

Sebald, M., Veron, M., 1963. Base DNA content and classification of Vibrios. Annales de l'Institut Pasteur 105, 897—910.

Silva, J., Leite, D., Fernandes, M., Mena, C., Gibbs, P.A., Teixeira, P., 2011. *Campylobacter* spp. as a foodborne pathogen: a review. Frontiers in Microbiology 2, 200.

Skjøt-Rasmussen, L., Ethelberg, S., Emborg, H.D., Agersø, Y., Larsen, L.S., Nordentoft, S., Olsen, S.S., Ejlertsen, T., Holt, H., Nielsen, E.M., Hammerum, A.M., 2009. Trends in occurrence of antimicrobial resistance in *Campylobacter jejuni* isolates from broiler chickens, broiler chicken meat, and human domestically acquired cases and travel associated cases in Denmark. International Journal of Food Microbiology 131 (2—3), 277—279.

Smith, T., 1919. The etiological relation of spirilla (Vibrio fetus) to bovine abortion. Journal of Experimental Medicine 30 (4), 313—323.

Tajada, P., Gomez-Graces, J.L., Alos, J.I., Balas, D., Cogollos, R., 1996. Antimicrobial susceptibilities of *Campylobacter jejuni* and *Campylobacter coli* to 12 beta-lactam agents and combinations with beta-lactamase inhibitors. Antimicrobial Agents and Chemotherapy 40 (8), 1924—1925.

Tenover, F.C., Gilbert, T., O'Hara, P., 1989. Nucleotide sequence of a novel kanamycin resistance gene, *aphA-7*, from *Campylobacter jejuni* and comparison to other kanamycin phosphotransferase genes. Plasmid 22 (1), 52—58.

Unicomb, L., Ferguson, J., Riley, T.V., Collignon, P., 2003. Fluoroquinolone resistance in *Campylobacter* absent from isolates, Australia. Emerging Infectious Diseases 9 (11), 1482.

Van der Auwera, P., Scorneaux, B., 1985. In vitro susceptibility of *Campylobacter jejuni* to 27 antimicrobial agents and various combinations of beta-lactams with clavulanic acid or sulbactam. Antimicrobial Agents and Chemotherapy 28 (1), 37—40.

Vandamme, P., 2000. Taxonomy of the family campylobacteraceae. In: Namchamkin, I., Blaser, M.J. (Eds.), Campylobacter. ASM, Washington, DC, pp. 3—27.

Waller, D.F., Ogata, S.A., 2000. Quantitative immunocapture PCR assay for detection of *Campylobacter jejuni* in foods. Applied and Environmental Microbiology 66 (9), 4115—4118.

Wang, G., Clark, C.G., Taylor, T.M., Pucknell, C., Barton, C., Price, L., Woodward, D.L., Rodgers, F.G., 2002. Colony multiplex PCR assay for identification and differentiation of *Campylobacter jejuni*, *C. coli*, *C. lari*, *C. upsaliensis*, and *C. fetus* subsp. *fetus*. Journal of Clinical Microbiology 40 (12), 4744—4747.

Wang, Y., Taylor, D.E., 1990. Chloramphenicol resistance in *Campylobacter coli*: nucleotide sequence, expression, and cloning vector construction. Gene 94 (1), 23—28.

Wang, Y., Dong, Y., Deng, F., Liu, D., Yao, H., Zhang, Q., Shen, J., Liu, Z., Gao, Y., Wu, C., Shen, Z., 2015. Species shift and multidrug resistance of *Campylobacter* from chicken and swine, China, 2008—14. Journal of Antimicrobial Chemotherapy 71 (3), 666—669.

Wilson, D.L., Bell, J.A., Young, V.B., Wilder, S.R., Mansfield, L.S., Linz, J.E., 2003. Variation of the natural transformation frequency of *Campylobacter jejuni* in liquid shake culture. Microbiology 149 (12), 3603—3615.

Wozniak, A., 2011. Fluoroquinolones resistance of *Campylobacter jejuni* and *Campylobacter coli* isolated from poultry in 1994—1996 and 2005—2008 in Poland. Bulletin of the Veterinary Institute in Pulawy 55 (1), 15—20.

Yan, M., Sahin, O., Lin, J., Zhang, Q., 2006. Role of the CmeABC efflux pump in the emergence of fluoroquinolone-resistant *Campylobacter* under selection pressure. Journal of Antimicrobial Chemotherapy 58 (6), 1154—1159.

Chapter 20

Clostridium

Chapter outline

The bacterium was first isolated from the newborn infant's intestinal flora by Hall and O'Toole (1935). It was described as *Bacillus difficilis* because of the 'difficulty' they faced during isolation. In 1978, *Clostridium difficile* was identified as the primary cause of pseudomembranous colitis in human (Bartlett et al., 1978). *C. difficile* infection (CDI) was found associated with antibiotic-induced diarrhoea (25%—33%) along with pseudomembranous enteritis (90%). In the United States, CDI alone causes 29,000 deaths (400,000 cases) each year with more than $1 billion economic burden (Lessa et al., 2015). A systematic review revealed categorization of CDI-associated excess cost in the United States and estimated $6774—$10212 for CDI-associated hospital admission (Gabriel and Beriot-Mathiot, 2014). Higher incidence rate of CDI (~ 17.1 cases/10,000) was observed in Europe (Sweden), Canada and China (Huang et al., 2008; Dubberke and Olsen, 2012). CDI is also observed as the most frequent aetiology of healthcare-associated infection even exceeding *Staphylococcus aureus* infections (Magill et al., 2014). In the United States, rate of hospitalizations with *C. difficile* tripled in 2011 (12.7/1000 discharges) in comparison to 2001 (5.6/1000 discharges) (Steiner et al., 2012).CDI is characterized by mild to severe diarrhoea causing toxic megacolon, fulminant colitis, piercing of intestine, sepsis and death (Rupnik et al., 2009).

Therapeutic use of certain antibiotics (clindamycin, erythromycin, aminopenicillins, third-generation cephalosporins and fluoroquinolones) promotes CDI because of disruption of intestinal commensal bacteria ('dysbiosis'), which favours the growth of ingested or resident *C. difficile* strains (Owens et al., 2008). Multidrug-resistant strains of *C. difficile* further aggravate the situation because of their growth in presence of antibiotics against which they are resistant. Antibiotic resistance or reduced susceptibility against moxifloxacin, metronidazole and vancomycin was correlated with epidemic spread of hypervirulent *C. difficile* strains such as polymerase chain reaction (PCR) ribotype (RT) 027 in the United States and European countries (He et al., 2013; Ofosu, 2016).

Properties of the genus

Morphology: *C. difficile* are Gram-positive rods, measuring 3—5 μm in length and 0.5 μm in width. They are capsulated, motile by peritrichous flagella and sporulating in nature. Some strains also contain S-layer. The spores are oval, subterminal or terminal in position, do not bulge the parent cells and are produced in artificial medium after 72 h of incubation during decline phase of the growth. Some strains may produce polar fimbriae.

Antimicrobial Resistance in Agriculture. https://doi.org/10.1016/B978-0-12-815770-1.00020-1

Classification: *C. difficile* belongs to class Clostridia, order Clostridiales, family Clostridiaceae and genus *Clostridium*. On the basis of 16S rRNA gene sequences, *C. difficile* are closely related with *Clostridium sordellii* and *Clostridium bifermentans* (Elsayed and Zhang, 2004).

Susceptibility to disinfectants: *C. difficile* spores are resistant to the solvents such as alcohol, enzymes, detergents, disinfectants and environmental stress conditions such as heat, ultraviolet light and ionizing radiation. Vegetative bacteria rapidly die during oxygen exposure.

Natural habitat: They are commonly found in the soil, sand, river, lake, swimming pools, human hospitals and veterinary clinics surroundings, marine sediments, river bank mud, raw vegetables and floor swabs of private houses. It is found as a part of the normal flora of the human intestine (2%−4% in young adults). The isolation rate increases with the advancement of age (10%−20% in elderly persons). It is isolated from the faeces of cattle, horses, donkey, domestic birds, ducks, geese, dog and cat (Hensgens et al., 2012).

Genome: The GC content of *C. difficile* genome is 29 mol%. Approximately 11% of the genome consists of mobile genetic elements (MGEs) (Sebaihia et al., 2006). The plasmids are detected in the bacterium with molecular weights ranging from 2.7×10^6 to 100×10^6, and the plasmids contain the genetic information required for their replication and maintenance only. A few bacteria may contain introns (group I/II) associated with MGEs. The first intron found in *C. difficile* was a group II intron detected within orf14 of a conjugative transposon (*Tn5397*), and the intron-encoded proteins are capable of splicing like eukaryotes (Mullany et al., 1996; Roberts et al., 2001). A combination of a group I intron and an insertion sequence ('IStrons') are widely distributed in *C. difficile* genome which can use alternative splice site to generate variant proteins (Braun et al., 2000). The varieties of conjugative transposons (CTns) and mobilisable transposons (MTns) are also detected in *C. difficile* genome which is transferred from donor to the recipient by a conjugation like process. The CTns and MTns carry genes for antibiotic resistance and ABC transporters (Brouwer et al., 2011). *Tn5397*, *Tn916* (originated from *Bacillus subtilis*), *Tn4453a* and *Tn4453b* of *C. difficile* are well-characterized CTns, which confer resistance to tetracycline (*Tn5397*, *Tn916*; Mullany et al., 1996) and chloramphenicol (*Tn4453a* and *Tn4453b*; Wren et al., 1988). *C. difficile Tn5398* confers resistance against macrolide, lincomycin and streptogramin B (Hächler et al., 1987).

Antigenic characteristics

S-layer protein (SLP) is the major antigen of *C. difficile* used in the typing. This organism unusually expresses two kinds of SLPs, i.e., high molecular weight and low molecular weight proteins. Both the proteins are encoded by *slpA* gene and are produced by posttransitional cleavage of a single precursor. Currently, *C. difficile* comprises of 14 serogroups based on S-layer protein. Serologically it can cross-react with other Clostridia such as *C. sordellii*, *C. bifermentans* and *Clostridium glycolicum*.

The virulence of *C. difficile* isolates is expressed by PCR ribotype (RT), North American pulsed field gel electrophoresis type (NAP) and restriction endonuclease analysis groups depending on the typing method used. PCR ribotyping is based on the differences in the spacer regions of 16S and 23S ribosomal RNA. RT027 and RT078 are the hypervirulent ribotypes, associated with high mortality and recurrence of infection, and have recently spread throughout the world (Collins et al., 2013). The RT027 was further characterized as toxinotype III, restriction endonuclease analysis group BI, North American pulsed-field gel electrophoresis type NAP1 and was designated as BI/NAP1/027 (O'Connor et al., 2009). The BI/NAP1/027 strains of *C. difficile* showed higher rate of sporulation, toxin production and marked antibiotic resistance (fluoroquinolone) (McDonald et al., 2005). A pan-European longitudinal surveillance study indicated RT356 (Italy) as antibiotic resistant and RT005 and RT087 as susceptible isolates in European countries during 2011−14 (Freeman et al., 2015). Distribution of *C. difficile* PCR ribotypes in different countries is described in Table 20.1.

Toxins and virulence factors produced

Toxins

C. difficile produces two large glycosylating toxins known as TcdA (308 KDa) and TcdB (270 KDa). They are glucosyl transferases that inactivate Rho, Rac and Cdc42 within target cells. The TcdA acts as enterotoxin causing accumulation of fluid in the intestine and the TcdB is a potent cytotoxin. On the basis of sequence variations of the toxins, there are 22 toxinotypes of the bacterium. These types are designated by roman numericals (I−XXII).

The genes encoding the toxins (*tcdA*, *tcdB*) are located in a pathogenicity island (19.6 Kb, PaLoc) within the chromosome (Rupnik, 2008). The genes are expressed during the late log and stationary phases of growth in response to a

TABLE 20.1 Distribution of *Clostridium difficile* polymerase chain reaction (PCR) ribotypes.

PCR ribotype	Distribution
001	China, Japan, Korea, Spain, Germany, Scotland
002	Japan, Hong Kong, Korea
014	United States, Spain, France, Japan, China, Korea
017	China, Japan, Korea, Netherlands, Scotland
018	Japan, Korea
027	United States, Canada, Netherlands, Ireland, Germany, Chile, Asia
078	Spain, Germany, France
244	Australia
356	Italy

variety of environmental stimuli. There are three other genes (*tcdC, tcdD* and *tcdE*) found within the same pathogenicity island which encode regulatory proteins. The TcdC and TcdD function as a negative and positive regulator of the toxin production, respectively. The TcdE helps in release of the toxins by increasing the cell wall permeability. The production of the toxins is correlated with the stress conditions such as antibiotic exposure and 'catabolite repression'.

The major toxins (TcdA, TcdB) enter the cell via receptor-mediated endocytosis. The receptor for TcdA is a disaccharide (Galβ1-4GlcNac) which is present in a variety of cells. Within the cell, TcdB glucosylates RhoA, Rac and cdc42 protein via transfer of a sugar moiety to Thr-37 of the GTPase with UDP-glucose as a co-substrate. TcdA can also glucosylate RhoA protein in a similar way (less active than TcdB). Thus both of the toxins inactivate small GTPases within the cell. It results in cellular actin filament condensation, rounding of the cells and membrane blebbing followed by apoptosis.

A binary toxin was described in a few strains of *C. difficile* associated with formation of microtubule protrusions from cell wall that facilitated bacterial adhesion (Schwan et al., 2009).

Virulence factors

Pili, capsule and degradative enzymes act as additional virulence factors. Enzymes such as hyaluronidase, neuraminidase, chondroitin-4-sulphatase and heparinase are detected. The hyaluronidase plays major role in degradation of connective tissues.

Transmission

C. difficile spores are major vehicle of transmission in human. After entry of the spores into the human host, bile acids containing a specific protease (CspC) take prime role in germination of bacteria from the spores (Sorg and Sonenshein, 2008). *C. difficile* spores are detected in the environment on inert surfaces of hospitals or households (shoe-swabs), animal faeces, soils, rivers, sea, lakes, inland drainage, swimming pools, wastewater treatment plants, tap water and puddle water (Båverud et al., 2003; Alam et al., 2014; Janezic et al., 2016). *C. difficile* ribotypes prevalent in human were also detected in the intestine of food animals such as cattle, pigs, sheep, poultry and companion animals such as dogs and cats (Hensgens et al., 2012; Koene et al., 2012). Virulent ribotypes of *C. difficile* (RT078, RT014/020, RT045) were isolated from dogs and exotic pet such as reptile (sequence type 347, negative for toxin genes) (Davies et al., 2014; Andrés-Lasheras et al., 2018). Transmission of *C. difficile* between farmed pigs and humans was documented in the Netherlands where high-density pig farms are located (Ziakas et al., 2015).

Occurrence of *C. difficile* was also detected in several raw food items such as retail vegetables, ready-to-eat salads, lettuce, eggplant, green pepper, uncooked meats, ground beef, ground pork, chicken meat, ready-to-eat summer sausage and ready-to-eat Braunschweiger (Songer et al., 2009; Bakri et al., 2009; Weese et al., 2009, 2010; Metcalf et al., 2010; Rodriguez-Palacios et al., 2014). The concentration of *C. difficile* spores in studied meats or their products is although quite low, the spores can survive cooking temperature (70–72°C) and may germinate if the cooked food is maintained at permissive temperatures. Consumption of beef was reported as a risk factor for CDI while no confirmed foodborne CDI was reported (Søes et al., 2014).

Prolonged antibiotic use (ampicillin, amoxicillin, cephalosporins, clindamycin, fluoroquinolones) causing reduction of commensal Bacteroides and Firmicutes, advanced age, antineoplastic chemotherapy, organ transplantation, malnutrition, female gender, underlying menaces such as inflammatory bowel disease and chronic renal insufficiency and exposure to a carrier are the major risk factors for human transmission of *C. difficile* (Leffler and Lamont, 2015). Owing to lack of commensal-associated 'colonization resistance', the infants act as healthy carriers of *C. difficile* during the first year of life and the serum immunoglobulin G and A antitoxins (IgG and IgA) bind with *C. difficile* toxins and prevent the progress of infection (Jangi and Lamont, 2010). Loss of toll-like receptor signalling, accumulation of proinflammatory Th-17 cells and increased epithelial permeability due to antibiotic-induced dysbiosis were correlated with CDI (Chakra et al., 2014).

Diagnosis

Diarrhoeic faeces, rectal swabs and tissues may be collected for diagnosis of CDI. Stool testing for *C. difficile* toxins is recommended for the patients with diarrhoea only. Posttreatment clinical samples may show positive reaction for several months in absence of clinical symptoms (Sethi et al., 2010).

Laboratory examinations

Isolation of C. difficile

C. difficile is a strict anaerobe and prefers enriched media such as blood agar for its growth. Selective media are cycloserine cefoxitin fructose agar, cefoxitin mannitol agar and cefoxitin mannitol blood agar. The colonies in blood agar are 3–5 mm in diameter with an irregular, lobate edge, grey in colour and nonhaemolytic. Young colonies produce yellow-green colour under long-wavelength ultraviolet illumination (365 nm). After 48–72 h of incubation, grey or white coloured centre develops in the middle of the colonies. The centre formation is associated with the sporulation of the bacteria. Colonies in CCFA are 4 mm in diameter, yellow or ground glass-like with filamentous edges and typical 'horse manure' smell. Isolation of *C. difficile* cannot differentiate between toxigenic and nontoxigenic strains.

Glutamate dehydrogenase assay (GDH)

The assay is sensitive but cannot differentiate between toxigenic and nontoxigenic strains of *C. difficile*.

Detection of toxin

C. difficile toxin in the processed samples (tissue, rectal swabs) can be detected by cell culture (cell cytotoxicity assay) or enzyme immunoassays. Cell culture in Chinese hamster ovary cell line is suitable for detection of the toxin from faecal samples. The cytotoxic activity of the toxin was confirmed by rounding of the cells and neutralization of the toxin by *C. difficile* antitoxin. The test is considered as 'gold standard' for *C. difficile* diagnosis as it can correlate with the clinical cases. Among the enzyme immunoassays, counterimmunoelectrophoresis, latex agglutination test and ELISA can be performed for detection of *C. difficile* toxins.

Molecular biology

Nucleic acid amplification test (NAAT) detects genes for *C. difficile* toxins (A and/or B). NAAT is a sensitive method compared with the cell cytotoxicity assay. Detection of toxin genes is clinically irrelevant although, as negative isolates were found to be associated with clinical infection, and sometimes, the strains positive for toxin genes did not produce any toxins (Elliott et al., 2014). Instead of relying on a single test, two-step algorithms for accurate diagnosis of CDI are currently recommended considering the cost, rapidity, sensitivity and specificity. NAAT/GDH followed by enzyme immunoassays (Tox A/B) is the most accurate method for diagnosis of CDI (Polage et al., 2015). Most of the laboratories in the Europe and other places use single test although to detect CDI.

Characteristics of antimicrobial resistance

Metronidazole and vancomycin are the drugs of choice for treatment of CDI, but reports of high recurrence rates and reduced susceptibility are increasing. The macrocyclic antimicrobial, fidaxomicin, is promising for treatment of CDI because of lower rates of recurrence and minimal commensal flora disruption (Eyre et al., 2013). The susceptibility testing

TABLE 20.2 Prevalence/Occurrence of antimicrobial-resistant *Clostridium difficile* isolates.

Continent/ country	Clindamycin	Moxifloxacin	Rifamycin/ Rifampicin	Metronidazole	Vancomycin	
Europe	49.6%	40%	13%	0.11%	—	
United States	30%	36%	7.9%	—	—	Freeman et al. (2015)
Canada	—	83%	7.9%	—	—	Tenover et al., 2012; Tickler et al., (2014)
United Kingdom	—	—	—	24.4% (reduced susceptibility)	—	Karlowsky et al., (2012); Tenover et al., 2012
Spain	74%	43%	40%	6.3%	—	Baines et al. (2008)
Poland	—	100%	80%	—	—	Peláez et al., (2008); Rodríguez-Pardo et al., (2013)
Czech Republic	—	—	63.6%	—	—	Obuch-Woszczatyński et al. (2014)
Denmark	—	—	56.5%	—	—	Freeman et al. (2015)
Italy	—	—	62.3%	—	—	Freeman et al. (2015)
New Zealand	61%	—	—	—	—	Freeman et al. (2015)
Germany	—	68%	—	—	—	Roberts et al. (2011)
Hungary	—	—	58.6%	—	—	Reil et al. (2012)
China	73.5%	—	19.8%	23% (Heteroresistance)	—	Freeman et al. (2015)
Japan	87.7%	—	—	—	—	Huang et al., (2010); Lee et al., (2014)
Korea	81%	—	19.8%	—	—	Oka et al. (2011)
Iran	89.3%	—	—	5.3%	—	Kim et al., (2012); Lee et al., (2014)
Brazil	—	8%	—	—	58%	Goudarzi et al. (2013)
Israel	—	4.7%	—	20%	31.5%	Fraga et al. (2016)
Australia	—	3.4%	—	—	—	Tkhawkho et al. (2017)
						Knight et al. (2015)

trial in Europe comprising 22 countries (*C. difficile* European resistance, ClosER) revealed the presence of the ribotypes 027, 014, 001/072 and 078 with multiple antimicrobial resistance against rifampicin, moxifloxacin and clindamycin (Table 20.2). Reduced susceptibility to metronidazole and vancomycin was scarce and no evidence of resistance against fidaxomicin was observed in most of the European *C. difficile* isolates (Freeman et al., 2015). Reduced susceptibility to metronidazole of clinical *C. difficile* isolates was although detected in Poland, Spain, Texas and China (Huang et al., 2008; Obuch-Woszczatyński et al., 2014; Norman et al., 2014; Reigadas et al., 2015). Resistance to clindamycin and moxifloxacin of clinical *C. difficile* isolates varied between different countries (Table 20.2).

Clindamycin and erythromycin (macrolide—lincosamide—streptogramin B) resistance

Resistance to macrolide—lincosamide—streptogramin B group of antibiotics is mediated through ribosomal target modifications or active efflux. The bacterial enzyme ribosomal methylase (*ermB* encoded) can modify ribosomal (23S) target to prevent the drug binding. *C. difficile* possessed the *ermB* (carried by *Tn5398*) or *erm(FS)* genes which conferred the ribosomal methylation (Farrow et al., 2001; Schmidt et al., 2007). There are 17 different genetic organisations of *erm*(B) (E1—E17) observed in *C. difficile* (Spigaglia et al., 2011). *C. difficile* strains negative for *ermB* can also show erythromycin/clindamycin resistance and the vice versa, i.e., possession of *ermB* without resistance against clindamycin was also revealed (Tang-Feldman et al., 2005; Schmidt et al., 2007). Mutation in 23S rDNA (C656T substitution) was found to be associated with high level of erythromycin and low level of clindamycin resistance in *ermB*-negative *C. difficile* isolates (Schmidt et al., 2007). Certain hypervirulent ribotypes such as 027, 078, 001 and 017 were detected to be associated with erythromycin resistance.

Fluoroquinolone (moxifloxacin) resistance

Fluoroquinolones inhibit bacterial DNA synthesis by producing a cleavage of enzyme (DNA gyrase and/or topoisomerase IV) DNA complexes. Mutational changes of GyrA and/or GyrB subunit of DNA gyrase induced by *C. difficile* is the mechanism of quinolone resistance (Oh and Edlund, 2003). The common sites of mutation are T82I (GyrA) and D71V, T82V, D81N, A83V, A118V and A118T (GyrB).

Rifamycin (rifampicin) resistance

Rifamycin and rifaximin are commonly used for the treatment of CDI. Point mutation in DNA-dependent RNA polymerase β subunit (RpoB) is associated with rifamycin resistance in *C. difficile* isolates. The common mutations identified in *C. difficile* RpoB are R505K (MIC ≥ 32 µg/mL), H502N and I548M (O'Connor et al., 2008).

Metronidazole resistance

Metronidazole and vancomycin are the drugs of choice for the treatment of CDI. Most of the clinical *C. difficile* isolates are still susceptible to metronidazole, a few instances of treatment failure and in vitro resistance were reported (Table 20.2; Debast et al., 2014). According to EUCAST and CLSI guidelines, anaerobic bacteria were classified as resistant to metronidazole at MIC ≥32 µg/mL, susceptible at MIC ≤8 µg/mL and intermediate at MIC = 16 µg/mL (CLSI, 2012). The metronidazole metabolites inhibit bacterial DNA synthesis and break the DNA strand to initiate bacterial death. The precise mechanism of metronidazole resistance or reduced susceptibility in *C. difficile* isolates is yet to be elucidated. Mutation in ferric uptake regulator (*fur*) and associated deficient iron storage in *C. difficile* isolates was correlated with metronidazole resistance (Lynch et al., 2013; Moura et al., 2014).

Vancomycin resistance

Reduced susceptibly to vancomycin of *C. difficile* isolates is defined as an MIC of >2 µg/mL. Resistance or reduced susceptibility to vancomycin in *C. difficile* isolates was reported from Poland, Brazil and Israel (Table 20.2; Dworczyński et al., 1991). Vancomycin binds with D-alanyl-D-alanine and inhibits bacterial peptidoglycan synthesis. The precise mechanism of vancomycin resistance or reduced susceptibility is unknown. Substitution of amino acid Pro108Leu in the MurG (helps in conversion of lipid I to lipid II during peptidoglycan synthesis) and biofilm formation in *C. difficile* isolates was found to be associated with vancomycin resistance (Đapa et al., 2012; Leeds et al., 2013).

Fidaxomicin resistance

Fidaxomicin (macrocyclic group of antibiotic) is used as an alternative drug of choice for CDI in the United States and Europe since 2011 (Obuch-Woszczatyński et al., 2014). Binding at a site distinct from rifamycin and inhibition of bacterial RNA polymerase is the major mechanism of action. Exceptional reports of fidaxomicin-reduced susceptibility (MIC 2–4 mg/L) (Leeds et al., 2013) or resistance (MIC 16 mg/L) are available (Goldstein et al., 2011). Mutation in *rpoC* (Glu→Arg at position 1073) and CD22120 (*marR* homologue) and associated target site modifications in the RNA polymerase were correlated with resistance against fidaxomicin in *C. difficile* isolates (Leeds et al., 2013).

Tetracycline resistance

C. difficile resistance to tetracyclines is uncommon in clinical isolates and few studies indicated the highly variable occurrence rate (2.4%–41.6%) between the countries (Spigaglia, 2016). Resistance to tetracyclines in *C. difficile* isolates is mostly mediated by ribosomal protective protein (TetM) present in *Tn916*-like element (Spigaglia et al., 2006).

Other resistance genes such as *tetW* and conjugative transposon (*Tn6164*) possessing *tet(44)* and *ant(6)-Ib* genes were also detected in *C. difficile* isolates (Corver et al., 2012; Fry et al., 2012).

Chloramphenicol resistance

Chloramphenicol resistance of *C. difficile* is also uncommon and only 3.7% of European clinical isolates showed the resistance (Freeman et al., 2015). The resistance is mediated by *catD* gene (*Tn4453a* and *Tn4453b*) encoding chloramphenicol acetyl transferase (Wren et al., 1988).

Cephalosporin resistance

Most of the *C. difficile* strains show constitutive resistance against cephalosporins and a few coding sequences present in the genome were identified to be associated with the resistance (Spigaglia, 2016).

References

Alam, M.J., Anu, A., Walk, S.T., Garey, K.W., 2014. Investigation of potentially pathogenic *Clostridium difficile* contamination in household environs. Anaerobe 27, 31−33.

Andrés-Lasheras, S., Martín-Burriel, I., Mainar-Jaime, R.C., Morales, M., Kuijper, E., Blanco, J.L., Chirino-Trejo, M., Bolea, R., 2018. Preliminary studies on isolates of *Clostridium difficile* from dogs and exotic pets. BMC Veterinary Research 14 (1), 77.

Baines, S.D., O'connor, R., Freeman, J., Fawley, W.N., Harmanus, C., Mastrantonio, P., Kuijper, E.J., Wilcox, M.H., 2008. Emergence of reduced susceptibility to metronidazole in *Clostridium difficile*. Journal of Antimicrobial Chemotherapy 62 (5), 1046−1052.

Bakri, M.M., Brown, D.J., Butcher, J.P., Sutherland, A.D., 2009. *Clostridium difficile* in ready-to-eat salads, Scotland. Emerging Infectious Diseases 15 (5), 817.

Bartlett, J.G., Moon, N., Chang, T.W., Taylor, N., Onderdonk, A.B., 1978. Role of *Clostridium difficile* in antibiotic-associated pseudomembranous colitis. Gastroenterology 75 (5), 778−782.

Båverud, V., Gustafsson, A., Franklin, A., Aspan, A., Gunnarsson, A., 2003. *Clostridium difficile*: prevalence in horses and environment, and antimicrobial susceptibility. Equine Veterinary Journal 35 (5), 465−471.

Braun, V., Mehlig, M., Moos, M., Rupnik, M., Kalt, B., Mahony, D.E., Von Eichel-Streiber, C., 2000. A chimeric ribozyme in *Clostridium difficile* combines features of group I introns and insertion elements. Molecular Microbiology 36 (6), 1447−1459.

Brouwer, M.S., Warburton, P.J., Roberts, A.P., Mullany, P., Allan, E., 2011. Genetic organization, mobility and predicted functions of genes on integrated, mobile genetic elements in sequenced strains of *Clostridium difficile*. PLoS One 6 (8), e23014.

Chakra, C.N.A., Pepin, J., Sirard, S., Valiquette, L., 2014. Risk factors for recurrence, complications and mortality in *Clostridium difficile* infection: a systematic review. PLoS One 9 (6), e98400.

Clinical and Laboratory Standards Institute (CLSI), 2012. Methods for Antimicrobial Susceptibility Testing of Anaerobic Bacteria; Approved Standard, eighth ed. CLSI document M11-A8, Wayne, PA.

Collins, D.A., Hawkey, P.M., Riley, T.V., 2013. Epidemiology of *Clostridium difficile* infection in Asia. Antimicrobial Resistance and Infection Control 2 (1), 21.

Corver, J., Bakker, D., Brouwer, M.S., Harmanus, C., Hensgens, M.P., Roberts, A.P., Lipman, L.J., Kuijper, E.J., van Leeuwen, H.C., 2012. Analysis of a *Clostridium difficile* PCR ribotype 078 100 kilobase island reveals the presence of a novel transposon, *Tn 6164*. BMC Microbiology 12 (1), 130.

Ðapa, T., Leuzzi, R., Ng, Y.K., Baban, S.T., Adamo, R., Kuehne, S.A., Scarselli, M., Minton, N.P., Serruto, D., Unnikrishnan, M., 2012. Multiple factors modulate biofilm formation by the anaerobic pathogen *Clostridium difficile*. Journal of Bacteriology.

Davies, K.A., Longshaw, C.M., Davis, G.L., Bouza, E., Barbut, F., Barna, Z., Delmée, M., Fitzpatrick, F., Ivanova, K., Kuijper, E., Macovei, I.S., 2014. Underdiagnosis of *Clostridium difficile* across Europe: the European, multicentre, prospective, biannual, point-prevalence study of *Clostridium difficile* infection in hospitalised patients with diarrhoea (EUCLID). The Lancet Infectious Diseases 14 (12), 1208−1219.

Debast, S.B., Bauer, M.P., Kuijper, E.J., Committee, 2014. European society of clinical microbiology and infectious diseases: update of the treatment guidance document for *Clostridium difficile* infection. Clinical Microbiology and Infections 20, 1−26.

Dubberke, E.R., Olsen, M.A., 2012. Burden of *Clostridium difficile* on the healthcare system. Clinical Infectious Diseases 55 (Suppl. 2), S88−S92.

Dworczyński, A., Sokół, B., Meisel-Mikołajczyk, F., 1991. Antibiotic resistance of *Clostridium difficile* isolates. Cytobios 65 (262−263), 149−153.

Elliott, B., Dingle, K.E., Didelot, X., Crook, D.W., Riley, T.V., 2014. The complexity and diversity of the pathogenicity locus in *Clostridium difficile* clade 5. Genome Biology and Evolution 6 (12), 3159−3170.

Elsayed, S., Zhang, K., 2004. Human infection caused by *Clostridium hathewayi*. Emerging Infectious Diseases 10 (11), 1950.

Eyre, D.W., Babakhani, F., Griffiths, D., Seddon, J., Del Ojo Elias, C., Gorbach, S.L., Peto, T.E., Crook, D.W., Walker, A.S., 2013. Whole-genome sequencing demonstrates that fidaxomicin is superior to vancomycin for preventing reinfection and relapse of infection with *Clostridium difficile*. The Journal of Infectious Diseases 209 (9), 1446−1451.

Farrow, K.A., Lyras, D., Rood, J.I., 2001. Genomic analysis of the erythromycin resistance element Tn5398 from *Clostridium difficile*. Microbiology 147 (10), 2717−2728.

Fraga, E.G., Nicodemo, A.C., Sampaio, J.L.M., 2016. Antimicrobial susceptibility of Brazilian *Clostridium difficile* strains determined by agar dilution and disk diffusion. Brazilian Journal of Infectious Diseases 20 (5), 476–481.

Freeman, J., Vernon, J., Morris, K., Nicholson, S., Todhunter, S., Longshaw, C., Wilcox, M.H., 2015. Pan-European longitudinal surveillance of antibiotic resistance among prevalent *Clostridium difficile* ribotypes. Clinical Microbiology and Infections 21 (3) pp.248-e9.

Fry, P.R., Thakur, S., Gebreyes, W.A., 2012. Antimicrobial resistance, toxinotype and genotypic profiling of *Clostridium difficile* of swine origin. Journal of Clinical Microbiology.

Gabriel, L., Beriot-Mathiot, A., 2014. Hospitalization stay and costs attributable to *Clostridium difficile* infection: a critical review. Journal of Hospital Infection 88 (1), 12–21.

Goldstein, E.J., Citron, D.M., Sears, P., Babakhani, F., Sambol, S.P., Gerding, D.N., 2011. Comparative susceptibilities of fidaxomicin (OPT-80) of isolates collected at baseline, recurrence, and failure from patients in two fidaxomicin phase III trials of *Clostridium difficile* infection. Antimicrobial Agents and Chemotherapy.

Goudarzi, M., Goudarzi, H., Alebouyeh, M., Rad, M.A., Mehr, F.S.S., Zali, M.R., Aslani, M.M., 2013. Antimicrobial susceptibility of *Clostridium difficile* clinical isolates in Iran. Iranian Red Crescent Medical Journal 15 (8), 704.

Hächler, H., Berger-Bächi, B., Kayser, F.H., 1987. Genetic characterization of a *Clostridium difficile* erythromycin-clindamycin resistance determinant that is transferable to *Staphylococcus aureus*. Antimicrobial Agents and Chemotherapy 31 (7), 1039–1045.

Hall, I., O.T, E., 1935. Intestinal flora in newborn infants with a description of a new pathogenic anaerobe, Bacillus difficilis. American Journal of Diseases of Children 49, 390.

He, M., Miyajima, F., Roberts, P., Ellison, L., Pickard, D.J., Martin, M.J., Connor, T.R., Harris, S.R., Fairley, D., Bamford, K.B., D'Arc, S., 2013. Emergence and global spread of epidemic healthcare-associated *Clostridium difficile*. Nature Genetics 45 (1), 109.

Hensgens, M.P., Keessen, E.C., Squire, M.M., Riley, T.V., Koene, M.G., de Boer, E., Lipman, L.J., Kuijper, E.J., 2012. *Clostridium difficile* infection in the community: a zoonotic disease? Clinical Microbiology and Infections 18 (7), 635–645.

Huang, H., Wu, S., Wang, M., Zhang, Y., Fang, H., Palmgren, A.C., Weintraub, A., Nord, C.E., 2008. Molecular and clinical characteristics of *Clostridium difficile* infection in a university hospital in Shanghai, China. Clinical Infectious Diseases 47 (12), 1606–1608.

Huang, H., Weintraub, A., Fang, H., Wu, S., Zhang, Y., Nord, C.E., 2010. Antimicrobial susceptibility and heteroresistance in Chinese *Clostridium difficile* strains. Anaerobe 16 (6), 633–635.

Janezic, S., Potocnik, M., Zidaric, V., Rupnik, M., 2016. Highly divergent *Clostridium difficile* strains isolated from the environment. PLoS One 11 (11), e0167101.

Jangi, S., Lamont, J.T., 2010. Asymptomatic colonization by *Clostridium difficile* in infants: implications for disease in later life. Journal of Pediatric Gastroenterology and Nutrition 51 (1), 2–7.

Karlowsky, J.A., Zhanel, G.G., Hammond, G.W., Rubinstein, E., Wylie, J., Du, T., Mulvey, M.R., Alfa, M.J., 2012. Multidrug-resistant north American pulsotype 2 *Clostridium difficile* was the predominant toxigenic hospital-acquired strain in the province of Manitoba, Canada, in 2006–2007. Journal of Medical Microbiology 61 (5), 693–700.

Kim, J., Kang, J.O., Pai, H., Choi, T.Y., 2012. Association between PCR ribotypes and antimicrobial susceptibility among *Clostridium difficile* isolates from healthcare-associated infections in South Korea. International Journal of Antimicrobial Agents 40 (1), 24–29.

Knight, D.R., Giglio, S., Huntington, P.G., Korman, T.M., Kotsanas, D., Moore, C.V., Paterson, D.L., Prendergast, L., Huber, C.A., Robson, J., Waring, L., 2015. Surveillance for antimicrobial resistance in Australian isolates of *Clostridium difficile*, 2013–14. Journal of Antimicrobial Chemotherapy 70 (11), 2992–2999.

Koene, M.G.J., Mevius, D., Wagenaar, J.A., Harmanus, C., Hensgens, M.P.M., Meetsma, A.M., Putirulan, F.F., Van Bergen, M.A.P., Kuijper, E.J., 2012. *Clostridium difficile* in Dutch animals: their presence, characteristics and similarities with human isolates. Clinical Microbiology and Infections 18 (8), 778–784.

Lee, J.H., Lee, Y., Lee, K., Riley, T.V., Kim, H., 2014. The changes of PCR ribotype and antimicrobial resistance of *Clostridium difficile* in a tertiary care hospital over 10 years. Journal of Medical Microbiology 63 (6), 819–823.

Leeds, J.A., Sachdeva, M., Mullin, S., Barnes, S.W., Ruzin, A., 2013. In vitro selection, via serial passage, of *Clostridium difficile* mutants with reduced susceptibility to fidaxomicin or vancomycin. Journal of Antimicrobial Chemotherapy 69 (1), 41–44.

Leffler, D.A., Lamont, J.T., 2015. *Clostridium difficile* infection. New England Journal of Medicine 372 (16), 1539–1548.

Lessa, F.C., Mu, Y., Bamberg, W.M., Beldavs, Z.G., Dumyati, G.K., Dunn, J.R., Farley, M.M., Holzbauer, S.M., Meek, J.I., Phipps, E.C., Wilson, L.E., 2015. Burden of *Clostridium difficile* infection in the United States. New England Journal of Medicine 372 (9), 825–834.

Lynch, T., Chong, P., Zhang, J., Hizon, R., Du, T., Graham, M.R., Beniac, D.R., Booth, T.F., Kibsey, P., Miller, M., Gravel, D., 2013. Characterization of a stable, metronidazole-resistant *Clostridium difficile* clinical isolate. PLoS One 8 (1), e53757.

Magill, S.S., Edwards, J.R., Bamberg, W., Beldavs, Z.G., Dumyati, G., Kainer, M.A., Lynfield, R., Maloney, M., McAllister-Hollod, L., Nadle, J., Ray, S.M., 2014. Multistate point-prevalence survey of health care–associated infections. New England Journal of Medicine 370 (13), 1198–1208.

McDonald, L.C., Killgore, G.E., Thompson, A., Owens Jr., R.C., Kazakova, S.V., Sambol, S.P., Johnson, S., Gerding, D.N., 2005. An epidemic, toxin gene-variant strain of *Clostridium difficile*. New England Journal of Medicine 353 (23), 2433–2441.

Metcalf, D.S., Costa, M.C., Dew, W.M.V., Weese, J.S., 2010. *Clostridium difficile* in vegetables, Canada. Letters in Applied Microbiology 51 (5), 600–602.

Moura, I., Monot, M., Tani, C., Spigaglia, P., Barbanti, F., Norais, N., Dupuy, B., Bouza, E., Mastrantonio, P., 2014. A multi-disciplinary analysis of a non-toxigenic *Clostridium difficile* strain stable-resistant to metronidazole. Antimicrobial Agents and Chemotherapy.

Mullany, P., Pallen, M., Wilks, M., Stephen, J.R., Tabaqchali, S., 1996. A group II intron in a conjugative transposon from the gram-positive bacterium, *Clostridium difficile*. Gene 174 (1), 145—150.

Norman, K.N., Scott, H.M., Harvey, R.B., Norby, B., Hume, M.E., 2014. Comparison of antimicrobial susceptibility among *Clostridium difficile* isolated from an integrated human and swine population in Texas. Foodborne Pathogens and Disease 11 (4), 257—264.

Obuch-Woszczatyński, P., Lachowicz, D., Schneider, A., Mól, A., Pawłowska, J., Ożdżeńska-Milke, E., Pruszczyk, P., Wultańska, D., Młynarczyk, G., Harmanus, C., Kuijper, E.J., 2014. Occurrence of *Clostridium difficile* PCR-ribotype 027 and it's closely related PCR-ribotype 176 in hospitals in Poland in 2008-2010. Anaerobe 28, 13—17.

O'Connor, J.R., Galang, M.A., Sambol, S.P., Hecht, D.W., Vedantam, G., Gerding, D.N., Johnson, S., 2008. Rifampin and rifaximin resistance in clinical isolates of *Clostridium difficile*. Antimicrobial Agents and Chemotherapy 52 (8), 2813—2817.

O'Connor, J.R., Johnson, S., Gerding, D.N., 2009. *Clostridium difficile* infection caused by the epidemic BI/NAP1/027 strain. Gastroenterology 136 (6), 1913—1924.

Ofosu, A., 2016. *Clostridium difficile* infection: a review of current and emerging therapies. Annals of Gastroenterology: Quarterly Publication of the Hellenic Society of Gastroenterology 29 (2), 147.

Oh, H., Edlund, C., 2003. Mechanism of quinolone resistance in anaerobic bacteria. Clinical Microbiology and Infection 9 (6), 512—517.

Oka, K., Osaki, T., Hanawa, T., Kurata, S., Okazaki, M., Manzoku, T., Takahashi, M., Tanaka, M., Taguchi, H., Watanabe, T., Inamatsu, T., 2011. Molecular and microbiological characterization of *Clostridium difficile* isolates from single, relapse, and re-infection cases. Journal of Clinical Microbiology. https://doi.org/10.1128/JCM.05588-11.

Owens Jr., R.C., Donskey, C.J., Gaynes, R.P., Loo, V.G., Muto, C.A., 2008. Antimicrobial-associated risk factors for *Clostridium difficile* infection. Clinical Infectious Diseases 46 (Suppl. 1), S19—S31.

Peláez, T., Cercenado, E., Alcalá, L., Marin, M., Martín-López, A., Martínez-Alarcón, J., Catalán, P., Sánchez-Somolinos, M., Bouza, E., 2008. Metronidazole resistance in *Clostridium difficile* is heterogeneous. Journal of Clinical Microbiology 46 (9), 3028—3032.

Polage, C.R., Gyorke, C.E., Kennedy, M.A., Leslie, J.L., Chin, D.L., Wang, S., Nguyen, H.H., Huang, B., Tang, Y.W., Lee, L.W., Kim, K., 2015. Overdiagnosis of *Clostridium difficile* infection in the molecular test era. JAMA Internal Medicine 175 (11), 1792—1801.

Reigadas, E., Alcalá, L., Marín, M., Peláez, T., Martin, A., Iglesias, C., Bouza, E., 2015. In vitro activity of surotomycin against contemporary clinical isolates of toxigenic *Clostridium difficile* strains obtained in Spain. Journal of Antimicrobial Chemotherapy 70 (8), 2311—2315.

Reil, M., Hensgens, M.P.M., Kuijper, E.J., Jakobiak, T., Gruber, H., Kist, M., Borgmann, S., 2012. Seasonality of *Clostridium difficile* infections in southern Germany. Epidemiology and Infection 140 (10), 1787—1793.

Roberts, A.P., Braun, V., von Eichel-Streiber, C., Mullany, P., 2001. Demonstration that the group II intron from the clostridial conjugative transposon Tn5397 undergoes splicing in vivo. Journal of Bacteriology 183 (4), 1296—1299.

Roberts, S., Heffernan, H., Al Anbuky, N., Pope, C., Paviour, S., Camp, T., Swager, T., 2011. Molecular epidemiology and susceptibility profiles of *Clostridium difficile* in New Zealand, 2009. The New Zealand Medical Journal 124 (1332), 45—51.

Rodriguez-Palacios, A., Ilic, S., LeJeune, J.T., 2014. *Clostridium difficile* with moxifloxacin/clindamycin resistance in vegetables in Ohio, USA, and prevalence meta-analysis. Journal of Pathogens 2014.

Rodríguez-Pardo, D., Almirante, B., Bartolomé, R.M., Pomar, V., Mirelis, B., Navarro, F., Soriano, A., Sorlí, L., Martínez-Montauti, J., Molins, M.T., Lung, M., 2013. Epidemiology of *Clostridium difficile* infection and risk factors for unfavorable clinical outcomes: results of a hospital-based study in Barcelona, Spain. Journal of Clinical Microbiology. https://doi.org/10.1128/JCM.03352-12.

Rupnik, M., 2008. Heterogeneity of large clostridial toxins: importance of *Clostridium difficile* toxinotypes. FEMS Microbiology Reviews 32 (3), 541—555.

Rupnik, M., Wilcox, M.H., Gerding, D.N., 2009. *Clostridium difficile* infection: new developments in epidemiology and pathogenesis. Nature Reviews Microbiology 7 (7), 526.

Schmidt, C., Löffler, B., Ackermann, G., 2007. Antimicrobial phenotypes and molecular basis in clinical strains of *Clostridium difficile*. Diagnostic Microbiology and Infectious Disease 59 (1), 1—5.

Schwan, C., Stecher, B., Tzivelekidis, T., van Ham, M., Rohde, M., Hardt, W.D., Wehland, J., Aktories, K., 2009. *Clostridium difficile* toxin CDT induces formation of microtubule-based protrusions and increases adherence of bacteria. PLoS Pathogens 5 (10), e1000626.

Sebaihia, M., Wren, B.W., Mullany, P., Fairweather, N.F., Minton, N., Stabler, R., Thomson, N.R., Roberts, A.P., Cerdeño-Tárraga, A.M., Wang, H., Holden, M.T., 2006. The multidrug-resistant human pathogen *Clostridium difficile* has a highly mobile, mosaic genome. Nature Genetics 38 (7), 779.

Sethi, A.K., Al-Nassir, W.N., Nerandzic, M.M., Bobulsky, G.S., Donskey, C.J., 2010. Persistence of skin contamination and environmental shedding of *Clostridium difficile* during and after treatment of *C. difficile* infection. Infection Control and Hospital Epidemiology 31 (1), 21—27.

Søes, L.M., Holt, H.M., Böttiger, B., Nielsen, H.V., Andreasen, V., Kemp, M., Olsen, K.E.P., Ethelberg, S., Mølbak, K., 2014. Risk factors for *Clostridium difficile* infection in the community: a case-control study in patients in general practice, Denmark, 2009-2011. Epidemiology and Infection 142 (7), 1437—1448.

Songer, J.G., Trinh, H.T., Killgore, G.E., Thompson, A.D., McDonald, L.C., Limbago, B.M., 2009. *Clostridium difficile* in retail meat products, USA, 2007. Emerging Infectious Diseases 15 (5), 819.

Sorg, J.A., Sonenshein, A.L., 2008. Bile salts and glycine as cogerminants for *Clostridium difficile* spores. Journal of Bacteriology 190 (7), 2505—2512.

Spigaglia, P., Barbanti, F., Mastrantonio, P., 2006. New variants of the *tet (M)* gene in *Clostridium difficile* clinical isolates harbouring *Tn 916*-like elements. Journal of Antimicrobial Chemotherapy 57 (6), 1205—1209.

Spigaglia, P., Barbanti, F., Mastrantonio, P., European Study Group on Clostridium difficile (ESGCD), Ackermann, G., Balmelli, C., Barbut, F., Bouza, E., Brazier, J., Delmée, M., Drudy, D., 2011. Multidrug resistance in European *Clostridium difficile* clinical isolates. Journal of Antimicrobial Chemotherapy 66 (10), 2227–2234.

Spigaglia, P., 2016. Recent advances in the understanding of antibiotic resistance in *Clostridium difficile* infection. Therapeutic Advances in Infectious Disease 3 (1), 23–42.

Steiner, C., Andrews, R., Barrett, M., Weiss, A., 2012. HCUP projections: mobility/orthopedic procedures 2003 to 2012. In: HCUP Projections Report# 2012-03. US Agency for Healthcare Research and Quality.

Tang-Feldman, Y.J., Henderson, J.P., Ackermann, G., Feldman, S.S., Bedley, M., Silva Jr., J., Cohen, S.H., 2005. Prevalence of the *ermB* gene in *Clostridium difficile* strains isolated at a university teaching hospital from 1987 through 1998. Clinical Infectious Diseases 40 (10), 1537–1540.

Tenover, F.C., Tickler, I.A., Persing, D.H., 2012. Antimicrobial resistant strains of *Clostridium difficile* from North America. Antimicrobial Agents and Chemotherapy. https://doi.org/10.1128/AAC.00220-12.

Tickler, I.A., Goering, R.V., Whitmore, J.D., Lynn, A.N., Persing, D.H., Tenover, F.C., 2014. Strain types and antimicrobial resistance patterns of *Clostridium difficile* isolates from the United States: 2011-2013. Antimicrobial Agents and Chemotherapy. https://doi.org/10.1128/AAC.02775-13.

Tkhawkho, L., Nitzan, O., Pastukh, N., Brodsky, D., Jackson, K., Peretz, A., 2017. Antimicrobial susceptibility of *Clostridium difficile* isolates in Israel. Journal of Global Antimicrobial Resistance 10, 161–164.

Weese, J.S., Avery, B.P., Rousseau, J., Reid-Smith, R.J., 2009. Detection and enumeration of *Clostridium difficile* spores in retail beef and pork. Applied and Environmental Microbiology 75 (15), 5009–5011.

Weese, J.S., Reid-Smith, R.J., Avery, B.P., Rousseau, J., 2010. Detection and characterization of *Clostridium difficile* in retail chicken. Letters in Applied Microbiology 50 (4), 362–365.

Wren, B.W., Mullany, P., Clayton, C., Tabaqchali, S., 1988. Molecular cloning and genetic analysis of a chloramphenicol acetyltransferase determinant from *Clostridium difficile*. Antimicrobial Agents and Chemotherapy 32 (8), 1213–1217.

Ziakas, P.D., Zacharioudakis, I.M., Zervou, F.N., Grigoras, C., Pliakos, E.E., Mylonakis, E., 2015. Asymptomatic carriers of toxigenic *C. difficile* in long-term care facilities: a meta-analysis of prevalence and risk factors. PLoS One 10 (2), e0117195.

Chapter 21

Pasteurella and *Mannheimia*

Chapter outline

Trevisan (1887) coined the generic name *Pasteurella* and Lignieres (1900) proposed the specific name for each bacterial species under the genus *Pasteurella* according to the species of animals or birds infected, such as *Pasteurella aviseptica* for fowls, *Pasteurella suiseptica* for pigs, *Pasteurella boviseptica* for cattle, *Pasteurella oviseptica* for sheep and *Pasteurella leptiseptica* for rabbits. Rosenbuch and Merchant (1939) proposed a single species *Pasteurella multocida*, which is still in use.

Mannheimia is an exclusive animal pathogen associated with 'shipping fever' or bovine respiratory disease (BRD) in cattle. Kitt (1885) first described the bacterium as *Bacterium bipolare multocidum* isolated from shipping fever in cattle. The nomenclature was further changed into *Bacillus boviseptica* and finally *Pasteurella haemolytica* (Jones, 1921; Newsom and Cross, 1932). Based on fermentation capability of arabinose and trehalose, *P. haemolytica* was subdivided into two biotypes (A and T) and several capsular serotypes. The biotype A (with 12 capsular serotypes) was classified under a new genus *Mannheimia* because of disparities in 16S rDNA sequence, cultural and pathological characteristics (Mutters et al., 1985).

P. multocida are zoonotic bacteria producing local wound infection due to animal bite or scratches, meningitis, pneumonia, endocarditis, pyelonephritis, abortion, sepsis and rarely urinary tract infection in immunocompromised patients (Brue and Chosidow, 1994; Costanzo et al., 2017).

BRD is a multifactorial menace associated with stress (transport, weaning, commingling), viral and concurrent bacterial infections such as *Mannheimia haemolytica*, *P. multocida* and *Mycoplasma bovis*. BRD has high economic burden estimated to be more than three billion US dollar per year due to high morbidity, mortality (>50%), treatment and labour costs (Watts and Sweeney, 2010). Administration of antibiotics is the major way for the treatment of BRD. Tetracycline, β-lactam, macrolide, amphenicol and fluoroquinolone are currently licenced in the United States for the treatment of BRD. Multiple drug resistance in *P. multocida* and *M. haemolytica* associated with BRD started to appear in 1976 (Chang and Carter, 1976).

Properties

Morphology: *P. multocida* are nonmotile, nonsporing short rod or coccobacillus, 0.2–0.4 by 0.6–2.5 μm in size. In tissues, exudates and recently isolated cultures, the organism shows the typical bipolar staining characteristics with Leishman or methylene blue stain. *M. haemolytica* is a small, nonmotile, non–spore-forming bacillus, often showing coccobacillary forms with occasional bipolar staining. It can be culturally differentiated from *P. multocida* because of their ability to produce a narrow zone of haemolysis on ovine or bovine blood agar, ability to grow on McConkey agar and inability to produce indole.

Classification: The family *Pasteurellaceae* (order *Pasteurellales*, class *Gammaproteobacteria*) is currently comprised of 25 genera such as *Actinobacillus*, *Avibacterium*, *Gallibacterium*, *Haemophilus*, *Histophilus*, *Lonepinella*, *Mannheimia*, *Pasteurella*, *Phocoenobacter*, *Vespertiliibacter* and *Volucribacter* (International Committee on Sytematics of Prokaryotes, 2017). A new genus *Rodentibacter* was proposed recently (Adhikary et al., 2017). *P. multocida* and *M. haemolytica* are the major pathogenic species of the concerned genera.

Susceptibility to disinfectants: *P. multocida* and *M. haemolytica* are sensitive to phenol (0.5%), bichloride mercury (1:5000), cresol (3.5%), sodium hypochlorite (1%), glutaraldehyde (2%) and ethanol (70%).

Natural habitat: *P. multocida* are most prevalent commensal in upper respiratory tract and oropharynx of domestic and wild animals (Harper et al., 2006). The studies also identified gastrointestinal tract, urinary tract and uterus as probable habitat of *P. multocida* in cattle and buffalo (Williams et al., 2005; Annas et al., 2014). The nasopharynx and tonsils of healthy ruminants are preferred habitat of *M. haemolytica* (Frank et al., 1995). In immunosuppressed or stressed animals, *M. haemolytica* are isolated from lower respiratory tract also (Lawrence et al., 2010).

Genome

The genome of *Haemophilus influenzae* (Rd KW20) was sequenced first among the members of *Pasteurellaceae* family (Fleischmann et al., 1995). *P. multocida* genome is 1.4–2.4 Mbp in size with GC content 37–41 mol%. The complete genome sequence of *P. multocida* (Pm70 strain) was published in 2001 (May et al., 2001). A recent comparative genomics between the pathogenic and nonpathogenic isolates of *P. multocida* type A identified five genes and two insertion sequences associated with the virulence (Du et al., 2016). The plasmids (ColE1) play a major role in transmission of antibiotic resistance in *Pasteurellaceae*. Recent study showed that a single-nucleotide polymorphism near the origin of replication of the plasmid pB1000 (ColE1) in a *P. multocida* clinical isolate produced more than one copies of the plasmid with increased level of antibiotic resistance. In absence of the inducer (antibiotic), the bacterial cells can revert back to the wild type with single copy of plasmid (Santos-Lopez et al., 2017). Other than plasmids, multiple antibiotic resistance determinants are also chromosomally encoded within integrative and conjugative elements (ICEs) present in the genome of *Pasteurellaceae*. The ICE*Pmu1* in *P. multocida* and ICE*Mh1* in *M. haemolytica* are 82 and 92 kb in size, respectively (Michael et al., 2012a; Eidam et al., 2014). The ICEs contain regulatory genes associated with excision, integration and transfer between different members of *Pasteurellaceae* in the core region. The accessory regions encode antibiotic resistance, metabolic capacities and metal fixation (Bi et al., 2011). The presence of 12 antibiotic resistance genes in a single ICE was demonstrated in a *P. multocida* isolate, which established the potentiality of ICEs during horizontal gene transfer (Michael et al., 2012a).

M. haemolytica harbours homologous and compatible plasmids such as pAB2 (Wood et al., 1995) and pYFC1 (Chang et al., 1992), which carry antibiotic resistance genes.

Antigenic characteristics

Roberts (1947) developed a system of serological classification based on passive protection tests in mice and classified *P. multocida* into four types designated as types I, II, III and IV. Carter (1955) developed precipitation and indirect haemagglutination test based to classify *P. multocida* into capsular types A, B, C, D and E. Rimler and Rhoades (1989) isolated a consistent type from turkeys and it was designated as serogroup 'F'. The capsular types of *P. multocida* associated with different clinical infections are described in Table 21.1. Namioka and Murata (1961) identified 11 somatic antigen-based serotypes of *P. multocida*. Heddleston et al. (1972) developed an agar gel precipitation test for somatic typing of avian strains from fowl cholera but is now extended to strains from all host species. Carter capsular typing and Heddleston somatic typing are used in combination to designate *P. multocida* serotypes. In the Carter-Heddleston system, the capsular type is expressed first, followed by the somatic type. In the Namioka-Carter system, the expression is made in the reverse order. Asian and African *P. multocida* serotypes designated as B:2 and E:2, respectively, causes haemorrhagic septicaemia.

P. multocida shares common antigens with *M. haemolytica*, *Haemophilus canis*, *H. influenzae*, *Actinobacillus lignieresii*, *Escherichia coli* and *Neisseria catarrhalis* (Bain and Knox, 1961).

M. haemolytica is currently comprised of more than 20 serotypes and two biotypes (A and T) (Oppermann et al., 2017). The serotype A1 and A2 are associated with infections in cattle and sheep, respectively, throughout the world

TABLE 21.1 Capsular types of *Pasteurella multocida.*

Capsular types	Clinical infection
A	Fowl cholera in poultry; pneumonia in cattle, sheep and pigs; mastitis in sheep; snuffles in rabbits
B	Haemorrhagic septicaemia of cattle and water buffaloes in Asia
D	Atrophic rhinitis and pneumonia in pigs
E	Haemorrhagic septicaemia of cattle and water buffaloes in Africa
F	Commensal in turkey and poultry; fatal peritonitis in calves

(Crouch et al., 2012). During viral infection or other stress conditions *M. haemolytica* serotype A2 commonly carried by healthy cattle is replaced with A1 (Frank, 1988). The serotype switching (A2 to A1) occurred due to capsular switching or horizontal transfer of A1 from the infected cattle.

Toxins and virulence factors produced

Toxins

Toxigenic capsular types A and D of *P. multocida* produce an AB protein toxin known as *P. multocida* toxin (PMT, 146 kDa, encoded by *toxA*). The PMT causes host cellular cytoskeletal rearrangement through deamidation of heterotrimeric G proteins ($G_{\alpha q}$, $G_{\infty 11}$, $G_{\infty 12/13}$, $G_{\infty 13}$ and $G_{\alpha i}$) and suppression of T cells (including T helper cells) (Hildebrand et al., 2015). The PMT plays a major role in pathogenesis of atrophic rhinitis caused by *P. multocida* type D in pigs. The PMT-mediated bone atrophy occurs through disruption of cell signalling processes in osteoblasts and osteoclasts (Martineau-Doize et al., 1993).

M. haemolytica produces leukotoxin (105 KDa, repeat-in-toxin family, RTX), which causes activation of neutrophils and increased release of inflammatory cytokines (at low concentration) and apoptosis of pulmonary cells through formation of transmembrane pores (at high concentration) (Singh et al., 2011). The four-gene polycistronic operon (*lktCABD*) encodes the leukotoxin. The lktA acts as inactive proLKT protein, lktB and lktD helps in secretion of the toxin and lktC activates the inactive form by acylation (Zecchinon et al., 2005). The lysis of cells by the leukotoxin is dependent on specific interaction with the lymphocyte function-associated antigen 1 (LFA-1) or β2 integrin present on the target cell membrane (Jeyaseelan et al., 2000). The LktA protein contains domains with hydrophobic helices which causes spanning of host cell membrane to generate pores (Forestier and Welch, 1991). The carboxy terminal of the leukotoxin consists of glycine and aspartate-rich repeats like other RTX toxins, which binds calcium and potentiates the toxin activity (Rowe et al., 1994). In vivo pathogenesis studies in bovine model with leukotoxin mutant *M. haemolytica* isolates although showed reduced mortality and pulmonary lesions, other factors were also found critical for the pathogenesis (Highlander et al., 2000).

Certain strains of *M. haemolytica* produce a zinc metalloglycoprotease (encoded by *gcp*), which can lyse *O*-sialo-glycoproteins. The enzyme can enhance bacterial adhesion with the host cellular membrane (Nyarko et al., 1998). Neuraminidase (150−200 kDa) produced by *M. haemolytica* helps in colonization of the bacteria in the upper respiratory tract. The enzyme is active against N-acetyl-neuramin lactose, fetuin, alpha-1-acid glycoprotein and colominic acid (Straus et al., 1998).

Virulence factors: Major virulence factors produced by *P. multocida* and *M. haemolytica* are described in Table 21.2.

Transmission

P. multocida are commensal in the upper respiratory tract of animals such as cats (70%−90%), dogs (50%−60%) and pigs (50%) and act as opportunistic pathogen (Orsini et al., 2013). During immunosuppression or physiological stress condition, the organisms penetrate the tissues and multiply. Exogenous transmission is possible either by direct contact or through contaminated aerosols.

In human, most of the *P. multocida* infection occurs through bite, scratch, licks on skin abrasions by the carrier animals predominantly dogs and cats but also pigs, rabbits, guinea pigs, rats, horses, as well as wild animals such as lions, tigers, cougars and opossums. Other than bite or scratches, direct contact of injured skin and upper respiratory mucosa with

TABLE 21.2 Major virulence factors produced by *Pasteurella multocida* and *Mannheimia haemolytica*.

Virulence factors	Function
Hyaluronidase, chondroitinase, neuraminidase	Hyaluronidase is produced by haemorrhagic septicaemia causing strains (B:2 serotype) of *P. multocida*. The enzymes help in nutrient acquisition, colonization and dissemination. Neuraminidase helps to evade host defences by blocking mucin action.
Lipopolysaccharide	Resistance to serum complement.
Capsule	Capsule expressed by *P. multocida* is antiphagocytic because of hyaluronic acid components (serotype A), which helps in colonization of the bacteria in human lower respiratory tract. The serotype B capsule consists of arabinose, mannose and galactose. Serotype D and F capsules are composed of heparin or heparin sulphate and chondroitin, respectively. 'Fis'-protein (transcriptional regulator) regulates capsule production in *P. multocida*.
Outer membrane proteins, lipoprotein B	Act as adhesin by binding with host cellular fibronectin and helps in iron acquisition (iron-regulated OMPs) by the bacteria.
Siderophore-independent iron acquisition systems, transferrin-binding receptor	Siderophore-independent iron acquisition systems (homologous to *Actinobacillus* AfeABCD system) of *P. multocida* and transferrin-binding receptors of *M. haemolytica* are associated with iron acquisition.
Filamentous haemagglutinin (FhaB1 and FhaB2 (PfhB1, PfhB2))	They act as adhesin. Precise role in virulence of *P. multocida* is unknown, although reduced expression was detected in nonmucoid strains of *P. multocida*.
DNA uptake	Uptake signal sequences identified in *P. multocida* and *M. haemolytica* are associated with acquisition of new virulence genes.
Type IV fimbriae (PtfA)	Possessed by *P. multocida* serotypes A, B:2, D and associated with adhesion.
DNA adenine methylase (*Dam*)	Regulate expression of *P. multocida* virulence genes.

contaminated animal secretions was also detected as a route of transmission, especially in children, pregnant and aged persons (Wilson and Ho, 2013). Human to human horizontal and vertical transmission of *P. multocida* was also reported (Hillery et al., 1993; Spadafora et al., 2011). Exposure to infected pets acts as a predisposing factor for clinical pasteurellosis in patients with immunosuppression such as HIV infection, renal insufficiency and liver cirrhosis.

M. haemolytica resides as commensal in nasopharynx and tonsils of healthy cattle and causes endogenous infection during stress conditions associated with weaning, adverse weather, changes in feed, transportation for long distances, concurrent viral and mycoplasmal infection (Radostits et al., 2006). *P. haemolytica* var. *urae* was isolated from sputum of elderly human patients, but the pathogenic role was not ascertained (Jones and O'connor, 1962).

Diagnosis: The swabs collected from tonsil, nasal swabs, whole blood or serum, bone marrow from carcasses and faecal sample from birds can be collected as antemortem samples. A blood sample or swab collected from the heart is satisfactory for clinical diagnosis if it is taken within a few hours of death.

Laboratory examinations

Direct examination: A smear can be prepared from collected blood sample or the swabs and stained by Leishman or methylene blue or Gram's stain. *Pasteurella* appears as Gram-negative nonsporing coccobacilli with typical bipolar staining characteristics.

Isolation of *P. multocida*: *P. multocida* can be isolated in dextrose starch agar, casein-sucrose-yeast medium with 5% blood (bovine or ovine), chocolate agar, Mueller-Hinton agar and brain heart infusion agar (Lariviere et al., 1993). No growth in MacConkey's agar is observed. The optimum growth temperature is 35–37°C for 18–24 h. The organism shows different types of colonies which are related to the capsular type. Capsular type A produces the largest colonies which are translucent, greyish in colour and mucoid in consistency. *P. multocida* type D and F strains also produce mucoid colonies. Colonies of types B and E vary in size, depending on the degree of capsulation. The colonies will range from larger greyish colonies, when freshly isolated or when grown in media containing blood or serum, to smaller colonies that give a yellowish-green or bluish-green iridescence, when viewed under transmitted light.

Animal inoculation test: A small volume (0.2 mL) of collected blood or portion of bone marrow in saline is inoculated subcutaneously or intramuscularly into mice. If viable *P. multocida* is present, the mice dies within 24—36 h following inoculation and a pure culture of *P. multocida* can be isolated.

Serological tests: The serological tests for detecting antibodies are not normally used for diagnosis of pasteurellosis. High titres (1/160—1/1280) detected by the Indirect haemagglutination assay (IHA) test are indicative of recent exposure to *P. multocida*. The serological tests such as rapid slide agglutination test (for capsular typing), indirect haemagglutination test (for capsular typing), agar gel immunodiffusion tests (for capsular and somatic typing) and counterimmunoelectrophoresis (for capsular typing) are performed for serotyping of *P. multocida* isolates.

Molecular biology: P6-like (PSL) protein of *P. multocida* was used as target for polymerase chain reaction (PCR) amplification developed by Kasten et al. (1997), but the PCR also produced a positive reaction with *H. influenzae*. The sensitive (100 cells) KMT PCR was developed later, which can detect *P. multocida* types A, B, D and F from tissue samples after enrichment (Townsend et al., 1998; Lee et al., 2000).

Characteristics of antimicrobial resistance

Chemotherapy is the major way to control BRD (*M. haemolytica*) and other infections (*P. multocida*) in domestic animals and birds (Brogden et al., 2007). In a large-scale study conducted over 10 years period (2000—09) in the United States and Canada, *M. haemolytica* and *P. multocida* isolated from bovine respiratory tract showed low level of resistance against enrofloxacin, florfenicol and tulathromycin (Portis et al., 2012). None of the *P. multocida* strains isolated from respiratory tract infections of dogs and cats investigated under BfT-GermVet program showed resistance against any of the antimicrobial agent except sulfonamides (Schwarz et al., 2007). The pan-European antibiotic sensitivity monitoring study (VetPath, 2002—06) incorporating *P. multocida* and *M. haemolytica* isolates from cattle and pigs showed absence or very low resistance (<2%) to amoxicillin/clavulanic acid, ceftiofur, enrofloxacin, florfenicol, tulathromycin, tiamulin and tilmicosin (de Jong et al., 2014). Another large-scale study with *M. haemolytica* isolates from feedlot cattle in Canada also documented low level of resistance (0%—4.5%) among the isolates (Noyes et al., 2015).

The studies conducted after 2011 observed increased occurrence (>35%) of the *M. haemolytica* strains resistant to different antibiotics in the United States. Significant relationship in coresistance patterns was observed against oxytetracycline and tilmicosin in the studied *M. haemolytica* isolates (Lubbers and Hanzlicek, 2013).

β-Lactam resistance

Resistance of *P. multocida* to β-lactam antibiotics is associated with production of β-lactamase, reduced outer membrane permeability and multidrug efflux systems (Kehrenberg et al., 2006). Certain β-lactamase genes such as bla_{TEM-1}, bla_{PSE-1}, bla_{ROB-1}, bla_{CMY-2} and bla_{OXA-2} were detected in *P. multocida* isolated from human (dog bite wound), birds, cattle and pigs (Livrelli et al., 1988; Naas et al., 2001; Wu et al., 2003; Chander et al., 2011; Michael et al., 2012a). The integrative conjugative element (ICE*Pmu1*) of *P. multocida* was detected to harbour ROB-1 gene (Michael et al., 2012a). The small plasmids (4.1 and 5.7 kb in *P. multocida* and 4.1 and 5.2 kb in *M. haemolytica*) were detected to carry most of the β-lactam resistance genes (Livrelli et al., 1988, 1991). The plasmid with >6 kb in size possessed bla_{ROB-1} and additional resistance genes.

Tetracycline resistance

Tetracycline resistance is associated with 'tet' proteins such as *tet(A)*, *tet(B)*, *tet(C)*, *tet(G)*, *tet(H)*, *tet(L)* and *tet(K)*, which help in export of tetracyclines from the bacterial cell. The tetracycline resistance was reported in *P. multocida* and *M. haemolytica* strains isolated from animals since 1970s (Berman and Hirsh, 1978). *Tet(H)* was identified as a major protein associated with tetracycline resistance in *P. multocida* and *M. haemolytica* strains isolated from cattle and pigs (Hansen et al., 1996). The transposon *Tn5706* (pPMT1 plasmid) of cattle originated *P. multocida* was identified to harbour *tet(H)* (Kehrenberg et al., 1998). Two insertion sequences (IS1596 and IS1597) enclose the *tetR-tet(H)* gene region in *Tn5706* (pPMT1). The sulfonamide (*sul2*) and streptomycin (*strA*, *strB*) resistance genes were found to enclose the *tetR-tet(H)* locus in pVM111 plasmid of *P. multocida* (Kehrenberg et al., 2003). One of the smallest plasmid (pMHT1) devoids of IS1596 and IS1597 was also detected to carry *tet(H)* in animal *P. multocida* and *M. haemolytica* isolates (Kehrenberg et al., 2001).

European *P. multocida* and *M. haemolytica* isolates from cattle and pigs possessed *tet(B)* in a nonconjugative transposon *Tn10* as the most widespread tetracycline resistance determinant (Chopra and Roberts, 2001). The integrative conjugative elements (ICE*Pmu1* in *P. multocida* and ICE*Mh1* in *M. haemolytica*) do not harbour *tet(B)* (Michael et al., 2012a; Eidam et al., 2014). The *tet(G)* gene was detected in avian *P. multocida* (pJR1 plasmid) and bovine *M. haemolytica* isolates (Wu et al., 2003). The possibility of *tet(G)* expression induced by tetracycline exposure is low, as the pJR1 plasmid does not possess *tet(R)* in the locus. The chromosomal and plasmidic *tet(L)* was detected in *M. haemolytica* and *P. multocida* strains isolated from cattle (Kehrenberg et al., 2005a). The studied plasmid (pCCK3259) from *M. haemolytica* possessed the elements required for constitutive expression of the *tet(L)* and mobABC operon for transfer of the plasmid. The *tet(M)* (*Tn916*) and *tet(O)* genes encoding ribosomal protective proteins were observed in *P. multocida* isolates with low frequency (Flannagan et al., 1994).

Macrolide resistance

The chromosomal gene *erm(42)* encoding monomethyltransferase (without dimethyltransferase activity) was found to be associated with high macrolide resistance in *M. haemolytica* and *P. multocida* isolates. The *erm(42)* sequence is different from other *erm* sequences described earlier and solely can confer resistance against macrolides, lincosamides and streptogramin group B. The chromosomal sequences present near the *erm(42)* indicated other members of the *Pasteurellaceae* family as a source (Desmolaize et al., 2011).

Mutations in 23S rRNA (A2058G or A2059G) were also correlated with high level of resistance (MICs > 64 mg/L) to macrolides such as erythromycin, tilmicosin, tildipirosin, tulathromycin and gamithromycin in *P. multocida* and *M. haemolytica* strains (Olsen et al., 2014). The macrolide resistance in *P. multocida* and *M. haemolytica* strains is also mediated by macrolide efflux and phosphotransferase proteins (encoded by chromosomal *mrs(E)* and *mph(E)*). In combination with *erm(42)*, the macrolide efflux and phosphotransferase proteins can produce highest level of resistance against tulathromycin, gamithromycin, tilmicosin and clindamycin (Michael et al., 2012b). The three genes (*erm(42)*, *mre(E)*, *mph(E)*) are located in the same integrative conjugative element (ICE*Pmu1*) (Michael et al., 2012a).

Aminoglycoside resistance

The streptomycin resistance in *P. multocida* strains was reported first in 1978 and the strains were isolated from the turkeys (Berman and Hirsh, 1978). The small (less than 15 kb) nonconjugative plasmids possessed the streptomycin resistance gene (*str*) along with *sul2* (sulfonamide resistance), *aphA1* (kanamycin/neomycin resistance), *catA3* (chloramphenicol resistance) and *bla*~ROB-1~ (ampicillin resistance) in *P. multocida* and *M. haemolytica* isolates. The streptomycin resistance genes (*strA* and *strB*) carried by *Tn5393* can encode aminoglycoside phosphotransferase enzymes (Chiou and Jones, 1993). Among the genes (*strA* and *strB*), the *strA* can confer functional resistance against streptomycin (Kehrenberg and Schwarz, 2001). The plasmid (pJR2) from avian *P. multocida* possessed *aadA1* gene encoding aminoglycoside-3-adenyltransferase, which can confer resistance against streptomycin and spectinomycin (aminocyclitol) (Wu et al., 2003). Another novel adenyltransferase (*aadA14*) was identified in bovine *P. multocida* isolates (Kehrenberg et al., 2005b). The integrative conjugative elements (ICE*Pmu1* and ICE*Mh1*) can carry *strA*, *strB*, *aadA1* and *aphA1* along with other resistance genes.

Kanamycin/neomycin resistance in *P. multocida* and *M. haemolytica* isolates is mediated by chromosomal *aphA1*, which encodes aminoglycoside phosphotransferase. The plasmid-mediated *aphA3* was also detected in pCCK411 (5.1 kb) in *P. multocida* strains (Kehrenberg and Schwarz, 2005a).

Mutations in 16SrRNA gene and *rpsE* (encoding ribosomal protein S5) in *P. multocida* isolates were associated with spectinomycin resistance because of prevention of spectinomycin binding with the bacterial ribosome (Kehrenberg and Schwarz, 2007). Recently a novel *aadA31* gene (ICE*Mh1*) encoding spectinomycin/streptomycin adenylyltransferase was detected in *M. haemolytica* strains isolated from pigs with pneumonia (Cameron et al., 2018).

Quinolone resistance

Resistance to quinolones in *P. multocida* is comparatively rare, and mutation in *gyrA* (Asp87Asn, Ala84Pro) and *parC* encoding DNA gyrase and topoisomerase IV, respectively, was found to be associated with quinolone resistance (Michael et al., 2012b; Kong et al., 2014). In *M. haemolytica* isolated from infected cattle, resistance to nalidixic acid was associated with two mutations in *gyrA* and one additional change in *parC* (Katsuda et al., 2009).

Sulphonamide and trimethoprim resistance

Resistance to sulphonamides in *P. multocida* and *M. haemolytica* is associated with type 2 dihydropteroate synthase, encoded by *sul2* gene. The small plasmids (3–15 kbp) and integrative conjugative elements (ICE*Pmu1*) can harbour *sul2* gene (Schwarz, 2008). The *sul2* was often detected with *strA* in *sul2-strA* orientation in *P. multocida* and *M. haemolytica* isolates, which explains the coresistance pattern observed against both of the antibiotics (Kehrenberg and Schwarz, 2001). In a few *P. multocida* and *Mannheimia* isolates, *tetR-tet(H)* (tetracycline resistance) and *catA3* (chloramphenicol resistance) were found to be inserted between *sul2* and *strA* orientation (Kehrenberg et al., 2003).

The trimethoprim resistance determinant (*dfrA20*) was detected in bovine *P. multocida* isolates (Kehrenberg and Schwarz, 2005b). The gene is carried by an 11-kb plasmid (pCCK154) and can encode dihydrofolate reductase responsible for trimethoprim resistance.

Chloramphenicol and florfenicol resistance

The *catA3* and *catB2* (chloramphenicol acetyltransferase) were detected to be associated with chloramphenicol resistance in *P. multocida* and *M. haemolytica* isolates (Yamamoto et al., 1990; Schwarz et al., 2004). The *catA3* was found to be plasmid-associated (5–6 kb) or chromosomal.

Resistance to florfenicol (structural analogue of thiamphenicol) in *P. multocida* and *M. haemolytica* strains isolated from respiratory tract of cattle, pigs, poultry, dogs and cats was not detected in earlier studies conducted throughout the world (Priebe and Schwarz, 2003; Kaspar et al., 2007). Florfenicol resistance in bovine *P. multocida* and *M. haemolytica* isolates became evident during 2005 in the United Kingdom, United States and Canada (Kehrenberg and Schwarz, 2005a, 2005b; Portis et al., 2012). The gene *floR* carried by a 10,874 bp plasmid (pCCK381) was found to be associated with florfenicol resistance. The plasmid pCCK381 was generated by interplasmid recombination between the plasmids of *Dichelobacter nodosus* (pDN1), *E. coli* (pMBSF1) and *Vibrio salmonicida* (pRVS1) (Kehrenberg and Schwarz, 2005a, 2005b). The *floR* was also detected in multiresistance plasmids (pCCK13698, pCCK1900) and integrative conjugative element (ICE*Pmu1*) (Kehrenberg et al., 2008). The *floR* is found as part of 'resistance region 1' in ICE*Pmu1*, enclosed by copies of ISApl1 (Tegetmeyer et al., 2008).

Characteristics of antimicrobial resistance in *P. multocida* and *M. haemolytica* isolates observed in cattle, pigs and poultry are discussed in the following section.

Cattle

M. haemolytica and *P. multocida* isolated from cattle with BRD were found resistant to dihydrostreptomycin, tetracycline, penicillin and chloramphenicol in Michigan (Chang and Carter, 1976). During 1989, *M. haemolytica* and *P. multocida* isolated from cattle in Texas revealed resistance against ceftiofur and tetracycline (Post et al., 1991). However, both of these early reports cannot be used for comparison because of lack of CLSI-approved interpretive criteria used in the studies. The significant resistance to tilmicosin was observed in *M. haemolytica* and *P. multocida* isolated from exclusively cattle lung lesions in the United States and Canada, although the CLSI breakpoints were not developed for tilmicosin during the study period (Watts et al., 1994). Another large study with 842 isolates from the cattle pneumonic lungs over the span of 1994–2002 in Oklahoma reported decline in florfenicol susceptibility in *P. multocida* isolates (Welsh et al., 2004). Low resistance was detected against oxytetracycline and tilmicosin (single isolate) in *M. haemolytica* isolated from nasal swabs of feedlot cattle selected randomly in Canada (Klima et al., 2014). Portis et al. (2012) conducted a study during the period of 2000–09 with samples from BRD and observed slow increase in occurrence of resistance against danofloxacin, enrofloxacin and florfenicol.

Pigs

High resistance to sulphadimethoxine, oxytetracycline, chlortetracycline and florfenicol was observed in *P. multocida* strains isolated from pigs in Korea during 2010–16 probably because of heavy use of antibiotics in pig industry. Antimicrobial susceptibility of all isolates was performed using broth microdilution method (Oh et al., 2018). Similar kind of higher resistance against tetracyclines in swine *P. multocida* isolates was also observed in North America (Sweeney et al., 2017). The resistance with lower frequency against tetracyclines and florfenicol in swine *P. multocida* strains was reported from Europe (El et al., 2016), Australia (Dayao et al., 2014) and Czech Republic (Nedbalcová and Kučerová, 2013).

Poultry

The study with *P. multocida* strains isolated from poultry in India revealed high resistance against sulfadiazine (100%), and <10% isolates showed resistance against chloramphenicol, ciprofloxacin, norfloxacin, enrofloxacin, gentamicin and lincomycin (Shivachandra et al., 2004). The authors did not use CLSI-approved interpretive criteria. In Brazil, avian *P. multocida* isolates also showed highest resistance against sulphaquinoxaline (Furian et al., 2016). In the United States, low resistance (<7%) was observed in avian *P. multocida* isolates against tilmicosin, tetracycline, spectinomycin, gentamicin and ampicillin (Huang et al., 2009).

References

Adhikary, S., Nicklas, W., Bisgaard, M., Boot, R., Kuhnert, P., Waberschek, T., Aalbæk, B., Korczak, B., Christensen, H., 2017. *Rodentibacter* gen. nov. including *Rodentibacter pneumotropicus* comb. nov., *Rodentibacter heylii* sp. nov., *Rodentibacter myodis* sp. nov., *Rodentibacter ratti* sp. nov., *Rodentibacter heidelbergensis* sp. nov., *Rodentibacter trehalosifermentans* sp. nov., *Rodentibacter rarus* sp. nov., *Rodentibacter mrazii* and two genomospecies. International Journal of Systematic and Evolutionary Microbiology 67, 1793–1806.

Annas, S., Zamri-Saad, M., Jesse, F.F.A., Zunita, Z., 2014. New sites of localisation of *Pasteurella multocida* B: 2 in buffalo surviving experimental haemorrhagic septicaemia. BMC Veterinary Research 10 (1), 88.

Bain, R.V.S., Knox, K.W., 1961. *Pasteurella multocida* type I: the antigens of Pasteurella multocida type 1. II. Lipopolysaccharides. Immunology 4 (2), 122.

Berman, S.M., Hirsh, D.C., 1978. Partial characterization of R-plasmids from *Pasteurella multocida* isolated from turkeys. Antimicrobial Agents and Chemotherapy 14 (3), 348–352.

Bi, D., Xu, Z., Harrison, E.M., Tai, C., Wei, Y., He, X., Jia, S., Deng, Z., Rajakumar, K., Ou, H.Y., 2011. ICEberg: a web-based resource for integrative and conjugative elements found in bacteria. Nucleic Acids Research 40 (D1), D621–D626.

Brogden, K.A., Nordholm, G., Ackermann, M., 2007. Antimicrobial activity of cathelicidins BMAP28, SMAP28, SMAP29, and PMAP23 against *Pasteurella multocida* is more broad-spectrum than host species specific. Veterinary Microbiology 119 (1), 76–81.

Brue, C., Chosidow, O., 1994. *Pasteurella multocida* wound infection and cellulitis. International Journal of Dermatology 33 (7), 471–473.

Cameron, A., Klima, C.L., Ha, R., Gruninger, R.J., Zaheer, R., McAllister, T.A., 2018. A novel aadA aminoglycoside resistance gene in bovine and porcine pathogens. mSphere 3 (1) pp.e00568-17.

Carter, G.R., 1955. Studies on *Pasteurella multocida*. I. A hemagglutination test for the identification of serological types. American Journal of Veterinary Research 16 (60), 481–484.

Chander, Y., Oliveira, S., Goyal, S.M., 2011. Characterisation of ceftiofur resistance in swine bacterial pathogens. The Veterinary Journal 187 (1), 139–141.

Chang, W.H., Carter, G.R., 1976. Multiple drug resistance in *Pasteurella multocida* and *Pasteurella haemolytica* from cattle and swine. Journal of the American Veterinary Medical Association 169 (7), 710–712.

Chang, Y.F., Ma, D.P., Bai, H.Q., Young, R., Struck, D.K., Shin, S.J., Lein, D.H., 1992. Characterization of plasmids with antimicrobial resistant genes in *Pasteurella haemolytica* A1. DNA Sequence 3 (2), 89–97.

Chiou, C.S., Jones, A.L., 1993. Nucleotide sequence analysis of a transposon (*Tn5393*) carrying streptomycin resistance genes in *Erwinia amylovora* and other gram-negative bacteria. Journal of Bacteriology 175 (3), 732–740.

Chopra, I., Roberts, M., 2001. Tetracycline antibiotics: mode of action, applications, molecular biology, and epidemiology of bacterial resistance. Microbiology and Molecular Biology Reviews 65 (2), 232–260.

Costanzo II, J.T., Wojciechowski, A.L., Bajwa, R.P., 2017. Urinary tract infection with *Pasteurella multocida* in a patient with cat exposure and abnormal urinary tract physiology: case report and literature review. IDCases 9, 109–111.

Crouch, C.F., LaFleur, R., Ramage, C., Reddick, D., Murray, J., Donachie, W., Francis, M.J., 2012. Cross protection of a *Mannheimia haemolytica* A1 Lkt-/*Pasteurella multocida* ΔhyaE bovine respiratory disease vaccine against experimental challenge with *Mannheimia haemolytica* A6 in calves. Vaccine 30 (13), 2320–2328.

Dayao, D.A.E., Gibson, J.S., Blackall, P.J., Turni, C., 2014. Antimicrobial resistance in bacteria associated with porcine respiratory disease in Australia. Veterinary Microbiology 171 (1–2), 232–235.

de Jong, A., Thomas, V., Simjee, S., Moyaert, H., El Garch, F., Maher, K., Morrissey, I., Butty, P., Klein, U., Marion, H., Rigaut, D., 2014. Antimicrobial susceptibility monitoring of respiratory tract pathogens isolated from diseased cattle and pigs across Europe: the VetPath study. Veterinary Microbiology 172 (1–2), 202–215.

Desmolaize, B., Rose, S., Warrass, R., Douthwaite, S., 2011. A novel *Erm* monomethyltransferase in antibiotic-resistant isolates of *Mannheimia haemolytica* and *Pasteurella multocida*. Molecular Microbiology 80 (1), 184–194.

Du, H., Fang, R., Pan, T., Li, T., Li, N., He, Q., Wu, R., Peng, Y., Zhou, Z., 2016. Comparative genomics analysis of two different virulent bovine *Pasteurella multocida* isolates. International Journal of Genomics. Article ID 4512493. https://doi.org/10.1155/2016/4512493.

Eidam, C., Poehlein, A., Leimbach, A., Michael, G.B., Kadlec, K., Liesegang, H., Daniel, R., Sweeney, M.T., Murray, R.W., Watts, J.L., Schwarz, S., 2014. Analysis and comparative genomics of ICEMh1, a novel integrative and conjugative element (ICE) of *Mannheimia haemolytica*. Journal of Antimicrobial Chemotherapy 70 (1), 93–97.

El, F.G., Simjee, S., Moyaert, H., Klein, U., Ludwig, C., Marion, H., Haag-Diergarten, S., Richard-Mazet, A., Thomas, V., Siegwart, E., 2016. Monitoring of antimicrobial susceptibility of respiratory tract pathogens isolated from diseased cattle and pigs across Europe, 2009-2012: VetPath results. Veterinary Microbiology 194, 11–22.

Flannagan, S.E., Zitzow, L.A., Su, Y.A., Clewell, D.B., 1994. Nucleotide sequence of the 18-kb conjugative transposon Tn916 from *Enterococcus faecalis*. Plasmid 32 (3), 350–354.

Fleischmann, R.D., Adams, M.D., White, O., Clayton, R.A., Kirkness, E.F., Kerlavage, A.R., Bult, C.J., Tomb, J.F., Dougherty, B.A., Merrick, J.M., 1995. Whole-genome random sequencing and assembly of *Haemophilus influenzae* Rd. Science 269 (5223), 496–512.

Forestier, C., Welch, R.A., 1991. Identification of RTX toxin target cell specificity domains by use of hybrid genes. Infection and Immunity 59 (11), 4212–4220.

Frank, G.H., 1988. When *Pasteurella haemolytica* colonizes the nasal passages of cattle. Veterinary Medicine 83, 1000–1064.

Frank, G.H., Briggs, R.E., Zehr, E.S., 1995. Colonization of the tonsils and nasopharynx of calves by a rifampicin-resistant *Pasteurella haemolytica* and its inhibition by vaccination. American Journal of Veterinary Research 56 (7), 866–869.

Furian, T.Q., Borges, K.A., Laviniki, V., Rocha, S.L.D.S., Almeida, C.N.D., Nascimento, V.P.D., Salle, C.T.P., Moraes, H.L.D.S., 2016. Virulence genes and antimicrobial resistance of *Pasteurella multocida* isolated from poultry and swine. Brazilian Journal of Microbiology 47 (1), 210–216.

Hansen, L.M., Blanchard, P.C., Hirsh, D.C., 1996. Distribution of *tet (H)* among *Pasteurella* isolates from the United States and Canada. Antimicrobial Agents and Chemotherapy 40 (6), 1558–1560.

Harper, M., Boyce, J.D., Adler, B., 2006. *Pasteurella multocida* pathogenesis: 125 years after Pasteur. FEMS Microbiology Letters 265 (1), 1–10.

Heddleston, K.L., Gallagher, J.E., Rebers, P.A., 1972. Fowl cholera: gel diffusion precipitin test for serotyping *Pasteurella multocida* from avian species. Avian Diseases 925–936.

Highlander, S.K., Fedorova, N.D., Dusek, D.M., Panciera, R., Alvarez, L.E., Rinehart, C., 2000. Inactivation of *Pasteurella (Mannheimia) haemolytica* leukotoxin causes partial attenuation of virulence in a calf challenge model. Infection and Immunity 68 (7), 3916–3922.

Hildebrand, D., Heeg, K., Kubatzky, K.F., 2015. *Pasteurella multocida* toxin manipulates T cell differentiation. Frontiers in Microbiology 6, 1273.

Hillery, S., Reiss-Levy, E.A., Browne, C., Au, T., Lemmon, J., 1993. *Pasteurella multocida* meningitis in a two-day old neonate. Scandinavian Journal of Infectious Diseases 25 (5), 655–658.

Huang, T.M., Lin, T.L., Wu, C.C., 2009. Antimicrobial susceptibility and resistance of chicken *Escherichia coli*, *Salmonella* spp., and *Pasteurella multocida* isolates. Avian Diseases 53 (1), 89–93.

International Committee on Sytematics of Prokaryotes, 2017. Available at: http://www.the-icsp.org/taxa-covered-family-pasteurellaceae.

Jeyaseelan, S., Hsuan, S.L., Kannan, M.S., Walcheck, B., Wang, J.F., Kehrli, M.E., Lally, E.T., Sieck, G.C., Maheswaran, S.K., 2000. Lymphocyte function-associated antigen 1 is a receptor for *Pasteurella haemolytica* leukotoxin in bovine leukocytes. Infection and Immunity 68 (1), 72–79.

Jones, D.M., O'connor, P.M., 1962. *Pasteurella haemolytica* var. *ureae* from human sputum. Journal of Clinical Pathology 15 (3), 247–248.

Jones, F.A., 1921. A study of *Bacillus bovisepticus*. Journal of Experimental Medicine 34, 561–577.

Kaspar, H., Schröer, U., Wallmann, J., 2007. Quantitative resistance level (MIC) of Pasteurella multocida isolated from pigs between 2004 and 2006: national resistance monitoring by the BVL. *Berliner und Munchener tierarztliche Wochenschrift* 120 (9-10), 442–451.

Kasten, R.W., Carpenter, T.E., Snipes, K.P., Hirsh, D.C., 1997. Detection of *Pasteurella multocida*-specific DNA in Turkey flocks by use of the polymerase chain reaction. Avian Diseases 676–682.

Katsuda, K., Kohmoto, M., Mikami, O., Uchida, I., 2009. Antimicrobial resistance and genetic characterization of fluoroquinolone-resistant *Mannheimia haemolytica* isolates from cattle with bovine pneumonia. Veterinary Microbiology 139 (1–2), 74–79.

Kehrenberg, C., Schwarz, S., 2001. Occurrence and linkage of genes coding for resistance to sulfonamides, streptomycin and chloramphenicol in bacteria of the genera *Pasteurella* and *Mannheimia*. FEMS Microbiology Letters 205 (2), 283–290.

Kehrenberg, C., Schwarz, S., 2005a. Molecular basis of resistance to kanamycin and neomycin in *Pasteurella* and *Mannheimia* isolates of animal origin. In: ASM Conference on Pasteurellaceae, p. 55.

Kehrenberg, C., Schwarz, S., 2005b. *dfrA20*, a novel trimethoprim resistance gene from *Pasteurella multocida*. Antimicrobial Agents and Chemotherapy 49 (1), 414–417.

Kehrenberg, C., Schwarz, S., 2007. Mutations in 16S rRNA and ribosomal protein S5 associated with high-level spectinomycin resistance in *Pasteurella multocida*. Antimicrobial Agents and Chemotherapy 51 (6), 2244–2246.

Kehrenberg, C., Werckenthin, C., Schwarz, S., 1998. *Tn5706*, a transposon-like element from *Pasteurella multocida* mediating tetracycline resistance. Antimicrobial Agents and Chemotherapy 42 (8), 2116–2118.

Kehrenberg, C., Salmon, S.A., Watts, J.L., Schwarz, S., 2001. Tetracycline resistance genes in isolates of *Pasteurella multocida*, *Mannheimia haemolytica*, *Mannheimia glucosida* and *Mannheimia varigena* from bovine and swine respiratory disease: intergeneric spread of the *tet (H)* plasmid pMHT1. Journal of Antimicrobial Chemotherapy 48 (5), 631–640.

Kehrenberg, C., Tham, N.T.T., Schwarz, S., 2003. New plasmid-borne antibiotic resistance gene cluster in *Pasteurella multocida*. Antimicrobial Agents and Chemotherapy 47 (9), 2978–2980.

Kehrenberg, C., Catry, B., Haesebrouck, F., De Kruif, A., Schwarz, S., 2005a. *Tet (L)*-mediated tetracycline resistance in bovine *Mannheimia* and *Pasteurella* isolates. Journal of Antimicrobial Chemotherapy 56 (2), 403–406.

Kehrenberg, C., Catry, B., Haesebrouck, F., de Kruif, A., Schwarz, S., 2005b. Novel spectinomycin/streptomycin resistance gene, *aadA14*, from *Pasteurella multocida*. Antimicrobial Agents and Chemotherapy 49 (7), 3046–3049.

Kehrenberg, C., Walker, R.D., Wu, C.C., 2006. Antimicrobial resistance in members of the family *Pasteurellaceae*. In: Antimicrobial Resistance in Bacteria of Animal Origin. American Society of Microbiology, pp. 167–186.

Kehrenberg, C., Wallmann, J., Schwarz, S., 2008. Molecular analysis of florfenicol-resistant *Pasteurella multocida* isolates in Germany. Journal of Antimicrobial Chemotherapy 62 (5), 951–955.

Kitt, T., 1885. Uber eine experimentelle, der Rinderseuche ahnliche Infektionskranheit. Sitzunbsber. Ges. Morphol. Physiol. Muenchen 140–168.

Klima, C.L., Alexander, T.W., Hendrick, S., McAllister, T.A., 2014. Characterization of *Mannheimia haemolytica* isolated from feedlot cattle that were healthy or treated for bovine respiratory disease. Canadian Journal of Veterinary Research 78 (1), 38–45.

Kong, L.C., Gao, D., Gao, Y.H., Liu, S.M., 2014. Fluoroquinolone resistance mechanism of clinical isolates and selected mutants of *Pasteurella multocida* from bovine respiratory disease in China. Journal of Veterinary Medical Science 76 (12), 1655–1657.

Lariviere, S., Leblanc, L., Mittal, K.R., Martineau, G.P., 1993. Comparison of isolation methods for the recovery of *Bordetella bronchiseptica* and *Pasteurella multocida* from the nasal cavities of piglets. Journal of Clinical Microbiology 31 (2), 364–367.

Lawrence, P.K., Kittichotirat, W., McDermott, J.E., Bumgarner, R.E., 2010. A three-way comparative genomic analysis of *Mannheimia haemolytica* isolates. BMC Genomics 11 (1), 535.

Lee, C.W., Wilkie, I.W., Townsend, K.M., Frost, A.J., 2000. The demonstration of *Pasteurella multocida* in the alimentary tract of chickens after experimental oral infection. Veterinary Microbiology 72 (1–2), 47–55.

Lignieres, J., 1900. Bull. soc. cent. med. vet. quoted from medical research council 1929. System of Bacteriology 4, 446.

Livrelli, V., Peduzzi, J., Joly, B., 1991. Sequence and molecular characterization of the ROB-1 beta-lactamase gene from *Pasteurella haemolytica*. Antimicrobial Agents and Chemotherapy 35 (2), 242–251.

Livrelli, V.O., Darfeuille-Richaud, A., Rich, C.D., Joly, B.H., Martel, J.L., 1988. Genetic determinant of the ROB-1 beta-lactamase in bovine and porcine *Pasteurella* strains. Antimicrobial Agents and Chemotherapy 32 (8), 1282–1284.

Lubbers, B.V., Hanzlicek, G.A., 2013. Antimicrobial multidrug resistance and coresistance patterns of *Mannheimia haemolytica* isolated from bovine respiratory disease cases-a three-year (2009–2011) retrospective analysis. Journal of Veterinary Diagnostic Investigation 25 (3), 413–417.

Martineau-Doize, B., Caya, I., Gagne, S., Jutras, I., Dumas, G., 1993. Effects of *Pasteurella multocida* toxin on the osteoclast population of the rat. Journal of Comparative Pathology 108 (1), 81–91.

May, B.J., Zhang, Q., Li, L.L., Paustian, M.L., Whittam, T.S., Kapur, V., 2001. Complete genomic sequence of *Pasteurella multocida*, Pm70. Proceedings of the National Academy of Sciences 98 (6), 3460–3465.

Michael, G.B., Kadlec, K., Sweeney, M.T., Brzuszkiewicz, E., Liesegang, H., Daniel, R., Murray, R.W., Watts, J.L., Schwarz, S., 2012a. *ICEPmu1*, an integrative conjugative element (ICE) of *Pasteurella multocida*: analysis of the regions that comprise 12 antimicrobial resistance genes. Journal of Antimicrobial Chemotherapy 67, 84–90.

Michael, G.B., Eidam, C., Kadlec, K., Meyer, K., Sweeney, M.T., Murray, R.W., Watts, J.L., Schwarz, S., 2012b. Increased MICs of gamithromycin and tildipirosin in the presence of the genes *erm(42)* and *msr(E)-mph(E)* for bovine *Pasteurella multocida* and *Mannheimia haemolytica*. Journal of Antimicrobial Chemotherapy 67 (6), 1555–1557.

Mutters, R., Ihm, P., Pohl, S., Frederiksen, W., Mannheim, W., 1985. Reclassification of the genus *Pasteurella* Trevisan 1887 on the basis of deoxyribonucleic acid homology, with proposals for the new species *Pasteurella dagmatis, Pasteurella canis, Pasteurella stomatis, Pasteurella anatis*, and *Pasteurella langaa*. International Journal of Systematic and Evolutionary Microbiology 35 (3), 309–322.

Naas, T., Benaoudia, F., Lebrun, L., Nordmann, P., 2001. Molecular identification of TEM-1 β-lactamase in a *Pasteurella multocida* isolate of human origin. European Journal of Clinical Microbiology and Infectious Diseases 20 (3), 210–213.

Namioka, S., Murata, M., 1961. Serological studies on *Pasteurella multocida*. I. A simplified method for capsule typing of the organism. Cornell Veterinarian 51, 498–507.

Nedbalcová, K., Kučerová, Z., 2013. Antimicrobial susceptibility of *Pasteurella multocida* and *Haemophilus parasuis* isolates associated with porcine pneumonia. Acta Veterinaria Brno 82 (1), 3–7.

Newsom, I.E., Cross, F., 1932. Some bipolar organisms found in pneumonia in sheep. Journal of the American Veterinary Medical Association 80, 711–719.

Noyes, N.R., Benedict, K.M., Gow, S.P., Booker, C.W., Hannon, S.J., McAllister, T.A., Morley, P.S., 2015. *Mannheimia haemolytica* in feedlot cattle: prevalence of recovery and associations with antimicrobial use, resistance, and health outcomes. Journal of Veterinary Internal Medicine 29 (2), 705–713.

Nyarko, K.A., Coomber, B.L., Mellors, A., Gentry, P.A., 1998. Bovine platelet adhesion is enhanced by leukotoxin and sialoglycoprotease isolated from *Pasteurella haemolytica* A1 cultures. Veterinary Microbiology 61 (1–2), 81–91.

Oh, Y.H., Moon, D.C., Lee, Y.J., Hyun, B.H., Lim, S.K., 2018. Antimicrobial resistance of *Pasteurella multocida* strains isolated from pigs between 2010 and 2016. Veterinary Record Open 5 (1), e000293.

Olsen, A.S., Warrass, R., Douthwaite, S., 2014. Macrolide resistance conferred by rRNA mutations in field isolates of *Mannheimia haemolytica* and *Pasteurella multocida*. Journal of Antimicrobial Chemotherapy 70 (2), 420–423.

Oppermann, T., Busse, N., Czermak, P., 2017. *Mannheimia haemolytica* growth and leukotoxin production for vaccine manufacturing-a bioprocess review. Electronic Journal of Biotechnology 28, 95–100.

Orsini, J., Perez, R., Llosa, A., Araguez, N., 2013. Non-zoonotic *Pasteurella multocida* infection as a cause of septic shock in a patient with liver cirrhosis: a case report and review of the literature. Journal of Global Infectious Diseases 5 (4), 176.

Priebe, S., Schwarz, S., 2003. In vitro activities of florfenicol against bovine and porcine respiratory tract pathogens. Antimicrobial Agents and Chemotherapy 47 (8), 2703–2705.

Portis, E., Lindeman, C., Johansen, L., Stoltman, G., 2012. A ten-year (2000–2009) study of antimicrobial susceptibility of bacteria that cause bovine respiratory disease complex-*Mannheimia haemolytica, Pasteurella multocida*, and *Histophilus somni*-in the United States and Canada. Journal of Veterinary Diagnostic Investigation 24 (5), 932–944.

Post, K.W., Cole, N.A., Raleigh, R.H., 1991. In vitro antimicrobial susceptibility of *Pasteurella haemolytica* and *Pasteurella multocida* recovered from cattle with bovine respiratory disease complex. Journal of Veterinary Diagnostic Investigation 3 (2), 124–126.

Radostits, O.M., Gay, C.C., Hinchcliff, K.W., Constable, P.D. (Eds.), 2006. Veterinary Medicine E-Book: A Textbook of the Diseases of Cattle, Horses, Sheep, Pigs and Goats. Elsevier Health Sciences.

Rimler, R.B., Rhoades, K.R., 1989. Pasteurella multocida. In: Adlam, C., Rutter, J.M. (Eds.), *Pasteurella* and Pasteurellosis. Academic Press, London, pp. 95–113.

Roberts, R.S., 1947. An immunological study of *Pasteurella septica*. Journal of Comparative Pathology and Therapeutics 57, 261–278.

Rosenbuch, C.T., Merchant, I.A., 1939. Journal of Bacteriology 37, 69.

Rowe, G.E., Pellett, S., Welch, R.A., 1994. Analysis of toxinogenic functions associated with the RTX repeat region and monoclonal antibody D12 epitope of *Escherichia coli* hemolysin. Infection and Immunity 62 (2), 579–588.

Santos-Lopez, A., Bernabe-Balas, C., Ares-Arroyo, M., Ortega-Huedo, R., Hoefer, A., San Millan, A., Gonzalez-Zorn, B., 2017. A Naturally occurring single nucleotide polymorphism in a multicopy plasmid produces a reversible increase in antibiotic resistance. Antimicrobial Agents and Chemotherapy 61 (2) e01735-16.

Schwarz, S., 2008. Mechanisms of Antimicrobial Resistance in *Pasteurellaceae*. Caister Academic Press, Norfolk, UK, pp. 199–228.

Schwarz, S., Alesík, E., Grobbel, M., Lübke-Becker, A., Werckenthin, C., Wieler, L.H., Wallmann, J., 2007. Antimicrobial susceptibility of *Pasteurella multocida* and *Bordetella bronchiseptica* from dogs and cats as determined in the BfT-GermVet monitoring program 2004-2006. Berliner und Münchener Tierärztliche Wochenschrift 120 (9–10), 423–430.

Schwarz, S., Kehrenberg, C., Doublet, B., Cloeckaert, A., 2004. Molecular basis of bacterial resistance to chloramphenicol and florfenicol. FEMS Microbiology Reviews 28 (5), 519–542.

Shivachandra, S.B., Kumar, A.A., Biswas, A., Ramakrishnan, M.A., Singh, V.P., Srivastava, S.K., 2004. Antibiotic sensitivity patterns among Indian strains of avian *Pasteurella multocida*. Tropical Animal Health and Production 36 (8), 743–750.

Singh, K., Ritchey, J.W., Confer, A.W., 2011. *Mannheimia haemolytica*: bacterial-host interactions in bovine pneumonia. Veterinary Pathology 48 (2), 338–348.

Spadafora, R., Pomero, G., Delogu, A., Gozzoli, L., Gancia, P., 2011. A rare case of neonatal sepsis/meningitis caused by *Pasteurella multocida* complicated with status epilepticus and focal cerebritis. La Pediatria medica e chirurgica: Medical and Surgical Pediatrics 33 (4), 199–202.

Straus, D.C., Purdy, C.W., Loan, R.W., Briggs, R.F., Frank, G.H., 1998. *In vivo* production of neuraminidase by *Pasteurella haemolytica* in market stressed cattle after natural infection. Current Microbiology 37 (4), 240–244.

Sweeney, M.T., Lindeman, C., Johansen, L., Mullins, L., Murray, R., Senn, M.K., Bade, D., Machin, C., Kotarski, S.F., Tiwari, R., Watts, J.L., 2017. Antimicrobial susceptibility of *Actinobacillus pleuropneumoniae, Pasteurella multocida, Streptococcus suis*, and *Bordetella bronchiseptica* isolated from pigs in the United States and Canada, 2011 to 2015. Journal of Swine Health and Production 25 (3), 106–120.

Tegetmeyer, H.E., Jones, S.C., Langford, P.R., Baltes, N., 2008. ISApl1, a novel insertion element of *Actinobacillus pleuropneumoniae*, prevents ApxIV-based serological detection of serotype 7 strain AP76. Veterinary Microbiology 128 (3–4), 342–353.

Townsend, K.M., Frost, A.J., Lee, C.W., Papadimitriou, J.M., Dawkins, H.J., 1998. Development of PCR assays for species-and type-specific identification of *Pasteurella multocida* isolates. Journal of Clinical Microbiology 36 (4), 1096–1100.

Trevisan, V., 1887. Rc. 1st lombardo sci. lett. piso. In: Quoted from Buchanan RE 1952 General Systematic Bacteriology. Williams and Wilkins, Baltimore, p. 94.

Watts, J.L., Yancey, R.J., Salmon, S.A., Case, C.A., 1994. A 4-year survey of antimicrobial susceptibility trends for isolates from cattle with bovine respiratory disease in North America. Journal of Clinical Microbiology 32 (3), 725–731.

Watts, J.L., Sweeney, M.T., 2010. Antimicrobial resistance in bovine respiratory disease pathogens: measures, trends, and impact on efficacy. Veterinary Clinics of North America: Food Animal Practice 26 (1), 79–88.

Welsh, R.D., Dye, L.B., Payton, M.E., Confer, A.W., 2004. Isolation and antimicrobial susceptibilities of bacterial pathogens from bovine pneumonia: 1994-2002. Journal of Veterinary Diagnostic Investigation 16 (5), 426–431.

Williams, E.J., Fischer, D.P., Pfeiffer, D.U., England, G.C., Noakes, D.E., Dobson, H., Sheldon, I.M., 2005. Clinical evaluation of postpartum vaginal mucus reflects uterine bacterial infection and the immune response in cattle. Theriogenology 63 (1), 102–117.

Wilson, B.A., Ho, M., 2013. *Pasteurella multocida*: from zoonosis to cellular microbiology. Clinical Microbiology Reviews 26 (3), 631–655.

Wood, A.R., Lainson, F.A., Wright, F., Baird, G.D., Donachie, W., 1995. A native plasmid of *Pasteurella haemolytica* serotype A1: DNA sequence analysis and investigation of its potential as a vector. Research in Veterinary Science 58 (2), 163–168.

Wu, J.R., Shieh, H.K., Shien, J.H., Gong, S.R., Chang, P.C., 2003. Molecular characterization of plasmids with antimicrobial resistant genes in avian isolates of *Pasteurella multocida*. Avian Diseases 47 (4), 1384–1392.

Yamamoto, J., Sakano, T., Shimizu, M., 1990. Drug resistance and R plasmids in *Pasteurella multocida* isolates from swine. Microbiology and Immunology 34 (9), 715–721.

Zecchinon, L., Fett, T., Desmecht, D., 2005. How *Mannheimia haemolytica* defeats host defence through a kiss of death mechanism. Veterinary Research 36 (2), 133–156.

Chapter 22

Vibrio

Chapter outline

Cholera-like syndrome was depicted in literature since the periods of Hippocrates and Lord Buddha. The first outbreak of cholera was described in India in 1817 (Barua, 1992). Filippo Pacini (1854), an Italian anatomist, observed a Gram-negative bacterium associated with human cholera. Robert Koch (1884) first isolated and confirmed the association of 'comma-shaped bacteria', later designated as *Vibrio cholerae* with the menace in Calcutta (Kolkata), India. In 1959, Sambhu Nath De, Professor of Pathology at Nilratan Sircar Medical College in Kolkata, discovered the exotoxin produced by *V. cholerae* and a simple method (rabbit ligated ileal loop assay) to study the in vitro effect of exotoxins (De, 1959). The global disease burden of human cholera is 1.3−4 million cases per year with 21,000−143,000 deaths (Ali et al., 2015).

The Ganges delta of India and Bangladesh is considered as the worst affected place with cholera, although the infection is widespread throughout the world. The spread of cholera in different continents occurred through six 'waves' ('pandemics') since 1817 (Pollitzer, 1959). The current seventh pandemic (7P) was originated in Indonesia (Sulawesi) in 1961 and spread throughout Asia, Africa and Latin America. The seventh pandemic is mostly caused by O1 serogroup of the El Tor biotype (7PET) with sporadic association of serogroup O139 (Albert, 1994). In 1963, the seventh pandemic reached South Asia and circulated for more than 50 years with intermittent transmission to other continents (Cvjetanovic and Barua, 1972). The pandemic reached Africa (1970) and Latin America (1991) causing major outbreaks in Peru and other countries. Within 1997, the pandemic in Latin America caused 1.2 million cases and 12,000 deaths (Kumate et al., 1998). Recent study indicated that Latin American *V. cholerae* isolates belonged to 7PET lineage circulating globally (Domman et al., 2017). China also experienced the seventh pandemic in 1980s and 1990s which were brought from Indonesia through the Chinese people living in the country (Liang et al., 2013). The most recent major seventh pandemic outbreak was detected in Haiti causing more than 9400 deaths in 2010 which was originated through patients from endemic countries (Katz et al., 2013; Pan American Health Organization, 2017). During 2008−10, two minor cholera outbreaks were detected in Hainan, Anhui and Jiangsu provinces of China (Mutreja et al., 2011). Recent analysis of *V. cholerae* strains isolated from China confirmed their position in clade 3.B in wave 3, which might be transmitted into China from South Asia (Pang et al., 2016).

Properties

Morphology: *V. cholerae* is a Gram-negative, curved bacillus, measuring 2−3 μm by 0.5 μm with a single polar flagellum and it shows a typical darting motility under dark-field or phase contrast microscopy.

Classification: *V. cholerae* belongs to the order Vibrionales and family Vibrionaceae.

Antimicrobial Resistance in Agriculture. https://doi.org/10.1016/B978-0-12-815770-1.00022-5

Susceptibility to disinfectants: *V. cholerae* is susceptible to common disinfectants such as 1% chlorine, 2% tincture of iodine and potassium aluminium sulphate (Clark, 1956).

Natural habitat: *V. cholerae* is common in aquatic environment (estuaries and brackish waters) as either free-living cells or associated with plants, green algae, copepods (crustaceans) and chironomids (nonbiting midges) (Huq et al., 1983). The copepods (crustaceans) and chironomids are considered as natural reservoir of *V. cholerae*, which are consumed by fishes and water birds present in the aquatic ecosystem (Halpern and Senderovich, 2015). A strong association between chitinous surface (copepods) and *V. cholerae* is observed. The major pathogenicity island of *V. cholerae* (*Vibrio* pathogenicity island 1, VPI-1/TCP) and type VI secretion system (T6SS) is induced by chitin, required for establishment of bacterial colony on the chitinous surface (Ho et al., 2014). *V. cholerae* O1 were isolated from the fishes such as sardines (*Stolephorus* sp.), mullet (*Liza* sp.), zebrafish (*Danio rerio*) and *Tilapia* sp. Non-O1/O139 *V. cholerae* were detected in lorna fish (*Sciaena deliciosa*), common St. Peter's fish (*Tilapia* sp. and *Tilapia zillii*), Josephus cichlid (*Astatotilapia flaviijosephi*), common carp (*Cyprinus carpio*), sea catfish (*Arius felis*), pinfish (*Lagodon rhomboides*), goldfish (*Carassius auratus*), guppy fish (*Poecilia reticulate*) and common nase (*Chondrostoma nasus*) (Halpern and Izhaki, 2017). Both healthy and diseased fishes were detected to possess *V. cholerae* in the intestines, gills, skin, kidney, liver and brain tissue. *V. cholerae* present in the fish gut secrete enzymes such as proteases and chitinases which help in digestion of chitinous zooplanktons (Senderovich et al., 2010).

In aquatic environment, occasionally due to deprivation of nutrients, *V. cholerae* is converted into quiescent cells which are reverted back to infectious form in favourable conditions (Reidl and Klose, 2002). Most of the environmental strains of *V. cholerae* are nontoxigenic, which can acquire the toxin genes in human gut. Sometimes environmental strains of *V. cholerae* are transduced with cholera toxin-encoding phage (CTXP) (Faruque et al., 1998). *V. cholerae* can also colonize yeast, amoeba, flies and mice other than human (Blow et al., 2005; Abd et al., 2007; Bankapalli et al., 2017).

In the life cycle of *V. cholerae*, both 'planktonic' and 'biofilm' forms are observed with different transcription profiles. Downregulation of motility gene expression and induction of genes associated with biofilm extracellular matrix can convert the planktonic cells into biofilm (Moorthy and Watnick, 2005). The conversion is controlled by intracellular concentration of secondary messenger cyclic diguanylic acid (Tischler and Camilli, 2004). The biofilm stage of *V. cholerae* was detected to express quorum-sensing regulator (HapR), stationary phase sigma factor (RpoS), *V. cholerae* exopolysaccharide matrix (vpsU, vpsA-K, vpsL-Q), adherence factor (Bap1), envelope protein (RbmC) and extracellular DNA (eDNA, providing stability of biofilm and act as source of phosphate) (Silva and Benitez, 2016). *V. cholerae* biofilm production is negatively regulated by quorum sensing through the regulators AphA and HapR. The AphA increases the expression of the biofilm activator VpsT in low bacterial cell density, and in high cell density HapR reduces biofilm formation by lowering intracellular c-di-GMP concentration and suppression of VpsT (Waters et al., 2008). Moreover, termination of motility enhances the expression of toxin and virulence factors (ctxA, tcpA) of *V. cholerae* required for establishment of infection (Wang et al., 2013).

Genome

V. cholerae is studied as a model bacterium in the field of bacterial study with multiple chromosomes. The two chromosomes comprising the *V. cholerae* genome are designated as chromosome 1 (Chr1, 3 Mb) and chromosome 2 (Chr2, 1 Mb) (Heidelberg et al., 2000). Acquisition of a large plasmid during ancient times was the origin of the *V. cholerae* chromosome 2. The similarities were detected between origin of replication in Chr2 (*ori2*) and iteron-like plasmids. The initiator protein (RctB) controls the Chr2 replication in a concentration-dependent manner (Jha et al., 2012). The RctB is conserved in the family *Vibrionaceae* but has no similarity with other regulatory proteins (Egan and Waldor, 2003). The origin of replication present in Chr1 (*ori1*) acts like other bacterial chromosome. The *ori1* contains DnaA boxes and GATC sites, which act as major replication initiator (Koch et al., 2010). Division of the genome into two replicons helps in faster replication of the bacteria. *V. cholerae* shows doubling times of 17 min, which is 5 min less than *E. coli* doubling time (Soler-Bistué et al., 2015). The Chr2 has more plasticity and evolves faster than Chr1. The Chr1 possesses the genes for growth and viability, DNA replication and repair, transcription, translation, cell wall biosynthesis and different metabolic pathways. The Chr2 harbours the genes encoding ribosomal proteins (L35, L20), initiation factor (IF3), D-serine dehydratase and threonyl-tRNA synthetase (Heidelberg et al., 2000).

Transfer of antibiotic resistance determinants in *V. cholerae* is facilitated with mobile genetic elements. *V. cholerae* integrons can incorporate antibiotic resistance cassettes by site-specific recombination in a site proximal to the promoter that controls their expression. Class 1 and class 2 integrons associated with *Tn402* and *Tn21* transposons, respectively, were detected in *V. cholerae*. The integrons carried antibiotic resistance genes such as *dfrA1*, which offered trimethoprim resistance (Opintan et al., 2008). Transfer of integrons is induced by exposure to antibiotics and related stress

(Beaber et al., 2004). One of the largest integron, known as 'superintegron' or '*Vibrio cholerae* repeats', is observed in Chr2. It is 126 kbp in size, contains 179 cassettes and is considered as the most variable region of the genome (Mazel et al., 1998). It contains several genes, function of which is mostly unknown. Few genes have significant similarity with antibiotic resistance genes such as *qnr* conferring resistance to quinolone (Kim et al., 2010). The integrating conjugative element (ICE) such as SXT (100 kb) was detected in *V. cholerae*, which offered resistance for sulfamethoxazole/trimethoprim, streptomycin and chloramphenicol (Burrus et al., 2006a, 2006b). The SXT was first detected in a *V. cholerae* O139 strain isolated from India and currently it is common in clinical and environmental isolates of *V. cholerae* in Asia and Africa (Waldor et al., 1996; Amita et al., 2003). The variant of SXT (ICEVchMex1) was first described in Mexico and it is found prevalent in Western world. The SXT element can integrate with *prfC*, a *V. cholerae* chromosomal gene which encodes peptide chain release factor (Hochhut and Waldor, 1999). After integration the SXT element can replicate along with the chromosome. During bacterial conjugation, the SXT element encodes the conjugation apparatus which facilitates transfer of SXT elements along with SXT-encoded antibiotic resistance genes into competent bacteria (Burrus et al., 2006). The exposure to antibiotics (ciprofloxacin) and associated stress acts as inducing factor for activating SXT-encoded repressor SetR, which can encourage conjugation of the SXT elements (Beaber et al., 2004). Other than integrons and ICEs, the plasmids belonged to incompatibility groups IncC and IncJ were detected in *V. cholerae* decades ago (Rahal et al., 1978). *V. cholerae* O139 isolated from India possessed 200 kb plasmid, which produced multidrug resistance to tetracycline, ampicillin, chloramphenicol, kanamycin, gentamicin, sulfamethoxazole and trimethoprim (Yamamoto et al., 1995).

Besides mobile genetic elements, the transformation acts as major way of gene transfer in *V. cholerae*. Other than chitin-induced T6SS, *V. cholerae* also uses contact-dependent killing for neighbouring bacteria and uptake their DNA by natural transformation. The transformation not only causes horizontal gene transfer but also repair of DNA and use of such DNA as food or building blocks (Redfield, 2001). Competence for DNA uptake in *V. cholerae* depends on presence of the polymer chitin and its nonmonomeric degradation products and species-specific auto-inducer molecules (Meibom et al., 2005). The biotic surface rich in chitin such as exoskeleton of copepods thus acts as a preferred bacterial niche for genetic exchange.

Antigenic characteristics

Based on O-antigen, more than 200 serovars is described in *V. cholerae*. All the cholera pandemics occurred so far are attributed to O1 serogroup. It is further classified into three serotypes (Ogawa, Inaba and Hikojima) based on O-antigen and two biotypes, i.e., 'classical' and 'El Tor', based on phenotypical characteristics. The six cholera pandemics (1899−1923) occurred by classical strains, and El Tor strain was associated with current seventh pandemic (Safa et al., 2010). The frequent switch between Ogawa and Inaba strains occurs associated with clinical infections, although no difference in symptoms is observed. In 1992, O139 serovar emerged and replaced El Tor strains as aetiology of cholera in India and Bangladesh (Albert et al., 1993). The strain O139 was originated from El Tor strains by horizontal gene transfer and replacement of serogroup-specific antigen and SXT-encoded resistance genes against sulfamethoxazole, trimethoprim and chloramphenicol (Waldor et al., 1996). In recent times, non-O1/non-O139 *V. cholerae* serogroups also emerged associated with gastroenteritis, wound infections and bacteraemia (Deshayes et al., 2015).

Toxins and virulence factors produced

Toxins: *V. cholerae* after colonization secrete cholera toxin, an AB_5 family ADP-ribosyltransferase, which causes profuse rice watery diarrhoea in the patients. The genes *ctxA* and *ctxB* encode cholera toxin and are carried by a filamentous phage (CTXF) (Waldor et al., 1996).

Virulence factors

Major virulence factor of *V. cholerae* is toxin-coregulated pilus (TCP), a type IV pilus required for adherence and intestinal colonization (proximal part of the small intestine) in mice and humans. The gene encoding TCP is located within *V. cholerae* pathogenicity island (VPI) or TCP island (Karaolis et al., 1998). Resistance nodulation division (RND) efflux system of *V. cholerae* helps in expression of both cholera toxin and TCP (Taylor et al., 2012).

The sheathed polar flagellum driven by sodium-motive force and alternative RNA polymerase subunits (σ54, σ28 and σ54-dependent transcriptional activators FlrA and FlrC) is another virulence factor (Prouty et al., 2001). Clockwise motility of *V. cholerae* depends on both the appendages.

TABLE 22.1 Major virulence factors produced by *Vibrio cholerae*.

Virulence factors	Function
V. cholerae biofilm-matrix cluster (VcBMC), which comprises *Vibrio* polysaccharide (encoded by *vps-1* and *vps-2* gene clusters) and rugosity and biofilm structure modulator A (*rbm*) cluster (*RbmA, Bap1, RbmC*)	Development of biofilm structure
galU and *gale*	UDP-glucose and UDP-galactose synthesis required for biofilm formation
ToxR-regulated porin (OmpU), transcriptional regulators (CadC, HepA), glutathione synthetase (GshB), DNA repair and recombination enzyme (RecO)	Acid tolerance in the intestinal tract
ToxR-regulated porin (OmpU)	Tolerance to bile acids and antimicrobial peptides
N-acetyl-L-cysteine, soluble mucinase (haemagglutinin/protease, Hap)	Mucolytic agent secreted by *V. cholerae* to penetrate mucin-rich barrier to colonize intestinal epithelium
TagA	A metalloprotease which specifically modifies mucin glycoproteins attached to the host cell surface. It helps in colonization during the later stages of movement through the intestinal mucosa
Neuraminidase (NanH)	It is an extracellular enzyme that cleaves two sialic acid groups from the GM1 ganglioside, present on the surface of epithelial cells and thus it unmasks the receptors for cholera toxin
Chitinase	Needed to utilize chitin
Multivalent adhesion molecule 7 (Mam7), GlcNAc-binding protein (GbpA), FrhA	Adhesin

Table 22.1 describes other important virulence factors produced by *V. cholerae*.

Transmission

Ingestion of contaminated water or food is the major way of *V. cholerae* transmission in human. The infection is more prevalent in the countries with restricted safe drinking water and sanitation facilities. Consumption of raw/salted/smoked or undercooked fishes such as Hilsa (*Hilsa ilisha*) and whitebait was found to be associated with cholera outbreaks (Pandit and Hora, 1951; Forssman et al., 2007). High bacterial concentration (10^8 cfu) is required for initiation of infection in the small intestine, as *V. cholerae* are sensitive to acidic pH. In children, aged and the persons using antacids for prolonged period, low concentration (10^4 cfu) of *V. cholerae* can produce the infection. Person to person spread is limited because of requirement of high infective dose to produce the disease.

Infected people shed *V. cholerae* through the faeces which further contaminate aquatic environment. In the waterbodies the bacteria can exist either in a planktonic state or in a biofilm. During the persistence stage in the waterbodies, *V. cholerae* cells become coccoid in shape and metabolically inactive. They are activated and act as seed to generate numerous progeny when they receive signals from active bacterial cells present in the environment or host cells.

Diagnosis

Fresh faeces or rectal swabs (2 swabs/patient) in transport medium are preferred clinical samples for detection of *V. cholerae*. The faecal samples should be collected within 4 days of onset and before beginning of antimicrobial therapy. Cary–Blair transport medium is commonly used because of high pH (8.4). Alkaline peptone water is an alternative transport medium if the culture is to be done within 6 hours. The buffered glycerol saline as transport medium is contraindicated for *V. cholerae*. Piece of sterile cotton or filter paper soaked with suspected stool sample can be collected in a sterile plastic bag (zipper) if transport medium is not available. The collected samples can be preserved at 4°C in refrigerator up to 48 hours. The samples are sent to the laboratory in insulated container or thermo flask with ice pack or dry ice (WHO and CDC, 1999).

Laboratory examinations

Direct examination: The collected faecal suspensions in normal saline can be microscopically examined for the presence of small, curved rods with 'darting motility' under phase contrast or dark-field microscopy. In Gram-stained smear prepared from isolated bacterial colony, *V. cholerae* appears as Gram-negative, small and curved rods.

Isolation of *V. cholerae*: The bacteria can be isolated in special media such as thiosulfate-citrate-bile salts-sucrose agar or taurocholate-tellurite-gelatin agar. Characteristic yellow and shiny colonies, 2–4 mm in diameter, sometimes with an elevated centre, appear after 18–24 hours incubation at 35–37°C. The suspected *V. cholerae* colonies are subcultured into heart infusion agar or tryptone soy agar at 35–37°C for up to 24 h. Gram staining and biochemical tests conducted on subcultured colonies such as oxidase test, string test, growth in triple sugar iron agar/Kligler iron agar/lysine iron agar can confirm the isolates. The string test can differentiate *V. cholerae* from *Aeromonas* (negative in string test) and other *Vibrio* sp. (weakly positive).

Serological tests: The slide agglutination test (SAT) with polyvalent O1 or O139 antiserum is available which can be conducted with fresh subculture (6 hours growth) of *V. cholerae* from a nonselective agar. The regional laboratories may send the cultures to national or international reference laboratory for confirmation of O1/O139 serotype during outbreaks. The culture positive for SAT with polyvalent O1 can be further typed with monovalent Ogawa and Inaba antiserum. If the culture shows positive reaction with both Ogawa and Inaba antisera, it should be sent to reference laboratory for identification of Hikojima serotype.

Molecular biology: Diagnostic polymerase chain reaction is developed for detection of *V. cholerae* DNA targeting the genes encoding cholera toxin (*ctx*), regulatory gene (*toxR*) and housekeeping genes *atpA*, *rpoB* and *dnaJ* (Kim et al., 2015).

Characteristics of antimicrobial resistance

Antibiotics directly do not help to cure cholera but are recommended with oral rehydration therapy to reduce the volume of diarrhoea, faecal shedding of the bacteria and duration of illness. Antimicrobial agents recommended by the WHO for treating cholera patients include tetracycline, doxycycline, furazolidone, trimethoprim/sulfamethoxazole, erythromycin, chloramphenicol, ciprofloxacin and norfloxacin (Perilla et al., 2003). The sporadic occurrence of multiple drug-resistant *V. cholerae* was detected in Philippines during 1964–65 (Kuwahara et al., 1967). However, *V. cholerae* remained pan-susceptible to different groups of antibiotics for a long period up to 1976 (O'grady et al., 1976). During 1980s, increasing trend of resistance in *V. cholerae* was observed in Tanzania and Bangladesh because of overuse of tetracycline (Mhalu et al., 1979; Glass et al., 1980). Resistance of *V. cholerae* against tetracycline and quinolones has restricted their use in severe dehydrated patients (Garg et al., 2001). Substantial death of patients occurred because of spread of resistant strains during cholera epidemic in the Rwandan refugee camps in Goma, Zaire, Africa in 1994 (Uganda, 1995). The resistance spread to several other countries (Table 22.2). The pattern of resistance also changed from trimethoprim/sulfamethoxazole (1980s) to tetracycline and furazolidone (1990s) to quinolones (2000s) in subsequent years.

Quinolone resistance

The chromosomal mutations initially in *gyrA* and later additionally in *parC* encoding DNA gyrase and topoisomerase IV, respectively, are found associated with quinolone resistance in *V. cholerae* (Baranwal et al., 2002). Substitutions of single amino acid (Ser-83; Ile in *gyrA* and Ser-85; Leu in *parC*) were responsible for quinolone resistance in *V. cholerae* isolates (Quilici et al., 2010). Other than chromosomal mutations, *V. cholerae* contain different efflux pumps under two major family, i.e., ATP-binding cassette (ABC) superfamily and proton-motive force (PMF) pump family. The PMF family includes major facilitator superfamily (MFS), multidrug and toxic compound extrusion (MATE) family, small multidrug resistance (SMR) family and the RND superfamily (Putman et al., 2000). The putative genes of MATE family such as *norM, vcrM, vcmB, vcmD, vcmH* and *vcmN27* associated with increased MIC against fluoroquinolones, aminoglycosides and ethidium bromide were detected in *V. cholerae* (Borges-Walmsley et al., 2005; Singh et al., 2006). MFS transporters associated with quinolone resistance were also described in *V. cholerae* (Baranwal et al., 2002). Four operons (VexAB, VexCD, VexGH and VexIJK) associated with RND efflux system were reported not only to produce antimicrobial resistance in *V. cholerae* but also to help in colonization in mice intestine (Bina et al., 2006).

Reduced expression of *vca0421* (encodes a hypothetical protein) in *V. cholerae* O1 was demonstrated to produce resistance to fluoroquinolones (Okuda et al., 2010).

Plasmids associated with multiple drug resistance (IncC, IncJ) were reported from *V. cholerae* in Africa (Finch et al., 1988). A new plasmid-associated intrinsic quinolone resistance gene (*qnrVC3*), homologue to *qnr*, was detected in *V. cholerae* isolates from Brazil and Bangladesh (Fonseca et al., 2008; Kim et al., 2010).

β-Lactam resistance

The extended-spectrum β-lactamase belonged to CTX-M class was detected in *V. cholerae*, which confer resistance against higher generation cephalosporins (cefotaxime) (Walther-Rasmussen and Høiby, 2004). Besides, other β-lactamases belonged to TEM-1 and PER-2 types were also reported in *V. cholerae* (Petroni et al., 2002).

Chloramphenicol and other antibiotic resistance

MFS transporters belonged to PMF pump family were detected in *V. cholerae* associated with chloramphenicol, nalidixic acid and bile salt resistance (Colmer et al., 1998). The MFS efflux protein (EmrD-3) was detected in El Tor strain (N16961) and non-O1/non-O139 strains (V51, V52, TMA 21), which offered resistance against chloramphenicol, linezolid, rifampicin and erythromycin (Smith et al., 2009).

Characteristics of antimicrobial resistance in *V. cholerae* isolates observed in human are discussed in the following section.

The analysis of data about trend of antimicrobial resistance in clinical *V. cholerae* isolates, generated by different surveillance centres in Kolkata (India) and Bangladesh, revealed that the resistance pattern is dependent on use of antibiotics, region and period. Resistance to trimethoprim/sulfamethoxazole and nalidixic acid thus appeared in Kolkata because of their heavy use as drug of choice during the said period (Jesudason and Saaya, 1997). The characteristics of antimicrobial resistance in *V. cholerae* strains reported from different countries are described in Table 22.2.

TABLE 22.2 Characteristics of antimicrobial resistance in *Vibrio cholerae* isolated from different countries.

V. cholerae strain	Antimicrobial resistance	Year	Country
—	Chloramphenicol, doxycycline, kanamycin, streptomycin, sulfonamides, tetracycline	1991	Ecuador
O1 Inaba/Ogawa	Chloramphenicol, co-trimoxazole	1993–2005	Pakistan
—	Sulfamethoxazole/trimethoprim, chloramphenicol, tetracycline, doxycycline, streptomycin	1994	Italy
O1/non-O1	Ampicillin, chloramphenicol, sulfamethoxazole/trimethoprim, tetracycline	1995–2001	Indonesia
O1	Streptomycin	1995	Vietnam
—	Tetracycline, trimethoprim-sulfamethoxazole, kanamycin, gentamicin, chloramphenicol, ampicillin	1997	Honduras
O1 El Tor Ogawa	Furazolidone, co-trimoxazole, amoxicillin, ciprofloxacin	1999–2007	India (Chandigarh)
O1 El Tor Ogawa, O139	Furazolidone	2000	India (Odissa)
—	Co-trimoxazole, streptomycin, tetracycline, ampicillin, chloramphenicol	2000	Madagascar
O1, O139, non-O1/non-O139	Fluoroquinolone	2000–04	India (Karnataka)
O1 El Tor Ogawa/Inaba	Nalidixic acid, co-trimoxazole	2001–06	India (Delhi)
O1 El Tor Ogawa, O139, non-O1/non-O139	Ampicillin, co-trimoxazole, nalidixic acid	2002	India (Karnataka)
O1 El Tor Ogawa	Chloramphenicol, co-trimoxazole, tetracycline	2002–04	Mozambique, Africa
O1	Ciprofloxacin	2002–08	Bangladesh

TABLE 22.2 Characteristics of antimicrobial resistance in *Vibrio cholerae* isolated from different countries.—cont'd

V. cholerae strain	Antimicrobial resistance	Year	Country
O1	Amoxicillin, erythromycin	2003	Vietnam
O139	Ampicillin, streptomycin, gentamicin, tetracycline, chloramphenicol, sulfamethoxazole/trimethoprim	2004	China
–	Sulfamethoxazole/trimethoprim, streptomycin, chloramphenicol	2004–06	Iran
O1 El Tor	Co-trimoxazole	2004–06	Senegal
O1	Sulfamethoxazole/trimethoprim, ampicillin	2004–05	Cameroon
O1 El Tor Inaba	Sulfamethoxazole/trimethoprim, streptomycin	2006–07	Namibia
O1 Inaba	Co-trimoxazole, ampicillin, chloramphenicol	2006–08	Ethiopia
O1 El Tor	Ampicillin, aztreonam, co-trimoxazole, erythromycin, metronidazole, nalidixic acid	2007	India
O1 El Tor Ogawa	Furazolidone, nalidixic acid, co-trimoxazole	2008–09	Nepal
O1 El Tor Ogawa/Inaba	Furazolidone, sulfamethoxazole/trimethoprim	2009	Zimbabwe
Ol El Tor	Ciprofloxacin	2010	India (Puducherry)
O1 El Tor Ogawa	Furazolidone, nalidixic acid, sulfisoxazole, streptomycin, trimethoprim/sulfamethoxazole	2010–11	Haiti
O1 El Tor/non-O1/non-O139	Sulfamethoxazole/trimethoprim, ampicillin ciprofloxacin	2011–14	Ghana
O1 El Tor Ogawa	Tetracycline, sulfamethoxazole/trimethoprim, chloramphenicol, nitrofurantoin	2012–15	Mozambique, Africa

References

Abd, H., Saeed, A., Weintraub, A., Nair, G.B., Sandström, G., 2007. *Vibrio cholerae* O1 strains are facultative intracellular bacteria, able to survive and multiply symbiotically inside the aquatic free-living amoeba *Acanthamoeba castellanii*. FEMS Microbiology Ecology 60 (1), 33–39.

Albert, M.J., 1994. *Vibrio cholerae* O139 Bengal. Journal of Clinical Microbiology 32 (10), 2345.

Albert, M.J., Ansaruzzaman, M., Bardhan, P.K., Faruque, A.S.G., Faruque, S.M., Islam, M.S., Mahalanabis, D., Sack, R.B., Salam, M.A., Siddique, A.K., Yunus, M.D., 1993. Large epidemic of cholera-like disease in Bangladesh caused by *Vibrio cholerae* O139 synonym Bengal. The Lancet 342 (8868), 387–390.

Ali, M., Nelson, A.R., Lopez, A.L., Sack, D.A., 2015. Updated global burden of cholera in endemic countries. PLoS Neglected Tropical Diseases 9 (6), e0003832.

Amita, M., Chowdhury, S.R., Thungapathra, M., Ramamurthy, T., Nair, G.B., Ghosh, A., 2003. Class I integrons and SXT elements in El Tor strains isolated before and after 1992 *Vibrio cholerae* O139 outbreak, Calcutta, India. Emerging Infectious Diseases 9 (4), 500.

Bankapalli, L.K., Mishra, R.C., Raychaudhuri, S., 2017. VopE, a *Vibrio cholerae* type III effector, attenuates the activation of CWI-MAPK pathway in yeast model system. Frontiers in Cellular and Infection Microbiology 7, 82.

Baranwal, S., Dey, K., Ramamurthy, T., Nair, G.B., Kundu, M., 2002. Role of active efflux in association with target gene mutations in fluoroquinolone resistance in clinical isolates of *Vibrio cholerae*. Antimicrobial Agents and Chemotherapy 46 (8), 2676–2678.

Barua, D., 1992. History of cholera. In: Cholera. Springer, Boston, MA, pp. 1–36.

Beaber, J.W., Hochhut, B., Waldor, M.K., 2004. SOS response promotes horizontal dissemination of antibiotic resistance genes. Nature 427 (6969), 72.

Bina, J.E., Provenzano, D., Wang, C., Bina, X.R., Mekalanos, J.J., 2006. Characterization of the *Vibrio cholerae* vexAB and vexCD efflux systems. Archives of Microbiology 186 (3), 171–181.

Blow, N.S., Salomon, R.N., Garrity, K., Reveillaud, I., Kopin, A., Jackson, F.R., Watnick, P.I., 2005. *Vibrio cholerae* infection of *Drosophila melanogaster* mimics the human disease cholera. PLoS Pathogens 1 (1), e8.

Borges-Walmsley, M.I., Du, D., McKeegan, K.S., Sharples, G.J., Walmsley, A.R., 2005. VceR regulates the *vceCAB* drug efflux pump operon of *Vibrio cholerae* by alternating between mutually exclusive conformations that bind either drugs or promoter DNA. Journal of Molecular Biology 349 (2), 387–400.

Burrus, V., Marrero, J., Waldor, M.K., 2006a. The current ICE age: biology and evolution of SXT-related integrating conjugative elements. Plasmid 55 (3), 173–183.

Burrus, V., Quezada-Calvillo, R., Marrero, J., Waldor, M.K., 2006b. SXT-related integrating conjugative element in New World *Vibrio cholerae*. Applied and Environmental Microbiology 72 (4), 3054–3057.

Clark, R.N., 1956. The purification of water on a small scale. Bulletin of the World Health Organization 14 (4), 820.

Colmer, J.A., Fralick, J.A., Hamood, A.N., 1998. Isolation and characterization of a putative multidrug resistance pump from *Vibrio cholerae*. Molecular Microbiology 27 (1), 63–72.

Cvjetanovic, B., Barua, D., 1972. The seventh pandemic of cholera. Nature 239 (5368), 137.

De, S.N., 1959. Enterotoxicity of bacteria-free culture-filtrate of *Vibrio cholerae*. Nature 183 (4674), 1533.

Deshayes, S., Daurel, C., Cattoir, V., Parienti, J.J., Quilici, M.L., de La Blanchardière, A., 2015. Non-O1, non-O139 *Vibrio cholerae* bacteraemia: case report and literature review. SpringerPlus 4 (1), 575.

Domman, D., Quilici, M.L., Dorman, M.J., Njamkepo, E., Mutreja, A., Mather, A.E., Delgado, G., Morales-Espinosa, R., Grimont, P.A., Lizárraga-Partida, M.L., Bouchier, C., 2017. Integrated view of *Vibrio cholerae* in the Americas. Science 358 (6364), 789–793.

Egan, E.S., Waldor, M.K., 2003. Distinct replication requirements for the two *Vibrio cholerae* chromosomes. Cell 114 (4), 521–530.

Faruque, S.M., Albert, M.J., Mekalanos, J.J., 1998. Epidemiology, genetics, and ecology of toxigenic *Vibrio cholerae*. Microbiology and Molecular Biology Reviews 62 (4), 1301–1314.

Finch, M.J., Morris Jr., J.G., Kaviti, J., Kagwanja, W., Levine, M.M., 1988. Epidemiology of antimicrobial resistant cholera in Kenya and east Africa. The American Journal of Tropical Medicine and Hygiene 39 (5), 484–490.

Fonseca, É.L., dos Santos Freitas, F., Vieira, V.V., Vicente, A.C., 2008. New *qnr* gene cassettes associated with superintegron repeats in *Vibrio cholerae* O1. Emerging Infectious Diseases 14 (7), 1129.

Forssman, B., Mannes, T., Musto, J., Gottlieb, T., Robertson, G., Natoli, J.D., Shadbolt, C., Biffin, B., Gupta, L., 2007. *Vibrio cholerae* O1 El Tor cluster in Sydney linked to imported whitebait. Medical Journal of Australia 187 (6), 345.

Garg, P., Sinha, S., Chakraborty, R., Bhattacharya, S.K., Nair, G.B., Ramamurthy, T., Takeda, Y., 2001. Emergence of fluoroquinolone-resistant strains of *Vibrio cholerae* O1 biotype El Tor among hospitalized patients with cholera in Calcutta, India. Antimicrobial Agents and Chemotherapy 45 (5), 1605–1606.

Glass, R.I., Huq, I., Alim, A.R.M.A., Yunus, M., 1980. Emergence of multiply antibiotic-resistant *Vibrio cholerae* in Bangladesh. Journal of Infectious Diseases 142 (6), 939–942.

Halpern, M., Izhaki, I., 2017. Fish as hosts of *Vibrio cholerae*. Frontiers in Microbiology 8, 282.

Halpern, M., Senderovich, Y., 2015. Chironomid microbiome. Microbial Ecology 70 (1), 1–8.

Heidelberg, J.F., Eisen, J.A., Nelson, W.C., Clayton, R.A., Gwinn, M.L., Dodson, R.J., Haft, D.H., Hickey, E.K., Peterson, J.D., Umayam, L., Gill, S.R., 2000. DNA sequence of both chromosomes of the cholera pathogen *Vibrio cholerae*. Nature 406 (6795), 477.

Ho, B.T., Dong, T.G., Mekalanos, J.J., 2014. A view to a kill: the bacterial type VI secretion system. Cell Host & Microbe 15 (1), 9–21.

Hochhut, B., Waldor, M.K., 1999. Site-specific integration of the conjugal *Vibrio cholerae* SXT element into *prfC*. Molecular Microbiology 32 (1), 99–110.

Huq, A., Small, E.B., West, P.A., Huq, M.I., Rahman, R., Colwell, R.R., 1983. Ecological relationships between *Vibrio cholerae* and planktonic crustacean copepods. Applied and Environmental Microbiology 45 (1), 275–283.

Jesudason, M.V., Saaya, R., 1997. Resistance of *Vibrio cholerae* 01 to nalidixic acid. The Indian Journal of Medical Research 105, 153–154.

Jha, J.K., Demarre, G., Venkova-Canova, T., Chattoraj, D.K., 2012. Replication regulation of *Vibrio cholerae* chromosome II involves initiator binding to the origin both as monomer and as dimer. Nucleic Acids Research 40 (13), 6026–6038.

Karaolis, D.K., Johnson, J.A., Bailey, C.C., Boedeker, E.C., Kaper, J.B., Reeves, P.R., 1998. A *Vibrio cholerae* pathogenicity island associated with epidemic and pandemic strains. Proceedings of the National Academy of Sciences 95 (6), 3134–3139.

Katz, L.S., Petkau, A., Beaulaurier, J., Tyler, S., Antonova, E.S., Turnsek, M.A., Guo, Y., Wang, S., Paxinos, E.E., Orata, F., Gladney, L.M., 2013. Evolutionary dynamics of *Vibrio cholerae* O1 following a single-source introduction to Haiti. mBio 4 (4) e00398-13.

Kim, H.B., Wang, M., Ahmed, S., Park, C.H., LaRocque, R.C., Faruque, A.S., Salam, M.A., Khan, W.A., Qadri, F., Calderwood, S.B., Jacoby, G.A., 2010. Transferable quinolone resistance in *Vibrio cholerae*. Antimicrobial Agents and Chemotherapy 54 (2), 799–803.

Kim, H.J., Ryu, J.O., Lee, S.Y., Kim, E.S., Kim, H.Y., 2015. Multiplex PCR for detection of the *Vibrio* genus and five pathogenic *Vibrio* species with primer sets designed using comparative genomics. BMC Microbiology 15 (1), 239.

Koch, B., Ma, X., Løbner-Olesen, A., 2010. Replication of *Vibrio cholerae* chromosome I in *Escherichia coli*: dependence on dam methylation. Journal of Bacteriology 192 (15), 3903–3914.

Koch, R., 1884. An address on cholera and its *bacillus*. British Medical Journal 2 (1236), 453.

Kumate, J., Sepúlveda, J., Gutiérrez, G., 1998. Cholera epidemiology in Latin America and perspectives for eradication. Bulletin de l'Institut Pasteur 96 (4), 217–226.

Kuwahara, S., Goto, S., Kimura, M., Abe, H., 1967. Drug-sensitivity of El tor vibrio strains isolated in the Philippines in 1964 and 1965. Bulletin of the World Health Organization 37 (5), 763.

Liang, W., Wang, L., Liang, P., Zheng, X., Zhou, H., Zhang, J., Zhang, L., Kan, B., 2013. Sequence polymorphisms of rfbT among the *Vibrio cholerae* O1 strains in the Ogawa and Inaba serotype shifts. BMC Microbiology 13 (1), 173.

Mazel, D., Dychinco, B., Webb, V.A., Davies, J., 1998. A distinctive class of integron in the *Vibrio cholerae* genome. Science 280 (5363), 605–608.

Meibom, K.L., Blokesch, M., Dolganov, N.A., Wu, C.Y., Schoolnik, G.K., 2005. Chitin induces natural competence in *Vibrio cholerae*. Science 310 (5755), 1824–1827.

Mhalu, F.S., Mmari, P.W., Ijumba, J., 1979. Rapid emergence of El Tor vibrio cholera resistant to antimicrobial agents during first six months of fourth cholera epidemic in Tanzania. The Lancet 313 (8112), 345–347.

Moorthy, S., Watnick, P.I., 2005. Identification of novel stage-specific genetic requirements through whole genome transcription profiling of *Vibrio cholerae* biofilm development. Molecular Microbiology 57 (6), 1623–1635.

Mutreja, A., Kim, D.W., Thomson, N.R., Connor, T.R., Lee, J.H., Kariuki, S., Croucher, N.J., Choi, S.Y., Harris, S.R., Lebens, M., Niyogi, S.K., 2011. Evidence for several waves of global transmission in the seventh cholera pandemic. Nature 477 (7365), 462.

O'grady, F., Lewis, M.J., Pearson, N.J., 1976. Global surveillance of antibiotic sensitivity of *Vibrio cholerae*. Bulletin of the World Health Organization 54 (2), 181.

Okuda, J., Hayashi, N., Wakahara, Y., Gotoh, N., 2010. Reduced expression of the *vca0421* gene of *Vibrio cholerae* O1 results in innate resistance to ciprofloxacin. Antimicrobial Agents and Chemotherapy 54 (11), 4917–4919.

Opintan, J.A., Newman, M.J., Nsiah-Poodoh, O.A., Okeke, I.N., 2008. *Vibrio cholerae* O1 from Accra, Ghana carrying a class 2 integron and the SXT element. Journal of Antimicrobial Chemotherapy 62 (5), 929–933.

Pacini, F., 1854. *Osservazioni microscopiche e deduzioni patologiche sul cholera asiatico*. tip. di F. Bencini.

Pan American Health Organization/World Health Organization, 2017. Cholera in the Americas – Situation Summary. Available at: www.paho.org/hq/index.php?option=com_docman&task=doc_download&Itemid=270&gid=38251&lang=fr;.

Pandit, C.G., Hora, S.L., 1951. The probable role of the Hilsa fish, *Hilsa ilisha* (Ham) in maintaining cholera endemicity in India. Indian Journal of Medical Sciences 5 (8), 343–356.

Pang, B., Du, P., Zhou, Z., Diao, B., Cui, Z., Zhou, H., Kan, B., 2016. The transmission and antibiotic resistance variation in a multiple drug resistance clade of *Vibrio cholerae* circulating in multiple countries in Asia. PLoS One 11 (3), e0149742.

Perilla, M.J., Bopp, C., Elliott, J., Facklam, R., Popovic, T., Wells, J., World Health Organization, 2003. Manual for the Laboratory Identification and Antimicrobial Susceptibility Testing of Bacterial Pathogens of Public Health Importance in the Developing World: *Haemophilus influenzae*, *Neisseria meningitidis*, *Streptococcus pneumoniae*, *Neisseria gonorrhoea*, *Salmonella* Serotype Typhi, *Shigella*, and *Vibrio cholerae*.

Petroni, A., Corso, A., Melano, R., Cacace, M.L., Bru, A.M., Rossi, A., Galas, M., 2002. Plasmidic extended-spectrum β-lactamases in *Vibrio cholerae* O1 El tor isolates in Argentina. Antimicrobial Agents and Chemotherapy 46 (5), 1462–1468.

Pollitzer, R., 1959. History of the disease. In: WHO Monograph Series No 43. Cholera. WHO, Geneva.

Prouty, M.G., Correa, N.E., Klose, K.E., 2001. The novel σ54-and σ28-dependent flagellar gene transcription hierarchy of *Vibrio cholerae*. Molecular Microbiology 39 (6), 1595–1609.

Putman, M., van Veen, H.W., Konings, W.N., 2000. Molecular properties of bacterial multidrug transporters. Microbiology and Molecular Biology Reviews 64 (4), 672–693.

Quilici, M.L., Massenet, D., Gake, B., Bwalki, B., Olson, D.M., 2010. *Vibrio cholerae* O1 variant with reduced susceptibility to ciprofloxacin, western Africa. Emerging Infectious Diseases 16 (11), 1804.

Rahal, K., Gerbaud, G.R., Bouanchaud, D.H., 1978. Stability of R plasmids belonging to different incompatibility groups in *Vibrio cholerae* "Eltor". In: Annales de microbiologie, vol. 129, pp. 409–414 (4).

Redfield, R.J., 2001. Do bacteria have sex? Nature Reviews Genetics 2 (8), 634.

Reidl, J., Klose, K.E., 2002. *Vibrio cholerae* and cholera: out of the water and into the host. FEMS Microbiology Reviews 26 (2), 125–139.

Safa, A., Nair, G.B., Kong, R.Y., 2010. Evolution of new variants of *Vibrio cholerae* O1. Trends in Microbiology 18 (1), 46–54.

Senderovich, Y., Izhaki, I., Halpern, M., 2010. Fish as reservoirs and vectors of *Vibrio cholerae*. PLoS One 5 (1), e8607.

Silva, A.J., Benitez, J.A., 2016. *Vibrio cholerae* biofilms and cholera pathogenesis. PLoS Neglected Tropical Diseases 10 (2), e0004330.

Singh, A.K., Haldar, R., Mandal, D., Kundu, M., 2006. Analysis of the topology of *Vibrio cholerae* NorM and identification of amino acid residues involved in norfloxacin resistance. Antimicrobial Agents and Chemotherapy 50 (11), 3717–3723.

Smith, K.P., Kumar, S., Varela, M.F., 2009. Identification, cloning, and functional characterization of EmrD-3, a putative multidrug efflux pump of the major facilitator superfamily from *Vibrio cholerae* O395. Archives of Microbiology 191 (12), 903–911.

Soler-Bistué, A., Mondotte, J.A., Bland, M.J., Val, M.E., Saleh, M.C., Mazel, D., 2015. Genomic location of the major ribosomal protein gene locus determines *Vibrio cholerae* global growth and infectivity. PLoS Genetics 11 (4), e1005156.

Taylor, D.L., Bina, X.R., Bina, J.E., 2012. *Vibrio cholerae* VexH encodes a multiple drug efflux pump that contributes to the production of cholera toxin and the toxin co-regulated pilus. PLoS One 7 (5), e38208.

Tischler, A.D., Camilli, A., 2004. Cyclic diguanylate (c-di-GMP) regulates *Vibrio cholerae* biofilm formation. Molecular Microbiology 53 (3), 857–869.

Uganda, K., 1995. Public health impact of Rwandan refugee crisis: what happened in Goma, Zaire, in July, 1994? Lancet 345, 339–344.

Waldor, M.K., Tschäpe, H., Mekalanos, J.J., 1996. A new type of conjugative transposon encodes resistance to sulfamethoxazole, trimethoprim, and streptomycin in *Vibrio cholerae* O139. Journal of Bacteriology 178 (14), 4157–4165.

Walther-Rasmussen, J., Høiby, N., 2004. Cefotaximases (CTX-M-ases), an expanding family of extended-spectrum β-lactamases. Canadian Journal of Microbiology 50 (3), 137–165.

Wang, H., Zhang, L., Silva, A.J., Benitez, J.A., 2013. A quinazoline 2, 4 diamino analog suppresses *Vibrio cholerae* flagellar motility by interacting with the motor protein PomB and induces envelope stress. Antimicrobial Agents and Chemotherapy pp.AAC-00473.

Waters, C.M., Lu, W., Rabinowitz, J.D., Bassler, B.L., 2008. Quorum sensing controls biofilm formation in *Vibrio cholerae* through modulation of cyclic di-GMP levels and repression of vpsT. Journal of Bacteriology 190 (7), 2527–2536.

World Health Organization and Centers for Disease Control and Prevention, 1999. Laboratory Methods for the Diagnosis of Epidemic Dysentery and Cholera. Available at: http://apps.who.int/iris/bitstream/handle/10665/66885/WHO_CDS_CSR_EDC_99.8.pdf;jsessionid=1A54AB90091EFF 600A1D269A5DE81DA9?sequence=1.

Yamamoto, T., Nair, G.B., Takeda, Y., 1995. Emergence of tetracycline resistance due to a multiple drug resistance plasmid in *Vibrio cholerae* O139. FEMS Immunology and Medical Microbiology 11 (2), 131–136.

Chapter 23

Pseudomonas

Chapter outline

Sédillot (1850) first detected that the discolouration of surgical wound dressings was associated with a 'germ' or 'transferrable agent'. Lucke (1862) described that the bluish-green pigmentation of surgical dressing is associated with the presence of small vibrio-like organisms (Pitt, 1998). Carle Gessard (1882) isolated the organism as *Pseudomonas* from cutaneous wounds of two patients with bluish-green pus (Gessard, 1984).

Pseudomonas aeruginosa is considered as the potent member of 'ESKAPE' group of pathogens, prepared by the Infectious Disease Society of America on the basis of increasing clinical occurrence and ineffective antibiotic treatment against the organisms (Boucher et al., 2009). *P. aeruginosa* are opportunistic pathogens and are associated with both acute and chronic eye, urinary and respiratory tract infections in human including otitis externa ('swimmer's ear'), folliculitis associated with skin damage (burn wounds) and high moisture content in the ears of the swimmers (Rice et al., 2012). *P. aeruginosa* also causes nosocomial infection (bloodstream infection) and ventilator-associated pneumonia in hospital settings by formation of biofilm on abiotic surfaces such as medical devices or on inpatient tissues (Chenoweth and Saint, 2013). The bloodstream infection (BSI) due to hospital-acquired *P. aeruginosa* infection causes a mortality of 20%−50% (Chatzinikolaou et al., 2000). Cystic fibrosis (CF) in the lungs is considered as a genetic disorder because of recessive mutations in the CF transmembrane regulator genes which reduce pulmonary mucociliary clearing of bacteria. Biofilm-producing *P. aeruginosa* is the most common inhabitant in a CF-associated lung, which is difficult to eliminate using antibiotics (Rudkjøbing et al., 2012).

The prevalence of multidrug-resistant (MDR) *P. aeruginosa* in patients in intensive care unit and tertiary hospitals shows an increasing trend throughout the world (United States, Europe, South America, Asia) for last one decade (Nathwani et al., 2014). MDR *P. aeruginosa* infection is associated with increased morbidity, mortality, hospital stay and associated costs. A US study estimated the cost as \$43,714−\$187,260 for MDR *P. aeruginosa* infection (Evans et al., 2007). The Centers for Disease Control (CDC) reported 6700 MDR *P. aeruginosa* infection in a year in the United States, which caused 440 deaths. A metaanalysis indicated more death associated with carbapenem-resistant *P. aeruginosa* infection than the carbapenem susceptible isolates (Zhang et al., 2016). Colistin was considered as a last resort for MDR *P. aeruginosa* infection, although colistin-resistant *P. aeruginosa* strains are reported from Denmark, United Kingdom and Australia (Johansen et al., 2008).

Antimicrobial Resistance in Agriculture. https://doi.org/10.1016/B978-0-12-815770-1.00023-7

Properties

Morphology: *Pseudomonas* is Gram-negative, straight or curved rod, motile by one or more polar flagella. The filamentous forms are sometimes observed. The bacteria are nonacid fast, nonsporulating and uncapsulated. Pili on the bacterial surface are detected. Environmental and tissue strains can produce slime, composed of glycolipoprotein and polysaccharide of lipopolysaccharide (LPS).

Classification: *Pseudomonas* belongs to class γ-proteobacteria, order Pseudomonadales and family *Pseudomonadaceae*. Earlier *Pseudomonas* included two groups of bacteria, viz. fluorescent group and pseudomallei group. Currently, the pseudomallei group is considered as a new genus known as *Burkholderia*. The genus *Pseudomonas* contains more than 120 numbers of species most of which are saprophytes. *P. aeruginosa*, *Pseudomonas fluorescens* and *Pseudomonas putida* are major pathogenic species (Peix et al., 2009).

Susceptibility to disinfectants: *P. aeruginosa* is relatively tolerant to chlorine, which may be the reason for the presence of the bacteria in treated swimming pools (Wheater et al., 1980).

Natural habitat: *P. aeruginosa* is commonly found in soil, plants, water (river, sewage treatment plant, untreated hospital wastewater, swimming pools and hot tubs), intestinal tract of man and animals, canine ear, uterus of mare, eye of horse, skin and mucous membrane of healthy animals, insects and nematodes because of its high environmental adaptability (Stover et al., 2000). Mucoid phenotype of *P. aeruginosa* can survive even in chlorinated water (Grobe et al., 2001). The untreated hospital wastewater acted as major source of MDR *P. aeruginosa* for environment (Fuentefria et al., 2008). In spite of poor carriage rate of *P. aeruginosa* in healthy man (2.6%−24%), faecal and nonfaecal shedding from human, birds and rodents are the major source of *P. aeruginosa* contamination in pool and tub water (Rusin et al., 1997). The pool structures and surrounding wet surfaces such as drains, decks and benches, shoes, towels and toys can also act as source of pool water contamination with *P. aeruginosa* (Fisher et al., 1985; Price and Ahearn, 1988).

Genome

The sequencing of *P. aeruginosa* genome revealed a genome size of 6,262,403 base pairs with 5570 open reading frames (ORF), one of the largest genomes among the bacteria. In total, approximately 372 ORFs are identified as functional, encoding proteins associated with cell adhesion, chemotaxis and motility (type IV pili and exopolysaccharides), enzymes for LPS synthesis, type III secretion system, outer membrane proteins (OprD porin family) and efflux systems generating antibiotic resistance (Stover et al., 2000). High environmental adaptability of *P. aeruginosa* occurs because of its large and complex genome (Silby et al., 2011).

Antigenic characteristics

Pseudomonas has two types of antigens, i.e., somatic and flagellar. Serotyping can be done using antisera against somatic antigen (O-typing) as well as flagellar antigen (H-typing). *P. aeruginosa* is routinely serotyped by 'Fisher immunotyping scheme' (based on LPS or high molecular weight polysaccharide), 'Homma scheme' (Japan) and 'International Antigenic Typing System'. Among several clonal types, clone C of *P. aeruginosa* is common in CF lungs in human and ST235 is considered as MDR phenotype spreading rapidly throughout the world (Tielen et al., 2011; Friedman et al., 2016).

Toxins and virulence factors produced

Toxins

(a) Exotoxins: Among the five protein secretion systems, type II (T2SS) and type III secretion systems (T3SS) of *P. aeruginosa* are associated with secretion of major toxins such as exotoxin-A (T2SS) and exotoxin-S, -T, -U and -Y (T3SS). These toxins can inhibit the cellular protein synthesis by blocking the activity of elongation factor (EF 2). Exo-A is ADP-ribosyltransferase which acts as cytotoxin. ExoS and ExoT are bifunctional enzymes that can disrupt Ras and Ras-like GTPase to disorder the cellular actin cytoskeleton and host cellular processes such as phagocytosis and wound healing (Galle et al., 2012). Exo-U has phospholipase A2-like activity causing cellular membrane damage and necrosis (Sato and Frank, 2004). Exo-Y is an adenylate cyclase associated with oedema formation.

(b) Endotoxin: *Pseudomonas* produces a specialized endotoxin, known as original endotoxic protein. It is structurally composed of LPS along with a protein. It acts as inducer for stimulation of innate immune system.

(c) Bacteriocin: *Pseudomonas* also produces bacteriocin, known as 'pyocin'. Like other bacteriocins, the pyocin can also inhibit the growth of similar natured bacteria.

(d) Pigment: Pyocyanin is a type of phenazine derivative (blue redox-active) and is secreted by *P. aeruginosa*. The pyocyanin is responsible for the production of a blue-green pigment which is used for rapid diagnosis of *P. aeruginosa*. It can generate reactive oxygen radicals (superoxide) with the exposure to oxygen. These radicals are toxic to the host cells. The bacteria itself protects from this toxicity by producing catalase and superoxide dismutase that can neutralize the radicals.

Virulence factors: Major virulence factors produced by *P. aeruginosa* are described in Table 23.1.

Transmission

P. aeruginosa enters the body through damaged mucosa (exogenous infection) or it is activated during immunocompromised condition (endogenous infection). Environment plays a significant role in transmission of *P. aeruginosa* and the studies indicated significant genotypic and functional similarities between the environmental and clinical strains (Coggan and Wolfgang, 2012). In health care facilities, infected patients, sinks and taps are the major source of exogenous infection. In intensive care unit, endogenous infection with *P. aeruginosa* mostly takes place (Blanc et al., 2007).

Transmission of *P. aeruginosa* in pools takes place through epidermal invasion causing folliculitis and otitis. Development of otitis depends on exposure time to the contaminated pool water, young age (>19 years) and existing ear infections (Schets et al., 2011). Inexperienced swimmers may receive *P. aeruginosa* from contaminated pool water through

TABLE 23.1 Major virulence factors produced by *Pseudomonas aeruginosa*.

Virulence factors	Function
Pseudocapsule (alginate), polysaccharide-encoding locus (*pel*) and polysaccharide synthesis locus (*psl*), which are also involved in forming the biofilm matrix embedded around microcolonies	Formation and maintenance of biofilm matrix The biofilm can inhibit polymorphonuclear chemotaxis and reduce the attack by antibiotics, reactive oxygen species and complement factors
Single polar flagellum (*FleR-FleS*), type IV pili (PilR—PilS), chitin-binding protein, LecA and LecB	Colonization and initial surface attachment Type IV pili also help in 'twitching motility', which causes bacterial movement along the host cell surface. It helps in development of a mature biofilm
RocA2	Fimbriae adhesin gene regulation
PhoP-PhoQ, GacA-GacS system	Swarming motility, biofilm formation
NarL-NarX system	Nitrate sensing and respiration, biofilm formation, swimming motility
CbrB-CbrA	Carbon and nitrogen storage, cytotoxicity, swarming motility, nematode virulence
RocR (SadR)	Cytotoxicity, regulation of fimbriae adhesins, biofilm formation
SadS (RocS1), LadS, RetS, pfpl, pyrB, PhoQ, sucC, clpP, lon, czcR, clpS, ureB, aroB	Biofilm formation and maturation
Elastase (LasB)	It can degrade the proteins such as immunoglobulins (Ig-A, Ig-G), cytokines, chemokines (IL-2, IL-8), complement and causes tissue damage by its attack on elastin
LasA protein	LasA also has elastase-like activity. It starts the damage of elastin by producing a 'nick' upon which other proteases act easily
Phospholipase C (haemolytic)	It can break down phosphatidylcholine and sphingomyelin, common in eukaryotic cell membranes and as lung surfactant. Degradation promotes lung injury
Pyochelin and pyoverdin, PfeR—PfeS system	They are siderophores that helps in assimilation of iron from the surrounding media or tissue for the bacterial growth

ingestion also. Formation of biofilm in the pools even in the presence of 1—3mg/lit of chlorine acts as a source of planktonic *P. aeruginosa* cells. Only the chlorine shock treatments with 10 mg/lit can reduce the biofilm numbers (Goeres et al., 2004).

Diagnosis

Pseudomonas is commonly found in the environment, often detected as contaminant in the laboratory. Detection of *Pseudomonas* should be clinically correlated.

Laboratory examination

Direct examination: A smear can be prepared from collected tissues to stain by Gram's method. *Pseudomonas* is Gram-negative medium-sized rods with no other distinctive features to identify.

Isolation of *P. aeruginosa*: *Pseudomonas* can be isolated in ordinary bacteriological media such as trypticase soy agar with or without blood, MacConkey agar. Incubation temperature is 20—42°C. Cetrimide agar is the selective medium for *P. aeruginosa*. On ordinary agar it produces convex glistening colonies with spreading edges. In blood agar haemolysis is found. It can produce different pigments in the ordinary medium that helps in identification of the bacteria. *P. aeruginosa* produces four type of pigments such as pyocyanin (blue), pyoverdin (yellow), pyorubin (red) and pyomelanin (black). Pyoverdin can fluoresce under ultraviolet light, previously known as 'fluorescein'. The cultures also develop a characteristic 'fruity' or 'grape-like' or 'corn taco-like' or 'corn tortillas' odour. *P. fluorescens* does not produce odour but may produce pyoverdin pigment in the artificial culture.

Molecular biology: Polymerase chain reaction is developed to detect *P. aeruginosa* from CF cases of human patients targeting *groES* and *groEL* genes.

Characteristics of antimicrobial resistance

Intrinsic resistance

Outer membrane present in Gram-negative bacteria has selective permeability which inhibits entry of antibiotic molecules, especially of greater size. *P. aeruginosa* has 12—100-fold lower outer membrane permeability than *Escherichia coli* (Nikaido and Hancock, 1986). Moreover, the major porin protein (OprF) present in *P. aeruginosa* outer membrane cannot uptake the antibiotics for passage because of inefficient channel architecture (Nikaido et al., 1991). The efflux system (MexA, MexB, OprM) of *P. aeruginosa* produces intrinsic resistance against quinolones, β-lactams (except imipenem), tetracycline and chloramphenicol (Poole et al., 1993). Resistance to triclosan (biocide) in *P. aeruginosa* is associated with production of additional enoyl-ACP reductase molecules (target of triclosan) (Blair et al., 2015).

β-Lactam resistance

Derepression of chromosomal β-lactamase (AmpC) is associated with β-lactam antibiotic resistance (ticarcillin, piperacillin, third-generation cephalosporins) in *P. aeruginosa*. The derepression is mediated by *blaI* mutation and the permanently derepressed strains produce excess amount of AmpC β-lactamase (Livermore, 1987). Loss of major porin protein (OprF), alteration in penicillin-binding protein structure, mutation of *tonB* (iron-regulated outer membrane protein) and possession of plasmid-encoded β-lactamase such as PSE-1,4; CARB-3,4; TEM-1,4,21,24,42; CTX-M-1,2,3,43; PME-1, LCR-1, NPS-1, SHV-2a, 5, 12; VEB, GES-1,9,13; IBC and OXA-1,2,3,5,6 are also described as mechanism for β-lactam resistance in *P. aeruginosa* (Malouin and Bryan, 1986; Curtis et al., 1988; Bush et al., 1995). The PSE-1 (most common in nature) and PSE-4 enzymes can inactivate penicillin and are inhibited by β-lactamase inhibitors. The PSEs are inactive against antipseudomonal cephalosporins, carbapenems or aztreonam, whereas OXA-type β-lactamases produced by *P. aeruginosa* can inactivate ceftazidime or aztreonam. The rare ESBLs (VEB, GES and IBC) are active against third-generation cephalosporins, penicillin and aztreonam. Overexpression of MexAB-OprM multidrug efflux pump due to a *NalB* mutation is another way of resistance against β-lactams detected in *P. aeruginosa* (Germ et al., 1999).

International clonal complex CC11 is correlated with wide dissemination of PER-1-producing *P. aeruginosa* in European (Turkey, Belgium, Italy, Spain, Poland, Hungary, Serbia, Tunisia, Greece) and Asian countries (China, Japan, Iran) (Potron et al., 2015). The VEB-1-producing *P. aeruginosa* was detected in Thailand, Kuwait, India, Iran, Bulgaria, United Kingdom and Denmark (Aubert et al., 2004; Potron et al., 2015).

Carbapenem resistance

Possession of certain β-lactamases (GES-2,5,18) by *P. aeruginosa* confers resistance to carbapenems. Earliest GES-type carbapenemase (GES-2) was detected in *P. aeruginosa* strains isolated from nosocomial pneumonia patient in South Africa (Poirel et al., 2001). KPC-producing *P. aeruginosa* are rare in occurrence, although reported from Colombia, Trinidad, United States and few other countries (Villegas et al., 2007; Poirel et al., 2010). Resistance to imipenem and reduced susceptibility to meropenem in *P. aeruginosa* is associated with loss of major porin protein (OprD) (Tamber and Hancock, 2003).

Aminoglycoside resistance

P. aeruginosa possesses different plasmid-encoded aminoglycoside modifying enzymes such as AAC(3)-I, AAC(3)-Ia, AAC(3)-II, AAC(6′)-I, AAC(6′)-II and ANT(2″), which can reduce the bacterial drug uptake or drug interaction with bacterial ribosome. Mutation of chromosomally encoded aminoglycoside resistance gene (*aphA*) is the secondary mechanism of aminoglycoside resistance (Okii et al., 1983). The class 1 integron (*In51*) encoding metallo-β-lactamase in *P. aeruginosa* was detected to harbour novel aminoglycoside resistance gene cassette (*aadA6*) (Naas et al., 1999). *P. aeruginosa* can also encode different 16S rRNA methylases (RmtA, RmtD, ArmA), which can produce the resistance by modifying the drug target (Yokoyama et al., 2003). *P. aeruginosa* isolates producing 16S rRNA methylases (RmtD, ArmA) are MDR through the coproduction of metallo-β-lactamase or extended spectrum β-lactamase and are found to be imipenem-resistant (Doi et al., 2007). Overexpression of the MexXY efflux pump because of a mutation in the regulatory gene *MexZ* is another way of resistance against aminoglycosides in *P. aeruginosa* isolates (Westbrock-Wadman et al., 1999).

Quinolone resistance

P. aeruginosa are intrinsically resistant to quinolones because of constitutive expression of efflux system (MexA, MexB, OprM) and reduced drug uptake. The expression of MexAB-OprM RND-type efflux system is also associated with reduced susceptibility to chloramphenicol, tetracycline and β-lactams (Li et al., 1995). Mutation in quinolone target enzymes topoisomerase II and IV (encoded by *gyrA* and *parC*) and regulator genes for the efflux system are described as mechanisms of acquired resistance in *P. aeruginosa* (Higgins et al., 2003). Recent study indicated upregulation of MexEF-OprN system and reduced OprD expression in *P. aeruginosa* is associated with resistance against both quinolone and imipenem and reduced susceptibility to meropenem (Morita et al., 2015).

Colistin resistance

Certain structural changes in outer membrane of *P. aeruginosa* such as increase in the palmitate content of lipid-A and replacement of 2-hydroxylaurate with 4-aminoarabinose are associated with resistance to colistin (Denton et al., 2002). The genes upregulated in colistin-resistant *P. aeruginosa* isolates encode cell wall–associated hydrolase, glycosyltransferase and arabinose efflux permease. Some two-component systems such as PmrAB (Mg^{++}-dependent), PhoPQ (Mg^{++}-dependent), ParRS, CprRS and ColRS regulate colistin (polymyxin) resistance in *P. aeruginosa* (Lee et al., 2014).

References

Aubert, D., Girlich, D., Naas, T., Nagarajan, S., Nordmann, P., 2004. Functional and structural characterization of the genetic environment of an extended-spectrum β-lactamase blaVEB gene from a *Pseudomonas aeruginosa* isolate obtained in India. Antimicrobial Agents and Chemotherapy 48 (9), 3284–3290.

Blair, J.M., Webber, M.A., Baylay, A.J., Ogbolu, D.O., Piddock, L.J., 2015. Molecular mechanisms of antibiotic resistance. Nature Reviews Microbiology 13 (1), 42.

Blanc, D.S., Francioli, P., Zanetti, G., 2007. Molecular epidemiology of *Pseudomonas aeruginosa* in the intensive care units-a review. The Open Microbiology Journal 1, 8.

Boucher, H.W., Talbot, G.H., Bradley, J.S., Edwards, J.E., Gilbert, D., Rice, L.B., Scheld, M., Spellberg, B., Bartlett, J., 2009. Bad bugs, no drugs: no ESKAPE! an update from the Infectious Diseases Society of America. Clinical Infectious Diseases 48 (1), 1–12.

Bush, K., Jacoby, G.A., Medeiros, A.A., 1995. A functional classification scheme for beta-lactamases and its correlation with molecular structure. Antimicrobial Agents and Chemotherapy 39 (6), 1211.

Chatzinikolaou, I., Abi-Said, D., Bodey, G.P., Rolston, K.V., Tarrand, J.J., Samonis, G., 2000. Recent experience with *Pseudomonas aeruginosa* bacteremia in patients with cancer: retrospective analysis of 245 episodes. Archives of Internal Medicine 160 (4), 501–509.

Chenoweth, C., Saint, S., 2013. Preventing catheter-associated urinary tract infections in the intensive care unit. Critical Care Clinics 29 (1), 19–32.

Coggan, K.A., Wolfgang, M.C., 2012. Global regulatory pathways and cross-talk control *Pseudomonas aeruginosa* environmental lifestyle and virulence phenotype. Current Issues in Molecular Biology 14 (2), 47.

Curtis, N.A., Eisenstadt, R.L., East, S.J., Cornford, R.J., Walker, L.A., White, A.J., 1988. Iron-regulated outer membrane proteins of *Escherichia coli* K-12 and mechanism of action of catechol-substituted cephalosporins. Antimicrobial Agents and Chemotherapy 32 (12), 1879–1886.

Denton, M., Kerr, K., Mooney, L., Keer, V., Rajgopal, A., Brownlee, K., Arundel, P., Conway, S., 2002. Transmission of colistin-resistant *Pseudomonas aeruginosa* between patients attending a pediatric cystic fibrosis center. Pediatric Pulmonology 34 (4), 257–261.

Doi, Y., Ghilardi, A.C., Adams, J., de Oliveira Garcia, D., Paterson, D.L., 2007. High prevalence of metallo-β-lactamase and 16S rRNA methylase coproduction among imipenem-resistant *Pseudomonas aeruginosa* isolates in Brazil. Antimicrobial Agents and Chemotherapy 51 (9), 3388–3390.

Evans, H.L., Lefrak, S.N., Lyman, J., Smith, R.L., Chong, T.W., McElearney, S.T., Schulman, A.R., Hughes, M.G., Raymond, D.P., Pruett, T.L., Sawyer, R.G., 2007. Cost of gram-negative resistance. Critical Care Medicine 35 (1), 89–95.

Fisher, M.C., Goldsmith, J.F., Gilligan, P.H., 1985. Sneakers as a source of *Pseudomonas aeruginosa* in children with osteomyelitis following puncture wounds. Journal of Pediatric Orthopaedics 5 (5), 626.

Friedman, N.D., Temkin, E., Carmeli, Y., 2016. The negative impact of antibiotic resistance. Clinical Microbiology and Infections 22 (5), 416–422.

Fuentefria, D.B., Ferreira, A.E., Gräf, T., Corção, G., 2008. *Pseudomonas aeruginosa*: spread of antimicrobial resistance in hospital effluent and surface water. Revista da Sociedade Brasileira de Medicina Tropical 41 (5), 470–473.

Galle, M., Jin, S., Bogaert, P., Haegman, M., Vandenabeele, P., Beyaert, R., 2012. The *Pseudomonas aeruginosa* type III secretion system has an exotoxin S/T/Y independent pathogenic role during acute lung infection. PLoS One 7 (7), e41547.

Germ, M., Yoshihara, E., Yoneyama, H., Nakae, T., 1999. Interplay between the efflux pump and the outer membrane permeability barrier in fluorescent dye accumulation in *Pseudomonas aeruginosa*. Biochemical and Biophysical Research Communications 261 (2), 452–455.

Gessard, C., 1984. On the blue and green coloration that appears on bandages. Reviews of Infectious Diseases 6 (Suppl. ment_3), S775–S776.

Goeres, D.M., Palys, T., Sandel, B.B., Geiger, J., 2004. Evaluation of disinfectant efficacy against biofilm and suspended bacteria in a laboratory swimming pool model. Water Research 38 (13), 3103–3109.

Grobe, S., Wingender, J., Flemming, H.C., 2001. Capability of mucoid *Pseudomonas aeruginosa* to survive in chlorinated water. International Journal of Hygiene and Environmental Health 204 (2–3), 139–142.

Higgins, P.G., Fluit, A.C., Milatovic, D., Verhoef, J., Schmitz, F.J., 2003. Mutations in GyrA, ParC, MexR and NfxB in clinical isolates of *Pseudomonas aeruginosa*. International Journal of Antimicrobial Agents 21 (5), 409–413.

Johansen, H.K., Moskowitz, S.M., Ciofu, O., Pressler, T., Høiby, N., 2008. Spread of colistin resistant non-mucoid *Pseudomonas aeruginosa* among chronically infected Danish cystic fibrosis patients. Journal of Cystic Fibrosis 7 (5), 391–397.

Lee, J.Y., Na, I.Y., Park, Y.K., Ko, K.S., 2014. Genomic variations between colistin-susceptible and -resistant *Pseudomonas aeruginosa* clinical isolates and their effects on colistin resistance. Journal of Antimicrobial Chemotherapy 69 (5), 1248–1256.

Li, X.Z., Nikaido, H., Poole, K., 1995. Role of mexA-mexB-oprM in antibiotic efflux in *Pseudomonas aeruginosa*. Antimicrobial Agents and Chemotherapy 39 (9), 1948–1953.

Livermore, D.M., 1987. Clinical significance of beta-lactamase induction and stable derepression in gram-negative rods. European Journal of Clinical Microbiology 6 (4), 439–445.

Malouin, F., Bryan, L.E., 1986. Modification of penicillin-binding proteins as mechanisms of beta-lactam resistance. Antimicrobial Agents and Chemotherapy 30 (1), 1.

Morita, Y., Tomida, J., Kawamura, Y., 2015. Efflux-mediated fluoroquinolone resistance in the multidrug-resistant *Pseudomonas aeruginosa* clinical isolate PA7: identification of a novel MexS variant involved in up regulation of the mexEF-oprN multidrug efflux operon. Frontiers in Microbiology 6, 8.

Naas, T., Poirel, L., Nordmann, P., 1999. Molecular characterisation of *In51*, a class 1 integron containing a novel aminoglycoside adenylyltransferase gene cassette, *aadA6*, in *Pseudomonas aeruginosa*. Biochimica et Biophysica Acta (BBA) – Gene Structure and Expression 1489 (2–3), 445–451.

Nathwani, D., Raman, G., Sulham, K., Gavaghan, M., Menon, V., 2014. Clinical and economic consequences of hospital-acquired resistant and multidrug-resistant *Pseudomonas aeruginosa* infections: a systematic review and meta-analysis. Antimicrobial Resistance and Infection Control 3 (1), 32.

Nikaido, H., Nikaido, K., Harayama, S., 1991. Identification and characterization of porins in *Pseudomonas aeruginosa*. Journal of Biological Chemistry 266 (2), 770–779.

Nikaido, H., Hancock, R., 1986. Outer membrane permeability of *Pseudomonas aeruginosa*. The Bacteria 10, 145–193.

Okii, M., Iyobe, S., Mitsuhashi, S., 1983. Mapping of the gene specifying aminoglycoside 3'-phosphotransferase II on the *Pseudomonas aeruginosa* chromosome. Journal of Bacteriology 155 (2), 643–649.

Peix, A., Ramírez-Bahena, M.H., Velázquez, E., 2009. Historical evolution and current status of the taxonomy of genus *Pseudomonas*. Infection, Genetics and Evolution 9 (6), 1132–1147.

Pitt, T.L., 1998. *Pseudomonas, Burkholderia* and related *Genera* (Chapter 47). In: Collier, L. (Ed.), Topley and Wilson's Microbiology and Microbial Infections, vol. 2. Systematic Bacteriology.

Poirel, L., Nordmann, P., Lagrutta, E., Cleary, T., Munoz-Price, L.S., 2010. Emergence of KPC-producing *Pseudomonas aeruginosa* in the United States. Antimicrobial Agents and Chemotherapy 54 (7), 3072, 3072.

Poirel, L., Weldhagen, G.F., Naas, T., De Champs, C., Dove, M.G., Nordmann, P., 2001. GES-2, a Class A β-lactamase from *Pseudomonas aeruginosa* with increased hydrolysis of imipenem. Antimicrobial Agents and Chemotherapy 45 (9), 2598–2603.

Poole, K., Krebes, K., McNally, C., Neshat, S., 1993. Multiple antibiotic resistance in *Pseudomonas aeruginosa*: evidence for involvement of an efflux operon. Journal of Bacteriology 175 (22), 7363—7372.

Potron, A., Poirel, L., Nordmann, P., 2015. Emerging broad-spectrum resistance in *Pseudomonas aeruginosa* and *Acinetobacter baumannii*: mechanisms and epidemiology. International Journal of Antimicrobial Agents 45 (6), 568—585.

Price, D., Ahearn, D.G., 1988. Incidence and persistence of *Pseudomonas aeruginosa* in whirlpools. Journal of Clinical Microbiology 26 (9), 1650—1654.

Rice, S.A., Van den Akker, B., Pomati, F., Roser, D., 2012. A risk assessment of *Pseudomonas aeruginosa* in swimming pools: a review. Journal of Water and Health 10 (2), 181—196.

Rudkjøbing, V.B., Thomsen, T.R., Alhede, M., Kragh, K.N., Nielsen, P.H., Johansen, U.R., Givskov, M., Høiby, N., Bjarnsholt, T., 2012. The microorganisms in chronically infected end-stage and non-end-stage cystic fibrosis patients. FEMS Immunology and Medical Microbiology 65 (2), 236—244.

Rusin, P.A., Rose, J.B., Haas, C.N., Gerba, C.P., 1997. Risk assessment of opportunistic bacterial pathogens in drinking water. In: Reviews of Environmental Contamination and Toxicology. Springer, New York, NY, pp. 57—83.

Sato, H., Frank, D.W., 2004. ExoU is a potent intracellular phospholipase. Molecular Microbiology 53 (5), 1279—1290.

Schets, F.M., Schijven, J.F., de Roda Husman, A.M., 2011. Exposure assessment for swimmers in bathing waters and swimming pools. Water Research 45 (7), 2392—2400.

Silby, M.W., Winstanley, C., Godfrey, S.A., Levy, S.B., Jackson, R.W., 2011. *Pseudomonas* genomes: diverse and adaptable. FEMS Microbiology Reviews 35 (4), 652—680.

Stover, C.K., Pham, X.Q., Erwin, A.L., Mizoguchi, S.D., Warrener, P., Hickey, M.J., Brinkman, F.S.L., Hufnagle, W.O., Kowalik, D.J., Lagrou, M., Garber, R.L., 2000. Complete genome sequence of *Pseudomonas aeruginosa* PAO1, an opportunistic pathogen. Nature 406 (6799), 959.

Tamber, S., Hancock, R.E., 2003. On the mechanism of solute uptake in *Pseudomonas*. Frontiers in Bioscience 8, s472—s483.

Tielen, P., Narten, M., Rosin, N., Biegler, I., Haddad, I., Hogardt, M., Neubauer, R., Schobert, M., Wiehlmann, L., Jahn, D., 2011. Genotypic and phenotypic characterization of *Pseudomonas aeruginosa* isolates from urinary tract infections. International Journal of Medical Microbiology 301 (4), 282—292.

Villegas, M.V., Lolans, K., Correa, A., Kattan, J.N., Lopez, J.A., Quinn, J.P., Colombian Nosocomial Resistance Study Group, 2007. First identification of *Pseudomonas aeruginosa* isolates producing a KPC-type carbapenem-hydrolyzing β-lactamase. Antimicrobial Agents and Chemotherapy 51 (4), 1553—1555.

Westbrock-Wadman, S., Sherman, D.R., Hickey, M.J., Coulter, S.N., Zhu, Y.Q., Warrener, P., Nguyen, L.Y., Shawar, R.M., Folger, K.R., Stover, C.K., 1999. Characterization of a *Pseudomonas aeruginosa* efflux pump contributing to aminoglycoside impermeability. Antimicrobial Agents and Chemotherapy 43 (12), 2975—2983.

Wheater, D.W.F., Mara, D.D., Jawad, L., Oragui, J., 1980. *Pseudomonas aeruginosa* and *Escherichia coli* in sewage and fresh water. Water Research 14 (7), 713—721.

Yokoyama, K., Doi, Y., Yamane, K., Kurokawa, H., Shibata, N., Shibayama, K., Yagi, T., Kato, H., Arakawa, Y., 2003. Acquisition of 16S rRNA methylase gene in *Pseudomonas aeruginosa*. The Lancet 362 (9399), 1888—1893.

Zhang, Y., Chen, X.L., Huang, A.W., Liu, S.L., Liu, W.J., Zhang, N., Lu, X.Z., 2016. Mortality attributable to carbapenem-resistant *Pseudomonas aeruginosa* bacteremia: a meta-analysis of cohort studies. Emerging Microbes and Infections 5 (3), e27.

Chapter 24

Aeromonas

Chapter outline

In 1891, a bacterial infection in frogs ('red leg disease') was associated with *Aeromonas*-like organisms. The genus *Aeromonas* was defined later (Stanier, 1943). Pathogenic significance of *Aeromonas* in human was described first in 1954 in a woman from Jamaica (Hill et al., 1954) and later in a series of cases in association with septicaemia and cirrhosis of liver (Laennec's cirrhosis) in patients (von Graevenitz and Mensch, 1968). In human, *Aeromonas* is associated with wound infections, septicaemia, especially during haematological malignancy, hepatobiliary menaces, meningitis, endocarditis, osteomyelitis, chronic diarrhoea and colitis in immunocompromised patients (Obi and Bessong, 2002; Figueras, 2005).

In 1984, *Aeromonas hydrophila* was introduced into the genus which can infect a wide range of animals and fresh or marine water fishes other than human (Popoff, 1984). In fishes, it causes hemorrhagic septicemia, epizootic ulcerative syndrome (EUS), infectious abnormal dropsy, exopthalmia and fin and tail rot. EUS is a major infection of fresh and brackish water fishes in Asian and the Indo-Pacific regions including India, Thailand, Bangladesh, Australia, Malaysia, Indonesia and Papua New Guinea (Harikrishnan and Balasundaram, 2005). Per capita consumption and supply of sea foods including fishes increased throughout the world in recent times as a source of proteins, omega-3 fatty acids, vitamin D, selenium and iodine. Approximately 56.6 million people all over the world are engaged in aquaculture and fishery sectors of which majority are from Asia (84%), Africa (10%) and Latin America (4%) (FAO, 2016). Antimicrobials (quinolones, chloramphenicol, nitrofuran, gentian violet) are used as therapy or prophylaxis in aquaculture through the feed or water immersion. The unused antibiotics are deposited and thus contaminate the water and increase the prevalence of resistant bacteria. Other than direct application, soil, sewage and sediments also act as source of contamination in river, sea and aquaculture (Kümmerer, 2009).

Properties

Morphology: *Aeromonas* are facultative anaerobic, chemoorganotrophic Gram-negative straight rods or coccobacilli which are motile with the help of a single flagellum. The bacterial measurement is 0.3–1.0 × 1.0–3.5 μm. Peritrichous flagella are observed in few *Aeromonas* strains adapted in solid media (United States Environmental Protection Agency, 2006). The bacteria can produce catalase, oxidase and nitrate reductase.

Classification: The phylogenetic analysis removed *Aeromonas* from Vibrionaceae family and placed it under the family Aeromonadaceae (Colwell et al., 1986). Other distinguishing characteristics include resistance to vibriostatic compound O/129 (150 μg), presence of ornithine decarboxylase, inability to tolerate 6.5% sodium chloride, incapability to ferment inositol, negative result in string test, capability to liquefy gelatin and ability to ferment D-mannitol and sucrose (United States Environmental Protection Agency, 2006).

Earlier the genus *Aeromonas* was subdivided into two major groups, i.e., motile-mesophilic (*A. hydrophila*) and non–motile-psychrophilic (*Aeromonas salmonicida*). Based on DNA relatedness, mesophilic group is further subdivided

Antimicrobial Resistance in Agriculture. https://doi.org/10.1016/B978-0-12-815770-1.00024-9

into 14 phenospecies and 17 DNA hybridization groups (HGs) or genomospecies. The term 'phenospecies' is used to describe a single heterogeneous species consisting of multiple HGs. Few HGs (HG-1/*A. hydrophila*, HG-4/*Aeromonas caviae*, HG-8/*Aeromonas veronii* biovar *sobria*, HG-9/*Aeromonas jandaei*, HG-10, HG-12/*Aeromonas schubertii*, HG-14/ *Aeromonas trota*) of *Aeromonas* are exclusive human pathogen and others are common in aquatic environment and animals (HG-2, HG-3, HG-5, HG-6, HG-7, HG-11, HG-15, HG-16, HG-17) (Janda and Abbott, 1998; Sinha et al., 2004).

Susceptibility to disinfectants: Aeromonads are sensitive to sodium hypochlorite, quaternary ammonium salts, iodoform, 2-chlorophenol and glutaraldehyde (Roberts et al., 1996).

Natural habitat: *Aeromonas* are found in the intestinal tract of human (healthy or diarrhoeic), fish (surface and gut), shellfish, shrimp, horse, pig, sheep, cattle, turtle, alligator, snake and frogs, and different foods such as meat, raw or pasteurized milk, cheese, fresh vegetables, smoked fish and mineral water (Gray, 1984; Agarwal et al., 2000; Cereser et al., 2013). In the environment, surface water, groundwater, sewage, effluents and activated sludge may act as source of Aeromonads (El-Taweel and Shaban, 2001; Chauret et al., 2001). The bacteria also survived chlorinated drinking water distribution system in several countries by producing biofilm (Figueras et al., 2005). *A. hydrophila* is enlisted as the 'contaminant candidate' by United States Environmental Protection Agency (USEPA, 2001).

Genome: The genome of *A. hydrophila* (ATCC 7966) is of 4.7 Mbp in size (GC: 61.5 mol%), which contains 31 rRNA, 128 tRNA, 4283 genes and 7 pseudogenes. The genome can encode 4118 proteins (Seshadri et al., 2006).

Antigenic characteristics

A. hydrophila has both somatic and flagellar antigens based on which the bacteria were classified into 12 O-antigen and 9 H-antigen groups (Ewing et al., 1961). Each serogroup consists of numerous serotypes.

Transmission

A. hydrophila can initiate infection in fishes during stress or with other pathogens (Leung et al., 1995). Overcrowding, low-dissolved oxygen, higher organic matter, fluctuation of temperature, mechanical injuries and spawning in susceptible fishes are the major predisposing factors. Accumulation of pesticides from agricultural fields and low temperature during monsoon favours *A. hydrophila* infection in fishes in tropical countries (Braaten and Hektoen, 1991).

In human, food- and water-borne outbreaks of *Aeromonas* were reported from Norfolk, United States and India (Holmberg et al., 1986; Morena et al., 1993; Taneja et al., 2004). Injury in contaminated aquatic environment or during handling fishes causes *Aeromonas*-associated cellulitis, myositis, septicaemia and wound infections (Joseph, 2000; Lehane and Rawlin, 2000).

Toxins and virulence factors

Enterotoxin: *Aeromonas* can produce chromosomally encoded several types of enterotoxins. The cytotoxic enterotoxins (Act) are heat-labile (56°C, 20 min) and type II-secretion system associated. They can destroy intestinal epithelium through activation of the arachidonic acid metabolism. Increased intracellular cAMP level was detected with activation of heat-labile (Alt) and the heat-stable (Ast) enterotoxins and various haemolysins such as AerA, HlyA, Ahh1, Asa1 and *A. sobria* haemolysin of *Aeromonas* (Brown et al., 1997; Wang et al., 2003). The cytotoxins, heat-labile (Alt) and the heat-stable (Ast) enterotoxins were found to be associated with severe diarrhoea (Albert et al., 2000; Bauab et al., 2003).

The virulence factors of *A. hydrophila* are described in Table 24.1.

Diagnosis

Isolation of *Aeromonas*: *Aeromonas* can be isolated in specific media at 22°C—35°C (although the growth can take place at 0—45°C), pH 5.5—9 and 0%—4% sodium chloride concentration (Ghenghesh et al., 2008). Earlier, Shotts and Rimler (1973) prepared a specific isolation medium for *Aeromonas* using certain ingredients such as L-lysine, L-ornithine, L-cystine, maltose, sodium thiosulfate, bromothymol blue, ferric ammonium citrate, sodium deoxycholate, novobiocin, yeast extract and sodium chloride. Currently, the specific media such as starch ampicillin agar, bile salts inositol brilliant green agar, tryptose broth containing ampicillin (30 mg/lit) and starch glutamate ampicillin penicillin (SGAP-10) medium are recommended for isolation of *Aeromonas* from foods and sewage sludge, respectively (Eaton et al., 2005). In clinical laboratories, blood agar is used for isolation of *Aeromonas*. After incubation of 24—48 h, distinctive colonies with

TABLE 24.1 Virulence factors of *A. hydrophila*.

Virulence factors	Function
Flagella	Movement in surface (lateral flagella) or suspension (polar)
Type IV pilus	It helps in adhesion of the bacteria. Biogenesis of type IV pilus is regulated by *tapABCD*. Type IV pilus is associated with gastroenteritis. The bundle forming pilus is (*bfp*) and also acts as colonization factor
TapD	Secretion of virulence factors such as aerolysin and proteases
Capsule, S-layer	Antiphagocytic, resistance to complement system, adherence
O-antigen of lipopolysaccharides	Colonization factor
Collagenase	Cytotoxic to Vero cells
Extracellular protease	Thermostable protease and can degrade casein and elastin
Enolase	Production of plasmin through degradation of blood plasma proteins, acts as heat shock protein
Lipase (Ast and Alt)	Cytotonic enterotoxins
Pore-forming RTX toxin (RtxA)	Rounding of cells and apoptosis
Phospholipase C/lecithinase (*plc*)	Cytotoxicity
Adhesin (*minD*)	Mucosal adherence, biofilm formation, cell division, motility
5-Enolpyruvylshikimate-3-phosphate synthase (*aroA*)	Folate availability and viability
Nuclease (*ahn*)	Precise role unknown
RNase R (*vacB*)	Exoribonuclease which helps in growth at 4°C and motility
Quorum-sensing response regulators (*ahyRI*, *N*-(butanoyl)-L-homoserine lactones (BHL), *N*-hexanoyl-L-homoserine lactones (AHL), QseB)	Biofilm formation

or without haemolysis are detected. In RS-agar, *A. hydrophila* produces yellow-coloured colonies. Enrichment broth such as alkaline peptone water is recommended for isolation of *Aeromonas* from highly contaminated samples.

Serological tests: Serological tests are not reliable for detection of *Aeromonas* because of antigenic diversity and ubiquitous presence of the bacteria.

Molecular biology: The crossover in ribosomal sequences and heterogeneity makes 16S ribosomal DNA of *Aeromonas* unsuitable as target gene in diagnostic polymerase chain reaction (PCR) (Morandi et al., 2005). Instead, nucleotide sequencing of *gyrB* gene was found as a better diagnostic option (Yanez et al., 2003). PCR was also used for detection of *Aeromonas* in food samples (Özbaş et al., 2000). Microarray assay was developed for detection of population dynamics of *A. hydrophila* in coastal water environment and pathogenicity in murine model (Galindo et al., 2003; Stine et al., 2003). Multilocus sequence typing using four genes such as 16S rDNA, *recA*, *gyrB* and *chiA* was found effective to detect the genetic relatedness between the isolates (Carnahan, 2001).

Characteristics of antimicrobial resistance

β-Lactam resistance

Aeromonas exhibits resistance to penicillins, ampicillin, carbenicillin and ticarcillin. Different *Aeromonas* species can produce diverse classes of plasmid encoded β-lactamases such as B, C and D (*A. hydrophila*), C and D (*A. caviae*), B and D (*A. veronii*), D (*A. schubertii*) and C (*A. trota*) (Fosse et al., 2003). Expression of β-lactamase genes in *Aeromonas* is highly coordinated and is controlled by a single mechanism (Walsh et al., 1997). Among the major integron classes (1, 2 and 3), majority of *A. hydrophila* isolates possess class 1 integron, not 2 and 3 (Lukkana et al., 2011).

TABLE 24.2 Antimicrobial resistance in *Aeromonas* isolated from fishes, meat, milk and environment.

Source	Major antibiotic resistance	References
Fishes (carp, Indian carp, rohu, grass carp)	Penicillin, ampicillin, bacitracin, cloxacillin, novobiocin	Hatha et al. (2005); Čížek et al. (2010)
Fish (tilapia)	Penicillin, ampicillin, carbenicillin, cephalothin, clindamycin, polymyxin-B, rifampicin, streptomycin	Castro-Escarpulli et al. (2003)
Prawn and finfish	Bacitracin, kanamycin, methicillin, novobiocin	Vivekanandhan et al. (2002); Thayumanavan et al. (2003)
Trouts	Amoxycillin/clavulanic acid, penicillin, gentamicin, oxytetracycline, sulfamethoxazole/trimethoprim, amoxicillin, ampicillin, clindamycin, erythromycin, imipenem, novobiocin	Kırkan et al. (2003); Stratev et al. (2013)
Milk	Penicillin, amoxicillin, ampicillin, cloxacillin, erythromycin, methicillin, trimethoprim/sulfamethoxazole, vancomycin	Yucel and Citak (2003)
Cheese (Kareish)	Penicillin, amoxicillin, ampicillin, cefadroxil, cloxacillin, erythromycin, trimethoprim/sulfamethoxazole	Enany et al. (2013)
Meat (lamb)	Ampicillin, bacitracin, kanamycin, novobiocin, polymyxin B, vancomycin	Rajakumar et al. (2012)
Meat (chicken)	Ampicillin, amoxicillin, bacitracin, erythromycin, polymyxin B	Rajakumar et al. (2012)
Salads	Augmentin, ceftriaxone, nitrofurantoin, gentamicin, co-trimoxazole, amoxicillin, ciprofloxacin, streptomycin	Adebayo et al. (2012)
Lettuce	Ampicillin, tetracycline, cefotaxime, ceftazidime, imipenem	Palú et al. (2006)
River water	Cephalothin, ticarcillin, sulfamethoxazole, ampicillin	Goñi-Urriza et al. (2000)

Tetracycline resistance

A. hydrophila isolated from catfish, aquaculture pond water and sediments possessed tetracycline resistance determinants (tetA, tetB, tetC, tetD, tetE and tetY) (DePaola et al., 1988).

Quinolone resistance

Mutation in *gyr*A and *par*C was correlated with quinolone resistance in *A. hydrophila* isolated from freshwater and *Aeromonas punctata* and *A. media* isolated from urban effluents (Alcaide et al., 2010; Figueira et al., 2011). The *qnr*-mediated quinolone resistance was detected in *Aeromonas allosaccarophila* and *A. punctata* isolated from aquatic environment (Picão et al., 2008; Xia et al., 2010).

Types of antimicrobial resistance of *A. hydrophila* isolates observed in fishes, meat, milk and environment are enumerated in Table 24.2.

References

Adebayo, E.A., Majolagbe, O.N., Ola, I.O., Ogundiran, M.A., 2012. Antibiotic resistance pattern of isolated bacteria from salads. Journal of Research in Biology 2, 136−142.

Agarwal, R.K., Kapoor, K.N., Kumar, A., Bhilegaonkar, K.N., 2000. Aeromonads in foods of animal origin. Indian Journal of Animal Sciences 70 (9), 942−943.

Albert, M.J., Ansaruzzaman, M., Talukder, K.A., Chopra, A.K., Kuhn, I., Rahman, M., Faruque, A.S.G., Islam, M.S., Sack, R.B., Mollby, R., 2000. Prevalence of enterotoxin genes in *Aeromonas* spp. isolated from children with diarrhea, healthy controls, and the environment. Journal of Clinical Microbiology 38 (10), 3785−3790.

Alcaide, E., Blasco, M.D., Esteve, C., 2010. Mechanisms of quinolone resistance in *Aeromonas* species isolated from humans, water and eels. Research in Microbiology 161 (1), 40−45.

Bauab, T.M., Levy, C.E., Rodrigues, J., Falcão, D.P., 2003. Niche-specific association of *Aeromonas* ribotypes from human and environmental origin. Microbiology and Immunology 47 (1), 7–16.

Braaten, B., Hektoen, H., 1991, June. The environmental impact of aquaculture. In: Report on a Regional Study and Workshop on Fish Disease and Fish Health Management, pp. 469–524.

Brown, R.L., Sanderson, K., Kirov, S.M., 1997. Plasmids and *Aeromonas* virulence. FEMS Immunology and Medical Microbiology 17 (4), 217–223.

Carnahan, A.M., 2001. Genetic Relatedness of *Aeromonas* Species Based on the DNA Sequences of Four Distinct Genomic Loci. PhD Dissertation. University of Maryland, College Park, Md, USA.

Castro-Escarpulli, G., Figueras, M.J., Aguilera-Arreola, G., Soler, L., Fernandez-Rendon, E., Aparicio, G.O., Guarro, J., Chacon, M.R., 2003. Characterization of *Aeromonas* spp. isolated from frozen fish intended for human consumption in Mexico. International Journal of Food Microbiology 84 (1), 41–49.

Cereser, N.D., Júnior, O.R., Martineli, T.M., Souza, V., Rodrigues, L.B., Kerkoff, J., 2013. Resistance profile of *Aeromonas* spp. isolated in dairy products industry/Perfil de resistência de *Aeromonas* spp. isolada no fluxograma de produção do queijo minas frescal industrial e artesanal. Ars Veterinaria 29 (1), 30–36.

Chauret, C., Volk, C., Creason, R., Jarosh, J., Robinson, J., Warnes, C., 2001. Detection of *Aeromonas hydrophila* in a drinking-water distribution system: a field and pilot study. Canadian Journal of Microbiology 47 (8), 782–786.

Čížek, A., Dolejská, M., Sochorová, R., Strachotová, K., Piačková, V., Veselý, T., 2010. Antimicrobial resistance and its genetic determinants in aeromonads isolated in ornamental (koi) carp (*Cyprinus carpio koi*) and common carp (*Cyprinus carpio*). Veterinary Microbiology 142 (3–4), 435–439.

Colwell, R.R., MacDonell, M.T., De Ley, J., 1986. Proposal to recognize the family Aeromonadaceae fam. nov. International Journal of Systematic and Evolutionary Microbiology 36 (3), 473–477.

DePaola, A., Flynn, P.A., McPhearson, R.M., Levy, S.B., 1988. Phenotypic and genotypic characterization of tetracycline-and oxytetracycline-resistant *Aeromonas hydrophila* from cultured channel catfish (*Ictalurus punctatus*) and their environments. Applied and Environmental Microbiology 54 (7), 1861–1863.

Eaton, A.D., Clesceri, L.S., Greenberg, A.E., Franson, M.A.H., 2005. Standard methods for the examination of water and wastewater. American public health association 1015, 49–51.

El-Taweel, G.E., Shaban, A.M., 2001. Microbiological quality of drinking water at eight water treatment plants. International Journal of Environmental Health Research 11 (4), 285–290.

Enany, M.E., Shalaby, A.M., Shabanaa, I.I., EL-Gammal, A.M., Hassan, M.E., 2013. Characterization of *Aeromonas hydrophila* complex isolated from foods of animal origin. Suez Canal Veterinary Medicine Journal 18 (2), 165–176.

Ewing, W.H., Hugh, R., Johnson, J.G., 1961. Studies on the Aeromonas Group. U.S. Dep. Health Educ. Welfare, Public Health Serv. Communicable Disease Center, Atlanta, Georgia, p. 37.

FAO, 2016. The State of World Fisheries and Aquaculture 2016. Contributing to Food Security and Nutrition for All, p. 200. Rome.

Figueira, V., Vaz-Moreira, I., Silva, M., Manaia, C.M., 2011. Diversity and antibiotic resistance of *Aeromonas* spp. in drinking and waste water treatment plants. Water Research 45 (17), 5599–5611.

Figueras, M.J., 2005. Clinical relevance of *Aeromonas* sM503. Reviews in Medical Microbiology 16 (4), 145–153.

Figueras, M.J., Suarez-Franquet, A., Chacon, M.R., Soler, L., Navarro, M., Alejandre, C., Grasa, B., Martinez-Murcia, A.J., Guarro, J., 2005. First record of the rare species *Aeromonas culicicola* from a drinking water supply. Applied and Environmental Microbiology 71 (1), 538–541.

Fosse, T., Giraud-Morin, C., Madinier, I., 2003. Phenotypes of beta-lactam resistance in the genus *Aeromonas*. Pathologie Biologie 51 (5), 290–296.

Galindo, C.L., Sha, J., Ribardo, D.A., Fadl, A.A., Pillai, L., Chopra, A.K., 2003. Identification of *Aeromonas hydrophila* cytotoxic enterotoxin-induced genes in macrophages using microarrays. Journal of Biological Chemistry 278 (41), 40198–40212.

Ghenghesh, K.S., Ahmed, S.F., El-Khalek, R.A., Al-Gendy, A., Klena, J., 2008. *Aeromonas*-associated infections in developing countries. The Journal of Infection in Developing Countries 2 (02), 081–098.

Goñi-Urriza, M., Pineau, L., Capdepuy, M., Roques, C., Caumette, P., Quentin, C., 2000. Antimicrobial resistance of mesophilic *Aeromonas* spp. isolated from two European rivers. Journal of Antimicrobial Chemotherapy 46 (2), 297–301.

Gray, S.J., 1984. *Aeromonas hydrophila* in livestock: incidence, biochemical characteristics and antibiotic susceptibility. Epidemiology and Infection 92 (3), 365–375.

Harikrishnan, R., Balasundaram, C., 2005. Modern trends in *Aeromonas hydrophila* disease management with fish. Reviews in Fisheries Science 13 (4), 281–320.

Hatha, M., Vivekanandhan, A.A., Joice, G.J., 2005. Antibiotic resistance pattern of motile aeromonads from farm raised fresh water fish. International Journal of Food Microbiology 98 (2), 131–134.

Hill, K.R., Caselitz, F.H., Moody, L.M., 1954. A case of acute, metastatic, myositis caused by a new organism of the family pseudomonadaceae: a preliminary report. West Indian Medical Journal 3 (1), 9–11.

Holmberg, S.D., Schell, W.L., Fanning, G.R., Wachsmuth, I.K., Hickman-brenner, F.W., Blake, P.A., Brenner, D.J., Farmer, J.3., 1986. *Aeromonas* intestinal infections in the United States. Annals of Internal Medicine 105 (5), 683–689.

Janda, J.M., Abbott, S.L., 1998. Evolving concepts regarding the genus *Aeromonas*: an expanding panorama of species, disease presentations, and unanswered questions. Clinical Infectious Diseases 27 (2), 332–344.

Joseph, S.W., 2000. Update on the genus *Aeromonas*. ASM news 66, 218–223.

Kırkan, Ş., Göksoy, E.Ö., Kaya, O., 2003. Isolation and antimicrobial susceptibility of *Aeromonas salmonicida* in rainbow trout (*Oncorhynchus mykiss*) in Turkey hatchery farms. Journal of Veterinary Medicine Series B 50 (7), 339–342.

Kümmerer, K., 2009. Antibiotics in the aquatic environment-a review-part I. Chemosphere 75 (4), 417—434.

Lehane, L., Rawlin, G.T., 2000. Topically acquired bacterial zoonoses from fish: a review. The Medical journal of Australia 173 (5), 256—259.

Leung, K.Y., Yeap, I.V., Lam, T.J., Sin, Y.M., 1995. Serum resistance as a good indicator for virulence in *Aeromonas hydrophila* strains isolated from diseased fish in South-East Asia. Journal of Fish Diseases 18 (6), 511—518.

Lukkana, M., Wongtavatchai, J., Chuanchuen, R., 2011. Class 1 integrons in *Aeromonas hydrophila* isolates from farmed Nile tilapia (*Oreochromis nilotica*). Journal of Veterinary Medical Science 74, 435—440.

Morandi, A., Zhaxybayeva, O., Gogarten, J.P., Graf, J., 2005. Evolutionary and diagnostic implications of intragenomic heterogeneity in the 16S rRNA gene in *Aeromonas* strains. Journal of Bacteriology 187 (18), 6561—6564.

Morena, M.L.D.L., Van, R., Singh, K., Brian, M., Murray, B.E., Pickering, L.K., 1993. Diarrhea associated with *Aeromonas* species in children in day care centers. Journal of Infectious Diseases 168 (1), 215—218.

Obi, C.L., Bessong, P.O., 2002. Diarrhoeagenic bacterial pathogens in HIV-positive patients with diarrhoea in rural communities of Limpopo province, South Africa. Journal of Health, Population and Nutrition 230—234.

Özbaş, Z.Y., Lehner, A., Wagner, M., 2000. Development of a multiplex and semi-nested PCR assay for detection of Yersinia enterocolitica and Aeromonas hydrophila in raw milk. Food Microbiology 17 (2), 197—203.

Palú, A.P., Gomes, L.M., Miguel, M.A.L., Balassiano, I.T., Queiroz, M.L.P., Freitas-Almeida, A.C., de Oliveira, S.S., 2006. Antimicrobial resistance in food and clinical *Aeromonas* isolates. Food Microbiology 23 (5), 504—509.

Picão, R.C., Poirel, L., Demarta, A., Silva, C.S.F., Corvaglia, A.R., Petrini, O., Nordmann, P., 2008. Plasmid-mediated quinolone resistance in *Aeromonas allosaccharophila* recovered from a Swiss lake. Journal of Antimicrobial Chemotherapy 62 (5), 948—950.

Popoff, M., 1984. Genus III: *Aeromonas* Kluyver and van Niel 1936. Bergey's manual of systematic bacteriology 1, 545—548.

Rajakumar, S., Ayyasamy, P.M., Shanthi, K., Song, Y.C., Lakshmanaperumalsamy, P., 2012. Incidence, survival and antibiotic resistance of *Aeromonas hydrophila* isolated from lamb and chicken meat retail outlets. Journal of Current Perspectives in Applied Microbiology ISSN 2278, 1250.

Roberts, T.A., Tompkin, R.B., Baird-Parker, A.C., 1996. Microorganisms in Foods 5: Microbiological Specifications of Food Pathogens. Chapman & Hall.

Seshadri, R., Joseph, S.W., Chopra, A.K., Sha, J., Shaw, J., Graf, J., Haft, D., Wu, M., Ren, Q., Rosovitz, M.J., Madupu, R., 2006. Genome sequence of *Aeromonas hydrophila* ATCC 7966T: jack of all trades. Journal of Bacteriology 188 (23), 8272—8282.

Shotts, E.B., Rimler, R., 1973. Medium for the isolation of *Aeromonas hydrophila*. Applied Microbiology 26 (4), 550—553.

Sinha, S., Shimada, T., Ramamurthy, T., Bhattacharya, S.K., Yamasaki, S., Takeda, Y., Nair, G.B., 2004. Prevalence, serotype distribution, antibiotic susceptibility and genetic profiles of mesophilic *Aeromonas* species isolated from hospitalized diarrhoeal cases in Kolkata, India. Journal of Medical Microbiology 53 (6), 527—534.

Stanier, R.Y., 1943. A note on the taxonomy of *Proteus hydrophilus*. Journal of Bacteriology 46 (2), 213.

Stine, O.C., Carnahan, A., Singh, R., Powell, J., Furuno, J.P., Dorsey, A., Silbergeld, E., Williams, H.N., Morris, J.G., 2003. Characterization of microbial communities from coastal waters using microarrays. Environmental Monitoring and Assessment 81 (1—3), 327—336.

Stratev, D., Vashin, I., Daskalov, H., 2013. Antimicrobial resistance of β-haemolytic *Aeromonas hydrophila* strains isolated from rainbow trouts (*Oncorhynchus mykiss*). Bulgarian Journal of Veterinary Medicine 16 (4), 289—296.

Taneja, N., Khurana, S., Trehan, A., Marwaha, R.K., Sharma, M., 2004. An outbreak of hospital acquired diarrhea due to *Aeromonas sobria*. Indian Pediatrics 41 (9), 912—916.

Thayumanavan, T., Vivekanandhan, G., Savithamani, K., Subashkumar, R., Lakshmanaperumalsamy, P., 2003. Incidence of haemolysin-positive and drug-resistant *Aeromonas hydrophila* in freshly caught finfish and prawn collected from major commercial fishes of coastal South India. FEMS Immunology and Medical Microbiology 36 (1—2), 41—45.

United States Environmental Protection Agency, 2001. Method 1605. Aeromonas in Finished Water by Membrane Filtration Using Ampicillin-Dextrin Agar with Vancomycin (ADA-V). United States Environmental Protection Agency, Washigton, DC, USA.

United States Environmental Protection Agency, 2006. *Aeromonas*: Human Health Criteria Document, Office of Science and Technology. United States Protection Agency, Washigton, DC, USA.

Vivekanandhan, G., Savithamani, K., Hatha, A.A.M., Lakshmanaperumalsamy, P., 2002. Antibiotic resistance of Aeromonas hydrophila isolated from marketed fish and prawn of South India. International Journal of Food Microbiology 76 (1—2), 165—168.

von Graevenitz, A., Mensch, A.H., 1968. The genus *Aeromonas* in human bacteriology: report of 30 cases and review of the literature. New England Journal of Medicine 278 (5), 245—249.

Walsh, T.R., Stunt, R.A., Nabi, J.A., MacGowan, A.P., Bennett, P.M., 1997. Distribution and expression of beta-lactamase genes among *Aeromonas* spp. Journal of Antimicrobial Chemotherapy 40 (2), 171—178.

Wang, G., Clark, C.G., Liu, C., Pucknell, C., Munro, C.K., Kruk, T.M., Caldeira, R., Woodward, D.L., Rodgers, F.G., 2003. Detection and characterization of the hemolysin genes in *Aeromonas hydrophila* and *Aeromonas sobria* by multiplex PCR. Journal of Clinical Microbiology 41 (3), 1048—1054.

Xia, R., Guo, X., Zhang, Y., Xu, H., 2010. qnrVC-like gene located in a novel complex class 1 integron harboring the ISCR1 element in an *Aeromonas punctata* strain from an aquatic environment in Shandong Province, China. Antimicrobial Agents and Chemotherapy 54 (8), 3471—3474.

Yanez, M.A., Catalán, V., Apraiz, D., Figueras, M.J., Martinez-Murcia, A.J., 2003. Phylogenetic analysis of members of the genus *Aeromonas* based on gyrB gene sequences. International Journal of Systematic and Evolutionary Microbiology 53 (3), 875—883.

Yucel, N., Çitak, S., 2003. The occurrence, hemolytic activity and antibiotic susceptibility of motile *Aeromonas spp.* isolated from meat and milk samples in Turkey. Journal of Food Safety 23 (3), 189—200.

Chapter 25

Mycobacterium

Chapter outline

Tuberculosis is considered as most deadly infection causing 10.4 million new cases in a year around the world with 1.4 million deaths in recent times (WHO, 2016). Koch (1882) isolated mycobacteria and established its etiologic relationship with tuberculosis. He stained the bacteria with alkaline methylene blue and vesuvin. Titford (2010) developed acid fast stain for better visualization of the bacteria. The staining technique was further modified by Ziehl and Neelsen, accordingly it is known as Z-N staining. Koch (1890) prepared a glycerine broth extract of the tubercle bacillus ('tuberculin') as a therapeutic agent which was later used in diagnosis.

The major pathogenic group *M. tuberculosis* complex was originated 40,000 years ago in East Africa which later subdivided into two different clades, one remained confined in human while the other spread from human to animals (Wirth et al., 2008). The earliest scientific documentation of tuberculosis both in human and animals was detected in 3000 B.C (Taylor et al., 2005). The animal related clade is associated with ruminants and is known as bovine tuberculosis. Bovine tuberculosis was originated in Italy (Europe) and spread to United Kingdom (UK) and throughout the world during export of infected cattle from UK to their colonies (Myers and Steele, 1969; Renwick et al., 2007). In post colonial era, Europe remained major exporter of livestock to different low- and middle-income group of countries such as Africa along with animal related lineage of tuberculosis bacilli. During 2015–16, 89 countries throughout the world declared the presence of tubercle bacilli in their animals (OIE, 2018).

The animal associated clade causing bovine tuberculosis (*M. bovis* and *M. caprae*) not only affects adversely the livestock health but also produces negative impact on profitability, trait and genetic improvement programs with an estimated economic loss of over $ three billion annually (Steele, 1995; Boland et al., 2010). It can also cause zoonosis (zoonotic tuberculosis) in human during close contact or consumption of contaminated animal products (Cosivi et al., 1998). Globally zoonotic tuberculosis caused 121,268 new cases with an estimated 10,545 deaths in 2010 (WHO, 2015). It is rare in occurrence in developed countries due to proper control of the infection in cattle. Presence of reservoir/spillover hosts, certain ethnic groups (Hispanics and Mexicans in United States) was correlated with maintenance of bovine tuberculosis in high income countries such as USA (median: 0.3%), Europe (Austria, Germany, Greece, Spain; median: 0.4%), Australia and New Zealand (median: 0.2%) (Torgerson and Torgerson, 2010; Müller et al., 2013). In San Diego

California (USA), *M. bovis* infection in human accounts for 45% of tuberculosis cases in children and 6% of adult cases (Rodwell et al., 2010). Lack of control measures (slaughter house inspection and milk pasteurization), human behavior and high prevalence of HIV was found responsible for higher occurrence of bovine tuberculosis in low income countries such as Africa (median: 2.8%; Michel et al., 2010; Müller et al., 2013). Zoonotic tuberculosis is primarily characterized by tuberculous lymphadenitis in the cervical region ('scrofula' or extrapulomanry tuberculosis). In ancient times, 'scrofula' was known as 'King's evil' due to the faith on King's touch in curing the menace. During 19th century, Bollinger, May and Demme first observed the role of *M. bovis* in causing 'scrofula' in human. Prevalence of extrapulmonary tuberculosis was 8.3%−13.1% throughout the world in 2002 and is increasing specially in immunosuppressed/HIV patients in low- and middle-income countries (Arora and Chopra, 2007).

Use of streptomycin as mono-therapeutic agent against tuberculosis since 1944 caused the emergence of drug resistance in clinical bacterial isolates (Wolinsky et al., 1948). To combat the menace successfully multi-drug therapy with different antibiotics was introduced. As a consequence, multidrug-resistant tuberculosis (MDR-TB) bacteria (resistant against rifampicin and isoniazid) and extensively drug-resistant tuberculosis (XDR-TB) bacteria (also resistant against fluoroquinolone and one of the three injectable drugs kanamycin, capreomycin and amikacin) appeared globally. The isoniazid resistance in *M. tuberculosis* was detected in 10.3% of new cases, 27.7% of treated cases and 13.3% in combined cases (Wright et al., 2009).

Properties

Morphology: *Mycobacterium* is gram positive, straight or slightly curved rods with occasional coccobacillary, club and branched forms. In the tissues, it measures 1−4 µm in length and 0.2−0.3 µm in width. It occurs singly, in pair or in bundle. They are non-motile, uncapsulated and non-sporing in nature. It is difficult to demonstrate their gram-positive nature due to high lipid content of the cell wall. The stains are relatively impermeable to the bacterial cell. They are better stained with Ziehl-Neelsen (ZN) or acid-fast stain.

The bacterial cell contains cytoplasmic membrane, periplasmic space, peptidoglycan and lipids. The outer most layer is made of a ribbon like structure, known as 'mycoside', composed of glycolipids and peptidoglycolipids. The mycoside determines the colony characteristics, serological properties, and helps in intracellular survival. The layer of long chain mycolic acid and their esters is present below mycoside. The mycolic acids are β hydroxy acids substituted at α-position with alipathic chain and are responsible for acid fastness. It is attached with the underlying peptidoglycan layer by arabinogalactans (arabinose and galactan). The peptidoglycan is composed of N-glycosyl muramic acid and N-glycosyl glucosamine. Mycobacterial peptidoglycan has adjuvant property.

Classification: The genus *Mycobacterium* (Actinomycetes family) consists of more than 100 species. Among them, some are pathogenic for man and animals which grow slowly in artificial media in laboratory than the others. Recent taxonomic classification shows that slow growing mycobacterial group (pathogenic) is composed of several species. Among them the most widespread is *M. tuberculosis* complex (MTBC), comprising of *M. tuberculosis, M. bovis, M. caprae, M. microrti, M.* africanum and others. The species/sub-species under MTBC is also referred as 'ecotype' based on 16S ribosomal RNA sequences and nucleotide similarity at whole-genome level. Human tuberculosis is caused by *M. tuberculosis sensu stricto* and *M. africanum* (restricted to Africa). Animal adapted species of MTBC include *M. bovis* (cattle), *M. caprae* (sheep and goats), *M. pinnipedii* (seals, see lions), *M. mungi* (mangoose), *M. orygis* (antelope) and *M. microti* (voles). *M. canettii* and other smooth tuberculosis bacilli were earlier included in this complex but later it was re-classified as 'environmental *Mycobacterium*' (Koeck et al., 2011).

M. tuberculosis and *M. africanum* are further subdivided into lineages based on molecular signatures and geographical locations. *M. tuberculosis* has four lineages such as lineage 1 (Indo-Oceanic), lineage 2 (East-Asian Lineage, including 'Beijing' family), lineage 3 (East African Indian, including 'Delhi/CAS' family) and lineage 4 (Euro-American) (Filliol et al., 2003; Gagneux et al., 2006). The 'Beijing' lineage of *M. tuberculosis* was created on characteristic IS*6110*-RFLP patterns (Van Soolingen et al., 1995). The 'Beijing' and 'Delhi/CAS' lineages were found to be associated with MDR/XDR TB in China, India, Pakistan and other South-Asian countries (Hasan et al., 2010). Similarly, *M. bovis* was classified into three clonal complexes viz. African 1 (Af1, Cameroon, Nigeria, Chad, Mali), African 2 (Af2, East Africa) and European 1 (Eu1, Republic of Ireland, UK, France, Portugal, Spain, USA, Canada, South Africa, Australia and New Zealand) (Berg et al., 2011; Smith et al., 2011). The specific chromosomal deletion was the basis for the creation of Af1 (absence of spacer 30 in spoligotype pattern) and Af2 (absence of spacers three to seven in spoligotype pattern) clonal complexes.

M. avium-intracellulare complex (MAC), composed of *M. avium* and *M. intracellulare* is the major group of environmental *Mycobacterium*. *M. avium* is subdivided into four subspecies (ssp.) i.e., ssp. *avium* (Maa), ssp. *paratuberculosis* (Map), ssp. *silvaticum* and ssp. *hominissuis*. Among non-tuberculous mycobacteria the MAC is the common cause of lymphadenitis in human patients (O'brien et al., 2000). *M. avium* ssp. *paratuberculosis* (Map) is the etiological agent of paratuberculosis or Johne's disease in ruminants and Crohn disease in human patients.

Susceptibility to disinfectants: Mycobacteria are susceptible to ionic detergents and phenolic disinfectants.

Natural habitat: Infected animals and human are the major sources of *Mycobacterium* in the environment. Survival of the bacteria in soil and water for prolonged period occurs due to impermeable cell wall and slow growth nature. Cattle, buffaloes and goats act as maintenance host (reservoir) of *M. bovis*, while pigs, cats, dogs, horses and sheep are considered as 'spillover'. The wildlife such as baboon, black bear, cheetah and lion are spillovers of *M. bovis* and the badger (*Meles meles*) in the United Kingdom and the Republic of Ireland, brushtail possum (*Trichosurus vulpecula*) in New Zealand, European wild boar (*Sus scrofa*) in Iberian Peninsula, and white-tailed deer (*Odocoileus virginianus*) in the United States are established maintenance hosts (Carstensen and DonCarlos, 2011).The demarcation of spillover or maintenance hosts as per the animal species is not precise as it varies with the ecosystem. For example, the same white-tailed deer acts as maintenance host in Michigan (USA) and as spillover in Minnesota (USA) (Schmitt et al., 2002; Carstensen and DonCarlos, 2011). The spillovers can maintain the infection in presence of maintenance hosts while it may or may not transmit the infection further. For maintenance hosts the bacteria can persist without the presence of re-infection source. The bovine tuberculosis control strategy thus is aimed against the maintenance hosts. Presence of wildlife spillovers such as elk and bison in USA, and possums in New Zealand has created difficulties in eradication program (Nishi et al., 2006; Ramsey et al., 2009).

MAC can be isolated from soil, wastewater, water tank, municipal water, aerosols, protozoa, deep litter, fresh tropical vegetation in addition to the animals and human. MAC can utilize variable nutrients for their growth. Natural reservoirs of MAC members include domestic birds, chickens, cattle, swine, farmed deer, sheep, goats, horses, dogs and cats. Wildlife like white tailed deer, bison, boar, wild rabbit act as reservoirs of *M. avium* ssp. *paratuberculosis* and wild boar, deer, kangaroo are the reservoirs of *M. avium* ssp. *avium*.

Genome

There are several databases available with information on genome of MTBC and its variations such as *M. tuberculosis* variome resource (tbvar), *M. tuberculosis* clinical isolates genetic polymorphism database (MTCID), Mycobacterial genome divergence database (MGDD) and tuberculosis database (TBDB). The complete genome sequences of *M. tuberculosis* H37Rv, *M. bovis* AF2122/97 and *M. bovis* BCG are published (Cole et al., 1998; Garnier et al., 2003; Brosch et al., 2007). The genome of *M. tuberculosis* (H37Rv) is 4,411,529 bp in size and it has very high guanine-cytosine (GC) content. The genome contains more than 4000 genes with biased amino-acid content of the proteins due to high GC content (Cole et al., 1998). Among several other proteins encoded by the MTBC genome, putative transmembrane proteins, known as MmpL (*Mycobacterium* membrane protein large) acts as efflux system and is associated with fatty acid transport. The MmpL7 is also associated with antibiotic efflux (isoniazid) in *M. smegmatis* generating resistance (Pasca et al., 2005). The genome plasticity of MTBC is attributed to gene deletion, duplication and single nucleotide polymorphism. The gene duplication occurs multiple times independently in different MTBC lineages (Weiner et al., 2012). *M. leprae* genome contains interrupted coding sequences (30% of the genome) which causes genome decay, pseudogenization and consequently reduction in genome size. The reduction in genome size makes *M. leprae* more pathogenic and dependent on the host (Cole et al., 2001).

Antigenic characteristics

The 'proteins from *M. bovis*' (MPB-70/83) and 'proteins from *M. tuberculosis*' (MPT-70/83) are major antigens. MPB83 is a glycosylated cell wall-associated protein while MPB-70 is a secreated protein. MPB-70 was originally extracted from *M. bovis* BCG strains and certain BCG strains such as Tokyo, Moreau, Russia, Sweden, Birkhaug (Bergen) and Romania (Cantacuzinho) express high level of the antigen. The vaccination with BCG strains producing high amount of MPB-70/83 was found to cause post vaccination complications such as osteitis (Lotte et al., 1984). Expression of MPB 70/83 was correlated with the virulence of the field strains (*M. bovis*) as it helps to adhere with osteoblasts through OSFII (Harboe and Nagai, 1984; Takeshita et al., 1993). MPBs are encoded by two genes within an operon of six genes.

Toxins and virulence factors produced

Major virulence factors produced by *Mycobacterium* are described in Table 25.1.

TABLE 25.1 Major virulence factors produced by *Mycobacterium*.

Virulence factors	Function
Mycoside	Antiphagocytic
Dimycolyl trehalose or Trehalose-6-6'-dimycolate (cord factor)	It stimulates the granuloma formation, used as an adjuvant. It can also inhibit chemotaxis by neutrophils and disrupts mitochondria causing inhibition of oxidative phosphorylation.
Sulfolipid and phospholipid (phosphatidylinositol mannoside)	It prevents respiratory burst, phagolysosome fusion, disrupts reactive oxygen intermediate function; thus helps in intracellular survival of the bacteria.
Phenolic glycolipid (PGL) e.g., Phthiocerol dimycocerosates (PDIMs) and glycosylphenol-PDIM	It prevents production of pro-inflammatory cytokines. It can detoxify oxygen radicals and helps bacteria in intracellular survival.
Heparin binding haemagglutinin (HBHA)	Adhesion with host cells
Glycopeptidolipid (Glycopeptidolipids typically consist of a lipopeptide core that is N-linked to a mono-or di-unsaturated long chain fatty acid)	It can activate antigen presenting cells as adjuvant that mediate CD1 expression through Toll-like receptor 2
Heat shock protein (α-crystalline, HSP 65)	It protects bacteria from the reactive oxygen intermediates, myeloperoxidase during respiratory burst of the macrophages. It helps in intracellular survival of the bacteria
Catalase (KATG)	It lyses reactive oxygen intermediates (ROI) and prevents phagocytosis.
Fibronectin binding protein	It binds fibronectin making it unavailable for binding and activation of T cells and macrophages.
ESAT-6, CFP 10	They are highly immunogenic T- cell antigen and help in phagosomal evasion. It is encoded by RD-1 region of the genome
Ag85A, Ag85B	Mycolyl transferase enzymes associated with coupling of mycolic acids with arabinogalactan
noxR1, noxR3, ahpC	Antioxidant enzymes and it helps in intracellular survival of the bacteria
The dosRS (also known as devRS)	Helps in survival of the bacteria under hypoxic condition

Transmission

M. bovis is excreted through urine, faeces, milk and semen of infected animals and thus it can contaminate the pastures. Even the ticks of the infected cattle can carry the infection. *M. bovis* is transmitted between cattle and other animals through inhalation, ingestion and vertical way. The inhalation is the most common route of transmission between the animals (Cassidy, 2006). Inhalation of droplets, eructation during rumination, infected dust particles can take place. Uninfected cattle can acquire the infection from pastures, where the infected cattle grazed even several weeks earlier. This survival of bacteria in pastures is increased during hot and humid weather. Pseudo-vertical transmission is another rare possible route that occurs through ingestion of tuberculous milk typically containing 10^3 cfu/mL of bacteria. Earlier studies in India and Uganda (Africa) indicated genetic resistance of zebu cattle against tuberculosis (Hutt, 1958). Later studies confirmed the association between the polymorphic variations in BoLA DRB allele/DC-SIGN and tuberculosis resistance in cattle (Casati et al., 1995; Yamakawa et al., 2008).

Currently more than 40 wildlife species can harbour *M. bovis* from where it can be transmitted into domestic animals through direct contact, inhalation and predation (Zanella et al., 2008). The recognized predisposing factors for transmission into cattle herd from wildlife are stocking density, grazing methods (rotational versus strip), farm habitat, sharing common feed and water in pasture or farm, spreading of slurry, use of silage clamps etc (Griffin et al., 1993; Ward et al., 2010).

In the ancient times, nodules ('TB-grapes') observed in the lungs and mesentery of tuberculous cattle were considered as potential source of infection. In human, *M. bovis* is mostly transmitted through ingestion of unpasteurized dairy products or direct contact during slaughter or post mortem (Robinson et al., 1988; Grange, 2001). Movement of infected cattle between the continents helps in spreading the infection globally. Implementation of strict control policy such as 'test-and-slaughter' is lacking in some countries due to high cost which helps in spread and establishment of the infection (Cosivi et al., 1998). Exposure to *M. bovis* infected wildlife such as white-tailed deer, possums and elk also produced human infection (Fanning and Edwards, 1991; Wilkins et al., 2003). Human to human transmission of *M. bovis* is rare in occurrence and is observed in immunocompromised persons (Sunder et al., 2009). Reverse transmission of *M. bovis* from human to cattle is also documented (Fritsche et al., 2004).

Diagnosis

Ante mortem clinical specimens from *M. bovis* suspected cattle include saliva, aspirates from cavities, lymph nodes, biopsies and milk. The organs such as lymph nodes (submandibular, retropharyngeal, tracheobronchial, mediastinal, mesenteric), lungs, liver and spleen in 10% formalin are collected aseptically as post mortem samples. All the specimens should be immediately sent to the laboratory following the authentic rules and regulations for sending biohazardous substances. If there is delay in sending, refrigeration (4–6°C) of the samples should be done to prevent the growth of contaminants (Comer, 1994). If the refrigerator is not available, addition of 0.5% boric acid can prevent the contamination for 1 week.

Laboratory examination

As *M. bovis* is an OIE risk group 3 organisms (organisms that cause severe human or animal diseases and may spread into the community or animal population but for which effective prophylaxis and treatment are available) the laboratory should have suitable facilities and permission from the competent authority to handle such types of organisms.

Direct examination: A smear can be prepared from collected samples or tissue and stained by Ziehl-Neelsen method. *Mycobacterium* appears as red coloured slender rods singly or in bundle. The auramine-O staining followed by fluorescence microscopy was detected as more specific and sensitive than ZN staining (Marais et al., 2008). Confirmation of tuberculosis by direct examination requires high bacterial load in the collected samples although it is fastest, cheapest and simplest way for primary identification.

Isolation of *Mycobacterium*: This is considered as 'gold standard' method for detection of *Mycobacterium* although isolation is difficult from blood, urine and cerebrospinal fluids and the procedure is time consuming. The collected tissue samples are homogenized for 4–16 h with hypochlorite solution (1:1000). It is decontaminated with 5% oxalic acid and sulphuric acid, 2%–4% sodium hydroxide or 0.375%–0.75% hexadecylpyridinium chloride (HPC, cetylpyridinium chloride) and benzylkonium chloride. The acid or alkali mixture is neutralized, centrifuged and the sediment is used for culture.

A slope of the solid medium is prepared into a tightly screw capped glass tube for inoculation. Minimum 8–12 weeks of incubation at 37°C is required (Corner et al., 2012). The commonly used media are Lowenstein-Jensen (LJ), Herrold's, tuberculosis blood-agar (B83) and Middlebrook's agar (7H10, 7H11). The recommended liquid medium is Middlebrook (7H9). Glycerol can stimulate the growth of *M. tuberculosis* (eugonic), not *M. bovis* (dysgonic). Stonebrink's medium, containing inspissated egg with malachite green to prevent the contaminant can be used for isolation of *M. bovis*. The smooth, non-pigmented buffy or off-white coloured colonies are produced by *M. bovis*. In liquid medium it forms fungus like pellicle at top layer unless tween-80 is added to reduce the surface tension. Broth based culture systems such as BACTEC, Mycobacteria growth indicator tube (BACTEC MGIT) and VersaTREK are used currently which can detect the bacteria precisely in shorter time. The detection is carried out by radiometric method (BACTEC), fluorescence (BACTEC MGIT) or pressure change due to production of gas (VersaTREK) (Gormley et al., 2014).

Postmortem examination: The bronchitis followed by formation of 'tubercle' in lungs, lymph nodes, spleen and female genitalia are detected in *M. bovis* infected cattle. The 'tubercle' is typical abscess with necrotic foci, yellowish in colour, caseous or calcified in consistency. The surveillance of slaughter house for detection of post mortem lesions can be used as an alternative cost-effective approach for detection of bovine tuberculosis. The sensitivity of surveillance is although low (28%, USDA, 2009) but can be improved with proper training of slaughterhouse workers or inspectors.

Immunological tests

(a) Tuberculin skin test (TST): Tuberculin skin test is commonly used as a herd test in bovine tuberculosis eradication program or international trade (Dawson and Trapp, 2004). Tuberculin is mycobacterial extract, protein in nature, originally prepared by Robert Koch for treatment of tuberculosis. The bacteria (*M. bovis* AN5 strains) are grown in synthetic glycerinated medium and the active principle is extracted by trichloro-acetic acid, known as 'purified protein derivative (PPD)'. The AN5 strain is selected for high yield of cell mass in glycerinated media. In genomic analysis, it is observed that this strain does not have any substantial difference with others in different parts of the globe. In suspected cattle, tuberculin is injected by intradermal route at mid neck (cervical intradermal test, CIT) or caudal fold of tail (caudal fold test, CFT) or two different sites at mid neck (comparative cervical test, CCT). The skin fold swelling is measured after 72 h to read the test result. In positive cases in cattle, skin fold is increased by 4 mm or more and there are clinical signs like extensive edema, exudation, necrosis, pain or inflammation of the lymphatic ducts in that region or of the lymph nodes. The sensitivity and specificity varies according to the sites of tuberculin injection, and CFT and CCT are detected as most sensitive and specific tests, respectively (Monaghan et al., 1994). Replacement of PPD with other antigen (ESAT-6) increased specificity of TST with reduced sensitivity (Pollock et al., 2003). Combined use of cocktail antigens (ESAT-6, CFP-10, Rv3615c, MPB83) produced comparable sensitivity like PPD injected TST in naturally infected cattle (Whelan et al., 2009).

In USA and New Zealand, the caudal fold test is used as primary screening test and comparative cervical test or IFN-γ release assay are used as confirmatory tests in bovine tuberculosis eradication program. In Europe (Ireland, United Kingdom, Spain, Germany, France, Italy), cervical intradermal test (CIT) or comparative cervical test (CCT) are the primary screening tests while IFN-γ release assay is considered as confirmatory (Schiller et al., 2010). In few countries such as in Spain, isolation of *M. bovis* or *M. caprae* is further required to confirm the presence of tuberculosis (OIE, 2014).

The major deficiencies of TST in cattle are false positive reaction due to infection with non-tuberculous mycobacteria, local inflammation, vaccination and human errors (De la Rua-Domenech et al., 2006). The false negative reaction takes place due to very early stage of infection, anergy, stress associated with poor nutrition, transportation, parturition, concurrent viral infection, and use of immunosuppressive drugs.

(b) Interferon-gamma (IFN-γ) release assay (IGRA): It is an OIE-recommended alternative test for international trade. T-lymphocytes from blood of *M. bovis*-infected animals are re-exposed to PPD for 16—24 h. The sensitized T-cells will release interferon gamma (IFN-γ) which is measured by ELISA. The IGRA is highly sensitive, can differentiate vaccinated and infected animals and there is no requirement for maintenance of animals. The test requires a sophisticated laboratory in the close vicinity of the collection area as rapid processing of the blood samples is required. Non-specific responses in animals (in <15 weeks old animals) due to natural killer cell activity was also detected (Olsen et al., 2005; De la Rua-Domenech et al., 2006). The specificity of the test can be improved with ESAT-6 and CFP-10 in place of PPD (Vordermeier et al., 2005).

(c) Lymphocyte proliferation assay: It is suitable for detection of *M. bovis* in whole blood freshly collected from wildlife and zoo animals.

(d) Immuno-magnetic separation (IMS): The technique selectively captures *M. bovis* cells in the clinical specimens maintaining the viability of the bacterial cells. It has comparatively higher sensitivity than TST and conventional culture techniques (Stewart et al., 2013).

Serological tests: The cell mediated immunity decreases in the later stage of *M. bovis* infection and the TST/IGRA may produce false-negative reactions. In the countries where bovine tuberculosis is not strictly controlled with proper treatment, the serological tests may be used for detection of the carriers. The MPB 70/83 is the serodominant antigen detected in *M. bovis*. No satisfactory serological test is developed due to high antigenic variations between *M. bovis* strains (Pheiffer et al., 2005). A lateral flow based test developed against various antigens showed promising results in elephants, not in buffaloes (Greenwald et al., 2009). Other serological tests developed for detection of bovine tuberculosis included fluorescence polarization assay, rapid immunochromatographic test, dual path platform assay and chemiluminescent platform assay.

Molecular Biology: Rapid identification of MTBC isolates can be made by polymerase chain reaction targeting the genes for 16S—23S rRNA, insertion sequences (IS*6110*, IS*1081*) and specific proteins (MPB70). *M. bovis* can be detected by PCR targeting a mutation in the nucleotide positions 285 in *oxy*R and 169 in *pnc*A genes. Several modifications of PCR such as ligase chain reaction, transcription mediated amplification, strand displacement amplification (SDA), nucleic acid sequence based amplification (NASBA), branched DNA (b-DNA) and line probe assay (LiPA) were developed for detection of MTBC isolates (Ganguly, 2002).

Molecular typing of MTBC is based on whole genome (restriction endonuclease analysis, PFGE) or partial genome analysis. The partial genome analysis includes the typing methods based on insertion sequences, direct repeat, polymorphic GC-rich sequences and tandem repeat; random sequences (RAPD); housekeeping genes (MLST); and single nucleotide polymorphism. Different typing methods and their troubleshootings are discussed in Table 25.2.

TABLE 25.2 Molecular typing methods of MTBC.

Typing methods	Troubleshootings
Restriction endonuclease analysis (REA)	The whole genomic DNA of *M. bovis* is cleaved with *Bst*EII, *Pvu*II and *Bcl*I enzymes into small fragments which are separated by conventional agarose gel electrophoresis. Comparison of fragment based profile can differentiate the strains. The method generates excess amount of fragments and the discrimination becomes difficult.
Pulsed field gel electrophoresis (PFGE)	Small numbers of fragments are produced which can be separated easily in a pulsed electric field. It is tedious process and it requires skilled persons to perform
Whole genome sequencing (WGS)	WGS offers highest discrimination in differentiating the isolates
Whole genome microarray	Suitable for research based work, not for routine diagnosis
Restriction fragment length polymorphism (RFLP)	The target regions include insertion sequences (IS*6110*), polymorphic GC-rich repeat sequences (PGRS), direct repeat (DR) sequences, and repetitive DNA element pUCD. The IS*6110* typing can differentiate *M. tuberculosis*, not *M. bovis* (due to low copy numbers), and it is difficult to standardize and time consuming. The PGRS-RFLP offers better discrimination in *M. bovis* due to low copy numbers of IS*6110* but the banding pattern is complex.
Spacer oligonucleotide typing (spoligotyping)	The direct repeat (DR) region of MTBC is unique and is also known as clustered regularly interspaced palindromic repeat (CRISPR). The region is interspersed with unique sequences, called spacers (25–41 bp in length). Presence or absence of spacers (43 in numbers currently) is used in spoligotyping for differentiation of MTBC strains. The data is converted into a binary code (0, 1) and is internationally accepted as a 'prefix SB/SIT' followed by four digits. Few spacers such as 14, 15, 18, 39 and 40 are erroneous. Spoligotyping has low discriminatory capacity than MIRU-VNTR typing.
Variable number tandem repeat (VNTR)/multilocus variable-number tandem repeat analysis (MLVA)	It is PCR amplification of targeted loci present in MTBC strains followed by gel electrophoresis. The first VNTR locus identified in *M. tuberculosis* was a tandem repeat. In MTBC genome, repeats are observed in intergenic regions, known as 'mycobacterial interspersed repetitive units' (MIRUs, 45–100 bp in size, 40–50 in numbers). The MIRUs are commonly used in VNTR typing currently (MIRU-VNTR typing). The technique is inexpensive, rapid, and easy to perform and produces definite results.
IS*6110*-ampliprinting	Discrimination capacity is low
Random amplified polymorphic deoxyribonucleic acid (RAPD)	Poor discriminatory capacity
Multilocus sequence typing (MLST)	It is based on sequence analysis of internal fragments (450–500 bp) present in house-keeping genes. Less variation is observed in MTBC house-keeping genes
Region of deletion (RD) typing	It is used for differentiation of species under MTBC
Single nucleotide polymorphism (SNP) typing	It is a two-step method (PCR and sequencing/PCR and REA) and time-consuming.

Characteristics of antimicrobial resistance

Intrinsic resistance

Mycolic acid containing cell wall of *Mycobacterium* is less permeable to antibiotics and chemotherapeutic agents. *M. bovis* is naturally resistant to pyrazinamide, one of the first antibiotics offered to the patients (Olea-Popelka et al., 2017). Higher degree of resistance observed in 'Beijing' lineage of *M. tuberculosis* was associated with 'intrinsic elevated mutation rate' which increased the possibilities of acquiring resistance genes (Dos Vultos et al., 2008). Elevated mutation rate is absent in lineage 1 of MTBC, although the lineage 1 possessed more *inhA* promoter regions associated with isoniazid resistance (Zhang and Yew, 2009). *M. avium-intracellulare* complex (MAC) is intrinsically resistant to macrolide (clarithromycin) due to low cell wall permeability and expression of *erm37* gene (Andini and Nash, 2006).

Isoniazid resistance

Isoniazid is a pro-drug and it requires activation through catalase/peroxidase. Activated isoniazid forms a complex with NAD and prevents InhA to synthesize mycolic acid of the bacterial cell wall. Mutation (missense/nonsense mutations, insertions, deletions, truncation, and rarely full gene deletion) in *katG*, *inhA* (or promoter regions of *katG* and *inhA*), *ahpC*, *kasA* and *ndh* are associated with isoniazid resistance in MTBC (Ramaswamy et al., 2003). Among all the studied genes, mutation in *katG* (mutation frequency 50%−95%), *inhA* (8%−43%) and *ahpC* was strongly correlated with isoniazid resistance (Hazbón et al., 2006). The fitness cost in MTBC is observed during over expression of *inhA*, not in the mutation (S315T) in *katG* (Van Doorn et al., 2006).

The common mutation observed was S315T (*katG*) which produced defective isoniazid lacking anti mycobacterial activities (Vilchèze and Jacobs, 2007). Mutation in *inhA* is common in promoter region (15C→T) specially in mono-resistant strains (Leung et al., 2006). Multidrug resistant strains (isoniazid and ethambutol) are although developed due to mutation in *inhA* in MTBC (Banerjee et al., 1994). The mutations in *ndh* (A13C and V18A) reduce the activity of NADH dehydrogenase and produce resistance against both isoniazid and ethionamide (Ramaswamy et al., 2003). Role of AhpC was elucidated as compensatory mutation and the AhpC can mimic the katG action in its absence. It helps in survival of resistant mycobacteria (Ameeruddin and Elizabeth, 2014).

The WGS indicated presence of mutations in *nat*, *accD6* and *fabD* in resistant tubercle bacilli although the precise role in unknown (Ali et al., 2015).

Rifampicin resistance

The drug binds with β-subunit of RNA polymerase in MTBC and prevents mRNA elongation. Mutation in *rpoB* (mutation frequency: 95%) in resistant bacteria changed the conformation of the enzyme and reduced its affinity for the drug (Telenti et al., 1993). Most of the mutations take place in an 81 bp 'hotspot' region (codons 507−533) which is known as 'rifampicin resistance-determining region' (RRDR). Mutations occur generally in codons 531 and 526 with few exceptions (Caws et al., 2006). Certain mutations in codons 516, 518, 522, 529 and 533 are associated with low-level resistance to rifampicin and susceptibility to rifabutin and rifalazil (Cavusoglu et al., 2004). Resistance against rifampicin in tubercle bacilli is also associated with resistance to other drugs (isoniazid).

Pyrazinamide resistance

It is also a pro drug and it needs activation by the enzyme pyrazinamidase/nicotinamidase (encoded by *pncA* in *M. tuberculosis*).The active drug (pyrazinoic acid) prevents mycobacterial membrane transport and fatty acid synthesis. Mutation in *pncA* (561 bp/82 bp region of promoter; mutation frequency: 72%−99%) or in regulatory genes is associated with pyrazinamide resistance in tubercle bacilli (Juréen et al., 2008). *M. bovis* are intrinsically resistant to pyrazinamide due to natural substitution (H57A) in *pncA* which produces non-functional pyrazinamidase/nicotinamidase enzyme (Scorpio and Zhang, 1996).

Streptomycin resistance

The drug acts on prokaryotic 16S rRNA and prevents the initiation of translation. Mutation in *rrs* or *rpsL* (K43R) producing alterations in the drug binding site is associated with streptomycin resistance (Gillespie, 2002). Low level of strteptomycin resistance was associated with mutation in *gidB* encoding methylguanosine methyltransferase for 16S rRNA (Okamoto et al., 2007).

Ethambutol resistance

The drug inhibits the synthesis of cell wall arabinogalactan in mycobacteria. Mutation in *embB* (codon 306; mutation frequency: 47%−65%) encoding mycobacterial arabinosyl transferase was associated with ethambutol resistance (Sreevatsan et al., 1997).

Fluoroquinolone resistance

The group (ciprofloxacin and ofloxacin) is the second-line of drug used in treatment of tuberculosis. Mutation in conserved region of *gyrA* (frequency: 75%−94%) and *gyrB* (quinolone resistance-determining region) in tubercle bacilli was associated with quinolone resistance. The mutation is frequent at the positions Ala-90, Asp-94, Ala-74, Gly-88 and Ser-91. Double point mutations in *gyrA* were more frequent in clinical strains of *M. tuberculosis* (Sun et al., 2008). Efflux system (ABC-type) detected in *M. tuberculosis* also contributes in resistance against quinolones (Pasca et al., 2004). A fluoroquinolone-resistance protein (MfpA) was described in *M. tuberculosis* which can bind DNA-gyrase and prevent its activity (Hegde et al., 2005).

Aminoglycoside and cyclic peptide resistance

Aminoglycosides (kanamycin and amikacin) and cyclic peptides (capreomycin and viomycin) are used as second-line of drugs in treatment of tuberculosis. Mutations (A1401G) in *rrs* (encoding 16S rRNA) and in *tlyA* (encoding rRNA methyltransferase) in tubercle bacilli were correlated with resistance against aminoglycosides and cyclic peptides, respectively (Johansen et al., 2006; Jugheli et al., 2009). The cross resistance was observed between kanamycin and amikacin or between kanamycin and capreomycin/viomycin.

Ethionamide resistance

It is a 'pro-drug' and like isoniazid it is activated to produce an adduct with NAD. The active form can inhibit NADH-dependent enoyl-ACP reductase InhA. Additionally the ethionamide also targets a glycosyl transferase (*msh*) associated with bacterial mycothiol biosynthesis (Vilchèze et al., 2008). Resistance to ethionamide is associated with mutation in *ethA* and *inhA* (Hazbón et al., 2006).

Clofazimine resistance

Clofazimine acts on mycobacteria through membrane disruption, production of reactive oxygen species and inhibition of energy production. Mutation in *rv0678* (transcription repressor for transporter MmpL5) is associated with clofazimine resistance in *M. tuberculosis* (Zhang et al., 2015).

Para-amino salicylic acid resistance

It is also a 'pro-drug' and is activated by thymidylate synthase A (ThyA). Mutation in *thyA* gene is associated with para-amino salicylic acid resistance (Rengarajan et al., 2004).

Linezolid resistance

The mutations (G2061T and G2576T) in the 23S rRNA gene were associated with linezolid resistance in *M. tuberculosis* (Hillemann et al., 2008).

Pretomanid and delamanid resistance

Pretomanid and delamanid acts on mycobacteria by inhibition of mycolic acid synthesis and production of reactive nitrogen species. Mutations in *ddn* (deazaflavin-dependent nitroreductase) and *fdg1* (F420-dependent glucose-6-phosphate dehydrogenase) are associated with resistance against pretomanid and delamanid in *M. tuberculosis* (Singh et al., 2008).

Bedaquiline resistance

Bedaquiline acts on mycobacteria by inhibition of ATP synthesis. Mutation in *atpE* (ATP synthase C chain) and *rv0678* (transcription repressor for transporter MmpL5) genes are associated with resistance against bedaquiline in *M. tuberculosis* (Andries et al., 2014).

N-geranyl-N′-(2-adamantyl) ethane-1,2-diamine (SQ109) resistance

SQ109 acts on tubercle bacilli through inhibition of mycolic acid synthesis. Mutation in *mmpL3* (membrane transporter) in *M. tuberculosis* is associated with resistance against SQ109 (Tahlan et al., 2012).

β-Lactam resistance

Association of *M. tuberculosis* penicillin-binding proteins (PBP) and broad-spectrum β-lactamase (*blaC*) and classical therapeutic failure with penicillin is recently explored (Gupta et al., 2010; Schoonmaker et al., 2014). Carbapenems and β-lactam combinations with clavulanate showed promising results due to its activity against *M. tuberculosis* PBPs and broad-spectrum β-lactamase (Kumar et al., 2012). Recent study indicates about emergence of clavulanate resistance in *M. tuberculosis* (Soroka et al., 2015).

References

Ali, A., Hasan, Z., McNerney, R., Mallard, K., Hill-Cawthorne, G., Coll, F., Nair, M., Pain, A., Clark, T.G., Hasan, R., 2015. Whole genome sequencing based characterization of extensively drug-resistant *Mycobacterium tuberculosis* isolates from Pakistan. PLoS One 10 (2), e0117771.

Ameeruddin, N.U., Elizabeth, H.L., 2014. Impact of isoniazid resistance on virulence of global and south Indian clinical isolates of *Mycobacterium tuberculosis*. Tuberculosis 94 (6), 557–563.

Andini, N., Nash, K.A., 2006. Intrinsic macrolide resistance of the *Mycobacterium tuberculosis* complex is inducible. Antimicrobial Agents and Chemotherapy 50 (7), 2560–2562.

Andries, K., Villellas, C., Coeck, N., Thys, K., Gevers, T., Vranckx, L., Lounis, N., de Jong, B.C., Koul, A., 2014. Acquired resistance of *Mycobacterium tuberculosis* to bedaquiline. PLoS One 9 (7), e102135.

Arora, V.K., Chopra, K.K., 2007. Extrapulmonary tuberculosis. Indian Journal of Tuberculosis 54, 165–167.

Banerjee, A., Dubnau, E., Quemard, A., Balasubramanian, V., Um, K.S., Wilson, T., Collins, D., de Lisle, G., Jacobs, W.R., 1994. *inhA*, a gene encoding a target for isoniazid and ethionamide in *Mycobacterium tuberculosis*. Science 263 (5144), 227–230.

Berg, S., Garcia-Pelayo, M.C., Müller, B., Hailu, E., Asiimwe, B., Kremer, K., Dale, J., Boniotti, M.B., Rodriguez, S., Hilty, M., Rigouts, L., 2011. African 2, a clonal complex of *Mycobacterium bovis* epidemiologically important in east Africa. Journal of Bacteriology 193 (3), 670–678.

Boland, F., Kelly, G.E., Good, M., More, S.J., 2010. Bovine tuberculosis and milk production in infected dairy herds in Ireland. Preventive Veterinary Medicine 93 (2–3), 153–161.

Brosch, R., Gordon, S.V., Garnier, T., Eiglmeier, K., Frigui, W., Valenti, P., Dos Santos, S., Duthoy, S., Lacroix, C., Garcia-Pelayo, C., Inwald, J.K., 2007. Genome plasticity of BCG and impact on vaccine efficacy. Proceedings of the National Academy of Sciences 104 (13), 5596–5601.

Carstensen, M., DonCarlos, M.W., 2011. Preventing the establishment of a wildlife disease reservoir: a case study of bovine tuberculosis in wild deer in Minnesota, USA. Veterinary Medicine International. https://doi.org/10.4061/2011/413240. Article ID 413240.

Casati, M.Z., Longeri, M., Polli, M., Ceriotti, G., Poli, G., 1995. BoLA class II polymorphism and immune response to *Mycobacterium bovis* antigens in vitro. Journal of Animal Breeding and Genetics 112 (1-6), 391–400.

Cassidy, J.P., 2006. The pathogenesis and pathology of bovine tuberculosis with insights from studies of tuberculosis in humans and laboratory animal models. Veterinary Microbiology 112 (2–4), 151–161.

Cavusoglu, C., Karaca-Derici, Y., Bilgic, A., 2004. In-vitro activity of rifabutin against rifampicin-resistant *Mycobacterium tuberculosis* isolates with known *rpoB* mutations. Clinical Microbiology and Infections 10 (7), 662–665.

Caws, M., Duy, P.M., Tho, D.Q., Lan, N.T.N., Farrar, J., 2006. Mutations prevalent among rifampin-and isoniazid-resistant *Mycobacterium tuberculosis* isolates from a hospital in Vietnam. Journal of Clinical Microbiology 44 (7), 2333–2337.

Cole, S., Brosch, R., Parkhill, J., Garnier, T., Churcher, C., Harris, D., Gordon, S.V., Eiglmeier, K., Gas, S., Barry III, C.E., Tekaia, F., 1998. Deciphering the biology of *Mycobacterium tuberculosis* from the complete genome sequence. Nature 393 (6685), 537.

Cole, S.T., Eiglmeier, K., Parkhill, J., James, K.D., Thomson, N.R., Wheeler, P.R., Honore, N., Garnier, T., Churcher, C., Harris, D., Mungall, K., 2001. Massive gene decay in the leprosy bacillus. Nature 409 (6823), 1007.

Comer, L.A., 1994. Post mortem diagnosis of *Mycobacterium bovis* infection in cattle. Veterinary Microbiology 40, 53–63.

Corner, L.A.L., Gormley, E., Pfeiffer, D.U., 2012. Primary isolation of *Mycobacterium bovis* from bovine tissues: conditions for maximising the number of positive cultures. Veterinary Microbiology 156 (1–2), 162–171.

Cosivi, O., Grange, J.M., Daborn, C.J., Raviglione, M.C., Fujikura, T., Cousins, D., Robinson, R.A., Huchzermeyer, H.F., De Kantor, I., Meslin, F.X., 1998. Zoonotic tuberculosis due to *Mycobacterium bovis* in developing countries. Emerging Infectious Diseases 4 (1), 59.

Dawson, B., Trapp, R.G., 2004. Basic and Clinical Biostatistics. Mcgraw-Hill Publications Company, New York.

De la Rua-Domenech, R., Goodchild, A.T., Vordermeier, H.M., Hewinson, R.G., Christiansen, K.H., Clifton-Hadley, R.S., 2006. Ante mortem diagnosis of tuberculosis in cattle: a review of the tuberculin tests, γ-interferon assay and other ancillary diagnostic techniques. Research in Veterinary Science 81 (2), 190–210.

Dos Vultos, T., Mestre, O., Rauzier, J., Golec, M., Rastogi, N., Rasolofo, V., Tonjum, T., Sola, C., Matic, I., Gicquel, B., 2008. Evolution and diversity of clonal bacteria: the paradigm of *Mycobacterium tuberculosis*. PLoS One 3 (2), e1538.

Fanning, A., Edwards, S., 1991. *Mycobacterium bovis* infection in human beings in contact with elk (*Cervus elaphus*) in Alberta, Canada. The Lancet 338 (8777), 1253–1255.

Filliol, I., Driscoll, J.R., van Soolingen, D., Kreiswirth, B.N., Kremer, K., Valétudie, G., Anh, D.D., Barlow, R., Banerjee, D., Bifani, P.J., Brudey, K., 2003. Snapshot of moving and expanding clones of *Mycobacterium tuberculosis* and their global distribution assessed by spoligotyping in an international study. Journal of Clinical Microbiology 41 (5), 1963–1970.

Fritsche, A., Engel, R., Buhl, D., Zellweger, J.P., 2004. *Mycobacterium bovis* tuberculosis: from animal to man and back. International Journal of Tuberculosis and Lung Disease 8 (7), 903–904.

Gagneux, S., DeRiemer, K., Van, T., Kato-Maeda, M., De Jong, B.C., Narayanan, S., Nicol, M., Niemann, S., Kremer, K., Gutierrez, M.C., Hilty, M., 2006. Variable host-pathogen compatibility in *Mycobacterium tuberculosis*. Proceedings of the National Academy of Sciences 103 (8), 2869–2873.

Ganguly, N.K., 2002. What is new in diagnosis of tuberculosis? part I: techniques for diagnosis of tuberculosis. ICMR Bulletin 32.

Garnier, T., Eiglmeier, K., Camus, J.C., Medina, N., Mansoor, H., Pryor, M., Duthoy, S., Grondin, S., Lacroix, C., Monsempe, C., Simon, S., 2003. The complete genome sequence of *Mycobacterium bovis*. Proceedings of the National Academy of Sciences of the United States of America 100 (13), 7877–7882.

Gillespie, S.H., 2002. Evolution of drug resistance in *Mycobacterium tuberculosis*: clinical and molecular perspective. Antimicrobial Agents and Chemotherapy 46 (2), 267–274.

Gormley, E., Corner, L.A.L., Costello, E., Rodriguez-Campos, S., 2014. Bacteriological diagnosis and molecular strain typing of *Mycobacterium bovis* and *Mycobacterium caprae*. Research in Veterinary Science 97, S30–S43.

Grange, J.M., 2001. *Mycobacterium bovis* infection in human beings. Tuberculosis 81 (1), 71–77.

Greenwald, R., Lyashchenko, O., Esfandiari, J., Miller, M., Mikota, S., Olsen, J.H., Ball, R., Dumonceaux, G., Schmitt, D., Moller, T., Payeur, J.B., 2009. Highly accurate antibody assays for early and rapid detection of tuberculosis in African and Asian elephants. Clinical and Vaccine Immunology 16 (5), 605–612.

Griffin, J.M., Hahesy, T., Lynch, K., Salman, M.D., McCarthy, J., Hurley, T., 1993. The association of cattle husbandry practices, environmental factors and farmer characteristics with the occurrence of chronic bovine tuberculosis in dairy herds in the republic of Ireland. Preventive Veterinary Medicine 17 (3–4), 145–160.

Gupta, R., Lavollay, M., Mainardi, J.L., Arthur, M., Bishai, W.R., Lamichhane, G., 2010. The *Mycobacterium tuberculosis* protein Ldt Mt2 is a non-classical transpeptidase required for virulence and resistance to amoxicillin. Nature Medicine 16 (4), 466.

Harboe, M., Nagai, S., 1984. MPB70, a unique antigen of *Mycobacterium bovis* BCG. American Review of Respiratory Disease 129 (3), 444–452.

Hasan, R., Jabeen, K., Ali, A., Rafiq, Y., Laiq, R., Malik, B., Tanveer, M., Groenheit, R., Ghebremichael, S., Hoffner, S., Hasan, Z., 2010. Extensively drug-resistant tuberculosis, Pakistan. Emerging Infectious Diseases 16 (9), 1473.

Hazbón, M.H., Brimacombe, M., del Valle, M.B., Cavatore, M., Guerrero, M.I., Varma-Basil, M., Billman-Jacobe, H., Lavender, C., Fyfe, J., García-García, L., León, C.I., 2006. Population genetics study of isoniazid resistance mutations and evolution of multidrug-resistant *Mycobacterium tuberculosis*. Antimicrobial Agents and Chemotherapy 50 (8), 2640–2649.

Hegde, S.S., Vetting, M.W., Roderick, S.L., Mitchenall, L.A., Maxwell, A., Takiff, H.E., Blanchard, J.S., 2005. A fluoroquinolone resistance protein from *Mycobacterium tuberculosis* that mimics DNA. Science 308 (5727), 1480–1483.

Hillemann, D., Rüsch-Gerdes, S., Richter, E., 2008. *In vitro*-selected linezolid-resistant *Mycobacterium tuberculosis* mutants. Antimicrobial Agents and Chemotherapy 52 (2), 800–801.

Hutt, F.B., 1958. Genetic Resistance to Disease in Domestic Animals. Constable & Company Ltd, London, UK, pp. 91–93.

Johansen, S.K., Maus, C.E., Plikaytis, B.B., Douthwaite, S., 2006. Capreomycin binds across the ribosomal subunit interface using *tlyA*-encoded 2′-O-methylations in 16S and 23S rRNAs. Molecular Cell 23 (2), 173–182.

Jugheli, L., Bzekalava, N., de Rijk, P., Fissette, K., Portaels, F., Rigouts, L., 2009. High level of cross-resistance between kanamycin, amikacin, and capreomycin among *Mycobacterium tuberculosis* isolates from Georgia and a close relation with mutations in the rrs gene. Antimicrobial Agents and Chemotherapy 53 (12), 5064–5068.

Juréen, P., Werngren, J., Toro, J.C., Hoffner, S., 2008. Pyrazinamide resistance and *pncA* gene mutations in *Mycobacterium tuberculosis*. Antimicrobial Agents and Chemotherapy 52 (5), 1852–1854.

Koch, R., 1882. Die aetiologie der tuberculose. Berliner Klinische Wochenschrift 19, 221–230.

Koch, R., 1890. I. Weitere Mittheilungen über ein Heilmittel gegen Tuberculose. DMW – Deutsche Medizinische Wochenschrift 16 (46), 1029–1032.

Koeck, J.L., Fabre, M., Simon, F., Daffe, M., Garnotel, E., Matan, A.B., Gérôme, P., Bernatas, J.J., Buisson, Y., Pourcel, C., 2011. Clinical characteristics of the smooth tubercle bacilli '*Mycobacterium canettii*' infection suggest the existence of an environmental reservoir. Clinical Microbiology and Infections 17 (7), 1013–1019.

Kumar, P., Arora, K., Lloyd, J.R., Lee, I.Y., Nair, V., Fischer, E., Boshoff, H.I., Barry III, C.E., 2012. Meropenem inhibits D, D-carboxypeptidase activity in *Mycobacterium tuberculosis*. Molecular Microbiology 86 (2), 367–381.

Leung, E.T.Y., Ho, P.L., Yuen, K.Y., Woo, W.L., Lam, T.H., Kao, R.Y., Seto, W.H., Yam, W.C., 2006. Molecular characterization of isoniazid resistance in *Mycobacterium tuberculosis*: identification of a novel mutation in *inhA*. Antimicrobial Agents and Chemotherapy 50 (3), 1075–1078.

Lotte, A., Wasz-Höckert, O., Poisson, N., Dumitrescu, N., Verron, M., Couvet, E., 1984. BCG complications. Estimates of the risks among vaccinated subjects and statistical analysis of their main characteristics. Advances in Tuberculosis Research. Fortschritte der Tuberkuloseforschung. Progres de l'exploration de la tuberculose 21, 107.

Marais, B.J., Brittle, W., Painczyk, K., Hesseling, A.C., Beyers, N., Wasserman, E., Soolingen, D.V., Warren, R.M., 2008. Use of light-emitting diode fluorescence microscopy to detect acid-fast bacilli in sputum. Clinical Infectious Diseases 47 (2), 203–207.

Michel, A.L., Müller, B., Van Helden, P.D., 2010. *Mycobacterium bovis* at the animal-human interface: a problem, or not? Veterinary Microbiology 140 (3–4), 371–381.

Monaghan, M.L., Doherty, M.L., Collins, J.D., Kazda, J.F., Quinn, P.J., 1994. The tuberculin test. Veterinary Microbiology 40 (1–2), 111–124.

Müller, B., Dürr, S., Alonso, S., Hattendorf, J., Laisse, C.J., Parsons, S.D., Van Helden, P.D., Zinsstag, J., 2013. Zoonotic *Mycobacterium bovis*-induced tuberculosis in humans. Emerging Infectious Diseases 19 (6), 899.

Myers, J.A., Steele, J.H., 1969. Bovine Tuberculosis Control in Man and Animals. Warren H. Green, Inc., St. Louis, Missouri, USA.

Nishi, J.S., Shury, T., Elkin, B.T., 2006. Wildlife reservoirs for bovine tuberculosis (*Mycobacterium bovis*) in Canada: strategies for management and research. Veterinary Microbiology 112 (2–4), 325–338.

O'brien, D.P., Currie, B.J., Krause, V.L., 2000. Nontuberculous mycobacterial disease in northern Australia: a case series and review of the literature. Clinical Infectious Diseases 31 (4), 958–967.

OIE, 2014. Manual of Diagnostic Tests and Vaccines for Terrestrial Animals: Mammals, Birds and Bees. Office international des âepizooties, Paris, p. 5.

OIE, 2018. Available at: http://www.oie.int/en/animal-health-in-the-world/animal-diseases/Bovine-tuberculosis/.

Okamoto, S., Tamaru, A., Nakajima, C., Nishimura, K., Tanaka, Y., Tokuyama, S., Suzuki, Y., Ochi, K., 2007. Loss of a conserved 7-methylguanosine modification in 16S rRNA confers low-level streptomycin resistance in bacteria. Molecular Microbiology 63 (4), 1096–1106.

Olea-Popelka, F., Muwonge, A., Perera, A., Dean, A.S., Mumford, E., Erlacher-Vindel, E., Forcella, S., Silk, B.J., Ditiu, L., El Idrissi, A., Raviglione, M., 2017. Zoonotic tuberculosis in human beings caused by *Mycobacterium bovis*-a call for action. The Lancet Infectious Diseases 17 (1), e21–e25.

Olsen, I., Boysen, P., Kulberg, S., Hope, J.C., Jungersen, G., Storset, A.K., 2005. Bovine NK cells can produce gamma interferon in response to the secreted mycobacterial proteins ESAT-6 and MPP14 but not in response to MPB70. Infection and Immunity 73 (9), 5628–5635.

Pasca, M.R., Guglierame, P., Arcesi, F., Bellinzoni, M., De Rossi, E., Riccardi, G., 2004. Rv2686c-Rv2687c-Rv2688c, an ABC fluoroquinolone efflux pump in *Mycobacterium tuberculosis*. Antimicrobial Agents and Chemotherapy 48 (8), 3175–3178.

Pasca, M.R., Guglierame, P., De Rossi, E., Zara, F., Riccardi, G., 2005. MmpL7 gene of *Mycobacterium tuberculosis* is responsible for isoniazid efflux in *Mycobacterium smegmatis*. Antimicrobial Agents and Chemotherapy 49 (11), 4775–4777.

Pheiffer, C., Betts, J.C., Flynn, H.R., Lukey, P.T., van Helden, P., 2005. Protein expression by a Beijing strain differs from that of another clinical isolate and *Mycobacterium tuberculosis* H37Rv. Microbiology 151 (4), 1139–1150.

Pollock, J.M., McNair, J., Bassett, H., Cassidy, J.P., Costello, E., Aggerbeck, H., Rosenkrands, I., Andersen, P., 2003. Specific delayed-type hypersensitivity responses to ESAT-6 identify tuberculosis-infected cattle. Journal of Clinical Microbiology 41 (5), 1856–1860.

Ramaswamy, S.V., Reich, R., Dou, S.J., Jasperse, L., Pan, X., Wanger, A., Quitugua, T., Graviss, E.A., 2003. Single nucleotide polymorphisms in genes associated with isoniazid resistance in *Mycobacterium tuberculosis*. Antimicrobial Agents and Chemotherapy 47 (4), 1241–1250.

Ramsey, D.S.L., Aldwell, F.E., Cross, M.L., De Lisle, G.W., Buddle, B.M., 2009. Protection of free-living and captive possums against pulmonary challenge with *Mycobacterium bovis* following oral BCG vaccination. Tuberculosis 89 (2), 163–168.

Rengarajan, J., Sassetti, C.M., Naroditskaya, V., Sloutsky, A., Bloom, B.R., Rubin, E.J., 2004. The folate pathway is a target for resistance to the drug para-aminosalicylic acid (PAS) in mycobacteria. Molecular Microbiology 53 (1), 275–282.

Renwick, A.R., White, P.C.L., Bengis, R.G., 2007. Bovine tuberculosis in southern African wildlife: a multi-species host–pathogen system. Epidemiology and Infection 135 (4), 529–540.

Robinson, P., Morris, D., Antic, R., 1988. *Mycobacterium bovis* as an occupational hazard in abattoir workers. Australian and New Zealand Journal of Medicine 18 (5), 701–703.

Rodwell, T.C., Kapasi, A.J., Moore, M., Milian-Suazo, F., Harris, B., Guerrero, L.P., Moser, K., Strathdee, S.A., Garfein, R.S., 2010. Tracing the origins of *Mycobacterium bovis* tuberculosis in humans in the USA to cattle in Mexico using spoligotyping. International Journal of Infectious Diseases 14, e129–e135.

Schiller, I., Oesch, B., Vordermeier, H.M., Palmer, M.V., Harris, B.N., Orloski, K.A., Buddle, B.M., Thacker, T.C., Lyashchenko, K.P., Waters, W.R., 2010. Bovine tuberculosis: a review of current and emerging diagnostic techniques in view of their relevance for disease control and eradication. Transboundary and Emerging Diseases 57 (4), 205–220.

Schmitt, S.M., O'brien, D.J., Bruning-Fann, C.S., Fitzgerald, S.D., 2002. Bovine tuberculosis in Michigan wildlife and livestock. Annals of the New York Academy of Sciences 969 (1), 262–268.

Schoonmaker, M.K., Bishai, W.R., Lamichhane, G., 2014. Non-classical transpeptidases of *Mycobacterium tuberculosis* alter cell size, morphology, cytosolic matrix, protein localization, virulence and resistance to β-lactams. Journal of Bacteriology 196 (7), 1394–1402.

Scorpio, A., Zhang, Y., 1996. Mutations in *pncA*, a gene encoding pyrazinamidase/nicotinamidase, cause resistance to the antituberculous drug pyrazinamide in tubercle bacillus. Nature Medicine 2 (6), 662.

Singh, R., Manjunatha, U., Boshoff, H.I., Ha, Y.H., Niyomrattanakit, P., Ledwidge, R., Dowd, C.S., Lee, I.Y., Kim, P., Zhang, L., Kang, S., 2008. PA-824 kills non-replicating *Mycobacterium tuberculosis* by intracellular NO release. Science 322 (5906), 1392–1395.

Smith, N.H., Berg, S., Dale, J., Allen, A., Rodriguez, S., Romero, B., Matos, F., Ghebremichael, S., Karoui, C., Donati, C., da Conceicao Machado, A., 2011. European 1: a globally important clonal complex of *Mycobacterium bovis*. Infection, Genetics and Evolution 11 (6), 1340–1351.

Soroka, D., de La Sierra-Gallay, I.L., Dubée, V., Triboulet, S., Van Tilbeurgh, H., Compain, F., Ballell, L., Barros, D., Mainardi, J.L., Hugonnet, J.E., Arthur, M., 2015. Hydrolysis of clavulanate by *Mycobacterium tuberculosis* β-lactamase BlaC harboring a canonic SDN motif. Antimicrobial Agents and Chemotherapy 59 (9), 5714–5720.

Sreevatsan, S., Stockbauer, K.E., Pan, X.I., Kreiswirth, B.N., Moghazeh, S.L., Jacobs, W.R., Telenti, A., Musser, J.M., 1997. Ethambutol resistance in *Mycobacterium tuberculosis*: critical role of *embB* mutations. Antimicrobial Agents and Chemotherapy 41 (8), 1677–1681.

Steele, J.H., 1995. Regional and country status report. In: Thoen, C.O., Steele, J.H. (Eds.), *Mycobacterium bovis* Infection in Animals and Humans. Iowa press, Ames, pp. 169–172.

Stewart, L.D., McNair, J., McCallan, L., Gordon, A., Grant, I.R., 2013. Improved detection of *Mycobacterium bovis* infection in bovine lymph node tissue using immunomagnetic separation (IMS)-based methods. PLoS One 8 (3), e58374.

Sun, Z., Zhang, J., Zhang, X., Wang, S., Zhang, Y., Li, C., 2008. Comparison of *gyrA* gene mutations between laboratory-selected ofloxacin-resistant *Mycobacterium tuberculosis* strains and clinical isolates. International Journal of Antimicrobial Agents 31 (2), 115–121.

Sunder, S., Lanotte, P., Godreuil, S., Martin, C., Boschiroli, M.L., Besnier, J.M., 2009. Human-to-human transmission of tuberculosis caused by *Mycobacterium bovis* in immunocompetent patients. Journal of Clinical Microbiology 47 (4), 1249−1251.

Tahlan, K., Wilson, R., Kastrinsky, D.B., Arora, K., Nair, V., Fischer, E., Barnes, S.W., Walker, J.R., Alland, D., Barry, C.E., Boshoff, H.I., 2012. SQ109 targets MmpL3, a membrane transporter of trehalose monomycolate involved in mycolic acid donation to the cell wall core of *Mycobacterium tuberculosis*. Antimicrobial Agents and Chemotherapy 56, 1797−1809.

Takeshita, S., Kikuno, R., Tezuka, K.I., Amann, E., 1993. Osteoblast-specific factor 2: cloning of a putative bone adhesion protein with homology with the insect protein fasciclin I. Biochemical Journal 294 (1), 271−278.

Taylor, G.M., Young, D.B., Mays, S.A., 2005. Genotypic analysis of the earliest known prehistoric case of tuberculosis in Britain. Journal of Clinical Microbiology 43 (5), 2236−2240.

Telenti, A., Imboden, P., Marchesi, F., Schmidheini, T., Bodmer, T., 1993. Direct, automated detection of rifampin-resistant *Mycobacterium tuberculosis* by polymerase chain reaction and single-strand conformation polymorphism analysis. Antimicrobial Agents and Chemotherapy 37 (10), 2054−2058.

Titford, M., 2010. Paul Ehrlich: Histological Staining, Immunology, Chemotherapy. Laboratory Medicine 41 (8), 497−498.

Torgerson, P.R., Torgerson, D.J., 2010. Public health and bovine tuberculosis: what's all the fuss about? Trends in Microbiology 18 (2), 67−72.

United States Department of Agriculture (USDA), 2009. Analysis of Bovine Tuberculosis Surveillance in Accredited Free States. Available at: https://www.aphis.usda.gov/vs/nahss/cattle/tb_2009_evaluation_of_tb_in_accredited_free_states_jan_09.pdf.

Van Doorn, H.R., De Haas, P.E.W., Kremer, K., Vandenbroucke-Grauls, C.M.J.E., Borgdorff, M.W., Van Soolingen, D., 2006. Public health impact of isoniazid-resistant *Mycobacterium tuberculosis* strains with a mutation at amino-acid position 315 of *katG*: a decade of experience in the Netherlands. Clinical Microbiology and Infections 12 (8), 769−775.

Van Soolingen, D., Qian, L., De Haas, P.E., Douglas, J.T., Traore, H., Portaels, F., Qing, H.Z., Enkhsaikan, D., Nymadawa, P., Van Embden, J.D., 1995. Predominance of a single genotype of *Mycobacterium tuberculosis* in countries of east Asia. Journal of Clinical Microbiology 33 (12), 3234−3238.

Vilchèze, C., Jacobs Jr., W.R., 2007. The mechanism of isoniazid killing: clarity through the scope of genetics. Annual Review of Microbiology 61, 35−50.

Vilchèze, C., Av-Gay, Y., Attarian, R., Liu, Z., Hazbón, M.H., Colangeli, R., Chen, B., Liu, W., Alland, D., Sacchettini, J.C., Jacobs Jr., W.R., 2008. Mycothiol biosynthesis is essential for ethionamide susceptibility in *Mycobacterium tuberculosis*. Molecular Microbiology 69 (5), 1316−1329.

Vordermeier, H.M., Pontarollo, R., Karvonen, B., Cockle, P., Hecker, R., Singh, M., Babiuk, L.A., Hewinson, R.G., van Drunen Littel-van Den, S., 2005. Synthetic peptide vaccination in cattle: induction of strong cellular immune responses against peptides derived from the *Mycobacterium bovis* antigen Rv3019c. Vaccine 23 (35), 4375−4384.

Ward, A.I., Judge, J., Delahay, R.J., 2010. Farm husbandry and badger behavior: opportunities to manage badger to cattle transmission of *Mycobacterium bovis*? Preventive Veterinary Medicine 93 (1), 2−10.

Weiner, B., Gomez, J., Victor, T.C., Warren, R.M., Sloutsky, A., Plikaytis, B.B., Posey, J.E., Van Helden, P.D., van Pittius, N.C.G., Koehrsen, M., Sisk, P., 2012. Independent large scale duplications in multiple *M. tuberculosis* lineages overlapping the same genomic region. PLoS One 7 (2), e26038.

Whelan, A., Clifford, D., Hewinson, R.G., Vordermeier, M., 2009. Development of defined skin-test reagents for diagnosis of bovine tuberculosis. In: Proceedings of M. bovis V Conference.

WHO, 2015. Estimates of the Global Burden of Foodborne Diseases. http://www.who.int/foodsafety/publications/foodborne_disease/fergreport/en/.

Wilkins, M.J., Bartlett, P.C., Frawley, B., O'Brien, D.J., Miller, C.E., Boulton, M.L., 2003. *Mycobacterium bovis* (bovine TB) exposure as a recreational risk for hunters: results of a Michigan Hunter survey, 2001. International Journal of Tuberculosis and Lung Disease 7 (10), 1001−1009.

Wirth, T., Hildebrand, F., Allix-Béguec, C., Wölbeling, F., Kubica, T., Kremer, K., van Soolingen, D., Rüsch-Gerdes, S., Locht, C., Brisse, S., Meyer, A., 2008. Origin, spread and demography of the *Mycobacterium tuberculosis* complex. PLoS Pathogens 4 (9), e1000160.

Wolinsky, E., Reginster, A., Steenken Jr., W., 1948. Drug-resistant tubercle bacilli in patients under treatment with streptomycin. American Review of Tuberculosis 58, 335−343.

World Health Organization (WHO), 2016. Global Tuberculosis Report 2016. Available at: http://apps.who.int/iris/bitstream/handle/10665/250441/97?sequence=1.

Wright, A., Zignol, M., Van Deun, A., Falzon, D., Gerdes, S.R., Feldman, K., Hoffner, S., Drobniewski, F., Barrera, L., van Soolingen, D., Boulabhal, F., 2009. Epidemiology of antituberculosis drug resistance 2002-07: an updated analysis of the global project on anti-tuberculosis drug resistance surveillance. The Lancet 373 (9678), 1861−1873.

Yamakawa, Y., Pennelegion, C., Willcocks, S., Stalker, A., MacHugh, N., Burt, D., Coffey, T.J., Werling, D., 2008. Identification and functional characterization of a bovine orthologue to DC-SIGN. Journal of Leukocyte Biology 83 (6), 1396−1403.

Zanella, G., Durand, B., Hars, J., Moutou, F., Garin-Bastuji, B., Duvauchelle, A., Fermé, M., Karoui, C., Boschiroli, M.L., 2008. *Mycobacterium bovis* in wildlife in France. Journal of Wildlife Diseases 44 (1), 99−108.

Zhang, S., Chen, J., Cui, P., Shi, W., Zhang, W., Zhang, Y., 2015. Identification of novel mutations associated with clofazimine resistance in *Mycobacterium tuberculosis*. Journal of Antimicrobial Chemotherapy 70 (9), 2507−2510.

Zhang, Y., Yew, W.W., 2009. Mechanisms of drug resistance in *Mycobacterium tuberculosis* [State of the art series. Drug-resistant tuberculosis. Edited by CY. Chiang. Number 1 in the series]. International Journal of Tuberculosis and Lung Disease 13 (11), 1320−1330.

Chapter 26

Candida

Chapter outline

Candida (previously known as *Monilia*) is imperfect unicellular dimorphic fungus which often reproduces by budding and it can produce hyphae or pseudohyphae depending on the environmental condition. Hippocrates (460–377 BC) first documented oral pseudomembranous candidiasis and he described it with the name of 'aphthae albae', which was later supported by Galen (130–200 BC). Berg and Wilkinson described oral candidiasis (1841) and vaginal candidiasis (1849), respectively, the most common clinical forms in human. *Candida albicans, Candida glabrata, Candida tropicalis* and *Candida dubliniensis* are associated with oropharyngeal and vulvovaginal candidiasis (Coleman et al., 1993; Sobel, 1998). The vulvovaginal form is more common in women infected with HIV. *C. albicans* is also associated with blood stream infection (BSI, 'candidemia'), which causes 14.5%–49% mortality in adults mostly in developed countries (Zaoutis et al., 2005; Brown et al., 2012). Mortality is correlated with biofilm-forming capabilities, resistance to antifungals of *C. albicans* and APACHE III scores (acute physiology and chronic health evaluation scores) (Tumbarello et al., 2007). In total, 2,50,000–4,00,000 deaths per annum worldwide are estimated to be associated with *C. albicans* (Kullberg and Arendrup, 2015).

Candida is one of the major (15%) nosocomial infections in intensive care unit of human health care settings (Eggimann et al., 2003). The species-wise shifting from *C. albicans* to non-albicans (non–*C. albicans Candida*, NCAC) category occurred in recent times because of use of prophylactic antifungal drugs such as azoles and echinocandins (Kullberg and Arendrup, 2015). Nosocomial fungaemia and treatment failure due to multidrug-resistant *Candida auris* is a current concern throughout the world because of higher minimum inhibitory concentration (MIC) shown against major antifungals such as fluconazole, voriconazole, echinocandin and amphotericin B (Kathuria et al., 2015). Since the first report of BSI by *C. auris* in Korea during 2011, several reports flared up from the United States, United Kingdom, South Africa, Kuwait, Brazil, Venezuela, India and Pakistan (Lee et al., 2011). Whole-genome analysis of *C. auris* indicated about low strain diversity and its recent emergence (Sharma et al., 2016). *C. glabrata* causing oral thrush to deep-seated organ infections is another NCAC which is responsible for 15% of all *Candida*-related BSIs (Bethea et al., 2010). Innate resistance of *C. glabrata* against azole group of antifungals makes the treatment difficult (Fidel et al., 1999).

Infection with multidrug-resistant *Candida* causes poor clinical outcomes, breakthrough infections in high-risk patients, prolonged length of stay in hospitals and increased treatment cost (Fridkin, 2005; Baixench et al., 2007; Pfaller et al., 2010).

Antimicrobial Resistance in Agriculture. https://doi.org/10.1016/B978-0-12-815770-1.00026-2

Properties

Morphology: There are three major morphological forms of *Candida* such as unicellular yeast, hyphae and pseudohyphae. The yeast form is oval (3.5–6µm × 6–10 µm) with axial or bipolar budding. The hyphae are long tubes consisting of the cells with parallel sides, uniform width and true septum without any constriction. The pseudohyphae are chains of elongated ellipsoidal cells with constriction between them. In the yeast and pseudohyphae, the nuclear division and septa formation takes place near the bud, whereas in hyphae both the procedures occur within the germ tube. The thick walled chlamydospores remain attached with hyphae or pseudohyphae by a suspensor cell.

The cell wall is present outside the cell membrane composed of inner and outer layers. The inner layer is a meshwork of chitin, β-(1,3)glucan and β-(1,6)glucan, which is more electron translucent. The outer layer is 150 nm width composed of mannoprotein. Three types of cell wall proteins (CWP) are present in the cell wall. The most abundant type is glyco-phosphatidylinositol (GPI) CWP, which is covalently attached with β-(1,6)glucan through GPI anchor.

The expression of morphological forms varies with the species of *Candida*. All the three forms are expressed by *C. albicans* and *C. tropicalis,* whereas other species such as *Candida parapsilosis* can express the yeast and pseudohyphae forms. *C. glabrata* can express the yeast and pseudohyphae forms but primarily a yeast form both in the environment and host tissue without any morphological switch.

The morphological switch between the yeast and filamentous form is correlated with the virulence. Several external (environmental cues) and internal factors regulate the morphological switch of *Candida*. The environmental cues include presence of serum, temperature (37°C), low levels of oxygen, high levels of CO_2 and poor nutrition. The internal factors include the filament-induced gene (*HGC1*), which encodes a cyclin-related protein required for septin phosphorylation and inhibition of cell separation. Several members of secreted aspartyl proteinase (SAP) gene family (*SAP4, SAP5, SAP6*) are also expressed during morphological switch required for invasion of host tissues. The transition from yeast to hyphal phase in *Candida* is regulated by the activation of mitogen-activated protein kinase and cAMP-protein kinase A (PKA) signal transduction pathways, which can also coordinately regulate the virulence gene expression associated with this transition. Three sensor histidine kinases (Sln1, Chk1, Nik1) also regulate the phase conversion and mutants are unable to produce hyphae. Quorum sensing (microbial communication) molecules such as farnesol, tyrosol and dodecanol are also associated with the transition.

Another type of morphological transition observed in *C. albicans* is known as white-opaque transition. In the laboratory, this switching is rare (one in every 10^4 cell division) and it is regulated by host environmental factors. The 'white' cells are relatively round and form smooth colonies on solid media, while 'opaque' cells are large and elongated and form flat and grey or opaque colonies. Certain phenotype-specific genes (*WH11, EFG1*) are expressed by white cells, while *OP4* and *SAP4* are expressed by opaque cells. White cells are more virulent and can easily colonize the host internal organs, whereas the opaque cells are associated with cutaneous infection probably because of expression of *SAP4* gene. Master regulator of this complex switching system is WOR1, which can convert the white cells into opaque cells. The host environmental factors regulating white-opaque transition are CO_2 and N-acetyl glucosamine (present in commensal bacterial cell wall and gastrointestinal tract mucus), which can produce stable opaque phenotype.

Classification: The genus *Candida* belongs to the class *Saccharomycetes* (Hemiascomycetes). It has more than 200 species. Among them 20 species are associated with candidiasis in human and animals. *C. albicans, C. tropicalis* and *C. glabrata* are the most frequently isolated from clinical specimens. The other pathogenic species are *C. parapsilosis, Candida stellatoidea, Candida guilliermondii, Candida krusei, Candida kefyr* and *Candida pseudotropicalis* (Arendrup et al., 2002).

Susceptibility to disinfectants: Crystal violet is highly effective against *C. albicans*. Among antiseptics, 4% chlorhexidine gluconate in alcohol and 10% povidone iodine have potential antifungal activity against *Candida*. The quaternary ammonium compounds (1:10,000) are lethal at short contact time.

Natural habitat: *Candida* inhabit in the mucosal layer of animals and human such as alimentary, upper respiratory and genital tracts and oral mucosa such as posterior dorsum of tongue. Same or different strains are harboured by the healthy human or animals in different body parts (Kam and Xu, 2002). The strains can undergo 'microevolution' with minor genotypical changes in a small number of cell generations or 'substrain shuffling' within the same individual over time (Lockhart et al., 1995). The strains can invade the deeper part of the tissues to establish the infection under immuno-suppressed conditions caused by prolonged antibiotic or steroid use, inflammation and breakage of epidermal layer by injury. In the intestine, yeast form of *Candida* predominates. Morphologically altered yeast cells ('gut phenotype') are also observed during passage of *C. albicans* through the intestine. These altered cells express a specialized transcriptome which helps to assimilate nutrients from the bowel (Pande et al., 2013). *Candida* is commonly found in the environment even in the hyper saline niche.

Genome: The whole genome sequence is known for *C. albicans* (SC5314), *C. glabrata* and *C. auris*. The genome is diploid in most of the pathogenic *Candida* species such as *C. albicans, C. tropicalis* and *C. parapsilosis*. The haploid genome is detected in C. *guilliermondii* and *Candida lusitaniae*. The size of *C. albicans* genome is 10.6−15.5 Mbp with the number of genes varying from 5733 to 6318. The genome contains major repeat sequence elements where the genetic recombination can take place (Jones et al., 2004). Other than recombination, high genetic diversity in *C. albicans* is also generated through chromosomal polymorphisms, gene replacement and cryptic mating (Selmecki et al., 2010). *C. auris* genome is diploid, comprising 12.3 Mb with a GC content of 44.8%. A total of 6675 coding sequences among all the isolates were found with one 5.8S rRNA, 184 tRNA and 3262 repetitive elements (Sharma et al., 2016). More genome information can be accessed on *Candida* genome database (CGD; http://www.candidagenome.org).

At the transcription level, the sexual mating of *Candida* is regulated by *MTL* (mating type locus) loci present in the genome. The transcription factors a2, α1 and a1/α2 are required for the expression of specific genes and generation of a, α and a/α heterodimer cells. The locus also contains the additional genes such as gene for phosphatidylinositol kinase (*PIK*), oxysterol-binding proteins (*OBP*) and poly(A) polymerases (*PAP*) with unknown role in mating. In some species of *Candida* homothallic mating between same sexes is detected where either the *MTL* is absent or both the loci are fused into a single locus.

Antigenic characteristics

Candida has two major groups of antigens such as heat-stable polysaccharides (glucan, mannan) and heat-labile glycoproteins. The mannan is a major antigen of *Candida* that circulates during infection and it comprises 7% dry weight of the cell wall. It is resistant to heat, proteinase and acidic pH. The antigenicity varies with the length of the polysaccharide side chain and position of the glycosidic linkages (α-man and β-man indicating the α/β-linked oligomannose residues). *C. albicans* has two serotypes (A and B) based on these variations.

Virulence factors

Formation of biofilm by *Candida* spp. is detected in tissues (oral/vaginal) and on medical devices such as catheters, haemodialysis and peritoneal dialysis units, intracardiac prosthetic valves, pacemakers, ventricular assist devices and central nervous system shunts. Biofilm is associated with virulence as it helps in evasion of immune response, generation of antifungal resistance and survival of the fungi with the competitive organisms. *C. albicans, C. parapsilosis, C. tropicalis* and *C. glabrata* strains are good biofilm formers (Desai et al., 2014). Catheter-associated *C. albicans* infections are one of the major causes of mortality (30%−40%) in human health centres (Finkel and Mitchell, 2011).

In *C. albicans*, the biofilm consists of two layers, i.e., a basal layer made of blastospores and a covering matrix composed of hyphae. Compared with *C. albicans*, biofilms of *C. parapsilosis* and *C. tropicalis* are thin in nature and consist of blastospores with yeast cells and hyphae or pseudohyphae (Silva et al., 2012). The biofilm of *C. glabrata* is composed of yeast cells only, not the hyphae (Silva et al., 2011). Adhesion with cells or solid objects and transition from yeast to hyphae are crucial in biofilm formation (Kruppa et al., 2004). Adhesion of *Candida* is mediated by adhesin−ligand interaction and nonspecific interactions such as hydrophobic and electrostatic forces (Chandra et al., 2005).

Composition of Candidal biofilm matrix (β-glucan, proteins, phosphorus and hexosamines) varies with medium composition, pH, oxygen and fungal strain. Farnesol (quorum sensing molecule) is one of the crucial regulators for *Candida* biofilm formation as the genes associated with cell wall maintenance, cell surface hydrophilicity, iron transport and hyphae formation are influenced (Albuquerque and Casadevall, 2012). In *C. albicans* cells having mating competent genotype penetrable biofilm is detected (Yi et al., 2011).

The factors required for biofilm formation and regulation, other virulence factors and mechanisms detected in *C. albicans* are described in Table 26.1.

Transmission

Candida causes the endogenous or opportunistic infection in most of the clinical cases during immunosuppression. Nosocomial transmission in susceptible patients is also detected (Ben Abdeljelil et al., 2011).

TABLE 26.1 Virulence mechanisms and factors possessed by *Candida albicans*.

Virulence factors	Functions
Yeast-hyphae transition	The hyphae are more invasive because of application of mechanical force and can easily penetrate both the individual cells and the space between them, whereas the yeast cells are easily disseminated into the blood circulation. The *Candida* hyphae can damage endothelial cells and lyse the macrophages after phagocytosis. Reverse transition (hyphae-yeast) is associated with expression of PES1 and UME6 proteins.
Thigmotropism (directional hyphal growth through contact sensing)	It is the contact sensing mechanism of *Candida* hyphae by which they can identify the crevices, grooves present in the host tissues for effective penetration. The contact sensing also triggers the biofilm formation over the solid surface. It is regulated by extracellular calcium uptake through the calcium channels Cch1 and Mid1.
Biofilm	*Candida* is able to produce biofilm in host mucosal cell surfaces and medical devices along with some bacterial species. Within biofilm the cells have reduced growth rate because of limited nutrition. The *CDR* and *MDR* genes encoding two types of efflux pumps, i.e., ATP-binding cassette (ABC) transporters and major facilitators, are upregulated in biofilm cells that are associated with antifungal resistance. Transcription factors such as BCR1, EFG1, TEC1, NDT80, ROB1, UME6 and CPH2 are associated with biofilm formation in *C. albicans*. Certain regulatory proteins such as ZAP1, CCR4, CSH1 and IFD6 act as negative regulator, while GCA1, GCA2, ADH5 and RLM1 act as positive regulator in biofilm matrix formation.
B-cell mitogenic protein (ISM p43)	It causes hyperstimulation of B-cells and immunosuppression and helps in survival of the fungi within the host.
HYR1 (hyphal protein)	It is associated with antifungal resistance.
pH-sensitive protein (PHR1 and PHR2)	They are cell wall β-glycosidases. The PHR1 and PHR2 are expressed in neutral-alkaline and acidic pH, respectively. So they are associated with systemic and vaginal infection, respectively.
Extracellular pH modulation	*Candida* can modulate the extracellular pH towards alkaline and autoinduce the hyphae formation. It is associated with starvation and uptake of amino acids, polyamine, etc. The amino acids are cleaved intracellularly by fungal urea amidolyase (Dur1,2) to generate ammonia, which is exported into the external environment through the Ato (ammonia transport outward) export proteins. The export of ammonia makes the environment alkaline, which promotes the hyphal growth.
Metabolic plasticity	In the hostile environment (within macrophage) *Candida* promptly switches glycolysis to gluconeogenesis where lipid and amino acids serve as a nutrient source
Iron acquisition	*Candida* can acquire iron through different mechanisms such as reduction of host ferritin (Als3-mediated), acquisition of iron from the siderophores produced by other organisms (xeno-siderophore) and uptake from haemoglobin and other haem proteins.
Zinc acquisition	It is mediated by 'micronutrient transporter/zinc-binding protein (Pra1: pH-regulated antigen 1), which acts as a zincophore by binding extracellular zinc.

Enzymes

Secreted aspartyl proteinases (Sap 1–8; Sap 9,10 cell bound)	The enzyme degrades immunoglobulin and complement of the hosts. Its help in penetration of host tissues is controversial as detected in the recent studies.
Phospholipase A, B, C, D; lysophospholipase and lysophospholipase transacetylase	They are associated with host cell membrane damage (PLB), adherence and penetration.
Haemolysin (mannoprotein)	They lyse the erythrocytes to release iron required for survival of the fungi.
Catalase and superoxide dismutase	It provides protection against oxidative stress.

Adhesins/Invasins

Glycolytic proteins (GAPDH, PGK, ADH, enolase), heat shock proteins (Hsp104, Hsp90, Hsp78, Hsp70, Hsp60) Small heat shock proteins (sHsp) (Hsp31, Hsp30, Hsp21, Hsp12, Hsp10)	(a) They act as adhesion factors and modulators of host antifungal immune response. (b) The heat shock proteins can further act as chaperones and prevent protein unfolding and aggregation under stress such as high temperature, starvation and oxidative stress. (c) The sHsp proteins are low molecular weight chaperones that prevent protein aggregation.
Lectin like molecules	They help in adhesion of *Candida* with L-fucose, N-acetylgalactosamine or N-acetylglucosamine containing glycosides present in the epithelial cell receptors. They also recognize salivary protein (mucin) and bacterial cell surface (*Staphylococcus*) which helps in oral colonization.
Fimbriae	It helps in adhesion of *Candida* with the erythrocytes mediated through the fimbrial protein (66 Kda) and glycosphingolipids present in the erythrocyte surface.
Integrin analogue (a protein that can bind RGD (arginine-glycine-aspartic acid) motif)	(a) They help in adhesion of *Candida* with the proteins having RGD motifs such as extracellular matrix protein, complement (C3), fibrinogen, heterodimeric transmembrane proteins. (b) They play major role in yeast-hyphae transition.
Mannan	They help in adhesion of *Candida* with epithelial and endothelial surfaces, erythrocytes, salivary components.
ALS protein (encoded by *ALS* gene (agglutinin-like sequence)) consisting of eight members (ALS 1–7, ALS 9)	The hyphae associated ALS protein (ALS3) adheres with host laminin, fibronectin, collagen through the recognition of certain amino acids (threonine, serine or alanine). The ALS3 also acts as invasin and is associated with induced endocytosis by the host epithelial cells.
Hwp1 (a hypha-associated GPI-linked protein)	It acts as a substrate for mammalian transglutaminases and this reaction may covalently link *Candida* hyphae to host cells.
Ssa1 (cell surface expressed protein belonged to HSP70 family)	It acts as invasion and is associated with induced endocytosis by the host epithelial cells.
Fibronectin adhesin	They help in adhesion of *Candida* with fibronectin and vitronectin receptors.
Glycoside binding adhesin	They help in adhesion of *Candida* with glycoside receptor.
EAP1, PGA10	Glycophosphatidylinositol (GPI) linked cell wall protein and help in cell adhesion/biofilm formation.
PBR1, CSH1	White cell α-factor induced protein and help in adherence/biofilm formation.
CZF1	Adherence

Diagnosis

The clinical specimens include skin scrapings, centrifuged milk samples, blood, serum and tissue samples in 10% formalin for biopsy.

Laboratory examination

Direct examination: The smear prepared from the clinical specimens can be observed under microscope either by 10% KOH preparation or by staining with Gram's Method. In the tissue section, *Candida* can be observed by PAS/haematoxylin or methenamine silver stain. They appear as unicellular budding yeast or pseudohyphae.

Isolation of *Candida* spp.: *Candida* can be isolated in general fungal or bacteriological media such as Sabouraud dextrose agar (with penicillin, streptomycin, chloramphenicol), potato dextrose agar, blood agar and brain heart infusion agar. They are obligate aerobe and they can grow within a wide range of temperature and pH. The plates are incubated at 25–30°C for 2–3 days. Pigmentation is detected in corn meal Tween agar. Currently, the media with resins are in use, which can absorb the residual antifungal or other inhibitory substances present in the clinical samples and significantly improve the recovery of *Candida*. Furthermore, *C. albicans* can grow in the presence of 0.04% cycloheximide.

The colonies are circular, white or opaque in colour (white-opaque transition) and creamy in consistency.

For identification of *Candida* at species level, a chromogenic medium (CHROMagar) can be used, in which different species such as *C. albicans*, *C. tropicalis* and *C. krusei* produce green/bluish green, blue/purple with halo and pink/ruffled coloured colonies, respectively. Oxoid chromogenic *Candida* agar (OCCA) can also differentiate the species with the colour of the colonies. The sunflower seed agar (Pal's medium) can differentiate between *C. albicans* and *C. dubliniensis*, where only *C. dubliniensis* isolates exhibited a hyphal fringe surrounding the colonies.

Histopathology: The presence of blastospores and pseudohyphae in the histochemically stained smear can be identified. A monoclonal antibody (3H8) is developed against *C. albicans* cell wall mannoprotein which can specifically recognize *C. albicans* in culture and in paraffin-embedded tissue sections using immunofluorescent and immunohistochemical staining. This antibody specifically detects the mycelial forms and to lesser extent blastospores of *C. albicans* and does not react with any other *Candida* spp. Fluorescence in situ hybridization (FISH) using oligonucleotide probes directed against 18S rRNA has been used to differentiate *C. albicans* from *C. parapsilosis* in tissues.

Immunological assays: ELISA-based tests are developed to detect Candidal antigens such as SAP, mannan and β-D-glucan. Dissociation of antigen–antibody complexes is necessary for the optimal detection of mannan in the circulation. The sensitivity and specificity of the mannan-based test is 58% and 93%, respectively. These immunological assays are useful in diagnosis of *Candida* in immunocompromised patients who produce negligible or undetectable amount of antibodies.

Serological tests: ELISA-based serological tests are developed for detection of antibodies against Candidal amino-peptidase, mannan and SAP in the suspected serum. Indirect immunofluorescence assay is also developed for detection of anti-Candidal antibody (IgG). The serological tests for detection of *Candida* are not so much reliable. The false positive reaction occurs because of superficial colonization and false negative reaction occurs in immunocompromised patients producing low or undetectable level of antibodies.

Molecular biology: Several types of polymerase chain reactions (PCRs) such as seminested and nested PCR, multiplex PCR followed by DNA sequencing or pyrosequencing are developed for detection of Candidal DNA. The target DNA includes rRNA genes (5.8S, 18S, 28S), internal transcribed spacer and intergenic spacer regions. The extraction of DNA from the cell is challenging because of presence of rigid cell wall which often produces false negative results. The false positive result is produced because of airborne fungal contamination. Confirmation of PCR amplicon by enzyme immune assay using colorimetric substrate is considered as easy and cheapest method. Real-time PCR is developed using Taqman probe or light cycler system for identification of *Candida*.

Typing of *C. albicans* strains: *C. albicans* strains were differentiated earlier by biotyping, serotyping, toxin profile, antifungal resistance and resistance to various chemicals. Currently several DNA-based methods are used for typing of *C. albicans* strains. Highest discriminatory techniques for *C. albicans* strains are exact DNA-based methods such as microsatellite length polymorphism (MLP) and multilocus sequence typing (MLST) (Bougnoux et al., 2003; Sampaio et al., 2005). MLP typing is based on variability in the repeat number of microsatellite sequences, and MLST is based on polymorphisms in the sequences of internal fragments present in 6–8 genes. MLST is the only typing method of *C. albicans* which shares the results in a public database (http://calbicans.mlst.net/). Macrorestriction analysis (restriction of the chromosome length DNA with rare-cutting endonucleases such as *SfiI* and *BssHII*), restriction enzyme analysis (restriction of genomic DNA with *EcoRI*, *MspI*, *BglII*, *HinFI* or *HindIII*) with southern blotting and amplified fragment length polymorphism (AFLP) have high discriminatory power for *C. albicans* strains, easy to interpret, although primary setup cost is high and require skilled technicians (Matthews and Burnie, 1989; Shin et al., 2004; Ball et al., 2004).

Characteristics of antifungal resistance

Intrinsic resistance

Low affinity for ERG11 was described as intrinsic resistance mechanism of *C. krusei* against fluconazole (Orozco et al., 1998). *C. glabrata* was found intrinsically resistant against imidazoles (miconazole) and triazoles (fluconazole, voriconazole) (Tscherner et al., 2011). Natural mutation in *FKS1* causes reduced susceptibility of *C. parapsilosis* against echinocandins (Beyda et al., 2012). Loss of heterozygosity is important mechanism associated with antifungal resistance. Mutation in genes associated with antifungal resistance can be substituted with the other as *Candida* has diploid genome with a pair of each gene. The recombination between pairs of chromosomes produces loss of heterozygosity which can expose the effect of mutation in genes associated with antifungal resistance or phenotype diversity (Rosenberg, 2011). Loss of heterozygosity is associated with not only exposure to antifungals but also to heat and oxidative stress (Forche et al., 2011). *Candida haemulonii* and phylogenetically correlated *C. auris* showed intrinsic resistance to fluconazole and amphotericin B (Kumar et al., 2016). Recently published draft genome of *C. auris* revealed the presence of single copy genes such as *ERG3*, *ERG11*, *FKS1*, *FKS2* and *FKS3* and upregulated expression of ABC transporters for drug efflux (Sharma et al., 2016).

Resistance to azole

Fluconazole and itraconazole were used extensively against candidiasis due to oral bioavailability and safety for last one decade. Resistance to azoles in *Candida* infection associated with HIV patients started to be reported later (Skiest et al., 2007). *Candida* uses several mechanisms of resistance to azole either separately or in combination (Kanafani and Perfect, 2008). Induction of multidrug efflux pumps is crucial for azole resistance in *C. albicans* (MDR1, CDR1 and CDR2), *C. glabrata* (CgCDR1, CgCDR2) and *C. dubliniensis* (CdMDR1, CdCDR1) (Sanglard et al., 1995). Induction of CDR is required for resistance against all types of azoles and MDR is associated with fluconazole resistance. The target enzyme of azole is lanosterol 14α-sterol demethylase, encoded by *ERG11*. Mutation in *ERG11* is a less common resistance mechanism in clinical isolates of *C. albicans* (more common in *C. glabrata*), which alters the binding of the drug with enzymatic site (Löffler et al., 1997; Henry et al., 2000). Toxic substance such as 14α-methyl-3,6-diol is accumulated during contact with azoles in *Candida*. Mutation in *ERG3* prevents the accumulation of toxic substance and is considered as another possible way of resistance (Kelly et al., 1997). Mitochondrial dysfunction in 'petite mutant' cells of *C. glabrata* upregulates several genes such as ABC transporters (pleiotropic drug resistance factors (*PDR5* and *PDR16*)) and the genes associated with activation of RNA polymerase II transcription, calcium homeostasis, ribosomal biogenesis and cell wall biosynthesis (Kaur et al., 2004). The activated ABC transporters act as efflux pump for azoles in *C. glabrata* (Noble et al., 2013). Upregulation of the aldo-keto reductase (*AKR*) gene in *C. glabrata* was found to be associated with azole resistance (Farahyar et al., 2013).

Resistance to echinocandins

Intensive use of caspofungin and micafungin as first-line treatment against invasive *Candida* spp. since 2000 resulted in emergence of echinocandin resistance (Fekkar et al., 2014). Coresistance to both echinocandins and azoles is common in *C. glabrata* (Alexander et al., 2013). Echinocandins prevent synthesis of β-glucan in fungal cell wall by inhibiting β-glucan synthase. Mutation in genes encoding FKS-1 (amino acid positions 641−649 and 1345−1365, known as hotspot-1 and hotspot-2, respectively) and FKS-2 subunits of β (1,3)-D-glucan synthase produces echinocandin resistance in *C. albicans*, *C. dubliniensis*, *C. krusei*, *C. tropicalis* and *C. glabrata* (Park et al., 2005; Perlin, 2007; Grosset et al., 2016). The mutations do not alter the substrate binding of β-D-glucan synthase but reduce Vmax values (Garcia-Effron et al., 2009).

    C. albicans can upregulate the synthesis of fungal cell wall components (chitin) as a compensatory mechanism when β-glucan synthesis is reduced because of exposure to echinocandins. This increased chitin synthesis is associated with protein kinase C activation, high-osmolarity glycerol response and calcium-dependent calcineurin signalling pathway (Walker et al., 2008). Certain strains of *C. albicans* can grow in presence of supra-MIC concentration of echinocandin (caspofungin) because of increased chitin content of the cell wall (paradoxical effect) (Shields et al., 2011).

Resistance to polyene

Nonsense mutation in *ERG6* gene (substitution of cysteine by phenyl alanine) produced low ergosterol content in the cell membrane of *C. glabrata* and reduced susceptibility to polyenes (Vandeputte et al., 2008).

Resistance to flucytosine

The flucytosine uptake is reduced in *Candida* because of mutation in *FCY2* gene encoding cytosine permease. Several point mutations in *FCY1* (cytosine deaminase) and *FUR1* (uracil phosphoribosyltransferase) in *C. albicans*, *C. glabrata* and *C. lusitaniae* are associated with resistance to flucytosine (Vandeputte et al., 2011).

Resistance to cationic proteins (histatin 5)

C. glabrata showed resistance to histatin 5(human salivary cationic protein) as the fungi can escape histatin 5 activity by using fermentative pathways (Oppenheim et al., 1988).

Role of biofilm

Formation of biofilm by *Candida* is typically associated with antifungal resistance. High density of cells within the biofilm (resistance of *C. glabrata* to azole due to quorum sensing in dense bacterial population), prevention in penetration of drugs due to biofilm matrix, overexpression of efflux proteins such as CDR1 and CDR2 (ABC membrane transport proteins) and MDR1 (major facilitator protein), decreased growth rate and nutrient limitation and generation of resistant persister *Candida* cells are considered as mechanisms of antifungal resistance associated with biofilm formation (La Fleur et al., 2006; Sardi et al., 2011; Nett et al., 2011). Low glucose concentration induces persistence and biofilm formation in *C. glabrata* cells associated with resistance to amphotericin B. The nutrient deprivation such as low glucose concentration induces *SNF3* gene, which helps the fungi to survive in the hostile environment (Ng et al., 2016).

References

Albuquerque, P., Casadevall, A., 2012. Quorum sensing in fungi—a review. Medical Mycology 50 (4), 337–345.

Alexander, B.D., Johnson, M.D., Pfeiffer, C.D., Jiménez-Ortigosa, C., Catania, J., Booker, R., Castanheira, M., Messer, S.A., Perlin, D.S., Pfaller, M.A., 2013. Increasing echinocandin resistance in *Candida glabrata*: clinical failure correlates with presence of FKS mutations and elevated minimum inhibitory concentrations. Clinical Infectious Diseases 56 (12), 1724–1732.

Arendrup, M., Horn, T., Frimodt-Møller, N., 2002. *In vivo* pathogenicity of eight medically relevant *Candida* species in an animal model. Infection 30 (5), 286–291.

Baixench, M.T., Aoun, N., Desnos-Ollivier, M., Garcia-Hermoso, D., Bretagne, S., Ramires, S., Piketty, C., Dannaoui, E., 2007. Acquired resistance to echinocandins in *Candida albicans*: case report and review. Journal of Antimicrobial Chemotherapy 59 (6), 1076–1083.

Ball, L.M., Bes, M.A., Theelen, B., Boekhout, T., Egeler, R.M., Kuijper, E.J., 2004. Significance of amplified fragment length polymorphism in identification and epidemiological examination of *Candida* species colonization in children undergoing allogeneic stem cell transplantation. Journal of Clinical Microbiology 42 (4), 1673–1679.

Ben Abdeljelil, J., Saghrouni, F., Emira, N., Valentin-Gomez, E., Chatti, N., Boukadida, J., Ben Saïd, M., Del Castillo Agudo, L., 2011. Molecular typing of *Candida albicans* isolates from patients and health care workers in a neonatal intensive care unit. Journal of Applied Microbiology 111 (5), 1235–1249.

Bethea, E.K., Carver, B.J., Montedonico, A.E., Reynolds, T.B., 2010. The inositol regulon controls viability in *Candida glabrata*. Microbiology 156 (2), 452–462.

Beyda, N.D., Lewis, R.E., Garey, K.W., 2012. Echinocandin resistance in *Candida* species: mechanisms of reduced susceptibility and therapeutic approaches. The Annals of Pharmacotherapy 46 (7–8), 1086–1096.

Bougnoux, M.E., Tavanti, A., Bouchier, C., Gow, N.A.R., Magnier, A., Davidson, A.D., Maiden, M.C.J., d'Enfert, C., Odds, F.C., 2003. Collaborative consensus for optimized multilocus sequence typing of *Candida albicans*. Journal of Clinical Microbiology 41 (11), 5265–5266.

Brown, G.D., Denning, D.W., Gow, N.A., Levitz, S.M., Netea, M.G., White, T.C., 2012. Hidden killers: human fungal infections. Science Translational Medicine 4 (165), 165rv13-165rv13.

Chandra, J., Zhou, G., Ghannoum, M.A., 2005. Fungal biofilms and antimycotics. Current Drug Targets 6 (8), 887–894.

Coleman, D.C., Bennett, D.E., Sullivan, D.J., Gallagher, P.J., Henman, M.C., Shanley, D.B., Russell, R.J., 1993. Oral *Candida* in HIV infection and AIDS: new perspectives/new approaches. Critical Reviews in Microbiology 19 (2), 61–82.

Desai, J.V., Mitchell, A.P., Andes, D.R., 2014. Fungal biofilms, drug resistance, and recurrent infection. Cold Spring Harbor Perspectives in Medicine 4 (10) pii:.a019729.

Eggimann, P., Garbino, J., Pittet, D., 2003. Epidemiology of *Candida* species infections in critically ill non-immunosuppressed patients. The Lancet Infectious Diseases 3 (11), 685−702.

Farahyar, S., Zaini, F., Kordbacheh, P., Rezaie, S., Safara, M., Raoofian, R., Heidari, M., 2013. Overexpression of aldo-keto-reductase in azole-resistant clinical isolates of *Candida glabrata* determined by cDNA-AFLP. Daru Journal of Pharmaceutical Sciences 21 (1), 1.

Fekkar, A., Dannaoui, E., Meyer, I., Imbert, S., Brossas, J.Y., Uzunov, M., Mellon, G., Nguyen, S., Guiller, E., Caumes, E., Leblond, V., 2014. Emergence of echinocandin-resistant *Candida spp.* in a hospital setting: a consequence of 10 years of increasing use of antifungal therapy? European Journal of Clinical Microbiology & Infectious Diseases 33 (9), 1489−1496.

Fidel, P.L., Vazquez, J.A., Sobel, J.D., 1999. *Candida glabrata*: review of epidemiology, pathogenesis, and clinical disease with comparison to *C. albicans*. Clinical Microbiology Reviews 12 (1), 80−96.

Finkel, J.S., Mitchell, A.P., 2011. Genetic control of *Candida albicans* biofilm development. Nature Reviews Microbiology 9 (2), 109.

Forche, A., Abbey, D., Pisithkul, T., Weinzierl, M.A., Ringstrom, T., Bruck, D., Petersen, K., Berman, J., 2011. Stress alters rates and types of loss of heterozygosity in *Candida albicans*. mBio 2 (4) e00129-11.

Fridkin, S.K., 2005. Candidemia is costly-plain and simple. Clinical Infectious Diseases 41, 1240−1241.

Garcia-Effron, G., Park, S., Perlin, D.S., 2009. Correlating echinocandin MIC and kinetic inhibition of fks1 mutant glucan synthases for *Candida albicans*: implications for interpretive breakpoints. Antimicrobial Agents and Chemotherapy 53 (1), 112−122.

Grosset, M., Desnos-Ollivier, M., Godet, C., Kauffmann-Lacroix, C., Cazenave-Roblot, F., 2016. Recurrent episodes of candidemia due to *Candida glabrata, Candida tropicalis* and *Candida albicans* with acquired echinocandin resistance. Medical Mycology Case Reports 14, 20−23.

Henry, K.W., Nickels, J.T., Edlind, T.D., 2000. Upregulation of ERG genes in Candida species by azoles and other sterol biosynthesis inhibitors. Antimicrobial Agents and Chemotherapy 44 (10), 2693−2700.

Jones, T., Federspiel, N.A., Chibana, H., Dungan, J., Kalman, S., Magee, B.B., Newport, G., Thorstenson, Y.R., Agabian, N., Magee, P.T., Davis, R.W., 2004. The diploid genome sequence of *Candida albicans*. Proceedings of the National Academy of Sciences 101 (19), 7329−7334.

Kam, A.P., Xu, J., 2002. Diversity of commensal yeasts within and among healthy hosts. Diagnostic Microbiology and Infectious Disease 43 (1), 19−28.

Kanafani, Z.A., Perfect, J.R., 2008. Resistance to antifungal agents: mechanisms and clinical impact. Clinical Infectious Diseases 46 (1), 120−128.

Kathuria, S., Singh, P.K., Sharma, C., Prakash, A., Masih, A., Kumar, A., Meis, J.F., Chowdhary, A., 2015. Multidrug resistant *Candida auris* misidentified as *C. haemulonii*: characterization by matrix assisted laser desorption ionization-time of flight mass spectrometry (MALDI-TOF MS), DNA sequencing and its antifungal susceptibility profile variability by VITEK-2, CLSI-broth microdilution and E-test method. Journal of Clinical Microbiology 53, 1823−1830.

Kaur, R., Castaño, I., Cormack, B.P., 2004. Functional genomic analysis of fluconazole susceptibility in the pathogenic yeast *Candida glabrata*: roles of calcium signaling and mitochondria. Antimicrobial Agents and Chemotherapy 48 (5), 1600−1613.

Kelly, S.L., Lamb, D.C., Kelly, D.E., Manning, N.J., Loeffler, J., Hebart, H., Schumacher, U., Einsele, H., 1997. Resistance to fluconazole and cross-resistance to amphotericin B in *Candida albicans* from AIDS patients caused by defective sterol $\Delta5$, 6-desaturation. FEBS Letters 400 (1), 80−82.

Kruppa, M., Krom, B.P., Chauhan, N., Bambach, A.V., Cihlar, R.L., Calderone, R.A., 2004. The two-component signal transduction protein Chk1p regulates quorum sensing in *Candida albicans*. Eukaryotic Cell 3 (4), 1062−1065.

Kullberg, B.J., Arendrup, M.C., 2015. Invasive candidiasis. New England Journal of Medicine 373 (15), 1445−1456.

Kumar, A., Prakash, A., Singh, A., Kumar, H., Hagen, F., Meis, J.F., Chowdhary, A., 2016. *Candida haemulonii species* complex: an emerging species in India and its genetic diversity assessed with multilocus sequence and amplified fragment-length polymorphism analyses. Emerging Microbes & Infections 5 (5), e49.

LaFleur, M.D., Kumamoto, C.A., Lewis, K., 2006. *Candida albicans* biofilms produce antifungal-tolerant persister cells. Antimicrobial Agents and Chemotherapy 50 (11), 3839−3846.

Lee, W.G., Shin, J.H., Young, U., Kang, M.G., Kim, S.H., Park, K.H., Jang, H.C., 2011. The first three reported cases of nosocomial fungemia caused by *Candida auris*. Journal of Clinical Microbiology 49 (9), 3139−3142.

Lockhart, S.R., Fritch, J.J., Meier, A.S., Schröppel, K., Srikantha, T., Galask, R., Soll, D.R., 1995. Colonizing populations of *Candida albicans* are clonal in origin but undergo microevolution through C1 fragment reorganization as demonstrated by DNA fingerprinting and C1 sequencing. Journal of Clinical Microbiology 33 (6), 1501−1509.

Löffler, J., Kelly, S.L., Hebart, H., Schumacher, U., Lass-Flörl, C., Einsele, H., 1997. Molecular analysis of cyp51 from fluconazole-resistant *Candida albicans* strains. FEMS Microbiology Letters 151 (2), 263−268.

Matthews, R., Burnie, J., 1989. Assessment of DNA fingerprinting for rapid identification of outbreaks of systemic candidiasis. BMJ 298 (6670), 354−357.

Nett, J.E., Sanchez, H., Cain, M.T., Ross, K.M., Andes, D.R., 2011. Interface of *Candida albicans* biofilm matrix-associated drug resistance and cell wall integrity regulation. Eukaryotic Cell 10 (12), 1660−1669.

Ng, T.S., Desa, M.N.M., Sandai, D., Chong, P.P., Than, L.T.L., 2016. Growth, biofilm formation, antifungal susceptibility and oxidative stress resistance of *Candida glabrata* are affected by different glucose concentrations. Infection, Genetics and Evolution 40, 331−338.

Noble, J.A., Tsai, H.F., Suffis, S.D., Su, Q., Myers, T.G., Bennett, J.E., 2013. STB5 is a negative regulator of azole resistance in *Candida glabrata*. Antimicrobial Agents and Chemotherapy 57 (2), 959−967.

Oppenheim, F.G., Xu, T., McMillian, F.M., Levitz, S.M., Diamond, R.D., Offner, G.D., Troxler, R.F., 1988. Histatins, a novel family of histidine-rich proteins in human parotid secretion. Isolation, characterization, primary structure, and fungistatic effects on *Candida albicans*. Journal of Biological Chemistry 263 (16), 7472−7477.

Orozco, A.S., Higginbotham, L.M., Hitchcock, C.A., Parkinson, T., Falconer, D., Ibrahim, A.S., Ghannoum, M.A., Filler, S.G., 1998. Mechanism of fluconazole resistance in *Candida krusei*. Antimicrobial Agents and Chemotherapy 42 (10), 2645—2649.

Pande, K., Chen, C., Noble, S.M., 2013. Passage through the mammalian gut triggers a phenotypic switch that promotes *Candida albicans* commensalism. Nature Genetics 45 (9), 1088.

Park, S., Kelly, R., Kahn, J.N., Robles, J., Hsu, M.J., Register, E., Li, W., Vyas, V., Fan, H., Abruzzo, G., Flattery, A., 2005. Specific substitutions in the echinocandin target Fks1p account for reduced susceptibility of rare laboratory and clinical *Candida* sp. isolates. Antimicrobial Agents and Chemotherapy 49 (8), 3264—3273.

Perlin, D.S., 2007. Resistance to echinocandin-class antifungal drugs. Drug Resistance Updates 10 (3), 121—130.

Pfaller, M.A., Castanheira, M., Messer, S.A., Moet, G.J., Jones, R.N., 2010. Variation in *Candida* spp. distribution and antifungal resistance rates among bloodstream infection isolates by patient age: report from the SENTRY antimicrobial surveillance program (2008—2009). Diagnostic Microbiology and Infectious Disease 68 (3), 278—283.

Rosenberg, S.M., 2011. Stress-induced loss of heterozygosity in *Candida*: a possible missing link in the ability to evolve. mBio 2 (5), e00200—e00211.

Sampaio, P., Gusmão, L., Correia, A., Alves, C., Rodrigues, A.G., Pina-Vaz, C., Amorim, A., Pais, C., 2005. New microsatellite multiplex PCR for *Candida albicans* strain typing reveals microevolutionary changes. Journal of Clinical Microbiology 43 (8), 3869—3876.

Sanglard, D., Kuchler, K., Ischer, F., Pagani, J.L., Monod, M., Bille, J., 1995. Mechanisms of resistance to azole antifungal agents in *Candida albicans* isolates from AIDS patients involve specific multidrug transporters. Antimicrobial Agents and Chemotherapy 39 (11), 2378—2386.

Sardi, J.C.O., Almeida, A.M.F., Giannini, M.J.S.M., 2011. New antimicrobial therapies used against fungi present in subgingival sites-a brief review. Archives of Oral Biology 56 (10), 951—959.

Selmecki, A., Forche, A., Berman, J., 2010. Genomic plasticity of the human fungal pathogen *Candida albicans*. Eukaryotic Cell 9 (7), 991—1008.

Sharma, C., Kumar, N., Pandey, R., Meis, J.F., Chowdhary, A., 2016. Whole genome sequencing of emerging multidrug resistant *Candida auris* isolates in India demonstrates low genetic variation. New Microbes and New Infections 13, 77—82.

Shields, R.K., Nguyen, M.H., Du, C., Press, E., Cheng, S., Clancy, C.J., 2011. Paradoxical effect of caspofungin against *Candida* bloodstream isolates is mediated by multiple pathways but eliminated in human serum. Antimicrobial Agents and Chemotherapy 55 (6), 2641—2647.

Shin, J.H., Park, M.R., Song, J.W., Shin, D.H., Jung, S.I., Cho, D., Kee, S.J., Shin, M.G., Suh, S.P., Ryang, D.W., 2004. Microevolution of *Candida albicans* strains during catheter-related candidemia. Journal of Clinical Microbiology 42 (9), 4025—4031.

Silva, S., Negri, M., Henriques, M., Oliveira, R., Williams, D.W., Azeredo, J., 2012. *Candida glabrata*, *Candida parapsilosis* and *Candida tropicalis*: biology, epidemiology, pathogenicity and antifungal resistance. FEMS Microbiology Reviews 36 (2), 288—305.

Silva, S., Negri, M., Henriques, M., Oliveira, R., Williams, D.W., Azeredo, J., 2011. Adherence and biofilm formation of non-*Candida albicans Candida* species. Trends in Microbiology 19 (5), 241—247.

Skiest, D.J., Vazquez, J.A., Anstead, G.M., Graybill, J.R., Reynes, J., Ward, D., Hare, R., Boparai, N., Isaacs, R., 2007. Posaconazole for the treatment of azole-refractory oropharyngeal and esophageal candidiasis in subjects with HIV infection. Clinical Infectious Diseases 44 (4), 607—614.

Sobel, J.D., 1998. Key note lecture review article vulvovaginitis due to *Candida glabrata*:an emerging problem: Vulvovaginitis bedingt durch *Candida glabrata*. Ein aufkommendes Problem. Mycoses 41, 18—22.

Tscherner, M., Schwarzmüller, T., Kuchler, K., 2011. Pathogenesis and antifungal drug resistance of the human fungal pathogen *Candida glabrata*. Pharmaceuticals 4 (1), 169—186.

Tumbarello, M., Posteraro, B., Trecarichi, E.M., Fiori, B., Rossi, M., Porta, R., de Gaetano Donati, K., La Sorda, M., Spanu, T., Fadda, G., Cauda, R., 2007. Biofilm production by *Candida* species and inadequate antifungal therapy as predictors of mortality for patients with candidemia. Journal of Clinical Microbiology 45 (6), 1843—1850.

Vandeputte, P., Pineau, L., Larcher, G., Noel, T., Brèthes, D., Chabasse, D., Bouchara, J.P., 2011. Molecular mechanisms of resistance to 5-fluorocytosine in laboratory mutants of *Candida glabrata*. Mycopathologia 171 (1), 11—21.

Vandeputte, P., Tronchin, G., Larcher, G., Ernoult, E., Bergès, T., Chabasse, D., Bouchara, J.P., 2008. A nonsense mutation in the *ERG6* gene leads to reduced susceptibility to polyenes in a clinical isolate of *Candida glabrata*. Antimicrobial Agents and Chemotherapy 52 (10), 3701—3709.

Walker, L.A., Munro, C.A., De Bruijn, I., Lenardon, M.D., McKinnon, A., Gow, N.A., 2008. Stimulation of chitin synthesis rescues *Candida albicans* from echinocandins. PLoS Pathogens 4 (4), e1000040.

Yi, S., Sahni, N., Daniels, K.J., Lu, K.L., Srikantha, T., Huang, G., Garnaas, A.M., Soll, D.R., 2011. Alternative mating type configurations (a/α versus a/a or α/α) of *Candida albicans* result in alternative biofilms regulated by different pathways. PLoS Biology 9 (8), e1001117.

Zaoutis, T.E., Argon, J., Chu, J., Berlin, J.A., Walsh, T.J., Feudtner, C., 2005. The epidemiology and attributable outcomes of candidemia in adults and children hospitalized in the United States: a propensity analysis. Clinical Infectious Diseases 41 (9), 1232—1239.

Chapter 27

Others

Chapter outline

Chlamydia

Chlamydiae are Gram-negative, obligate intracellular bacteria with a complex developmental cycle consisting of two stages such as elementary body (infectious) and reticulate body (RB). During exposure to antibiotics or other stress factors, growth of *Chlamydia* is arrested and it is known as aberrant RB/aberrant bodies (AB). Chlamydial infection is common in human and animals. Human-associated pathogenic species such as *Chlamydia trachomatis* and *Chlamydia pneumoniae* cause urethritis, epididymitis in men, cervicitis, infertility, ectopic pregnancy in women and atypical pneumonia, respectively (Eick et al., 2011; Marrazzo and Suchland, 2014). *Chlamydia suis* causes respiratory distress, conjunctivitis, diarrhoea and reproductive disorders in farmed pigs and wild boars (Schautteet and Vanrompay, 2011). Direct zoonotic transmission of *C. suis* is not confirmed. Genetic material of *C. suis* is although detected in human clinical samples (Dean et al., 2013; De Puysseleyr et al., 2014).

Tetracyclines are recommended for treatment of chlamydiosis in human and livestock. Tetracycline-resistant *Chlamydia* were started to be reported from pigs in the United States since 1998 and later from European countries such as Italy, Belgium and Switzerland (Andersen and Rogers, 1998; Di Francesco et al., 2008; Schautteet and Vanrompay, 2011; Borel et al., 2012). Tetracycline resistance gene (*tetC*) present in a genomic island (Tet^R) was found to be associated with resistance, which encodes a tetracycline efflux pump (Dugan et al., 2004). The genomic island (Tet^R) of *C. suis* is the first identified acquired resistance factor in a bacterium through horizontal gene transfer. Majority of *C. suis* genomic island (Tet^R) also carries IScs605 originated from *Laribacter hongkongensis*, a fish pathogen (Sandoz and Rockey, 2010). Use of fish meal was correlated with the origin of IScs605 in *C. suis* although not confirmed.

In human, treatment failure (5%−23%) due to infection with azithromycin- and doxycycline-resistant *C. trachomatis* and *C. pneumoniae* was reported from several countries (Horner, 2012). Heterotypic resistance was detected in clinical isolates of *Chlamydia* associated with phenotypic changes in a stressed bacterial population (AB) (Bhengraj et al., 2010).

Estrella lausannensis

Estrella lausannensis belongs to the family *Criblamydiaceae* under the order *Chlamydiales* (Lienard et al., 2011). It can infect amoeba, fish cell lines and is associated with tubal pathology in women. Quinolone resistance in *E. lausannensis* was associated with amino acid substitutions in the quinolone resistance-determining region (QRDR) of GyrA (Ser83Gln and Val70Ser) and ParC (Ser80Ala and Glu84Asp) (de Barsy et al., 2014).

Parachlamydia acanthamoebae

Parachlamydia acanthamoebae, a kind of *Chlamydia*, is found to be associated with varieties of respiratory tract infections in human such as community-acquired pneumonia, ventilator-associated pneumonia, nosocomial pneumonia, lower

TABLE 27.1 Antimicrobial resistance genes detected in *Bacteroides fragilis*.

Genes	Resistance
cfiA (metallo-β-lactamase)	Carbapenem
nimA-H, nimJ (nitroimidazole)	Metronidazole
ermB, ermF, ermG	Clindamycin
msrSA, mefA	Macrolide, lincosamide
linAn2	Lincomycin, erythromycin
tetQ, tetX, tetX1	Tetracycline, tigecycline
bexA, bexB	Fluoroquinolone

respiratory tract infections and bronchitis (Greub et al., 2003; Lamoth et al., 2011). Resistance to quinolones was detected in *Parachlamydia* due to a mutation (position 70 and 83) in the QRDR of *gyrA* (Casson et al., 2006).

Bacteroides fragilis

Bacteroides fragilis are common cause of blood stream infections in human, neonatal diarrhoea in calves, lambs and mastitis in cattle. Resistance to penicillins, cephalosporins (except cefoxitin) and cefoxitin is associated with possession of *cepA* and *cfxA*, respectively (Eitel et al., 2013). Other antimicrobial resistance genes detected in *B. fragilis* are described in Table 27.1.

Aspergillus fumigatus

Aspergillus fumigatus causes a spectrum of human and animal infections including invasive aspergillosis (IA) with an estimated mortality rate of 28.5% in human (Bitar et al., 2014). The studies indicated about more than 1.2 million patients suffer with chronic pulmonary aspergillosis and another 4.8 million people are infected with allergic bronchopulmonary aspergillosis throughout the world annually (Denning et al., 2013). Recent emergence of IA is associated with tuberculosis, asthma, chronic obstructive pulmonary disease, therapy in malignancy, organ transplantation and autoimmune diseases (Brown et al., 2012).

Different azole compounds such as itraconazole, voriconazole, posaconazole and isavuconazole are common in therapy and prophylaxis of aspergillosis. The azoles act by inhibiting lanosterol 14-alpha-demethylase (*cyp51A* in *A. fumigatus*) required for synthesis of ergosterol (Bossche et al., 1995). Resistance to azole in *A. fumigatus* was restricted earlier to individual patients receiving azoles for prolonged period (Camps et al., 2012). A global emergence of azole resistance in *A. fumigatus* is current concern even in patients who did not receive azole therapy (azole-naïve) with a mortality rate as high as 88% in culture-positive patients (Van Der Linden et al., 2013; Steinmann et al., 2015). The resistance mechanisms such as presence of a 34 bp tandem repeat (TR) along with leucine to histidine substitution in codon 98 in *cyp51A* gene (TR34/L98H associated with itraconazole resistance) and a 46 bp tandem repeat associated with tyrosine to phenylalanine substitution in codon 121 and threonine to alanine substitution in codon 289 in *cyp51A* gene (TR46/Y121F/T289A causing voriconazole and other azole resistance) are described (Snelders et al., 2008; Van Der Linden et al., 2013). Recent study revealed the role of TR46/Y121F in destabilization of CYP51A protein, which produces high azole resistance in *A. fumigatus* (Snelders et al., 2015).

In European countries such as Denmark, TR34/L98H was found as the predominant mechanism of azole resistance in clinical isolates of *A. fumigatus* (Jensen et al., 2016). The TR34/L98H-mediated azole resistance in *A. fumigatus* is although spreading into other non-European countries such as China, India, Middle East, Africa and Australia probably through dispersal of fungal spores (Chowdhary et al., 2013).

Cryptococcus neoformans

Cryptococcus neoformans causes more than 600,000 deaths annually throughout the world associated with meningitis (Park et al., 2009). The infection is common in HIV patients and currently non-HIV patients are also infected who receive transplanted organs or prolonged anticancer therapy. Amphotericin B (polyene) and fluconazole are the antifungals of choice to treat cryptococcosis. Fluconazole is also recommended as a prophylactic drug to avoid cryptococcosis (Gullo et al., 2013).

Mutation in *ERG11* (encoding lanosterol 14-alpha-demethylase) and active efflux of the drug through ABC transporter (encoded by *AFR1*) in *C. neoformans* are associated with azole resistance (Rodero et al., 2003; Sanguinetti et al., 2006). The resistance genes (*ERG11* and *AFR1*) are encoded by chromosome 1 (Chr1). Aneuploidies increasing the numbers of chromosome (Chr1) may cause overexpression of the resistance genes and transcription factors (Cn Yap1) with enhanced fluconazole resistance ('heteroresistance') (Sionov et al., 2010; Paul et al., 2015). Cation transporters (Ena1 and Nha1) of *C. neoformans* regulate membrane stability and cation homeostasis, and it plays a redundant role in resistance against polyene and azoles (Jung et al., 2012).

Scedosporium spp.

Scedosporium apiospermum complex, *S. apiospermum* and *S. minutisporum* are ubiquitous saprophytic fungi commonly found in sewage, brackish water, salt water, swaps, coastal tidelands, soil, manure of poultry, cattle and bat guano (Samanta, 2015). *Scedosporium* is associated with cutaneous infection (mycetoma) in healthy human infected through inhalation or direct contact. In immunocompromised patients with malignancy/HIV/solid organ transplant, *Scedosporium apiospermum* complex causes disseminated infection throughout the body including central nervous system (Nesky et al., 2000; Balandin et al., 2016). Voriconazole is recommended for treatment of *Scedosporium*, although *Scedosporium* are increasingly become resistant against azoles and echinocandins (Tortorano et al., 2014).

References

Andersen, A.A., Rogers, D.G., 1998. Resistance to tetracycline and sulfadiazine in swine *C. trachomatis* isolates. In: Chlamydial Infections. Proceedings of the Ninth International Symposium on Human Chlamydial Infection. International Chlamydia Symposium, San Francisco, CA, pp. 313−316.

Balandin, B., Aguilar, M., Sánchez, I., Monzón, A., Rivera, I., Salas, C., Valdivia, M., Alcántara, S., Pérez, A., Ussetti, P., 2016. *Scedosporium apiospermum* and *S. prolificans* mixed disseminated infection in a lung transplant recipient: an unusual case of long-term survival with combined systemic and local antifungal therapy in intensive care unit. Medical Mycology Case Reports 11, 53−56.

Bhengraj, A.R., Vardhan, H., Srivastava, P., Salhan, S., Mittal, A., 2010. Decreased susceptibility to azithromycin and doxycycline in clinical isolates of *Chlamydia trachomatis* obtained from recurrently infected female patients in India. Chemotherapy 56 (5), 371−377.

Bitar, D., Lortholary, O., Le Strat, Y., Nicolau, J., Coignard, B., Tattevin, P., Che, D., Dromer, F., 2014. Population-based analysis of invasive fungal infections, France, 2001−2010. Emerging Infectious Diseases 20 (7), 1149.

Borel, N., Regenscheit, N., Di Francesco, A., Donati, M., Markov, J., Masserey, Y., Pospischil, A., 2012. Selection for tetracycline-resistant *Chlamydia suis* in treated pigs. Veterinary Microbiology 156 (1−2), 143−146.

Bossche, H.V., Koymans, L., Moereels, H., 1995. P450 inhibitors of use in medical treatment: focus on mechanisms of action. Pharmacology & Therapeutics 67 (1), 79−100.

Brown, G.D., Denning, D.W., Gow, N.A., Levitz, S.M., Netea, M.G., White, T.C., 2012. Hidden killers: human fungal infections. Science Translational Medicine 4, 165rv13.

Camps, S.M., van der Linden, J.W., Li, Y., Kuijper, E.J., van Dissel, J.T., Verweij, P.E., Melchers, W.J., 2012. Rapid induction of multiple resistance mechanisms in *Aspergillus fumigatus* during azole therapy: a case study and review of the literature. Antimicrobial Agents and Chemotherapy 56 (1), 10−16.

Casson, N., Greub, G., 2006. Resistance of different *Chlamydia*-like organisms to quinolones and mutations in the quinoline resistance-determining region of the DNA gyrase A-and topoisomerase-encoding genes. International Journal of Antimicrobial Agents 27 (6), 541−544.

Chowdhary, A., Kathuria, S., Xu, J., Meis, J.F., 2013. Emergence of azole-resistant *Aspergillus fumigatus* strains due to agricultural azole use creates an increasing threat to human health. PLoS Pathogens 9 (10), e1003633.

de Barsy, M., Bottinelli, L., Greub, G., 2014. Antibiotic susceptibility of *Estrella lausannensis*, a potential emerging pathogen. Microbes and Infection 16 (9), 746−754.

De Puysseleyr, K., De Puysseleyr, L., Dhondt, H., Geens, T., Braeckman, L., Morré, S.A., Cox, E., Vanrompay, D., 2014. Evaluation of the presence and zoonotic transmission of *Chlamydia suis* in a pig slaughterhouse. BMC Infectious Diseases 14 (1), 560.

Dean, D., Rothschild, J., Ruettger, A., Kandel, R.P., Sachse, K., 2013. Zoonotic *Chlamydiaceae* species associated with trachoma, Nepal. Emerging Infectious Diseases 19 (12), 1948.

Denning, D.W., Pleuvry, A., Cole, D.C., 2013. Global burden of allergic bronchopulmonary aspergillosis with asthma and its complication chronic pulmonary aspergillosis in adults. Medical Mycology 51 (4), 361−370.

Di Francesco, A., Donati, M., Rossi, M., Pignanelli, S., Shurdhi, A., Baldelli, R., Cevenini, R., 2008. Tetracycline-resistant *Chlamydia suis* isolates in Italy. The Veterinary Record 163, 251−252.

Dugan, J., Rockey, D.D., Jones, L., Andersen, A.A., 2004. Tetracycline resistance in *Chlamydia suis* mediated by genomic islands inserted into the chlamydial *inv*-like gene. Antimicrobial Agents and Chemotherapy 48 (10), 3989−3995.

Eick, A.A., Faix, D.J., Tobler, S.K., Nevin, R.L., Lindler, L.E., Hu, Z., Sanchez, J.L., MacIntosh, V.H., Russell, K.L., Gaydos, J.C., 2011. Serosurvey of bacterial and viral respiratory pathogens among deployed US service members. American Journal of Preventive Medicine 41 (6), 573—580.

Eitel, Z., Sóki, J., Urbán, E., Nagy, E., 2013. The prevalence of antibiotic resistance genes in *Bacteroides fragilis* group strains isolated in different European countries. Anaerobe 21, 43—49.

Greub, G., Berger, P., Papazian, L., Raoult, D., 2003. *Parachlamydiaceae* as rare agents of pneumonia. Emerging Infectious Diseases 9 (6), 755.

Gullo, F.P., Rossi, S.A., de CO Sardi, J., Teodoro, V.L.I., Mendes-Giannini, M.J.S., Fusco-Almeida, A.M., 2013. Cryptococcosis: epidemiology, fungal resistance, and new alternatives for treatment. European Journal of Clinical Microbiology & Infectious Diseases 32 (11), 1377—1391.

Horner, P.J., 2012. Azithromycin antimicrobial resistance and genital *Chlamydia trachomatis* infection: duration of therapy may be the key to improving efficacy. Sexually Transmitted Infections 88, 154—156.

Jensen, R.H., Hagen, F., Astvad, K.M.T., Tyron, A., Meis, J.F., Arendrup, M.C., 2016. Azole-resistant *Aspergillus fumigatus* in Denmark: a laboratory-based study on resistance mechanisms and genotypes. Clinical Microbiology and Infections 22 (6), 570-e1.

Jung, K.W., Strain, A.K., Nielsen, K., Jung, K.H., Bahn, Y.S., 2012. Two cation transporters Ena1 and Nha1 cooperatively modulate ion homeostasis, antifungal drug resistance, and virulence of *Cryptococcus neoformans* via the HOG pathway. Fungal Genetics and Biology 49 (4), 332—345.

Lamoth, F., Jaton, K., Vaudaux, B., Greub, G., 2011. *Parachlamydia* and *Rhabdochlamydia*: emerging agents of community-acquired respiratory infections in children. Clinical Infectious Diseases 53 (5), 500—501.

Lienard, J., Croxatto, A., Prod'hom, G., Greub, G., 2011. *Estrella lausannensis*, a new star in the *Chlamydiales* order. Microbes and Infection 13 (14—15), 1232—1241.

Marrazzo, J., Suchland, R., 2014. Recent advances in understanding and managing *Chlamydia trachomatis* infections. F1000prime Reports 6.

Nesky, M.A., McDougal, E.C., Peacock Jr., J.E., 2000. *Scedosporium apiospermum* complex brain abscess successfully treated with voriconazole and surgical drainage: case report and literature review of central nervous system pseudallescheriasis. Clinical Infectious Diseases 31 (3), 673—677.

Park, B.J., Wannemuehler, K.A., Marston, B.J., Govender, N., Pappas, P.G., Chiller, T.M., 2009. Estimation of the current global burden of cryptococcal meningitis among persons living with HIV/AIDS. AIDS 23 (4), 525—530.

Paul, S., Doering, T.L., Moye-Rowley, W.S., 2015. *Cryptococcus neoformans* Yap1 is required for normal fluconazole and oxidative stress resistance. Fungal Genetics and Biology 74, 1—9.

Rodero, L., Mellado, E., Rodriguez, A.C., Salve, A., Guelfand, L., Cahn, P., Cuenca-Estrella, M., Davel, G., Rodriguez-Tudela, J.L., 2003. G484S amino acid substitution in lanosterol 14-α demethylase (ERG11) is related to fluconazole resistance in a recurrent *Cryptococcus neoformans* clinical isolate. Antimicrobial Agents and Chemotherapy 47 (11), 3653—3656.

Samanta, I., 2015. Veterinary Mycology. Springer.

Sandoz, K.M., Rockey, D.D., 2010. Antibiotic resistance in chlamydiae. Future Microbiology 5 (9), 1427—1442.

Sanguinetti, M., Posteraro, B., La Sorda, M., Torelli, R., Fiori, B., Santangelo, R., Delogu, G., Fadda, G., 2006. Role of *AFR1*, an ABC transporter-encoding gene, in the in vivo response to fluconazole and virulence of *Cryptococcus neoformans*. Infection and Immunity 74 (2), 1352—1359.

Schautteet, K., Vanrompay, D., 2011. *Chlamydiaceae* infections in pig. Veterinary Research 42 (1), 29.

Sionov, E., Lee, H., Chang, Y.C., Kwon-Chung, K.J., 2010. *Cryptococcus neoformans* overcomes stress of azole drugs by formation of disomy in specific multiple chromosomes. PLoS Pathogens 6 (4), e1000848.

Snelders, E., Van Der Lee, H.A., Kuijpers, J., Rijs, A.J.M., Varga, J., Samson, R.A., Mellado, E., Donders, A.R.T., Melchers, W.J., Verweij, P.E., 2008. Emergence of azole resistance in *Aspergillus fumigatus* and spread of a single resistance mechanism. PLoS Medicine 5 (11), e219.

Snelders, E., Camps, S.M., Karawajczyk, A., Rijs, A.J., Zoll, J., Verweij, P.E., Melchers, W.J., 2015. Genotype—phenotype complexity of the TR46/Y121F/T289A cyp51A azole resistance mechanism in *Aspergillus fumigatus*. Fungal Genetics and Biology 82, 129—135.

Steinmann, J., Hamprecht, A., Vehreschild, M.J.G.T., Cornely, O.A., Buchheidt, D., Spiess, B., Koldehoff, M., Buer, J., Meis, J.F., Rath, P.M., 2015. Emergence of azole-resistant invasive aspergillosis in HSCT recipients in Germany. Journal of Antimicrobial Chemotherapy 70 (5), 1522—1526.

Tortorano, A.M., Richardson, M., Roilides, E., van Diepeningen, A., Caira, M., Munoz, P., Johnson, E., Meletiadis, J., Pana, Z.D., Lackner, M., Verweij, P., 2014. ESCMID and ECMM joint guidelines on diagnosis and management of hyalohyphomycosis: *Fusarium* spp., *Scedosporium* spp. and others. Clinical Microbiology and Infections 20, 27—46.

Van Der Linden, J.W., Camps, S.M., Kampinga, G.A., Arends, J.P., Debets-Ossenkopp, Y.J., Haas, P.J., Rijnders, B.J., Kuijper, E.J., Van Tiel, F.H., Varga, J., Karawajczyk, A., 2013. Aspergillosis due to voriconazole highly resistant *Aspergillus fumigatus* and recovery of genetically related resistant isolates from domiciles. Clinical Infectious Diseases 57 (4), 513—520.

Chapter 28

Cross-resistance between biocides and antimicrobials

Chapter outline

Biocides are defined as active substances or a preparation consisting of more than one active substance used to kill or reduce the virulence of pathogens (SCENIHR, 2009). Widespread use of biocides such as triclosan and quaternary ammonium compounds increases the selection of antimicrobial-resistant bacteria such as *Escherichia coli* and *Staphylococcus aureus* in the environment (Mcmurry et al., 1998; Russell, 2000; Wesgate et al., 2016). The heavy metal-based biocides (copper, zinc) are commonly used in livestock farms and aquaculture as footbath or antifouling paints in the cages and nets (Thomsen et al., 2008; Burridge et al., 2010). Use of heavy metals can maintain or increase the antimicrobial resistance in certain bacteria. The United States Food and Drug Administration (FDA) and European Union Biocidal Products Regulation make it mandatory for the manufacturers to declare the level of resistance generated in commensal bacteria after use of their biocidal products.

Classification of biocides

The biocides belong to several chemical groups such as alcohol, aldehyde, phenols, biguanide, peroxide, organic acids, metallic salts, halogens, etc. (Table 28.1).

Use of biocides in animal farm, agricultural field and fishery sector

In commercial animal or poultry farms, biocides are used for cleaning of farm premises, vehicles, utensils and buildings, foot dips at the entry of animal/poultry houses, teat dips, decontamination of carcasses and preservation of eggs or semen. Disinfection of farm premises, buildings, vehicles and utensils are carried out with hydrogen peroxide, acetic acid, sodium dichloroisocyanurate, quaternary ammonium compounds (didecyldimethylammonium chloride, alkyldimethylbenzylammonium chloride), glutaraldehyde, formaldehyde and isopropanol. The farm boots and tools are disinfected with sodium-p-toluene-sulfonchloramide and hydrogen peroxide. Copper sulphate is used for foot dips to prevent or cure foot rot in sheep and cattle, although banned in European countries (Thomsen et al., 2008). Teat dip with quaternary ammonium compounds, iodine (0.25%−1.0%), chlorine-based compounds [chloroisocyanurate, chlorhexidine (>0.5%), chlorine dioxide (0.32%), sodium hypochlorite] and bronopol is a common practice before or after milking to prevent the entry of organisms and to reduce the bacterial count for at least log 3. The organic acids are added in animal feed or silage as preservatives to reduce the concentration of spoilage bacteria. Certain heavy metals such as zinc oxide (2000−3000 ppm)

Antimicrobial Resistance in Agriculture. https://doi.org/10.1016/B978-0-12-815770-1.00028-6

TABLE 28.1 Classification, mechanism of action and usage of biocides.

Biocide	Mechanism of action	Usage	Remarks
Alcohols [ethanol (0.1% −99.9%), methanol (0.03%−15%), phenoxyethanol, propanol, propylene glycol, isopropanol (0.1%−77.22%)]	Inhibition of cell wall and nucleic acid synthesis of bacteria; protein denaturation; proton translocation (phenoxyethanol in *Escherichia coli*)	a. Used as antiseptic/ disinfectant in health care b. Used as preservative in pharmaceutical/ cosmetic industry	Ethanol/isopropanol (70%−90%) is approved by the US FDA for health care settings
Aldehyde [formaldehyde (0.03%−15.7%), glutaraldehyde (2%)]	Lysis of bacterial cell wall as alkylating agent	a. Used as disinfectant in health care b. Used as preservative in pharmaceutical/ cosmetic/paper industry	Glutaraldehyde ($\geq$2%) is approved by the US FDA for health care settings
Anionic surfactants (diethylamine)	As a part of a preparation it can lyse bacterial cell wall	a. Used as disinfectant in household products b. Used as preservative in pharmaceutical/ cosmetic industry	−
Biguanides (chlorhexidine digluconate, alexidine, polymeric biguanides)	Chlorhexidine specifically inhibits bacterial cytoplasmic membrane-bound ATPase	Used as disinfectant/antiseptic in household products, health care	−
Diamidines (hexamidine)	Lysis of bacterial cytoplasmic membrane	Used as antiseptic	−
Dyes (acridines, triphenylmethane, quinones)	Lysis of bacterial nucleic acids	Used as antiseptic	−
Halogens (sodium hypochlorite, chloramine, povidone-iodine)	Act as oxidizing agent	Used as disinfectant/ antiseptic in household products, health care, water treatment, industrial products, teat dip in livestock farms	Sodium hypochlorite (5.25% −6.15% household bleach diluted, 1:100, $\approx$500 ppm available chlorine) is approved by the US FDA for health care settings
Iodophors	Enzymatic interactions with thiol group	Used as disinfectant/ antiseptic in health care	−
Hydrogen peroxide (0.5% −29%)	Act as oxidizing agent	Used as disinfectant in household products, health care, industrial products	Hydrogen peroxide (1%−7.5%) is approved by the US FDA for health care settings
Pentamidine	Inhibition of bacterial nucleic acid synthesis	Used as disinfectant in medical devices (catheter)	−
Metals (silver nitrate, mercury)	Enzymatic interactions with thiol group	a. Used as disinfectant in health care b. Used as preservative in pharmaceutical industry	−
Chelated metal (copper, mercuric chloride, phenyl mercury, thiomersal)	Bacterial nucleotides act as target of chelated metals	Used as disinfectant in health care, livestock farm, aquaculture	−
Limonene	Unknown interaction with bacterial cytoplasmic membrane	Used as disinfectant in household products and industry	−
Organic acids and esters [parabens, propionic acid, potassium sorbate, sodium	Dissipation of proton motive force in cytoplasmic membrane of Gram-positive	a. Used as disinfectant in health care	−

Continued

TABLE 28.1 Classification, mechanism of action and usage of biocides.—cont'd

Biocide	Mechanism of action	Usage	Remarks
benzoate, acetic acid (0.4%—52%)]	bacteria; inhibition of amino acids uptake in Gram-negative bacteria	**b.** Used as preservative in pharmaceutical/ cosmetic/food industry	
Phenolics [triclosan (2,4,4′-trichloro-2′-hydroxy-diphenyl ether, 0.5%); dinitrophenol]	Triclosan binds with enoyl-acyl reductase required for bacterial fatty acid synthesis and acts as bacteriostatic agent Dinitrophenol reduces ATP synthesis in bacterial membrane	**c.** Used as disinfectant in health care, domestic products such as hand washes	—
Isothiazolinone	Reduces active transport and oxidation of glucose in *Staphylococcus aureus*	Used as disinfectant in personal care products, household products and industrial products	—
Quaternary ammonium compounds (benzalkonium chloride, cetrimide, cetylpyridinium, dequalinium chloride)	Aggregation of bacterial cytoplasmic membrane proteins and destabilization of the membrane	**a.** Used as disinfectant in health care, household products, teat dip in livestock farm **b.** Used as preservative in pharmaceutical/ cosmetic/food industry	—

and copper sulphate (125—250 ppm) are added in pig feed to improve the growth, performance and to prevent scour (Hill et al., 2000). Furthermore, chromium, tin, vanadium, nickel and molybdenum are also added in animal or poultry feed. Owing to lack of knowledge about their precise concentration to be used, most of the commercial animal or poultry feeds contain high concentration of the minerals which are not absorbed through the gut and are excreted directly into the environment (Ao and Pierce, 2013).

In agricultural field, biocides are used as insecticide, rodenticide, molluscicide and acaricide to control the pest infestation. Bordeaux mixture [$CuSO_4$ and $Ca(OH)_2$] is applied into vineyards and organic potato farming to control vine downy mildew and potato blight, respectively (Gisi et al., 2009).

In aquaculture, iodine, halogens, metallic salts, aldehydes, hydrogen peroxide, quaternary ammonium compounds and dyes are used for disinfection of equipments, ponds and waterbodies and fish eggs (Burridge et al., 2010).

In the United States, use of many biocides is regulated by Federal Pesticide Law (FIFRA) and Federal Food, Drugs and Cosmetic Act. In Europe, since 2012—13, biocide use is controlled by Biocidal Products Regulation 528/2012 (BPR) in place of Biocidal Products Directive (BPD, 98/8/EC). Few member countries of European Union and Asian countries have their own published lists of authorized substances to be used as biocide. For example, in Taiwan, use of biocides in animals and plants is regulated by Veterinary Drug Administration Law and Pesticide Management Act. Central Insecticide Board and Registration Committee of India have recently published guidelines for the registration of biocides used in paints.

How biocides work

Unlike the antimicrobials, the biocides use vivid mechanisms by which it can kill the organisms or inhibit their growth (Table 28.1, Meyer and Cookson, 2010).

Mechanism of resistance against biocides

Since 1950, resistance to biocides was reported in bacterial strains (Davin-Regli and Pagès, 2012). The clinical isolates of *E. coli*, *S. aureus*, *Mycobacterium chelonae*, *Burkholderia cepacia* and *Pseudomonas aeruginosa* were detected to be associated with reduced susceptibility to the biocides such as quaternary ammonium compounds, triclosan, paraben, and glutaraldehyde (Greenberg and Demple, 1989; Bamber and Neal, 1999; Manzoor et al., 1999; Fraud et al., 2001; Hutchinson et al., 2004; Romão et al., 2005). Intrinsic and acquired resistance mechanisms against biocides are observed in clinical bacterial isolates.

Intrinsic resistance

Modification of outer membrane proteins and phospholipids/lipopolysaccharide (LPS) structure in bacterial cell wall is associated with reduced permeability of biocides into the bacterial cell (Guerin-Mechin et al., 2000; Braoudaki and Hilton, 2005). Change in LPS structure increases positive charge of the bacterial outer membrane and the electrostatic repulsion prevents the entry of positively charged quaternary ammonium compounds (Bruinsma et al., 2006). Recent study elucidates the role of UDP-glucose 4-epimerase (*galE*) in increasing the positive charge of LPS in Gram-negative bacteria (*E. coli*), which repulses the positively charged biocides (quaternary ammonium compounds) (Tansirichaiya et al., 2018). Sugar composition of mycobacterial cell wall also reduces the penetration of biocides (Walsh and Fanning, 2008). In Gram-negative bacteria, reduced synthesis of porins is also detected to decrease the entry of biocides (Nikaido, 2003).

Expression of efflux pumps such as QacA-D, Smr, QacG and QacH in *S. aureus*, MexAB-OprM, MexCD-OprJ, MexEF-OprN and MexJK in *P. aeruginosa* and AcrAB-TolC, AcrEF-TolC and EmrE in *E. coli* is associated with reduced intracellular concentration and resistance to quaternary ammonium compounds, triclosan, phenolic parabens and intercalating agents (Littlejohn et al., 1992; Heir et al., 1999; Nishino and Yamaguchi, 2001; Morita et al., 2003). Exposure to biocide (triclosan) in *Stenotrophomonas maltophilia* can also induce efflux pump which helps in expulsion of antibiotics (quinolones) (Hernández et al., 2011).

Resistance to parabens, aldehydes, heavy metals and peroxygens is associated with enzymatic modification of biocides. For example, modification of the enzyme (enoyl-acyl reductase) structure produces reduced susceptibility to triclosan in *S. aureus* (Heath et al., 2000). In Gram-negative bacteria (*E. coli*), triclosan inhibits FabI-dependent fatty acid synthesis and FabI mutant bacteria are intrinsically triclosan resistant (Zhu et al., 2010).

Acquired resistance

Acquisition of mobile genetic elements (transposons, plasmids) encoding the resistance factors can induce acquired resistance to biocides in bacteria. Experimental introduction of genetic inserts containing *fabI* causes overexpression of enoyl-acyl reductase in *E. coli* and reduces the inhibitory effect of triclosan (Tansirichaiya et al., 2018).

Cross-resistance, co-resistance and co-regulation between biocides and antimicrobials

Cross-resistance

Use of biocides at suboptimal concentration for a prolonged period can induce multiple drug-resistant bacteria. Few biocides and antibiotics share common mechanism such as disruption of bacterial membrane integrity, inhibition of synthesis of enzymes and nucleic acids. For survival, the bacteria use similar defence mechanisms which may confer cross-resistance against structurally unrelated molecules. The efflux pump (MdrL) detected in *Listeria* is active to expel both the antibiotics (cefotaxime, clindamycin, erythromycin and josamycin) and metals (zinc, cobalt and chromium) from the bacterial cell (Mata et al., 2000). Presence of zinc can select a resistant phenotype of *Listeria* which confers co-resistance to any of the stated antibiotics. Oethinger et al. (1998) observed the association between cyclohexane tolerance and fluoroquinolones resistance in clinical isolates of *E. coli*. *Salmonella* serovars isolated from animals showed cross-resistance to multiple antibiotics and biocides (ethidium bromide, cetrimide, cyclohexane, triclosan, acridine orange) (Randall et al., 2001). Other studies also observed cross-resistance to antibiotics and disinfectants in *E. coli* strains associated with overexpression of AcrAB efflux pump (Ma et al., 1996; Moken et al., 1997). Exposure to quaternary ammonium compounds and tar oil phenol in *Salmonella* serovars of poultry caused overexpression of efflux pumps (AcrAB, TolC) and reduced susceptibility to multiple antibiotics (Baucheron et al., 2005). Exposure to biocide also increased expression of antibiotic resistance genes in clinical isolates of *S. aureus* (Huet et al., 2008).

Co-resistance

Biofilm is one of the defence mechanisms which induce co-resistance in bacteria to both biocides and antibiotics. Resistance in biofilm-producing bacteria is associated with decreased metabolism, reduced penetration of biocide/antibiotic through extracellular polymeric matrix, enzymatic inactivation and the induction of multidrug-resistant operons (*marA*) and efflux pumps (*acrB*) (Huang et al., 1995; Maira-Litran et al., 2000; Pan et al., 2006; Tabak et al., 2007). The diffusion of biocides through extracellular matrix is the major contributing factor identified to produce resistance against biocides in *Pseudomonas*-associated biofilms (Bridier et al., 2011). During exposure to metal-based biocides, the metals are chelated with the bacterial dead cells and metabolism end products to generate the biofilm matrix. This kind of matrix prevents further entry of metal ions into the deeper part of the structure (Harrison et al., 2007).

In Gram-negative bacteria (*E. coli*, *Salmonella*) *mar* and *soxS* regulons induce the overlapping genes associated with co-resistance to multiple antibiotics (ampicillin, nalidixic acid, chloramphenicol and tetracycline) and biocides (paraquat, organic solvent) (Poole, 2007). Some biocide/metal resistance genes (*mer*, *qac*) are present in the same mobile genetic elements (Tn*21*, Tn*5045*, class 1 integron) of bacteria along with antimicrobial resistance genes which may produce co-resistance even in absence of the antibiotic selection pressure (Liebert et al., 1999; Levy and Marshall, 2004; Petrova et al., 2011). The transposon (Tn*21*) present in *Salmonella typhimurium* carried mercury resistance gene along with resistance factors against sulfonamide, quaternary ammonium compounds, streptomycin, spectinomycin and penicillin (Summers et al., 1993).

A correlation between presence of heavy metal and antibiotic resistance in bacteria even in absence and weakly presence of antibiotic selection pressure was noted since 1970 (Timoney et al., 1978; Ji et al., 2012). Co-resistance of heavy metals (zinc, cadmium and copper) and antibiotics (β-lactams, erythromycin, kanamycin, novobiocin, ofloxacin and sulphanilamide) was reported in *B. cepacia* associated with DsbA-DsbB system and copper-resistant soil bacteria (Hayashi et al., 2000; Berg et al., 2005). Multidrug-resistant plasmid/transposon was detected in the bacteria possessing the genes for various antibiotics, heavy metals and other biocides, and the plasmids are carried by the bacteria with a fitness cost (Ghosh et al., 2000). The minimal selective concentration (MSC) of a drug or heavy metal is defined as the concentration in which advantage of being resistant is equal to the fitness cost of the bacteria. If the antibiotic or heavy metal is maintained in the concentration higher than MSC, more resistant bacteria emerge in the nature. Moreover, when an individual element (antibiotic or metal biocide) is not present in sufficient concentration (below MSC level) in the environment to select resistant bacteria, their combined concentration can do the same. Experimentally, various concentrations of arsenic, tetracycline and trimethoprim result in selection and maintenance of multidrug-resistant plasmid in *Klebsiella pneumoniae* and *E. coli* (Gullberg et al., 2014). However, the network constructed with the sequences of antibiotic/metal/biocide resistance genes revealed limited connections between the heavy metal and antibiotic resistance genes (Pal et al., 2015).

Co-regulation

Exposure to heavy metals can alter the expression of antibiotic resistance genes in bacteria, which is known as co-regulation. In presence of zinc, a two-component regulatory system (cscRS) is activated in *P. aeruginosa*, which encodes an efflux pump (RND) to confer resistance against zinc, cadmium and cobalt. Simultaneously the regulatory system also reduces expression of a porin (OprD) used by the antibiotic (imipenem) to enter the cell (Caille et al., 2007). The two-component regulatory system encodes the efflux pump through the transcription of the czcCBA operon. Mutation in czcS operon (GTG to TTG) in zinc-exposed *P. aeruginosa* was correlated with reduced expression of OprD (Perron et al., 2004).

References

Ao, T., Pierce, J., 2013. The replacement of inorganic mineral salts with mineral proteinates in poultry diets. World's Poultry Science Journal 69 (1), 5—16.

Bamber, A.I., Neal, T.J., 1999. An assessment of triclosan susceptibility in methicillin-resistant and methicillin-sensitive *Staphylococcus aureus*. Journal of Hospital Infection 41 (2), 107—109.

Baucheron, S., Mouline, C., Praud, K., Chaslus-Dancla, E., Cloeckaert, A., 2005. TolC but not AcrB is essential for multidrug-resistant *Salmonella enterica* serotype Typhimurium colonization of chicks. Journal of Antimicrobial Chemotherapy 55 (5), 707−712.

Berg, J., Tom-Petersen, A., Nybroe, O., 2005. Copper amendment of agricultural soil selects for bacterial antibiotic resistance in the field. Letters in Applied Microbiology 40 (2), 146−151.

Braoudaki, M., Hilton, A.C., 2005. Mechanisms of resistance in *Salmonella enterica* adapted to erythromycin, benzalkonium chloride and triclosan. International Journal of Antimicrobial Agents 25 (1), 31−37.

Bridier, A., Dubois-Brissonnet, F., Greub, G., Thomas, V., Briandet, R., 2011. Dynamics of the action of biocides in *Pseudomonas aeruginosa* biofilms. Antimicrobial Agents and Chemotherapy 55 (6), 2648−2654.

Bruinsma, G.M., Rustema-Abbing, M., van der Mei, H.C., Lakkis, C., Busscher, H.J., 2006. Resistance to a polyquaternium-1 lens care solution and isoelectric points of *Pseudomonas aeruginosa* strains. Journal of Antimicrobial Chemotherapy 57 (4), 764−766.

Burridge, L., Weis, J.S., Cabello, F., Pizarro, J., Bostick, K., 2010. Chemical use in salmon aquaculture: a review of current practices and possible environmental effects. Aquaculture 306 (1−4), 7−23.

Caille, O., Rossier, C., Perron, K., 2007. A copper-activated two-component system interacts with zinc and imipenem resistance in *Pseudomonas aeruginosa*. Journal of Bacteriology 189 (13), 4561−4568.

Davin-Regli, A., Pagès, J.M., 2012. Cross-resistance between biocides and antimicrobials: an emerging question. Revue Scientifique et Technique-OIE 31 (1), 89.

Fraud, S., Maillard, J.Y., Russell, A.D., 2001. Comparison of the mycobactericidal activity of ortho-phthalaldehyde, glutaraldehyde and other dialdehydes by a quantitative suspension test. Journal of Hospital Infection 48 (3), 214−221.

Ghosh, A., Singh, A., Ramteke, P.W., Singh, V.P., 2000. Characterization of large plasmids encoding resistance to toxic heavy metals in *Salmonella abortus equi*. Biochemical and Biophysical Research Communications 272 (1), 6−11.

Gisi, U., Chet, I., Gullino, M.L., 2009. Recent Developments in Management of Plant Diseases, vol. 1. Springer Dordrecht Heidelberg, London, New York.

Greenberg, J.T., Demple, B.R.U.C.E., 1989. A global response induced in *Escherichia coli* by redox-cycling agents overlaps with that induced by peroxide stress. Journal of Bacteriology 171 (7), 3933−3939.

Guerin-Mechin, L., Dubois-Brissonnet, F., Heyd, B., Leveau, J.Y., 2000. Quaternary ammonium compound stresses induce specific variations in fatty acid composition of *Pseudomonas aeruginosa*. International Journal of Food Microbiology 55 (1−3), 157−159.

Gullberg, E., Albrecht, L.M., Karlsson, C., Sandegren, L., Andersson, D.I., 2014. Selection of a multidrug resistance plasmid by sublethal levels of antibiotics and heavy metals. mBio 5 (5) e01918-14.

Harrison, J.J., Ceri, H., Turner, R.J., 2007. Multimetal resistance and tolerance in microbial biofilms. Nature Reviews Microbiology 5 (12), 928.

Hayashi, S., Abe, M., Kimoto, M., Furukawa, S., Nakazawa, T., 2000. The dsbA-dsbB disulfide bond formation system of Burkholderia cepacia is involved in the production of protease and alkaline phosphatase, motility, metal resistance, and multi-drug resistance. Microbiology and Immunology 44 (1), 41−50.

Heath, R.J., Li, J., Roland, G.E., Rock, C.O., 2000. Inhibition of the *Staphylococcus aureus* NADPH-dependent enoyl-acyl carrier protein reductase by triclosan and hexachlorophene. Journal of Biological Chemistry 275 (7), 4654−4659.

Heir, E., Sundheim, G., Holck, A.L., 1999. The *qacG* gene on plasmid pST94 confers resistance to quaternary ammonium compounds in staphylococci isolated from the food industry. Journal of Applied Microbiology 86 (3), 378−388.

Hernández, A., Ruiz, F.M., Romero, A., Martínez, J.L., 2011. The binding of triclosan to SmeT, the repressor of the multidrug efflux pump SmeDEF, induces antibiotic resistance in *Stenotrophomonas maltophilia*. PLoS Pathogens 7 (6), e1002103.

Hill, G.M., Cromwell, G.L., Crenshaw, T.D., Dove, C.R., Ewan, R.C., Knabe, D.A., Lewis, A.J., Libal, G.W., Mahan, D.C., Shurson, G.C., Southern, L.L., 2000. Growth promotion effects and plasma changes from feeding high dietary concentrations of zinc and copper to weanling pigs (regional study). Journal of Animal Science 78 (4), 1010−1016.

Huang, C.T., Yu, F.P., McFeters, G.A., Stewart, P.S., 1995. Non uniform spatial patterns of respiratory activity within biofilms during disinfection. Applied and Environmental Microbiology 61 (6), 2252−2256.

Huet, A.A., Raygada, J.L., Mendiratta, K., Seo, S.M., Kaatz, G.W., 2008. Multidrug efflux pump overexpression in *Staphylococcus aureus* after single and multiple in vitro exposures to biocides and dyes. Microbiology 154 (10), 3144−3153.

Hutchinson, J., Runge, W., Mulvey, M., Norris, G., Yetman, M., Valkova, N., Villemur, R., Lepine, F., 2004. *Burkholderia cepacia* infections associated with intrinsically contaminated ultrasound gel: the role of microbial degradation of parabens. Infection Control & Hospital Epidemiology 25 (4), 291−296.

Ji, X., Shen, Q., Liu, F., Ma, J., Xu, G., Wang, Y., Wu, M., 2012. Antibiotic resistance gene abundances associated with antibiotics and heavy metals in animal manures and agricultural soils adjacent to feedlots in Shanghai; China. Journal of Hazardous Materials 235, 178−185.

Levy, S.B., Marshall, B., 2004. Antibacterial resistance worldwide: causes, challenges and responses. Nature Medicine 10 (12s), S122.

Liebert, C.A., Hall, R.M., Summers, A.O., 1999. Transposon Tn21, flagship of the floating genome. Microbiology and Molecular Biology Reviews 63 (3), 507−522.

Littlejohn, T.G., Paulsen, I.T., Gillespie, M.T., Tennent, J.M., Midgley, M., Jones, I.G., Purewal, A.S., Skurray, R.A., 1992. Substrate specificity and energetics of antiseptic and disinfectant resistance in *Staphylococcus aureus*. FEMS Microbiology Letters 95 (2−3), 259−265.

Ma, D., Alberti, M., Lynch, C., Nikaido, H., Hearst, J.E., 1996. The local repressor AcrR plays a modulating role in the regulation of acrAB genes of *Escherichia coli* by global stress signals. Molecular Microbiology 19 (1), 101−112.

Maira-Litran, T., Allison, D.G., Gilbert, P., 2000. An evaluation of the potential of the multiple antibiotic resistance operon (*mar*) and the multidrug efflux pump acrAB to moderate resistance towards ciprofloxacin in *Escherichia coli* biofilms. Journal of Antimicrobial Chemotherapy 45 (6), 789−795.

Manzoor, S.E., Lambert, P.A., Griffiths, P.A., Gill, M.J., Fraise, A.P., 1999. Reduced glutaraldehyde susceptibility in *Mycobacterium chelonae* associated with altered cell wall polysaccharides. Journal of Antimicrobial Chemotherapy 43 (6), 759−765.

Mata, M.T., Baquero, F., Perez-Diaz, J.C., 2000. A multidrug efflux transporter in *Listeria monocytogenes*. FEMS Microbiology Letters 187 (2), 185−188.

Mcmurry, L.M., Oethinger, M., Levy, S.B., 1998. Overexpression of *marA*, *soxS*, or *acrAB* produces resistance to triclosan in laboratory and clinical strains of *Escherichia coli*. FEMS Microbiology Letters 166 (2), 305−309.

Meyer, B., Cookson, B., 2010. Does microbial resistance or adaptation to biocides create a hazard in infection prevention and control? Journal of Hospital Infection 76 (3), 200−205.

Moken, M.C., McMurry, L.M., Levy, S.B., 1997. Selection of multiple-antibiotic-resistant (mar) mutants of *Escherichia coli* by using the disinfectant pine oil: roles of the *mar* and *acrAB* loci. Antimicrobial Agents and Chemotherapy 41 (12), 2770−2772.

Morita, Y., Murata, T., Mima, T., Shiota, S., Kuroda, T., Mizushima, T., Gotoh, N., Nishino, T., Tsuchiya, T., 2003. Induction of mexCD-oprJ operon for a multidrug efflux pump by disinfectants in wild-type *Pseudomonas aeruginosa* PAO1. Journal of Antimicrobial Chemotherapy 51 (4), 991−994.

Nikaido, H., 2003. Molecular basis of bacterial outer membrane permeability revisited. Microbiology and Molecular Biology Reviews 67 (4), 593−656.

Nishino, K., Yamaguchi, A., 2001. Analysis of a complete library of putative drug transporter genes in *Escherichia coli*. Journal of Bacteriology 183 (20), 5803−5812.

Oethinger, M., Kern, W.V., Goldman, J.D., Levy, S.B., 1998. Association of organic solvent tolerance and fluoroquinolone resistance in clinical isolates of *Escherichia coli*. Journal of Antimicrobial Chemotherapy 41 (1), 111−114.

Pal, C., Bengtsson-Palme, J., Kristiansson, E., Larsson, D.J., 2015. Co-occurrence of resistance genes to antibiotics, biocides and metals reveals novel insights into their co-selection potential. BMC Genomics 16 (1), 964.

Pan, Y., Breidt, F., Kathariou, S., 2006. Resistance of *Listeria monocytogenes* biofilms to sanitizing agents in a simulated food processing environment. Applied and Environmental Microbiology 72 (12), 7711−7717.

Perron, K., Caille, O., Rossier, C., Van Delden, C., Dumas, J.L., Köhler, T., 2004. CzcR-CzcS, a two-component system involved in heavy metal and carbapenem resistance in *Pseudomonas aeruginosa*. Journal of Biological Chemistry 279 (10), 8761−8768.

Petrova, M., Gorlenko, Z., Mindlin, S., 2011. Tn*5045*, a novel integron-containing antibiotic and chromate resistance transposon isolated from a permafrost bacterium. Research in Microbiology 162 (3), 337−345.

Poole, K., 2007. Efflux pumps as antimicrobial resistance mechanisms. Annals of Medicine 39 (3), 162−176.

Randall, L.P., Cooles, S.W., Sayers, A.R., Woodward, M.J., 2001. Association between cyclohexane resistance in *Salmonella* of different serovars and increased resistance to multiple antibiotics, disinfectants and dyes. Journal of Medical Microbiology 50 (10), 919−924.

Romão, C.M.C.P.A., Faria, Y.N.D., Pereira, L.R., Asensi, M.D., 2005. Susceptibility of clinical isolates of multiresistant *Pseudomonas aeruginosa* to a hospital disinfectant and molecular typing. Memorias Do Instituto Oswaldo Cruz 100 (5), 541−548.

Russell, A.D., 2000. Do biocides select for antibiotic resistance? Journal of Pharmacy and Pharmacology 52 (2), 227−233.

SCENIHR (Scientific Committee on Emerging and Newly Identified Health Risks, 2009. Assessment of the Antibiotic Resistance Effects of Biocides. Available at: http://ec.europa.eu/health/ph_risk/committees/04_scenihr/docs/scenihr_o_021.pdf.

Summers, A.O., Wireman, J., Vimy, M.J., Lorscheider, F.L., Marshall, B., Levy, S.B., Bennett, S., Billard, L., 1993. Mercury released from dental" silver" fillings provokes an increase in mercury-and antibiotic-resistant bacteria in oral and intestinal floras of primates. Antimicrobial Agents and Chemotherapy 37 (4), 825−834.

Tabak, M., Scher, K., Hartog, E., Romling, U., Matthews, K.R., Chikindas, M.L., Yaron, S., 2007. Effect of triclosan on *Salmonella typhimurium* at different growth stages and in biofilms. FEMS Microbiology Letters 267 (2), 200−206.

Tansirichaiya, S., Reynolds, L.J., Cristarella, G., Wong, L.C., Rosendahl, K., Roberts, A.P., 2018. Reduced susceptibility to antiseptics is conferred by heterologous housekeeping genes. Microbial Drug Resistance 24 (2), 105−112.

Thomsen, P.T., Sørensen, J.T., Ersbøll, A.K., 2008. Evaluation of three commercial hoof-care products used in footbaths in Danish dairy herds. Journal of Dairy Science 91 (4), 1361−1365.

Timoney, J.F., Port, J., Giles, J., Spanier, J., 1978. Heavy-metal and antibiotic resistance in the bacterial flora of sediments of New York Bight. Applied and Environmental Microbiology 36 (3), 465−472.

Walsh, C., Fanning, S., 2008. Antimicrobial resistance in foodborne pathogens-a cause for concern? Current Drug Targets 9 (9), 808−815.

Wesgate, R., Grasha, P., Maillard, J.Y., 2016. Use of a predictive protocol to measure the antimicrobial resistance risks associated with biocidal product usage. American Journal of Infection Control 44 (4), 458−464.

Zhu, L., Lin, J., Ma, J., Cronan, J.E., Wang, H., 2010. Triclosan resistance of *Pseudomonas aeruginosa* PAO1 is due to FabV, a triclosan-resistant enoyl-acyl carrier protein reductase. Antimicrobial Agents and Chemotherapy 54 (2), 689−698.

Chapter 29

Antimicrobial stewardship

Chapter outline

Definition

Inappropriate use of costly and higher generation antibiotics is common both in human health care settings and community, especially in Southern Europe and United States (Goossens et al., 2007; Bell et al., 2014). Competitions in practices, fear of postoperative infections, improper diagnosis, and self-medication are major causes of antibiotic misuse in hospital and community although guidelines for judicious antibiotic use are available for the human physicians (Denes et al., 2012; Venekamp et al., 2012). In contrast, in low- and middle-income group of countries (LMIC) such as in Vietnam, lower generation and cheaper antibiotics are preferred for common cold or other respiratory tract infections as the people cannot afford the cost (Nguyen et al., 2013).

Society for Healthcare Epidemiology of America (SHEA) and Infectious Diseases Society of America (IDSA) first published the guidelines for human hospitals incorporating the antimicrobial stewardship (Shlaes et al., 1997). In the preceding year, John E. McGowan and Dale N. Gerding coined the term 'antimicrobial stewardship' (McGowan and Gerding, 1996). European Society of Clinical Microbiology and Infectious Diseases study group for antimicrobial stewardship (ESGAP) was established in 1998 under the leadership of Ian Gould and Jos van der Meer who spread the message of stewardship worldwide (Gould, 1999). During 1990—2000, the United States and European countries ('Strama' in Sweden) took the initiatives to promote antimicrobial stewardship in national level (Mölstad et al., 2008). During the same period (1990), restriction of antibiotic use was also introduced in animals and birds (as growth promoter) in Denmark and Sweden (Bengtsson and Greko, 2014).

'Antimicrobial stewardship' can be defined as a 'coherent set of actions' that confirms effective therapeutic availability of antimicrobials during necessity (Dyar et al., 2017). The circumference of the 'coherent set of actions' has moved from the therapeutical knowhow (selection, dose, route of administration and duration of antibiotics) to a concept of responsibility (Goff, 2011). The aim of the stewardship program earlier included an evidence-based approach to judicious antimicrobial use in patients minimizing the toxicity and favourable conditions for the generation of resistant bacteria. Currently, it encompasses a multifaceted approach taken by the Government, which includes policies, guidelines, surveillance of resistant organisms, mass awareness campaign and audit of practice.

Necessity

In human health care facilities, antimicrobial stewardship can decrease the occurrence of resistance, antibiotic-associated adverse effects and health care costs and improve patient care quality with more clinical success and frequency of correct prescribing for therapy and prophylaxis (Deuster et al., 2010; Toth et al., 2010; Davey et al., 2013). The study also revealed decreased hospital stay and duration of antibiotic therapy with stewardship intervention in surgical ward of human health care (Fernández-Morato et al., 2016). Similar kinds of benefits are expected in animal health care both in hospitals and in practice.

Antimicrobial Resistance in Agriculture. https://doi.org/10.1016/B978-0-12-815770-1.00029-8

Approaches and techniques

The 'stewardship intervention' in human healthcare settings includes the attempts to use antibiotics judiciously supported by decision-making tools (sensitivity testing) and to restrict unnecessary use (Septimus and Owens, 2011). The whole procedure to influence the prescribers is controlled by a multidisciplinary team attached with the healthcare system. The techniques used for stewardship intervention are making a guideline for physicians, limited advertisement of antimicrobials by the pharmaceuticals, restricted issue of antimicrobials by the hospital authority to the prescribers, rotational use of antimicrobials in intensive care unit ('antibiotic cycling'), persuading the prescribers to use alternate therapy, public awareness campaigns organized by Government and non-Government organizations (NGO), establishment of national surveillance system to receive the authentic data on current resistance pattern of the organisms, quality of antibiotics used and total antibiotic consumption in a stipulated period (MacDougall and Polk, 2005; Pulcini et al., 2017).

The suggested stewardship intervention in veterinary sector includes formation of a national stewardship policy with species-wise therapeutic guidelines, formulation of online and offline courses for veterinarians (continuing veterinary education program) and paraveterinarians, monitoring of antibiotic use with legal support and surveillance of current resistance pattern in animal pathogens and commensals (Hardefeldt et al., 2018). However, the stewardship intervention in veterinary sector is difficult to implement because of insufficient numbers of veterinarians (specially in low- and middle-income countries), limited access to education and training to the veterinarians and informal service providers, limited communication between academic and community veterinarians, restricted diagnostic tools and laboratory support, competition between practitioners and sales of antibiotics without consultation and prescription (in food animals). In the United States, although the companion animal practitioners are aware of antimicrobial resistance, little laboratory support is available for stewardship program (Grayzel et al., 2015). Even in developed countries, precise data of antibiotic consumption demarcated separately for companion and food animals are not available. In food animal industry in the United States, antimicrobial stewardship is somehow considered as a threat to affordability of meat, consistency of supply chain and, moreover, the profits (D'Angeli et al., 2016).

Good stewardship practice (GSP) is collection of active and motivated exercises for judicious antimicrobial use with a mindset for constant improvement (Prescott and Boerlin, 2016). The GSP consists of '5R', i.e., responsibility, reduction, refinement, replacement and review. 'Responsibility' is the first core element of a successful '5R' framework and in human healthcare setting it consists of a collaborative approach encompassing all the stakeholders starting from the physician to nurses and other healthcare staffs (Sanchez et al., 2016). The social interaction and cohesiveness between the physicians and the staffs can convert a conservative physician into an early adopter and improve the patient safety (Kwok et al., 2017). In veterinary practices also, 'responsibility' is a mutual approach between the practitioner with the selection of a proper antibiotic and the owner by following the instructions for proper use of the antibiotic and other management practices (Page et al., 2014). 'Reduction' in veterinary practice is defined as improvement of biosecurity strategy, use of vaccine, providing balanced feed, maintenance of proper hygiene, selection of genetically disease-resistant flock which can minimize the infectious diseases and subsequent use of antibiotics (Swaggerty et al., 2014; Murphy et al., 2017). Introduction of biosecurity practices among the backyard poultry farmers in India reduced the infection rate in birds and improved the egg production (Samanta et al., 2015, 2018). 'Refinement' is the accurate diagnosis of an infection of bacterial origin followed by prescription of the appropriate drug in proper dose and route and for the exact period. In animal practices, accurate diagnosis is difficult in several instances such as respiratory disease in feedlot cattle (Timsit et al., 2016). Recent development in diagnosis of animal diseases includes remote automatic sensing of animal behaviour (Colles et al., 2016), computer-aided lung auscultation in cattle (Mang et al., 2015), infrared thermography (Schaefer et al., 2012), etc. The approaches to improve the treatment protocol with minimizing the generation of resistance include use of drugs in appropriate dose during early stage of the infection, topical therapy in place of systemic approach where applicable and use of plant-based adjunct therapy to reduce the persistence time of antibiotics in the tissues (Martinez et al., 2012; Bajwa, 2016; Sar et al., 2018). 'Replacement' is the use of alternative approach in place of antibiotics if sufficient evidence is there for efficacy and safety. The alternative approach in livestock and poultry includes use of yeast or bacteria-based probiotics, prebiotics, synbiotics, bacteriophages, essential oils, antimicrobial peptides, immunoglobulins, spray-dried immune plasma, teat sealing paste during dry period to prevent the entry of pathogens in mastitis prone area and artificial bovine cytokines (Torrallardona, 2009; Ghosh et al., 2012; Ducatelle et al., 2015; Gadde et al., 2015; Vohra et al., 2016; Wang et al., 2016; Carvalho et al., 2017; McDougall et al., 2017; Ruiz et al., 2017; Chowdhury et al., 2018). 'Review' is the last and most crucial element of '5R', which is a continuous process of evaluation for all the interventions taken. Progress is measured for each objective with the available data associated with antibiotic consumption in food or companion animals, correlation between the consumption and resistance pattern in the bacteria, quality of antibiotics used, control of infectious diseases and, moreover, improvement of each intervention (Dunn and

Dunn, 2012; Kallen and Prins, 2017). The example of GSP was detected in the Netherlands, which reported 58% decrease in antibiotic sales in animal sector during 2009—15 and it was associated with reduced antimicrobial resistance in broilers, veal calves and pigs (ECDGHFS, 2017).

Pitfalls

Implementation of antimicrobial stewardship is easier in a well-equipped human hospital setting because of sufficient numbers of physicians, nurses, infectious disease specialists and other health care staffs and availability of microbiology laboratory. The prescriber can switch into a narrow spectrum antibiotic after receiving sufficient information about the pathogen from the laboratory. Thus, hospital stay, cost of treatment and possibility of resistance generation are reduced. The long-term care facilities may act as source of resistant organisms because of close contact with the patients receiving antibiotics for prolonged period (Toubes et al., 2003). Several human hospitals cannot implement the stewardship due to lack of funds, time and sufficient staffs (Doron and Davidson, 2011).

Such kind of stewardship intervention is difficult in the community as the dose and duration of antibiotics cannot be monitored in outdoor patients. Vaccines for all kinds of infectious diseases are not available in the market such as for prevention of urinary tract infections. People including clinicians are not always fully aware of the problem and they do not participate in the awareness campaigns. Implementation of stewardship program in community is not supported with a stringent law in several countries.

Sometimes stewardship intervention reduces the use of a specific group of antibiotic (cephalosporin) and increases the use of others (carbapenem) along with the resistance (Rahal et al., 1998).

WHO list of priority antimicrobial-resistant pathogens

Following the recommendation of the United Nations, World Health Organization (WHO) took the initiative to prepare a list of antimicrobial-resistant bacteria according to the priority in 2016. The list was prepared to guide the funding agencies and researchers and to create a global network for development of novel molecules against the resistant bacteria. The coordinating group for preparation of the list was selected through open tender launched by WHO and it consisted of WHO staff and international experts in infectious diseases, clinical microbiology, public health and pharmaceutical research. The coordinating group prepared the list on the basis of 10 criteria such as all-cause mortality, healthcare and community burden, prevalence of resistance, 10-year trend of resistance, transmissibility, preventability in hospital and community settings, treatability and current pipeline. Drug-resistant *Mycobacterium tuberculosis* is not included in the ranking list as it is already a globally established priority for which innovative treatment strategy is urgently needed. The complete list can be downloaded from the website of WHO (https://www.who.int).

International guidelines to minimize antimicrobial resistance

In 2016, United Nations called for a high-level meeting and established Interagency Coordination Group on Antimicrobial Resistance (IACG) to make a guideline to address the issue. In the World Health Assembly (May 2018) hosted by the Republic of Korea and Sweden, discussions were held on resistance surveillance throughout the world and the difficulties faced in surveillance program in LMIC (Jee et al., 2018). The first effort for the resistance surveillance program was initiated by the WHO as Global Antimicrobial Resistance Surveillance System (GLASS). The program is based on a standardized approach by all the member countries (71) for the collection, analysis, and sharing of AMR data. GLASS works with all the regional networks such as 'central Asian and eastern European surveillance of antimicrobial resistance (CAESAR)', 'European antimicrobial resistance surveillance network (EARS-Net)' and 'Latin American network for antimicrobial resistance surveillance (ReLAVRA)'. Antibiotic sensitivity of the bacterial isolates under GLASS program is performed following the standard protocols of European Committee on Antimicrobial Susceptibility Testing (EUCAST) or Clinical and Laboratory Standards Institute (CLSI) (GLASS, 2017—18).

The US Food and Drug Administration (FDA), Centers for Disease Control and Prevention (CDC) and United States Department of Agriculture (USDA) jointly established a similar kind of surveillance network in the national level for detection of antibiotic-resistant bacteria present in food animals in 1996, known as National Antimicrobial Resistance Monitoring System (NARMS). Based on the activities and reports of NARMS, FDA issued several guidelines and regulations in the United States such as #152, #209 and #213 for judicious use of antibiotics in food animal and poultry industry. The decision to ban the use of enrofloxacin and sarafloxacin in poultry industry was taken by the FDA (Karp et al., 2017). These FDA regulatory mandates were implemented in a phase-wise manner to provide sufficient time for the pharmaceutical companies to change label indications. The national surveillance network is also developed in human health care settings in Europe (European strategic action plan on antibiotic resistance) and Canada (Canadian Antimicrobial Resistance Surveillance System, CARSS). The European strategic action plan coordinates the national plans of 13 European countries to support the antimicrobial stewardship program (European Centre for Disease Prevention and Control, 2016). Antimicrobial resistance 'Dashboard' is being developed for geospatial mapping of resistance genes, mobile genetic elements and occurrence of resistant bacteria in clinical samples and the environment (Stedtfeld et al., 2016).

Asian Network for Surveillance of Resistant Pathogens (ANSORP) was established in 1996 to develop the guidelines for prevention and control of resistance. The network consists of 14 member countries and the prospective surveillance studies conducted with *Streptococcus pneumoniae* strains isolated from human patients in 11 countries revealed high prevalence rates of penicillin and erythromycin resistance especially in Vietnam (Kim et al., 2012). Subsequently in Vietnam, a surveillance network was developed to strengthen antimicrobial stewardship, known as Viet Nam Resistance (VINARES) project by Vietnamese healthcare professionals in collaboration with Oxford University Clinical Research Unit, Wellcome Trust major overseas programme and Linköping University (Wertheim et al., 2013). An expert panel comprising of different professional healthcare societies was established in Singapore to address the issue of resistance in human health care settings focussing on the conservation of antibiotics (Hsu et al., 2008).

In India, a network of microbiology laboratories in medical colleges was established during 2009–12, known as Indian Network for Surveillance of Antimicrobial Resistance (INSAR) with support from WHO to review the magnitude of the problem (Ray et al., 2013). Indian Council of Medical Research (ICMR) initiated the Antimicrobial Resistance Surveillance and Research Network (AMRSN) in 2013 for effective development of a stewardship program throughout the country (Walia et al., 2015). In the 12th 5-year plan (2012–17), Government of India launched 'National Programme on Containment of Antimicrobial Resistance' in 20 state medical college laboratories with National Center for Disease Control (NCDC) as the focal point. The ministry of health and family welfare, Government of India formed a core working group on antimicrobial resistance to draft the national action plan on antimicrobial resistance (NAP-AMR) in 2017 with a one health approach. The national action plan identified several priority areas such as awareness campaign, surveillance studies, effective infection prevention, optimizing the use of antimicrobials in human, animals and food, investments for more research and innovations and strengthening the country leadership on AMR by forming effective network (NAP-AMR, 2017–21).

Agriculture/veterinary stewardship guidelines

The United States Food and Agricultural Organization (FAO) in collaboration with World Organization for Animal Health (OIE) and WHO released a manual for developing national action plans on agriculture or veterinary stewardship including terrestrial and aquatic animal health and production, crop production and food safety standards (World health organization, food and agriculture organization, world organization for animal health, 2016). FAO developed the Codex Alimentarius, which is a collection of internationally adopted food standards to protect the consumers' health. According to Codex principles, assessing the risk to human health from foodborne-resistant bacteria is essential. FAO further developed the guidelines to determine the risk of human health from resistant bacteria present in food, animal feed and aquaculture (FAO/WHO Codex Alimentarius, 2015).

'European Platform for the Responsible Use of Medicines in Animals (EPRUMA, http://www.epruma.eu/)' was established in 2005 to promote the guidelines on judicious use of antimicrobials in food animals. In the United Kingdom, 'Responsible Use of Medicines in Agriculture Alliance (RUMA)' similarly published guidelines on effective antimicrobial use and vaccination in poultry, pigs, cattle, sheep and fish. To reduce the usage of antibiotics in food animals, vaccination, use of probiotics, immunostimulants, balanced feed with adequate trace minerals and improved husbandry practices such as buying animals from healthy herds, quarantine after arrival in farms and exclusion of contaminated feed and water was recommended by the US department of agriculture (USDA, 2007). In 2014, the Washington state department of health established a statewide 'one health steering committee' to develop a strategy to combat the resistance with one health focus (D'Angeli et al., 2016). American veterinary medicine association has developed guidelines on judicious therapeutic use of antibiotics to educate the veterinarians (www.avma.org).

'International Society for Companion Animal Infectious Disease (ISCAID)' has made guidelines for treatment of urinary tract infections, respiratory tract infections and superficial bacterial folliculitis in dogs and cats encompassing isolation of the etiological bacteria, antimicrobial susceptibility testing, selection of the drugs, therapeutic protocols and advice on infection control (Weese et al., 2011; Hillier et al., 2014). Antibiotics for use in companion animals are classified into three categories: tier 1, tire 2 and tier 3. Tier 1 drugs are selected when the diagnosis of the infection is accurate and possibility of resistance development is nil. For the use of tier 2 drugs sensitivity test is mandatory. Tier 3 drugs are used for highly resistant bacteria with consultation from specialists (Hillier et al., 2014).

In India, Prevention of Food Adulteration Rules, 1995, part XVIII, prescribed limit for antibiotics to be used in fisheries. Food Safety and Standards Authority of India (FSSAI) has framed the regulations to ban the use of certain antibiotics and pharmacologically active substances in fisheries (NAP-AMR, 2017—21). Indian Council of Agriculture Research (ICAR) in collaboration with FAO framed a national network of veterinary laboratories to generate data on antimicrobial resistance specific to livestock and fisheries. Provisionally, the network is known as 'Indian Network for Fishery and Animals Antimicrobial Resistance (INFAAR)'. Currently, the network has 21 members from ICAR institutions and agricultural/veterinary universities including both the authors of this book.

References

Bajwa, J., 2016. Canine superficial pyoderma and therapeutic considerations. Canadian Veterinary Journal 57 (2), 204.

Bell, B.G., Schellevis, F., Stobberingh, E., Goossens, H., Pringle, M., 2014. A systematic review and meta-analysis of the effects of antibiotic consumption on antibiotic resistance. BMC Infectious Diseases 14 (1), 13.

Bengtsson, B., Greko, C., 2014. Antibiotic resistance-consequences for animal health, welfare, and food production. Upsala Journal of Medical Sciences 119 (2), 96—102.

Carvalho, C., Costa, A.R., Silva, F., Oliveira, A., 2017. Bacteriophages and their derivatives for the treatment and control of food-producing animal infections. Critical Reviews in Microbiology 43 (5), 583—601.

Chowdhury, S., Mandal, G.P., Patra, A.K., Kumar, P., Samanta, I., Pradhan, S., Samanta, A.K., 2018. Different essential oils in diets of broiler chickens: 2. Gut microbes and morphology, immune response, and some blood profile and antioxidant enzymes. Animal Feed Science and Technology 236, 39—47.

Colles, F.M., Cain, R.J., Nickson, T., Smith, A.L., Roberts, S.J., Maiden, M.C., Lunn, D., Dawkins, M.S., 2016. Monitoring chicken flock behaviour provides early warning of infection by human pathogen *Campylobacter*. Proceedings of the Royal Society B: Biological Sciences 283 (1822), 20152323.

D'Angeli, M.A., Baker, J.B., Call, D.R., Davis, M.A., Kauber, K.J., Malhotra, U., Matsuura, G.T., Moore, D.A., Porter, C., Pottinger, P., Stockwell, V., 2016. Antimicrobial stewardship through a one health lens: observations from Washington State. International Journal of Health Governance 21 (3), 114—130.

Davey, P., Brown, E., Charani, E., Fenelon, L., Gould, I.M., Holmes, A., Ramsay, C.R., Wiffen, P.J., Wilcox, M., 2013. Interventions to improve antibiotic prescribing practices for hospital inpatients. Cochrane Database of Systematic Reviews 30 (4), CD003543.

Denes, E., Prouzergue, J., Ducroix-Roubertou, S., Aupetit, C., Weinbreck, P., 2012. Antibiotic prescription by general practitioners for urinary tract infections in outpatients. European Journal of Clinical Microbiology and Infectious Diseases 31 (11), 3079—3083.

Deuster, S., Roten, I., Muehlebach, S., 2010. Implementation of treatment guidelines to support judicious use of antibiotic therapy. Journal of Clinical Pharmacy and Therapeutics 35 (1), 71—78.

Doron, S., Davidson, L.E., 2011. Antimicrobial stewardship. In: Mayo Clinic Proceedings, vol. 86. Elsevier, pp. 1113—1123. No. 11.

Ducatelle, R., Eeckhaut, V., Haesebrouck, F., Van Immerseel, F., 2015. A review on prebiotics and probiotics for the control of dysbiosis: present status and future perspectives. Animal 9 (1), 43—48.

Dunn, F., Dunn, J., 2012. Clinical audit: application in small animal practice. In: Practice, vol. 34, pp. 243—245, 4.

Dyar, O.J., Huttner, B., Schouten, J., Pulcini, C., 2017. What is antimicrobial stewardship? Clinical Microbiology and Infection 23 (11), 793—798.

European Centre for Disease Prevention and Control, 2016. Antibiotic Resistance Strategies and Action Plans. Available at: https://ecdc.europa.eu/en/publications-data/directory-guidance-prevention-and-control/antimicrobial-resistance-strategies.

European Commission Directorate-General for Health and Food Safety (ECDGHFS), 2017. Final Report of a Fact-Finding Mission Carried Out in The Netherlands from 13 September 2016 to 20 September 2016 in Order to Gather Information on the Prudent Use of Antimicrobials in Animals. Audit number 2016-8889. http://ec.europa.eu/food/audits-analysis/audit_reports/details.cfm?rep_id=3753.

FAO/WHO Codex Alimentarius, 2015. Codex Texts on Foodborne Antimicrobial Resistance. Available at: http://www.fao.org/3/a-i4296t.pdf.

Fernández-Morato, J., Moro, L., Sancho, J., Grande, L., Clará, A., Grau, S., Horcajada, J.P., 2016. An antimicrobial stewardship program reduces antimicrobial therapy duration and hospital stay in surgical wards. Uimioterapia Uimioterapia 29, 119—122.

Gadde, U., Rathinam, T., Lillehoj, H.S., 2015. Passive immunization with hyperimmune egg-yolk IgY as prophylaxis and therapy for poultry diseases—a review. Animal Health Research Reviews 16 (2), 163—176.

Ghosh, T.K., Haldar, S., Bedford, M.R., Muthusami, N., Samanta, I., 2012. Assessment of yeast cell wall as replacements for antibiotic growth promoters in broiler diets: effects on performance, intestinal histo-morphology and humoral immune responses. Journal of Animal Physiology and Animal Nutrition 96 (2), 275—284.

Goff, D.A., 2011. Antimicrobial stewardship: bridging the gap between quality care and cost. Current Opinion in Infectious Diseases 24, S11—S20.

Goossens, H., Ferech, M., Coenen, S., Stephens, P., European Surveillance of Antimicrobial Consumption Project Group, 2007. Comparison of outpatient systemic antibacterial use in 2004 in the United States and 27 European countries. Clinical Infectious Diseases 44 (8), 1091—1095.

Gould, I.M., 1999. Stewardship of antibiotic use and resistance surveillance: the international scene. Journal of Hospital Infection 43, S253—S260.

Grayzel, S.E., Bender, J.B., Glore, R.P., Gumley, N., Sykes, J.E., Whichard, J.M., Papich, M.G., Watts, J.L., Barlam, T.F., Murphy, M.J., Hoang, C., 2015. Understanding companion animal practitioners' attitudes toward antimicrobial stewardship. Journal of the American Veterinary Medical Association 247 (8), 883–884.

Hardefeldt, L.Y., Gilkerson, J.R., Billman-Jacobe, H., Stevenson, M.A., Thursky, K., Bailey, K.E., Browning, G.F., 2018. Barriers to and enablers of implementing antimicrobial stewardship programs in veterinary practices. Journal of Veterinary Internal Medicine 32 (3), 1092–1099.

Hillier, A., Lloyd, D.H., Weese, J.S., Blondeau, J.M., Boothe, D., Breitschwerdt, E., Guardabassi, L., Papich, M.G., Rankin, S., Turnidge, J.D., Sykes, J.E., 2014. Guidelines for the diagnosis and antimicrobial therapy of canine superficial bacterial folliculitis (antimicrobial guidelines working group of the international society for companion animal infectious diseases). Veterinary Dermatology 25 (3) pp.163-e43.

Hsu, L.Y., Kwa, A.L., Lye, D.C., Chlebicki, M.P., Tan, T.Y., Ling, M.L., Wong, S.Y., Goh, L.G., 2008. Reducing antimicrobial resistance through appropriate antibiotic usage in Singapore. Singapore Medical Journal 49 (10), 749–755.

Jee, Y., Carlson, J., Rafai, E., Musonda, K., Huong, T.T.G., Daza, P., Sattayawuthipong, W., Yoon, T., 2018. Antimicrobial resistance: a threat to global health. The Lancet Infectious Diseases 18 (9), 939–940.

Kallen, M.C., Prins, J.M., 2017. A systematic review of quality indicators for appropriate antibiotic use in hospitalized adult patients. Infectious Disease Reports 9 (1).

Karp, B.E., Tate, H., Plumblee, J.R., Dessai, U., Whichard, J.M., Thacker, E.L., Hale, K.R., Wilson, W., Friedman, C.R., Griffin, P.M., McDermott, P.F., 2017. National antimicrobial resistance monitoring system: two decades of advancing public health through integrated surveillance of antimicrobial resistance. Foodborne Pathogens and Disease 14 (10), 545–557.

Kim, S.H., Song, J.H., Chung, D.R., Thamlikitkul, V., Yang, Y., Wang, H., Lu, M., So, T.M.K., Hsueh, P.R., Yasin, R.M., Carlos, C.C., 2012. Changing trends in antimicrobial resistance and serotypes of *Streptococcus pneumoniae* isolates in Asian countries: an Asian Network for Surveillance of Resistant Pathogens (ANSORP) study. Antimicrobial Agents and Chemotherapy 56 (3), 1418–1426.

Kwok, Y.L.A., Harris, P., McLaws, M.L., 2017. Social cohesion: the missing factor required for a successful hand hygiene program. American Journal of Infection Control 45 (3), 222–227.

MacDougall, C., Polk, R.E., 2005. Antimicrobial stewardship programs in health care systems. Clinical Microbiology Reviews 18 (4), 638–656.

Mang, A.V., Buczinski, S., Booker, C.W., Timsit, E., 2015. Evaluation of a computer-aided lung auscultation system for diagnosis of bovine respiratory disease in feedlot cattle. Journal of Veterinary Internal Medicine 29 (4), 1112–1116.

Martinez, M.N., Papich, M.G., Drusano, G.L., 2012. Dosing regimen matters: the importance of early intervention and rapid attainment of the pharmacokinetic/pharmacodynamic target. Antimicrobial Agents and Chemotherapy 56 (6), 2795–2805.

McDougall, S., Compton, C.W.R., Botha, N., 2017. Factors influencing antimicrobial prescribing by veterinarians and usage by dairy farmers in New Zealand. New Zealand Veterinary Journal 65 (2), 84–92.

McGowan, J.J., Gerding, D.N., 1996. Does antibiotic restriction prevent resistance? New Horizons (Baltimore, Md.) 4 (3), 370–376.

Mölstad, S., Cars, O., Struwe, J., 2008. Strama-a Swedish working model for containment of antibiotic resistance. Euro Surveillance 13 (46), 19041.

Murphy, D., Ricci, A., Auce, Z., Beechinor, J.G., Bergendahl, H., Breathnach, R., Bureš, J., Da Silva, D., Pedro, J., Hederová, J., Hekman, P., 2017. EMA and EFSA joint scientific opinion on measures to reduce the need to use antimicrobial agents in animal husbandry in the European Union, and the resulting impacts on food safety (RONAFA). EFSA Journal 15 (1).

National Action Plan on Antimicrobial Resistance (NAP-AMR 2017-21), 2017. Available at: http://www.searo.who.int/india/topics/antimicrobial_resistance/nap_amr.pdf.

Page, S., Prescott, J., Weese, S., 2014. The 5Rs approach to antimicrobial stewardship. The Veterinary Record 175 (8), 207.

Prescott, J.F., Boerlin, P., 2016. Antimicrobial use in companion animals and good stewardship practice. The Veterinary Record 179 (19), 486–488.

Pulcini, C., Morel, C.M., Tacconelli, E., Beovic, B., Goossens, H., Harbarth, S., Holmes, A., Howard, P., Morris, A.M., Nathwani, D., Sharland, M., 2017. Human resources estimates and funding for antibiotic stewardship teams are urgently needed. Clinical Microbiology and Infection 23 (11), 785–787.

Rahal, J.J., Urban, C., Horn, D., Freeman, K., Segal-Maurer, S., Maurer, J., Mariano, N., Marks, S., Burns, J.M., Dominick, D., Lim, M., 1998. Class restriction of cephalosporin use to control total cephalosporin resistance in nosocomial *Klebsiella*. Journal of the American Medical Association 280 (14), 1233–1237.

Ray, P., Manchanda, V., Bajaj, J., Chitnis, D.S., Gautam, V., Goswami, P., Gupta, V., Harish, B.N., Kagal, A., Kapil, A., Rao, R., 2013. Methicillin resistant *Staphylococcus aureus* (MRSA) in India: prevalence & susceptibility pattern. The Indian Journal of Medical Research 137 (2), 363.

Ruiz, R., Tedeschi, L.O., Sepúlveda, A., 2017. Investigation of the effect of pegbovigrastim on some periparturient immune disorders and performance in Mexican dairy herds. Journal of Dairy Science 100 (4), 3305–3317.

Samanta, I., Joardar, S.N., Das, P.K., 2018. Biosecurity strategies for backyard poultry: a controlled way for safe food production. In: Food Control and Biosecurity. Academic Press, pp. 481–517.

Samanta, I., Joardar, S.N., Ganguli, D., Das, P.K., Sarkar, U., 2015. Evaluation of egg production after adoption of biosecurity strategies by backyard poultry farmers in West Bengal. Veterinary World 8 (2), 177.

Sanchez, G.V., Fleming-Dutra, K.E., Roberts, R.M., Hicks, L.A., 2016. Core elements of outpatient antibiotic stewardship. Morbidity and Mortality Weekly Report Recommendations and Reports 65, 1–12.

Sar, T.K., Samanta, I., Mahanti, A., Akhtar, S., Dash, J.R., 2018. Potential of a polyherbal drug to prevent antimicrobial resistance in bacteria to antibiotics. Scientific Reports 8 (1), 10899.

Schaefer, A.L., Cook, N.J., Bench, C., Chabot, J.B., Colyn, J., Liu, T., Okine, E.K., Stewart, M., Webster, J.R., 2012. The non-invasive and automated detection of bovine respiratory disease onset in receiver calves using infrared thermography. Research in Veterinary Science 93 (2), 928–935.

Septimus, E.J., Owens Jr., R.C., 2011. Need and potential of antimicrobial stewardship in community hospitals. Clinical Infectious Diseases 53 (Suppl. 1_1), S8–S14.

Shlaes, D.M., Gerding, D.N., John, J.F., Craig, W.A., Bornstein, D.L., Duncan, R.A., Eckman, M.R., Farrer, W.E., Greene, W.H., Lorian, V., Levy, S., 1997. Society for healthcare epidemiology of America and infectious diseases society of America joint committee on the prevention of antimicrobial resistance guidelines for the prevention of antimicrobial resistance in hospitals. Infection Control and Hospital Epidemiology 18 (4), 275–291.

Stedtfeld, R.D., Williams, M.R., Fakher, U., Johnson, T.A., Stedtfeld, T.M., Wang, F., Khalife, W.T., Hughes, M., Etchebarne, B.E., Tiedje, J.M., Hashsham, S.A., 2016. Antimicrobial resistance dashboard application for mapping environmental occurrence and resistant pathogens. FEMS Microbiology Ecology 92 (3).

Swaggerty, C.L., Pevzner, I.Y., Kogut, M.H., 2014. Selection for pro-inflammatory mediators yields chickens with increased resistance against *Salmonella enterica* serovar enteritidis. Poultry Science 93 (3), 535–544.

Timsit, E., Dendukuri, N., Schiller, I., Buczinski, S., 2016. Diagnostic accuracy of clinical illness for bovine respiratory disease (BRD) diagnosis in beef cattle placed in feedlots: a systematic literature review and hierarchical Bayesian latent-class meta-analysis. Preventive Veterinary Medicine 135, 67–73.

Torrallardona, D., 2009. Spray dried animal plasma as an alternative to antibiotics in weanling pigs-a review. Asian-Australasian Journal of Animal Sciences 23 (1), 131–148.

Toth, N.R., Chambers, R.M., Davis, S.L., 2010. Implementation of a care bundle for antimicrobial stewardship. American Journal of Health-System Pharmacy 67 (9), 746–749.

Toubes, E., Singh, K., Yin, D., Lyu, R., Glick, N., Russell, L., Mohapatra, S., Saghal, N., Weinstein, R.A., Trenholme, G., 2003. Risk factors for antibiotic-resistant infection and treatment outcomes among hospitalized patients transferred from long-term care facilities: does antimicrobial choice make a difference? Clinical Infectious Diseases 36 (6), 724–730.

USDA, 2007. Antimicrobial Resistance Issues in Animal Agriculture available at: https://www.aphis.usda.gov/animal_health/emergingissues/downloads/antiresist2007update.pdf.

Van Nguyen, K., Do, N.T.T., Chandna, A., Nguyen, T.V., Van Pham, C., Doan, P.M., Nguyen, A.Q., Nguyen, C.K.T., Larsson, M., Escalante, S., Olowokure, B., 2013. Antibiotic use and resistance in emerging economies: a situation analysis for Viet Nam. BMC Public Health 13 (1), 1158.

Venekamp, R.P., Rovers, M.M., Verheij, T.J., Bonten, M.J., Sachs, A.P., 2012. Treatment of acute rhinosinusitis: discrepancy between guideline recommendations and clinical practice. Family Practice 29 (6), 706–712.

Vohra, A., Syal, P., Madan, A., 2016. Probiotic yeasts in livestock sector. Animal Feed Science and Technology 219, 31–47.

Walia, K., Ohri, V.C., Mathai, D., 2015. Antimicrobial stewardship programme (AMSP) practices in India. The Indian Journal of Medical Research 142 (2), 130.

Wang, S., Zeng, X., Yang, Q., Qiao, S., 2016. Antimicrobial peptides as potential alternatives to antibiotics in food animal industry. International Journal of Molecular Sciences 17 (5), 603.

Weese, J.S., Blondeau, J.M., Boothe, D., Breitschwerdt, E.B., Guardabassi, L., Hillier, A., Lloyd, D.H., Papich, M.G., Rankin, S.C., Turnidge, J.D., Sykes, J.E., 2011. Antimicrobial use guidelines for treatment of urinary tract disease in dogs and cats: antimicrobial guidelines working group of the international society for companion animal infectious diseases. Veterinary Medicine International 2011.

Wertheim, H.F., Chandna, A., Vu, P.D., Van Pham, C., Nguyen, P.D.T., Lam, Y.M., Van Nguyen, C.V., Larsson, M., Rydell, U., Nilsson, L.E., Farrar, J., 2013. Providing impetus, tools, and guidance to strengthen national capacity for antimicrobial stewardship in Viet Nam. PLoS Medicine 10 (5), e1001429.

World Health Organization, Food and Agriculture Organization, World Organisation for Animal Health, 2016. Antimicrobial Resistance. A Manual for Developing National Action Plans, Version 1. Available at: http://apps.who.int/iris/bitstream/10665/204470/1/9789241549530_eng.pdf?ua=1.

Chapter 30

Alternative antiinfective therapy

Chapter outline

Bacterial diseases are considered as a global burden to cause loss of disability-adjusted life years throughout the world and a major cause for mortality in low- and middle-income group of countries. Protection against the infectious diseases is based on four pillars such as immunization, nutrition, personal hygiene and antibacterial drugs. After the introduction of antibiotics in the community during the golden era, the US Surgeon General addressed the Congress in 1969 that the time had come to 'close the books on infectious diseases'. Unfortunately in the following years, the fourth pillar of protection became weak because of emergence of resistance as discussed in previous chapters. Much of the pharmaceutical giants also withdrew their efforts to develop a new drug molecule which can fight successfully the resistant bacterial population. Since 1990, restriction of antibiotic use was introduced in Denmark and Sweden, and since 2006, it is banned by the European Union as growth promoter in animals and birds (Bengtsson and Greko, 2014). Many countries have forbidden the use of certain antimicrobials in fishery and also refuse to import the aquaculture products treated with antibiotics. The situation made it imperative to search for alternative treatment strategies. Several approaches such as phage therapy, feed additives based on beneficial bacteria, yeast, enzymes, essential oils and others are common in use in animal and poultry industry. Feed additives are defined as ingredients or group of ingredients used for improving the digestibility of feed and animal or bird welfare and performances (Murphy et al., 2017). The feed additives are always used in healthy animals or birds. It is the major difference with veterinary medicinal products, used for treatment or prevention of infections and restoring or modification of physiological functions in animals and birds.

Some new strategies such as nanomaterial-based antiinfective particles, enzymes, antimicrobial peptides (AMPs), quorum sensing quenchers, efflux pump inhibitors, clay, predatory bacteria, teat sealants and antimicrobial photodynamic therapy (APDT) are being explored.

Bacteriophage therapy

Bacteriophages are species-specific viruses that can lyse the bacteria through the production of endolysin. Ernest Hankin (1896) and Bardell (1982) observed the antibacterial activity of unidentified 'entity' against *Vibrio cholerae* and *Bacillus subtilis*, respectively. Twort (1915) and d'Herelle (1917) identified the 'entity' as a virus and coined the term 'bacteriophage' (Twort, 1915; d'Herelle, 1917). Therapeutic attempt of bacteriophage to treat dysentery was initiated by the discoverer himself (d'Herelle) in 1919, which was transformed later into phage therapy centres in several countries (Guttman et al., 2005). The period between 1920 and 1950 was considered as golden era of phage therapy, especially during Second World

Antimicrobial Resistance in Agriculture. https://doi.org/10.1016/B978-0-12-815770-1.00030-4

War, it was used profusely by the German, Soviet and US armies. With the introduction of antibiotics in the market, the phage therapy became abandoned.

The phages are commonly used to prevent and treat many animal or human infections even caused by resistant bacteria because of nontoxic nature to the eukaryotic cells, specificity without altering host commensal microbiota, self-replicating and least probability to develop resistance (Miller et al., 2010; Loc-Carrillo and Abedon, 2011). The efficacy of phages MPK1, MPK6 and PAK-P1 against *Pseudomonas* was evaluated in mice model (Heo et al., 2009). The phages can adhere with the surface of biofilm and produce alginase enzyme to depolymerize the biofilm matrix (Hraiech et al., 2015). Combination therapy of phages and antibiotics (streptomycin) can control *Pseudomonas* infection more efficiently than single antibiotic therapy in the population (Torres-Barceló et al., 2014). Genetically engineered phages can reduce the host inflammatory response observed during treatment with lytic phages because of release of bacterial cell wall components after lysis (Hagens et al., 2004). Human clinical trials with phages against *Pseudomonas* infection (chronic otitis, venous leg ulcers), one of the most potent antibiotic-resistant bacteria, showed promising results (Wright et al., 2009; Rhoads et al., 2009).

Experiments with phages were performed to reduce the foodborne pathogens in agricultural and poultry products (Huff et al., 2005). Supplementation of diets with bacteriophages (0.035%–0.15%) increased body weight gain and reduced feed conversion ratio in broilers (Zhao et al., 2012; Kim et al., 2013). *Salmonella*, the major pathogen of day-old chicken, was successfully treated with the application of bacteriophages in drinking water of birds or through the coarse spray in the sheds (Borie et al., 2008; Lima et al., 2016). Effective synergism was detected in broilers between phages and probiotics during combined application (Borie et al., 2009). The bacteriophage was also used successfully to prevent horizontal transmission of *Salmonella* from infected to healthy chicken (Lim et al., 2012).

The phage therapy has several limitations. The complete information of the infecting bacteria should be known before the initiation of therapy because of specificity of the phages. The phages are ineffective against the infection caused by multiple bacterial strains owing to narrow host range (Hurley et al., 2012). The phage preparation should be free of contaminant bacterial cell wall components, while sterilization of the phage preparation can reduce the potency (Thiel, 2004). The study indicated the production of antiphage antibodies can neutralize the phages during therapy (Łusiak-Szelachowska et al., 2014). The pharmacokinetics of phage treatments are more complicated than the drugs. The phages can introduce antibiotic resistance or virulence genes into the bacteria instead of lysis. So purified virion or phage endolysins are evaluated for their potency (López et al., 2004).

Enzybiotics

Enzybiotics are enzymes used to control pathogenic bacterial infections in replacement of antibiotics. It is a combination of the words 'enzyme' and 'antibiotics' and the term was first used in 2001 (Nelson et al., 2001). Bacteriophage endolysin can recognize (cell wall–binding domain) and degrade (catalytic domain) bacterial cell wall peptidoglycan and it is now considered as an alternative enzymatic approach for resistant bacteria. The endolysin can be classified into several categories such as muramidase, glucosaminidase, transglycosylase, amidase and endopeptidase based on their catalytic domain (Schmelcher et al., 2012). The endolysins can avoid the different mechanisms used by the bacteria for development of resistance, as the enzymes are applied exogenously and they act on bacterial cell wall situated outside the cell. Moreover, it has no reported toxicity and the immune response generated in the host cannot neutralize the enzyme (Loeffler et al., 2003). Polycationic agents and chelators increase the potency of endolysin against Gram-negative bacteria with lysis of outer membrane, which is not penetrated by the endolysins as such (except a few such as *Salmonella* phage endolysin SPN9CC) (Briers et al., 2011). Effective synergism with phage-encoded holin proteins (permeabilization of bacterial membrane) was detected against multidrug-resistant *Streptococcus suis* and *Staphylococcus aureus* (Shi et al., 2012). Genetically engineered endolysins (Artilysin) comprising lipopolysaccharide-destabilizing peptides or AMPs were found effective against Gram-negative bacteria (Briers et al., 2014). The Artilysin was found effective in a clinical trial in dogs with chronic otitis caused by *Pseudomonas* (Briers and Lavigne, 2015). Antibacterial effect of endolysins (Cpl-1, Pal, Ply-G) was detected against mastitis-associated *S. aureus*, *Streptococcus uberis, Streptococcus agalactiae* and *Streptococcus dysgalactiae* in cattle (Horgan et al., 2009; Schmelcher et al., 2015); mixed multidrug-resistant *S. aureus* (MRSA) and *Streptococcus pyogenes* infection in mice (Gilmer et al., 2013); *S. pneumoniae* in rat/mice (Loeffler et al., 2003) and *Bacillus anthracis* in mice (Schuch et al., 2002).

Few bacteriophages encode exolysin or virion-associated peptidoglycan hydrolase for degradation of bacterial peptidoglycan during injection of phage nucleic acid. The exolysin has several beneficial properties such as stability, specificity, less chance for development of resistance and multiple domains, which can be used for improvement of antimicrobial properties during construction of chimeric proteins (Lavigne et al., 2004). Antimicrobial activity of artificial phage exolysin (HydH5) in combination with endolysin (LysH5) was detected against mastitis-associated *S. aureus* (Rodríguez-Rubio et al., 2013). Depolymerases are phage-encoded proteins that can also lyse the bacterial polysaccharides (Oliveira et al., 2013). A depolymerase with endosialidase activity decreased systemic *Escherichia coli* infection in experimental rats (Mushtaq et al., 2005).

The enzymes commonly used in poultry and pig feed industry are phytase, xylanase, cellulase, α-galactosidase, β-mannanase, α-amylase, pectinase and proteases. Dietary enzymes used in animal or poultry feed can help in breakdown of nutrients to smaller compounds for better digestion and absorption which are not degraded by the host enzymes (e.g., phytic acid) (Thacker, 2013). The enzymes can also increase the availability of starches, amino acids and minerals from the plant-based feed ingredients by breaking the cell wall carbohydrates, eliminate antinutritional factors such as phytic acids, nonstarch polysaccharides (NSP), reduce intestinal viscosity and activate caecal fermentation. The dietary enzymes also influence the composition of gut commensal bacteria due to production of short-chain oligosaccharides from cell wall NSP, which acts as prebiotics (Kiarie et al., 2013; Cheng et al., 2014). Supplementation of enzyme complex (phytase, NSP enzymes, β-mannanase, xylanase, amylase, protease) can improve the body weight (3.7%—4.2%) and reduce the feed conversion ratio (2.6%—4.8%) in broilers as an effective alternative to antibiotic-based growth promoters (Bedford, 2000; Hooge et al., 2010; Jackson and Hanford, 2014). The performance of broilers varies with differences in the enzyme category, dosage of enzyme, diet composition and genetic variations among the birds (Cheng et al., 2014).

Phytobiotics and essential oils

Phytogenic feed additives (phytobiotics) are defined as plant-derived or biological origin feed ingredients used in the diets to improve the productivity of livestock or poultry. It can be classified into four categories such as herbs obtained from flowering, nonwoody and nonpersistent plants; botanicals comprising of entire or processed parts of a plant (roots, leaves, bark); essential oils (hydrodistilled extracts of volatile plant compounds) and oleoresins, i.e., nonaqueous solvent—based plant extracts (Windisch and Kroismayr, 2006). Presence of certain chemicals in phytobiotics such as terpenoids, steroids, alkaloids, flavonoids and glucosinolates is associated with improved digestibility because of enhanced digestive enzyme secretion and absorption (Wang et al., 2008). The phytobiotics can reduce the concentration of microbial toxic metabolite and relief the body from immune stress. It can also act as antioxidant and reduce oxidative stress (Liu et al., 2014). Other beneficial effects include increased proliferation of immune cells, phagocytic activity of chicken heterophils, enhanced cytokine expression, increased antibody titres, inhibition of tumour growth (Pourhossein et al., 2015; Islam et al., 2016; Chowdhury et al., 2018); enhanced intestinal and pancreatic enzyme production and bile flow (Hashemipour et al., 2014); increased villi height and absorptive surface of the intestine (Ghazanfari et al., 2015) and maintenance of intestinal barrier (Placha et al., 2014). Thus the health and performance of the animals or birds is improved.

Addition of oregano (herb), garlic and horseradish (spice) in diets improved the weight gain and feed conversion of pigs and reduced the pre and postweaning mortality of piglets (Bilkei et al., 2011a, 2011b). Berberine is a plant-derived quaternary ammonium salt from the protoberberine group of isoquinoline alkaloids, with a long history of medicinal use both in Indian Ayurvedic and Chinese medicine. It is generally found in the roots, rhizomes and stem bark of varieties of medicinal plants such as *Berberis aquifolium* (Oregon grape), *Berberis vulgaris* (Barberry), *Berberis aristata* (tree turmeric), *Hydrastis canadensis* (goldenseal), *Phellodendron amurense* (Amur cork tree), *Coptis chinensis* (Chinese goldthread) and *Tinospora cordifolia* (guduchi) (Amritpal et al., 2010). The berberine showed potential antimicrobial activity against multidrug-resistant shiga toxin—producing *E. coli*, enterotoxin-producing *E. coli* and enteropathogenic *E. coli* isolated from yaks in India. The study detected the minimum inhibitory concentration (MIC) value of berberine against the multi drug resistant (MDR) isolates with binding kinetics to DNA and proteins (Bandyopadhyay et al., 2013). Berberine inhibits the protein synthesis and blocks the bacterial division and development. It can also induce pyknosis in the cytoplasm and bacterial death (Kang et al., 2015). Other antimicrobial compounds present in different medicinal plants include protocatechuic acid, gallic acid, ellagic acid, rutin and myricetin (Jayaraman et al., 2010).

In vivo use of tannins (chestnut and quebracho) in broilers experimentally infected with *Clostridium perfringens* showed reduced occurrence and severity of gross lesions with enhancement of body weight (Redondo et al., 2014). Several other plants, herbs and spices, for example, thyme, oregano, stevia, rosemary, marjoram, yarrow, garlic, ginger, sugar cane, green tea, *Scrophularia striata*, *Ferulago angulata*, *Forsythia suspensa*, *Portulaca oleracea* and coriander were used successfully in poultry diet to improve feed conversion and gain body weight (El-Abasy et al., 2002; Florou-Paneri et al., 2006; Atteh et al., 2008; Wang et al., 2008; Zhao et al., 2013; Rostami et al., 2015).

The garlic (*Allium sativum*), red clover (*Trifolium pratense*), caraway (*Carum carvi*), basil (*Ocimum basilium*), green tea (*Camellia sinensis*) and ginger (*Zingiber officinale*) were found as appetizer and growth stimulant in several fishes and aquatic animals such as Oriental weather loach (*Misgurnus anguillicaudatus*), Japanese amberjack (*Seriola quinqueradiata*), grass carp (*Ctenopharyngodon idellus*), Chinese soft-shelled turtle (*Pelodiscus sinensis*), black rockfish (*Sebastes schlegelii*), tiger shrimp (*Penaeus monodon*) and Nile tilapia (*Oreochromis niloticus*) (Harada, 1990; Venkatramalingam et al., 2007; Ahmad and Abdel-Tawwab, 2011; Lee and Gao, 2012; Hwang et al., 2013). The active compound allicin present in garlic is identified as the appetizing factor. The beneficial effect of phytobiotics is dose- and time-dependent, not fully established in aquaculture and animals or poultry. High cost and lack of availability are other constraints.

Essential oils

Essential oils are antimicrobial compounds present in aromatic plants, herbs and spices to protect the plants from bacteria and insects (Patra, 2012). Active compounds present in essential oils and antimicrobial property differ with plant species, plant genotypes and parts used, geographical origin, harvesting season, concentration of the ingredient used and period of storage. The essential oils have short half-life because of rapid clearance through the kidneys (glucuronates) and are better absorbed through oral, pulmonary and topical routes as detected in human study (Kohlert et al., 2002). Animal data are lacking regarding toxicity, optimum dosage and preferred route of application for better absorption.

The aromatic plant *Nigella sativa* L. (black cumin) is routinely used in traditional medicine as antibacterial, immune stimulant and antioxidants (Bourgou et al., 2012). The active constituents of the seeds include the essential oils consisting of carvone, terpene or D-limonene (carvene) and *p*-cymene. Supplementation of black cumin seed in broiler diet improved growth performance, immunity and nutrient utilization with linear decrease of *Salmonella* count in gut (Kumar et al., 2017).

Cinnamaldehyde has greater antimicrobial activity than other essential oils of phenolic nature. It can prevent the action of essential bacterial enzymes such as amino decarboxylases (Burt, 2004). It can produce synergism with organic acids as it changes bacterial membrane fatty acid profile and helps in penetration of organic acids into the bacterial cell (Di Pasqua et al., 2006). The organic acids act better in the upper part of poultry intestine (crop, gizzard) and the essential oils act on the lower segments (Langhout, 2000). The combination of essential oils and organic acids thus can cover the whole poultry intestine. In vivo supplementation in broilers with cinnamaldehyde and organic acid (formic acid) combination reduced the *Clostridium* count in the small intestine and caecum and increased the villi height and protective immunity against Newcastle disease (Pathak et al., 2017). In another study, supplementation of cinnamon bark oil in broiler diets was detected to improve immune response, gut health (reduced *E. coli* and *Clostridium* count), antioxidant status and blood cholesterol in broiler chickens (Chowdhury et al., 2018).

Improved body weight gain and feed efficiency was detected in broilers with other essential oils such as thymol and cinnamaldehyde, essential oils present in oregano, coriander, clove and star anise (Amerah et al., 2011; Hashemipour et al., 2014; Ghazanfari et al., 2015; Kim et al., 2016). The commercial phytobiotic product comprising of carvacrol, cinnamaldehyde and capsicum oleoresin was approved by the European Union, which showed improvement in growth and feed efficiency in birds (Pirgozliev et al., 2015).

Limitations of essential oils include narrow host specificity, i.e., more activity against Gram-positive bacteria only (Burt, 2004), reduction in antibacterial activity when mixed with animal or poultry feed because of poor solubility of its active components (Si et al., 2006).

Nanomaterial-based antiinfective particles

Nano-sized materials (1−100 nm) can be used in effective ways for treatment of infectious diseases. It can be classified into two broad categories, i.e., naturally occurring ultrafine particles and artificially produced particles. Several particles such as nanospheres, quantum dots, nanocapsules, nanobubbles, nanoclusters, liposomes, dendrimers, carbon nanotubes and polymeric nanoparticles are used in medicine as a means of drug delivery or as anticancer and antimicrobials or for tissue regeneration (De Jong and Borm, 2008).

Silver nanoparticles are the most common form of antimicrobial used. It acts in several ways and thus can prevent the generation of resistance. The silver ions released from the particle can disrupt bacterial membrane, damage cytochrome and nucleic acids, inhibit cell division and cause bacterial death (Lara et al., 2010). It also increases collagen expression from dermal fibroblasts and improves surgical wound healing with antibacterial accomplishment (Chowdhury et al., 2014). In vitro antibacterial property of silver nanoparticles was reported against multidrug-resistant isolates such as MRSA, *Edwardsiella tarda*, *Pseudomonas*, *Proteus*, *Flavobacterium* and *Vibrio* in shrimp (Ayala-Núñez et al., 2009;

Vaseeharan et al., 2010; Swain et al., 2014). The plant extracts are used to synthesize silver nanoparticles ('green' nano) having antibacterial property (Umashankari et al., 2012).

Owing to low toxicity, gold nanoparticles are currently preferred as antimicrobial molecules against multidrug-resistant bacterial isolates from animals and fishes (Li et al., 2014; Velmurugan et al., 2014). The gold nanoparticles exert antibacterial properties through reduction of ATP synthesis, interference with binding of tRNA to ribosome subunits and enhanced chemotaxis (Cui et al., 2012). Zinc oxide nanoparticles were detected to possess antibacterial properties against several fish pathogens such as *Aeromonas hydrophila*, *Flavobacterium branchiophilum*, *S. aureus*, *E. tarda*, *Citrobacter* spp., *Vibrio* spp., *Bacillus cereus*, *Enterococcus faecalis* and *Pseudomonas aeruginosa* associated with bacterial membrane damage (Jayaseelan et al., 2012; Swain et al., 2014). Titanium dioxide nanoparticles after photoactivation produced antibacterial effects on *Streptococcus iniae*, *E. tarda* and *Photobacterium damselae* (Cheng et al., 2011). Other nanoparticles such as copper oxide, iron (III) oxide, lanthanum calcium manganite (De et al., 2010), ceria (CeO2), gold-functionalized magnetic (Bonev et al., 2008), silver-gold alloy (Salehi et al., 2015), dextrose reduced gelatin-capped silver (Mohan et al., 2014) and nitric oxide—releasing silica nanoparticles (Carpenter et al., 2012) showed antibacterial activities against *Pseudomonas*. So far no literature has described the development of resistance against metallic nanoparticles, although most of the efficacy studies are conducted under laboratory conditions.

Chitosan and poly-D, L-lactide-co-glycolic acid (PLGA, FDA-approved)—based nanoparticles are used for drug delivery because of their easy penetration through blood—brain barrier, biodegradable, mucoadhesive and nontoxic nature, excretion through kidney and high surface area to volume ratio, which helps in compatible reactivity with other molecules present in the delivery system (De Jong and Borm, 2008). Chitosan-based nanoparticles were used for delivery of vitamin C and hormones in rainbow trout (*Oncorhynchus mykiss*) and common carp (*Cyprinus carpio*) (Rather et al., 2013). PLGA as a delivery system of rifampicin showed better therapeutic response against *Mycobacterium marinum* in zebrafish (Fenaroli et al., 2014). Polymeric nanoparticles, virus-like particles, liposomes, immunostimulant complex and metal nanoparticles are also used for vaccine delivery because of slow release of antigen in the body maintaining the immunogenicity (Zhao et al., 2014).

Others

Probiotics/prebiotics/synbiotics

Probiotics ('for life') can be defined as 'live microorganisms that, when administered in adequate amounts, confer a health benefit on the host' (Hill et al., 2014). Probiotics act through 'competitive exclusion' of pathogenic bacteria associated with inhibition of bacterial adherence by occupying the host cell receptors, secretion of bacteriocins (*Lactobacillus*, *Bacillus*) and competition for nutrients (Nurmi and Rantala, 1973). Different bacteria and yeasts/yeast cell wall products such as *Bacillus*, *Bifidobacterium*, *Enterococcus*, *Lactobacillus*, *Streptococcus*, *Lactococcus* and *Saccharomyces* were detected to act as growth stimulant with daily weight gain (because of increased digestive enzyme activity), decreased feed conversion ratio and reduction in pathogenic bacterial population in poultry, which is *at par* with the antibiotics (Simon et al., 2001; Griggs and Jacob, 2005; Faria Filho et al., 2006; Ghosh et al., 2012). The probiotic effect varies with the type of strains and mode of application (feed/water) but does not significantly vary with application of mono or multispecies/strains of the bacteria (Blajman et al., 2014). Addition of probiotics including edible mushroom (*Pleurotus florida*) in diet can also enhance immunoglobulin levels, antibody titres to pathogens, immune cell numbers (macrophages), cytokine production by intraepithelial lymphocytes, increased villi height and crypt depth, augmented beneficial bacterial population and enhancement of epithelial cell regeneration through production of cytokines in broilers (Ng et al., 2008; Paul et al., 2012; Sen et al., 2012; Muthusamy et al., 2013; Bai et al., 2013; Zhang and Kim, 2014; Ahmed et al., 2014). In layers, supplementation of probiotics improves egg production and egg mass (Lei et al., 2013). In aquaculture, bacteria (*Pediococcus acidilactici* (approved by European Commission), *Lactobacillus plantarum*, *Vibrio alginolyticus*, *Phaeobacter gallaeciensis*, *Pseudomonas aestumarina*), yeasts and moulds (*Aspergillus*, *Saccharomyces*) and microalgae (*Tetraselmis suecica*) are used as probiotics (Newaj-Fyzul and Austin, 2015). The probiotics in fish act through similar mechanisms such as production of bacteriocins, enzymes (protease, amylase, lysozyme), hydrogen peroxide and organic acids. In human medicine, a clinical trial conducted with *Lactobacillus* in ICU patients delayed the occurrence of respiratory tract infection caused by *Pseudomonas* (Forestier et al., 2008). The probiotic bacterial strains can also carry antimicrobial resistance genes or may acquire them from pathogenic or commensal bacteria which are serious safety issues for using probiotics in animals, birds and fishes (Muñoz-Atienza et al., 2013).

Prebiotics are 'non-digestible food ingredients that beneficially affect the host by selectively stimulating the growth of limited number of bacteria in the colon, and thus improve host health' (Roberfroid, 2007). Prebiotics also prevent the colonization of pathogens by stimulating the growth of beneficial bacteria secreting bacteriocins and direct binding with the pathogens to prevent their adhesion with host cells (Spring et al., 2000). Microbial fermentation of prebiotics produces short-chain fatty acids, which are used by the intestinal epithelial cells as a source of energy. Different nonstarch oligosaccharides or polysaccharides are used as prebiotics including mannan oligosaccharide (MOS), fructooligosaccharide (FOS), galactooligosaccharide, maltooligosaccharide, glucooligosaccharide, xylooligosaccharide, isomaltooligosaccharide (IOS), soya-oligosaccharide, inulin, oligofructose, lactulose, lactitol and pyrodextrins. Application of MOS (*Saccharomyces cerevisiae*), FOS (plants), IOS and lactulose enhanced growth, feed conversion efficiency, intestinal villi height and immune competence, *Lactobacillus* population and goblet cell numbers in broilers (Benites et al., 2008; Kim et al., 2011; Mookiah et al., 2014; Cho and Kim, 2014).

Synbiotics are application of probiotics along with prebiotics that stimulate the growth and metabolism of the applied probiotic cultures (Hume, 2011). Application of synbiotic products can improve body weight, average daily gain, feed efficiency, villi height and crypt depth and carcass yield percentage in broilers (Awad et al., 2009; Mookiah et al., 2014).

Organic acids

The organic acids are naturally found in animal and plant tissues and few of them are synthesised by microbes in the hind gut of human and animals. Organic acids and their sodium, potassium or calcium salts (short-chain fatty acids, medium-chain fatty acids (C6—C12, lauric acid), formic acid, acetic acid, lactic acid, propionic acid, butyric acid, sorbic acid, benzoic acid) are used in the diet of pigs and poultry, which reduces the upper gut pH and acid-intolerant bacterial population (*E. coli*, *Salmonella*, *Campylobacter*), increases villi height, width of the duodenum, depth of crypts, epithelial cell metabolism, proliferation and differentiation, body weight gain, acid-tolerant beneficial bacteria (*Lactobacillus*) and strengthens gut mucosal barrier (Peng et al., 2007; Dalmasso et al., 2008; Broom, 2015; Banday et al., 2015). The beneficial effects of organic acids depend on buffering capacity of other feed ingredients, source and purity of organic acids and their rate of inclusion in diet. The study with organic acids in poultry diet could not reveal any curative effect against necrotic enteritis induced with *Clostridium perfringens* (Geier et al., 2010). In shrimps and fishes administration of organic acids reduced infection rate (Lückstädt, 2006).

Antimicrobial peptides

AMPs contain 12—100 amino acids and are cationic and amphipathic in nature, which can interact with negatively charged membranes of microbes or host cells (Wang et al., 2014). The peptides are produced by bacteria, fungi, plants, invertebrates and vertebrates in nature. The peptides can prevent the growth of various pathogens (*Clostridium* and coliform) through formation of pores in the membrane, degradation of peptidoglycan and lysis of the cells. Few studies with cecropin A (1—11)-D(12—37)-Asn (CADN), AMP-P5 and naturally occurring peptides showed increased growth performance, better absorption through the intestine and enhanced mucosal immunity in poultry (Wang et al., 2009; Wen and He, 2012; Choi et al., 2013). Bacteriocin is a kind of AMP which has limited antibacterial action against similar group of bacteria from which it is synthesized. The well-studied bacteriocin in poultry diet is divercin AS7, which can modulate gut bacterial population with increased digestibility and growth performance (Józefiak et al., 2010). Major shortcomings of using AMPs in poultry or animal feed to replace antibiotics include high production cost, instability in the gut and possibility of resistance generation.

Predatory bacteria

Bdellovibrio and related group of bacteria can prevent the growth of Gram-negative multidrug-resistant pathogens including the biofilm producers through the secretion of DNAse and other enzymes (Kadouri et al., 2013). Limitations include destruction of host natural microbiome and reduction in predatory activity in presence of Gram-positive bacteria (Hobley et al., 2006).

Clay (phyllosilicates)

Clay particles (bentonite, zeolite, kaolin) are stratified tetrahedral and octahedral layers of minerals composed of silicon, aluminium and oxygen which can absorb pathogens, toxins, heavy metals and plant metabolites (Vondruskova et al., 2010). Addition of clay minerals in poultry diet can improve growth performance, reduce pathogen load (*E. coli*, *Clostridium*) and increase the activity of digestive enzymes (Xia et al., 2004; Lemos et al., 2015).

Teat sealants

Internal teat sealants (bismuth subnitrate) are used in dairy cows during dry or periparturient period to prevent the occurrence of mastitis. The metaanalysis showed that use of internal teat sealant can reduce the occurrence of new intramammary infection mostly caused by *Streptococcus* (73%) and clinical mastitis (29%) (Halasa et al., 2009; Rabiee and Lean, 2013). Use of teat sealants and common hygienic practices such as disinfection of teats before milking can reduce antimicrobial usage in dairy.

Antimicrobial photodynamic therapy

APDT is an effective alternative treatment approach for topical infections. In the presence of oxygen, the activated photosensitizer can react with neighbouring molecules to generate reactive oxygen species, which can lyse the pathogens. Several Gram-positive and Gram-negative bacteria, fungi and protozoa are found to be susceptible to APDT. Recently in veterinary medicine it was applied to treat caseous lymphadenitis in sheep (Sellera et al., 2016).

Quorum sensing quencher

Bacterial quorum sensing, consisting of acyl-homoserine lactones, autoinducing peptides and autoinducers, is required to communicate between compatible bacterial population for production of biofilm and synthesis of virulence factors such as lectin, exotoxin, pyocyanin, elastase, etc. (Carnes et al., 2010). Quorum sensing quenchers are inhibitors of signalling pathways and it can inhibit the expression of virulence genes and biofilm formation and reduce the risk of drug resistance. Several human clinical trials although showed toxicity and unstable therapeutic effects of the quencher molecules (Walz et al., 2010; Van Delden et al., 2012).

Hypothiocyanite

Hypothiocyanite is produced by the immune cells present in the respiratory tract to destroy the invading bacteria. A hypothiocyanite-based inhalation formulation is recently approved as orphan drug by the European medicines agency and the US FDA against *Pseudomonas*-associated cystic fibrosis (Hurley et al., 2012).

Efflux pump inhibitor

The access of the antibiotics to the target is prevented by increasing the efflux of the drug from the bacterial cell. The efflux is carried out by efflux pumps as discussed in details in earlier chapters. It has been shown that efflux of antibiotics can be mediated by more than one pump in a single bacterium. Phenyl-arginine-β-naphthylamide (PAβN) inhibits the efflux pumps and increases the sensitivity of *Pseudomonas* isolates to the antibiotics (Gill et al., 2015). The synergistic application of efflux pump inhibitors and iron chelators inhibits growth and biofilm formation of *P. aeruginosa* (Liu et al., 2010).

References

Ahmad, M.H., Abdel-Tawwab, M., 2011. The use of caraway seed meal as a feed additive in fish diets: growth performance, feed utilization, and whole-body composition of Nile tilapia, *Oreochromis niloticus* (L.) fingerlings. Aquaculture 314 (1−4), 110−114.

Ahmed, S.T., Islam, M.M., Mun, H.S., Sim, H.J., Kim, Y.J., Yang, C.J., 2014. Effects of *Bacillus amyloliquefaciens* as a probiotic strain on growth performance, cecal microflora, and fecal noxious gas emissions of broiler chickens. Poultry Science 93 (8), 1963−1971.

Amerah, A.M., Péron, A., Zaefarian, F., Ravindran, V., 2011. Influence of whole wheat inclusion and a blend of essential oils on the performance, nutrient utilisation, digestive tract development and ileal microbiota profile of broiler chickens. British Poultry Science 52 (1), 124−132.

Amritpal, S., Sanjiv, D., Navpreet, K., Jaswinder, S., 2010. Berberine: alkaloid with wide spectrum of pharmacological activities. Journal of Natural Products (India) 3, 64−75.

Atteh, J.O., Onagbesan, O.M., Tona, K., Decuypere, E., Geuns, J.M.C., Buyse, J., 2008. Evaluation of supplementary stevia (*Stevia rebaudiana*, bertoni) leaves and stevioside in broiler diets: effects on feed intake, nutrient metabolism, blood parameters and growth performance. Journal of Animal Physiology and Animal Nutrition 92 (6), 640−649.

Awad, W.A., Ghareeb, K., Abdel-Raheem, S., Böhm, J., 2009. Effects of dietary inclusion of probiotic and synbiotic on growth performance, organ weights, and intestinal histomorphology of broiler chickens. Poultry Science 88 (1), 49−56.

Ayala-Núñez, N.V., Villegas, H.H.L., Turrent, L.D.C.I., Padilla, C.R., 2009. Silver nanoparticles toxicity and bactericidal effect against methicillin-resistant *Staphylococcus aureus*: nanoscale does matter. NanoBiotechnology 5 (1−4), 2−9.

Bai, S.P., Wu, A.M., Ding, X.M., Lei, Y., Bai, J., Zhang, K.Y., Chio, J.S., 2013. Effects of probiotic-supplemented diets on growth performance and intestinal immune characteristics of broiler chickens. Poultry Science 92 (3), 663−670.

Banday, M.T., Adil, S., Khan, A.A., Untoo, M., 2015. A study on efficacy of fumaric acid supplementation in diet of broiler chicken. International Journal of Poultry Science 14 (11), 589.

Bandyopadhyay, S., Patra, P.H., Mahanti, A., Mondal, D.K., Dandapat, P., Bandyopadhyay, S., Samanta, I., Lodh, C., Bera, A.K., Bhattacharyya, D., Sarkar, M., 2013. Potential antibacterial activity of berberine against multi drug resistant enterovirulent *Escherichia coli* isolated from yaks (*Poephagus grunniens*) with haemorrhagic diarrhoea. Asian Pacific Journal of Tropical Medicine 6 (4), 315−319.

Bardell, D., 1982. An 1898 report by Gamaleya for a lytic agent specific for Bacillus anthracis. Journal of the history of medicine and allied sciences 37 (2), 222−225.

Bedford, M., 2000. Removal of antibiotic growth promoters from poultry diets: implications and strategies to minimise subsequent problems. World's Poultry Science Journal 56 (4), 347−365.

Bengtsson, B., Greko, C., 2014. Antibiotic resistance-consequences for animal health, welfare, and food production. Upsala Journal of Medical Sciences 119 (2), 96−102.

Benites, V., Gilharry, R., Gernat, A.G., Murillo, J.G., 2008. Effect of dietary mannan oligosaccharide from Bio-Mos or SAF-Mannan on live performance of broiler chickens. The Journal of Applied Poultry Research 17 (4), 471−475.

Bilkei, G., Bille, G., Bilkei, V., Bilkei, M., 2011a. Influence of phytogenic feed additives on production and mortality of pigs-part I: prophylactic effect of oregano in a pig fatting unit. Tierärztliche Umschau 66 (4), 157−162.

Bilkei, G., Bille, G., Bilkei, V., Bilkei, M., 2011b. Influence of phytogenic feed additives on production and mortality of pigs-part II: effect of garlic (*Allium sativum*), horseradish (*Aromatica rusticana*) and doxycycline in prevention of postparturient diseases of the sows and pre-and postweaning mortality in piglets. Tierärztliche Umschau 66 (6), 253−257.

Blajman, J.E., Frizzo, L.S., Zbrun, M.V., Astesana, D.M., Fusari, M.L., Soto, L.P., Rosmini, M.R., Signorini, M.L., 2014. Probiotics and broiler growth performance: a meta-analysis of randomised controlled trials. British Poultry Science 55 (4), 483−494.

Bonev, B., Hooper, J., Parisot, J., 2008. Principles of assessing bacterial susceptibility to antibiotics using the agar diffusion method. Journal of Antimicrobial Chemotherapy 61 (6), 1295−1301.

Borie, C., Albala, I., Sánchez, P., Sánchez, M.L., Ramírez, S., Navarro, C., Morales, M.A., Retamales, J., Robeson, J., 2008. Bacteriophage treatment reduces *Salmonella* colonization of infected chickens. Avian Diseases 52 (1), 64−67.

Borie, C., Sánchez, M.L., Navarro, C., Ramírez, S., Morales, M.A., Retamales, J., Robeson, J., 2009. Aerosol spray treatment with bacteriophages and competitive exclusion reduces *Salmonella* enteritidis infection in chickens. Avian Diseases 53 (2), 250−254.

Bourgou, S., Pichette, A., Marzouk, B., Legault, J., 2012. Antioxidant, anti-inflammatory, anticancer and antibacterial activities of extracts from *Nigella sativa* (black cumin) plant parts. Journal of Food Biochemistry 36 (5), 539−546.

Briers, Y., Lavigne, R., 2015. Breaking barriers: expansion of the use of endolysins as novel antibacterials against gram-negative bacteria. Future Microbiology 10 (3), 377−390.

Briers, Y., Walmagh, M., Lavigne, R., 2011. Use of bacteriophage endolysin EL188 and outer membrane permeabilizers against *Pseudomonas aeruginosa*. Journal of Applied Microbiology 110 (3), 778−785.

Briers, Y., Walmagh, M., Van Puyenbroeck, V., Cornelissen, A., Cenens, W., Aertsen, A., Oliveira, H., Azeredo, J., Verween, G., Pirnay, J.P., Miller, S., 2014. Engineered endolysin-based "Artilysins" to combat multidrug-resistant gram-negative pathogens. mBio 5 (4) e01379−14.

Broom, L.J., 2015. Organic acids for improving intestinal health of poultry. World's Poultry Science Journal 71 (4), 630−642.

Burt, S., 2004. Essential oils: their antibacterial properties and potential applications in foods-a review. International Journal of Food Microbiology 94 (3), 223−253.

Carnes, E.C., Lopez, D.M., Donegan, N.P., Cheung, A., Gresham, H., Timmins, G.S., Brinker, C.J., 2010. Confinement-induced quorum sensing of individual *Staphylococcus aureus* bacteria. Nature Chemical Biology 6 (1), 41.

Carpenter, A.W., Worley, B.V., Slomberg, D.L., Schoenfisch, M.H., 2012. Dual action antimicrobials: nitric oxide release from quaternary ammonium-functionalized silica nanoparticles. Biomacromolecules 13 (10), 3334−3342.

Cheng, T.C., Yao, K.S., Yeh, N., Chang, C.I., Hsu, H.C., Gonzalez, F., Chang, C.Y., 2011. Bactericidal effect of blue LED light irradiated TiO_2/Fe_3O_4 particles on fish pathogen in seawater. Thin Solid Films 519 (15), 5002−5006.

Cheng, G., Hao, H., Xie, S., Wang, X., Dai, M., Huang, L., Yuan, Z., 2014. Antibiotic alternatives: the substitution of antibiotics in animal husbandry? Frontiers in Microbiology 5, 217.

Cho, J.H., Kim, I.H., 2014. Effects of lactulose supplementation on performance, blood profiles, excreta microbial shedding of *Lactobacillus* and *Escherichia coli*, relative organ weight and excreta noxious gas contents in broilers. Journal of Animal Physiology and Animal Nutrition 98 (3), 424−430.

Choi, S.C., Ingale, S.L., Kim, J.S., Park, Y.K., Kwon, I.K., Chae, B.J., 2013. An antimicrobial peptide-A3: effects on growth performance, nutrient retention, intestinal and faecal microflora and intestinal morphology of broilers. British Poultry Science 54 (6), 738−746.

Chowdhury, S., De, M., Guha, R., Batabyal, S., Samanta, I., Hazra, S.K., Ghosh, T.K., Konar, A., Hazra, S., 2014. Influence of silver nanoparticles on post-surgical wound healing following topical application. European Journal of Nanomedicine 6 (4), 237−247.

Chowdhury, S., Mandal, G.P., Patra, A.K., Kumar, P., Samanta, I., Pradhan, S., Samanta, A.K., 2018. Different essential oils in diets of broiler chickens: 2. Gut microbes and morphology, immune response, and some blood profile and antioxidant enzymes. Animal Feed Science and Technology 236, 39−47.

Cui, Y., Zhao, Y., Tian, Y., Zhang, W., Lü, X., Jiang, X., 2012. The molecular mechanism of action of bactericidal gold nanoparticles on *Escherichia coli*. Biomaterials 33 (7), 2327−2333.

Dalmasso, G., Nguyen, H.T.T., Yan, Y., Charrier-Hisamuddin, L., Sitaraman, S.V., Merlin, D., 2008. Butyrate transcriptionally enhances peptide transporter PepT1 expression and activity. PLoS One 3 (6), e2476.

De, D., Mandal, S.M., Gauri, S.S., Bhattacharya, R., Ram, S., Roy, S.K., 2010. Antibacterial effect of lanthanum calcium manganate (La0. 67Ca0. 33MnO₃) nanoparticles against *Pseudomonas aeruginosa* ATCC 27853. Journal of Biomedical Nanotechnology 6 (2), 138−144.

De Jong, W.H., Borm, P.J., 2008. Drug delivery and nanoparticles: applications and hazards. International Journal of Nanomedicine 3 (2), 133.

Di Pasqua, R., Hoskins, N., Betts, G., Mauriello, G., 2006. Changes in membrane fatty acids composition of microbial cells induced by addiction of thymol, carvacrol, limonene, cinnamaldehyde, and eugenol in the growing media. Journal of Agricultural and Food Chemistry 54 (7), 2745−2749.

d'Herelle, F., 1917. Sur un microbe invisible antagoniste des bacilles dysentériques. Comptes rendus de l'Académie des Sciences 165, 373−375.

El-Abasy, M., Motobu, M., Shimura, K., Na, K.J., Kang, C.B., Koge, K., Onodera, T., Hirota, Y., 2002. Immunostimulating and growth-promoting effects of sugar cane extract (SCE) in chickens. Journal of Veterinary Medical Science 64 (11), 1061−1063.

Faria Filho, D.E., Torres, K.A.A., Faria, D.E., Campos, D.M.B., Rosa, P.S., 2006. Probiotics for broiler chickens in Brazil: systematic review and meta-analysis. Brazilian Journal of Poultry Science 8 (2), 89−98.

Fenaroli, F., Westmoreland, D., Benjaminsen, J., Kolstad, T., Skjeldal, F.M., Meijer, A.H., van der Vaart, M., Ulanova, L., Roos, N., Nyström, B., Hildahl, J., 2014. Nanoparticles as drug delivery system against tuberculosis in zebrafish embryos: direct visualization and treatment. ACS Nano 8 (7), 7014−7026.

Florou-Paneri, P., Giannenas, I., Christaki, E., Govaris, A., Botsoglou, N., 2006. Performance of chickens and oxidative stability of the produced meat as affected by feed supplementation with oregano, vitamin C, vitamin E and their combinations. Archiv für Geflügelkunde 70 (5), 232−239.

Forestier, C., Guelon, D., Cluytens, V., Gillart, T., Sirot, J., De Champs, C., 2008. Oral probiotic and prevention of *Pseudomonas aeruginosa* infections: a randomized, double-blind, placebo-controlled pilot study in intensive care unit patients. Critical Care 12 (3), R69.

Geier, M.S., Mikkelsen, L.L., Torok, V.A., Allison, G.E., Olnood, C.G., Boulianne, M., Hughes, R.J., Choct, M., 2010. Comparison of alternatives to in-feed antimicrobials for the prevention of clinical necrotic enteritis. Journal of Applied Microbiology 109 (4), 1329−1338.

Ghazanfari, S., Mohammadi, Z., Adib Moradi, M., 2015. Effects of coriander essential oil on the performance, blood characteristics, intestinal microbiota and histological of broilers. Brazilian Journal of Poultry Science 17 (4), 419−426.

Ghosh, T.K., Haldar, S., Bedford, M.R., Muthusami, N., Samanta, I., 2012. Assessment of yeast cell wall as replacements for antibiotic growth promoters in broiler diets: effects on performance, intestinal histo-morphology and humoral immune responses. Journal of Animal Physiology and Animal Nutrition 96 (2), 275−284.

Gill, E.E., Franco, O.L., Hancock, R.E., 2015. Antibiotic adjuvants: diverse strategies for controlling drug-resistant pathogens. Chemical Biology and Drug Design 85 (1), 56−78.

Gilmer, D.B., Schmitz, J.E., Euler, C.W., Fischetti, V.A., 2013. Novel bacteriophage lysin with broad lytic activity protects against mixed infection by *Streptococcus pyogenes* and methicillin-resistant *Staphylococcus aureus*. Antimicrobial Agents and Chemotherapy 57 (6), 2743−2750.

Griggs, J.P., Jacob, J.P., 2005. Alternatives to antibiotics for organic poultry production. The Journal of Applied Poultry Research 14 (4), 750−756.

Guttman, B., Raya, R., Kutter, E., Sulakvelidze, A., 2005. Bacteriophages: Biology and Applications, pp. 29−66.

Hagens, S., Habel, A., Von Ahsen, U., Von Gabain, A., Bläsi, U., 2004. Therapy of experimental *Pseudomonas* infections with a nonreplicating genetically modified phage. Antimicrobial Agents and Chemotherapy 48 (10), 3817−3822.

Halasa, T., Østerås, O., Hogeveen, H., van Werven, T., Nielen, M., 2009. Meta-analysis of dry cow management for dairy cattle. Part 1. Protection against new intramammary infections. Journal of Dairy Science 92 (7), 3134−3149.

Hankin, E.H., 1896. L'action bactericide des eaux de la Jumna et du Gange sur le vibrion du cholera. Ann. Inst. Pasteur 10 (5) p. ll.

Harada, K., 1990. Attraction activities of spices for oriental weather fish and yellowtail. Bulletin of the Japanese Society of Scientific Flsheries 56, 2029−2033.

Hashemipour, H., Kermanshahi, H., Golian, A., Khaksar, V., 2014. Effects of carboxy methyl cellulose and thymol+ carvacrol on performance, digesta viscosity and some blood metabolites of broilers. Journal of Animal Physiology and Animal Nutrition 98 (4), 672−679.

Heo, Y.J., Lee, Y.R., Jung, H.H., Lee, J., Ko, G., Cho, Y.H., 2009. Antibacterial efficacy of phages against *Pseudomonas aeruginosa* infections in mice and *Drosophila melanogaster*. Antimicrobial Agents and Chemotherapy 53 (6), 2469−2474.

Hill, C., Guarner, F., Reid, G., Gibson, G.R., Merenstein, D.J., Pot, B., Morelli, L., Canani, R.B., Flint, H.J., Salminen, S., Calder, P.C., 2014. The international scientific association for probiotics and prebiotics consensus statement on the scope and appropriate use of the term probiotic. Nature Reviews Gastroenterology and Hepatology 11 (8), 506−514.

Hobley, L., King, J.R., Sockett, R.E., 2006. *Bdellovibrio* predation in the presence of decoys: three-way bacterial interactions revealed by mathematical and experimental analyses. Applied and Environmental Microbiology 72 (10), 6757−6765.

Hooge, D.M., Pierce, J.L., McBride, K.W., Rigolin, P.J., 2010. Meta-analysis of broiler chicken trials using diets with or without Allzyme® SSF enzyme complex. International Journal of Poultry Science 9 (9), 819−823.

Horgan, M., O'Flynn, G., Garry, J., Cooney, J., Coffey, A., Fitzgerald, G.F., Ross, R.P., McAuliffe, O., 2009. Phage lysin LysK can be truncated to its CHAP domain and retain lytic activity against live antibiotic-resistant staphylococci. Applied and Environmental Microbiology 75 (3), 872−874.

Hraiech, S., Brégeon, F., Rolain, J.M., 2015. Bacteriophage-based therapy in cystic fibrosis-associated *Pseudomonas aeruginosa* infections: rationale and current status. Drug Design, Development and Therapy 9, 3653.

Huff, W.E., Huff, G.R., Rath, N.C., Balog, J.M., Donoghue, A.M., 2005. Alternatives to antibiotics: utilization of bacteriophage to treat colibacillosis and prevent foodborne pathogens. Poultry Science 84 (4), 655−659.

Hume, M.E., 2011. Historic perspective: prebiotics, probiotics, and other alternatives to antibiotics. Poultry Science 90 (11), 2663−2669.

Hurley, M.N., Cámara, M., Smyth, A.R., 2012. Novel approaches to the treatment of *Pseudomonas aeruginosa* infections in cystic fibrosis. European Respiratory Journal 40 (4), 1014−1023.

Hwang, J.H., Lee, S.W., Rha, S.J., Yoon, H.S., Park, E.S., Han, K.H., Kim, S.J., 2013. Dietary green tea extract improves growth performance, body composition, and stress recovery in the juvenile black rockfish, *Sebastes schlegeli*. Aquaculture International 21 (3), 525−538.

Islam, M.R., Oomah, D.B., Diarra, M.S., 2016. Potential immunomodulatory effects of non-dialyzable materials of cranberry extract in poultry production. Poultry Science 96 (2), 341−350.

Jackson, M.E., Hanford, K., 2014. Statistical meta-analysis of pen trials conducted testing heat-sensitive β-mannanase (Hemicell) feed enzyme in male broilers grown to market age. Poultry Science 93, 66.

Jayaraman, P., Sakharkar, M.K., Lim, C.S., Tang, T.H., Sakharkar, K.R., 2010. Activity and interactions of antibiotic and phytochemical combinations against *Pseudomonas aeruginosa in vitro*. International Journal of Biological Sciences 6 (6), 556.

Jayaseelan, C., Rahuman, A.A., Kirthi, A.V., Marimuthu, S., Santhoshkumar, T., Bagavan, A., Gaurav, K., Karthik, L., Rao, K.B., 2012. Novel microbial route to synthesize ZnO nanoparticles using *Aeromonas hydrophila* and their activity against pathogenic bacteria and fungi. Spectrochimica Acta Part A: Molecular and Biomolecular Spectroscopy 90, 78−84.

Józefiak, D., Sip, A., Kaczmarek, S., Rutkowski, A., 2010. The effects of *Carnobacterium* divergens AS7 bacteriocin on gastrointestinal microflora in vitro and on nutrient retention in broiler chickens. Journal of Animal and Feed Sciences 19 (3).

Kadouri, D.E., To, K., Shanks, R.M., Doi, Y., 2013. Predatory bacteria: a potential ally against multidrug-resistant gram-negative pathogens. PLoS One 8 (5), e63397.

Kang, S., Li, Z., Yin, Z., Jia, R., Song, X., Li, L., Chen, Z., Peng, L., Qu, J., Hu, Z., Lai, X., 2015. The antibacterial mechanism of berberine against *Actinobacillus pleuropneumoniae*. Natural Product Research 29 (23), 2203−2206.

Kiarie, E., Romero, L.F., Nyachoti, C.M., 2013. The role of added feed enzymes in promoting gut health in swine and poultry. Nutrition Research Reviews 26 (1), 71−88.

Kim, G.B., Seo, Y.M., Kim, C.H., Paik, I.K., 2011. Effect of dietary prebiotic supplementation on the performance, intestinal microflora, and immune response of broilers. Poultry Science 90 (1), 75−82.

Kim, S.C., Kim, J.W., Kim, J.U., Kim, I.H., 2013. Effects of dietary supplementation of bacteriophage on growth performance, nutrient digestibility, blood profiles, carcass characteristics and fecal microflora in broilers. Korean Journal of Poultry Science 40 (1), 75−81.

Kim, S.J., Lee, K.W., Kang, C.W., An, B.K., 2016. Growth performance, relative meat and organ weights, cecal microflora, and blood characteristics in broiler chickens fed diets containing different nutrient density with or without essential oils. Asian-Australasian Journal of Animal Sciences 29 (4), 549.

Kohlert, C., Schindler, G., März, R.W., Abel, G., Brinkhaus, B., Derendorf, H., Gräfe, E.U., Veit, M., 2002. Systemic availability and pharmacokinetics of thymol in humans. The Journal of Clinical Pharmacology 42 (7), 731−737.

Kumar, P., Patra, A.K., Mandal, G.P., Samanta, I., Pradhan, S., 2017. Effect of black cumin seeds on growth performance, nutrient utilization, immunity, gut health and nitrogen excretion in broiler chickens. Journal of the Science of Food and Agriculture 97 (11), 3742−3751.

Langhout, P., 2000. New additives for broiler chickens. World Poultry 16 (3), 22−27.

Lara, H.H., Ayala-Núñez, N.V., Turrent, L.D.C.I., Padilla, C.R., 2010. Bactericidal effect of silver nanoparticles against multidrug-resistant bacteria. World Journal of Microbiology and Biotechnology 26 (4), 615−621.

Lavigne, R., Briers, Y., Hertveldt, K., Robben, J., Volckaert, G., 2004. Identification and characterization of a highly thermostable bacteriophage lysozyme. Cellular and Molecular Life Sciences CMLS 61 (21), 2753−2759.

Lee, J.Y., Gao, Y., 2012. Review of the application of garlic, *Allium sativum*, in aquaculture. Journal of the World Aquaculture Society 43 (4), 447−458.

Lei, K., Li, Y.L., Yu, D.Y., Rajput, I.R., Li, W.F., 2013. Influence of dietary inclusion of *Bacillus licheniformis* on laying performance, egg quality, antioxidant enzyme activities, and intestinal barrier function of laying hens. Poultry Science 92 (9), 2389−2395.

Lemos, M.J.D., Calixto, L.F.L., Alves, O.D.S., Souza, D.S.D., Moura, B.B., Reis, T.L., 2015. Kaolin in the diet and its effects on performance, litter moisture and intestinal morphology of broiler chickens. Ciência Rural 45 (10), 1835−1840.

Li, X., Robinson, S.M., Gupta, A., Saha, K., Jiang, Z., Moyano, D.F., Sahar, A., Riley, M.A., Rotello, V.M., 2014. Functional gold nanoparticles as potent antimicrobial agents against multi-drug-resistant bacteria. ACS Nano 8 (10), 10682−10686.

Lim, T.H., Kim, M.S., Lee, D.H., Lee, Y.N., Park, J.K., Youn, H.N., Lee, H.J., Yang, S.Y., Cho, Y.W., Lee, J.B., Park, S.Y., 2012. Use of bacteriophage for biological control of *Salmonella* enteritidis infection in chicken. Research in Veterinary Science 93 (3), 1173−1178.

Lima, D.A.D., Furian, T.Q., Pillati, R.M., Silva, G.L., Morgam, R.B., Borges, K.A., Fortes, F.B.B., Moraes, H.L.D.S., Brito, B.G.D., Brito, K.C.T., Salle, C.T.P., 2016. Establishment of a pathogenicity index in *Salmonella* enteritidis and *Salmonella* typhimurium strains inoculated in one-day-old broiler chicks. Arquivo Brasileiro de Medicina Veterinária e Zootecnia 68 (2), 257−264.

Liu, Y., Yang, L., Molin, S., 2010. Synergistic activities of an efflux pump inhibitor and iron chelators against *Pseudomonas aeruginosa* growth and biofilm formation. Antimicrobial Agents and Chemotherapy 54 (9), 3960−3963.

Liu, H.N., Liu, Y., Hu, L.L., Suo, Y.L., Zhang, L., Jin, F., Feng, X.A., Teng, N., Li, Y., 2014. Effects of dietary supplementation of quercetin on performance, egg quality, cecal microflora populations, and antioxidant status in laying hens. Poultry Science 93 (2), 347−353.

Loc-Carrillo, C., Abedon, S.T., 2011. Pros and cons of phage therapy. Bacteriophage 1 (2), 111−114.

Loeffler, J.M., Djurkovic, S., Fischetti, V.A., 2003. Phage lytic enzyme Cpl-1 as a novel antimicrobial for pneumococcal bacteremia. Infection and Immunity 71 (11), 6199−6204.

López, R., García, E., García, P., 2004. Enzymes for anti-infective therapy: phage lysins. Drug Discovery Today: Therapeutic Strategies 1 (4), 469−474.

Łusiak-Szelachowska, M., Żaczek, M., Weber-Dąbrowska, B., Miedzybrodzki, R., Kłak, M., Fortuna, W., Letkiewicz, S., Rogóż, P., Szufnarowski, K., Jończyk-Matysiak, E., Owczarek, B., 2014. Phage neutralization by sera of patients receiving phage therapy. Viral Immunology 27 (6), 295−304.

Lückstädt, C., 2006. Use of organic acids as feed additives-sustainable aquaculture production the non-antibiotic way. International Aquafeed 9 (2), 21−26.

Miller, R.W., Skinner, J., Sulakvelidze, A., Mathis, G.F., Hofacre, C.L., 2010. Bacteriophage therapy for control of necrotic enteritis of broiler chickens experimentally infected with *Clostridium perfringens*. Avian Diseases 54 (1), 33−40.

Mohan, S., Oluwafemi, O.S., George, S.C., Jayachandran, V.P., Lewu, F.B., Songca, S.P., Kalarikkal, N., Thomas, S., 2014. Completely green synthesis of dextrose reduced silver nanoparticles, its antimicrobial and sensing properties. Carbohydrate Polymers 106, 469−474.

Mookiah, S., Sieo, C.C., Ramasamy, K., Abdullah, N., Ho, Y.W., 2014. Effects of dietary prebiotics, probiotic and synbiotics on performance, caecal bacterial populations and caecal fermentation concentrations of broiler chickens. Journal of the Science of Food and Agriculture 94 (2), 341−348.

Muñoz-Atienza, E., Gómez-Sala, B., Araújo, C., Campanero, C., Del Campo, R., Hernández, P.E., Herranz, C., Cintas, L.M., 2013. Antimicrobial activity, antibiotic susceptibility and virulence factors of lactic acid bacteria of aquatic origin intended for use as probiotics in aquaculture. BMC Microbiology 13 (1), 15.

Murphy, D., Ricci, A., Auce, Z., Beechinor, J.G., Bergendahl, H., Breathnach, R., Bureš, J., Da Silva, D., Pedro, J., Hederová, J., Hekman, P., 2017. EMA and EFSA joint scientific opinion on measures to reduce the need to use antimicrobial agents in animal husbandry in the European union, and the resulting impacts on food safety (RONAFA). EFSA Journal 15 (1).

Mushtaq, N., Redpath, M.B., Luzio, J.P., Taylor, P.W., 2005. Treatment of experimental *Escherichia coli* infection with recombinant bacteriophage-derived capsule depolymerase. Journal of Antimicrobial Chemotherapy 56 (1), 160−165.

Muthusamy, G., Joardar, S.N., Samanta, I., Isore, D.P., Roy, B., Kumar, T., 2013. β−Glucan from edible mushroom (*Pleurotus florida*) enhances mucosal immunity in poultry. Advances in Animal and Veterinary Sciences 1 (1), 116−119.

Nelson, D., Loomis, L., Fischetti, V.A., 2001. Prevention and elimination of upper respiratory colonization of mice by group A streptococci by using a bacteriophage lytic enzyme. Proceedings of the National Academy of Sciences 98 (7), 4107−4112.

Newaj-Fyzul, A., Austin, B., 2015. Probiotics, immunostimulants, plant products and oral vaccines, and their role as feed supplements in the control of bacterial fish diseases. Journal of Fish Diseases 38 (11), 937−955.

Ng, S.C., Hart, A.L., Kamm, M.A., Stagg, A.J., Knight, S.C., 2008. Mechanisms of action of probiotics: recent advances. Inflammatory Bowel Diseases 15 (2), 300−310.

Nurmi, E., Rantala, M., 1973. New aspects of *Salmonella* infection in broiler production. Nature 241 (5386), 210.

Oliveira, H., Melo, L.D., Santos, S.B., Nóbrega, F.L., Ferreira, E.C., Cerca, N., Azeredo, J., Kluskens, L.D., 2013. Molecular aspects and comparative genomics of bacteriophage endolysins. Journal of Virology 87 (8), 4558−4570.

Pathak, M., Mandal, G.P., Patra, A.K., Samanta, I., Pradhan, S., Haldar, S., 2017. Effects of dietary supplementation of cinnamaldehyde and formic acid on growth performance, intestinal microbiota and immune response in broiler chickens. Animal Production Science 57 (5), 821−827.

Patra, A.K., 2012. An overview of antimicrobial properties of different classes of phytochemicals. In: Dietary Phytochemicals and Microbes. Springer, Dordrecht, pp. 1−32.

Paul, I., Isore, D.P., Joardar, S.N., Samanta, I., Biswas, U., Maiti, T.K., Mukhopadhyay, S.K., 2012. Orally administered β-glucan of edible mushroom (*Pleurotus florida*) origin upregulates innate immune response in broiler. Indian Journal of Animal Sciences 82 (7), 745−748.

Peng, L., He, Z., Chen, W., Holzman, I.R., Lin, J., 2007. Effects of butyrate on intestinal barrier function in a Caco-2 cell monolayer model of intestinal barrier. Pediatric Research 61 (1), 37.

Pirgozliev, V., Bravo, D., Mirza, M.W., Rose, S.P., 2015. Growth performance and endogenous losses of broilers fed wheat-based diets with and without essential oils and xylanase supplementation. Poultry Science 94 (6), 1227−1232.

Placha, I., Takacova, J., Ryzner, M., Cobanova, K., Laukova, A., Strompfova, V., Venglovska, K., Faix, S., 2014. Effect of thyme essential oil and selenium on intestine integrity and antioxidant status of broilers. British Poultry Science 55 (1), 105−114.

Pourhossein, Z., Qotbi, A.A.A., Seidavi, A., Laudadio, V., Centoducati, G., Tufarelli, V., 2015. Effect of different levels of dietary sweet orange (*Citrus sinensis*) peel extract on humoral immune system responses in broiler chickens. Animal Science Journal 86 (1), 105−110.

Rabiee, A.R., Lean, I.J., 2013. The effect of internal teat sealant products (Teatseal and Orbeseal) on intramammary infection, clinical mastitis, and somatic cell counts in lactating dairy cows: a meta-analysis. Journal of Dairy Science 96 (11), 6915−6931.

Rather, M.A., Sharma, R., Gupta, S., Ferosekhan, S., Ramya, V.L., Jadhao, S.B., 2013. Chitosan-nanoconjugated hormone nanoparticles for sustained surge of gonadotropins and enhanced reproductive output in female fish. PLoS One 8 (2), e57094.

Redondo, L.M., Chacana, P.A., Dominguez, J.E., Fernandez Miyakawa, M.E.D., 2014. Perspectives in the use of tannins as alternative to antimicrobial growth promoter factors in poultry. Frontiers in Microbiology 5, 118.

Rhoads, D.D., Wolcott, R.D., Kuskowski, M.A., Wolcott, B.M., Ward, L.S., Sulakvelidze, A., 2009. Bacteriophage therapy of venous leg ulcers in humans: results of a phase I safety trial. Journal of Wound Care 18 (6), 237−243.

Roberfroid, M., 2007. Prebiotics: the concept revisited. Journal of Nutrition 137 (3), 830S−837S.

Rodríguez-Rubio, L., Martínez, B., Donovan, D.M., García, P., Rodríguez, A., 2013. Potential of the virion-associated peptidoglycan hydrolase HydH5 and its derivative fusion proteins in milk biopreservation. PLoS One 8 (1), e54828.

Rostami, F., Ghasemi, H.A., Taherpour, K., 2015. Effect of *Scrophularia striata* and *Ferulago angulata*, as alternatives to virginiamycin, on growth performance, intestinal microbial population, immune response, and blood constituents of broiler chickens. Poultry Science 94 (9), 2202−2209.

Salehi, A.H., Montazer, M., Toliyat, T., Mahmoudi-Rad, M., 2015. A new route for synthesis of silver: gold alloy nanoparticles loaded within phosphatidylcholine liposome structure as an effective antibacterial agent against *Pseudomonas aeruginosa*. Journal of Liposome Research 25 (1), 38−45.

Schmelcher, M., Donovan, D.M., Loessner, M.J., 2012. Bacteriophage endolysins as novel antimicrobials. Future Microbiology 7 (10), 1147−1171.

Schmelcher, M., Powell, A.M., Camp, M.J., Pohl, C.S., Donovan, D.M., 2015. Synergistic streptococcal phage λSA2 and B30 endolysins kill streptococci in cow milk and in a mouse model of mastitis. Applied Microbiology and Biotechnology 99 (20), 8475−8486.

Schuch, R., Nelson, D., Fischetti, V.A., 2002. A bacteriolytic agent that detects and kills *Bacillus anthracis*. Nature 418 (6900), 884.

Sellera, F.P., Gargano, R.G., Libera, A.M., Benesi, F.J., Azedo, M.R., de Sa, L.R., Ribeiro, M.S., da Silva Baptista, M., Pogliani, F.C., 2016. Antimicrobial photodynamic therapy for caseous lymphadenitis abscesses in sheep: report of ten cases. Photodiagnosis and Photodynamic Therapy 13, 120−122.

Sen, S., Ingale, S.L., Kim, Y.W., Kim, J.S., Kim, K.H., Lohakare, J.D., Kim, E.K., Kim, H.S., Ryu, M.H., Kwon, I.K., Chae, B.J., 2012. Effect of supplementation of *Bacillus subtilis* LS 1-2 to broiler diets on growth performance, nutrient retention, caecal microbiology and small intestinal morphology. Research in Veterinary Science 93 (1), 264−268.

Shi, Y., Li, N., Yan, Y., Wang, H., Li, Y., Lu, C., Sun, J., 2012. Combined antibacterial activity of phage lytic proteins holin and lysin from *Streptococcus suis* bacteriophage SMP. Current Microbiology 65 (1), 28−34.

Si, W., Gong, J., Tsao, R., Zhou, T., Yu, H., Poppe, C., Johnson, R., Du, Z., 2006. Antimicrobial activity of essential oils and structurally related synthetic food additives towards selected pathogenic and beneficial gut bacteria. Journal of Applied Microbiology 100 (2), 296−305.

Simon, O., Jadamus, A., Vahjen, W., 2001. Probiotic feed additives-effectiveness and expected modes of action. Journal of Animal and Feed Sciences 10, 51−68.

Spring, P., Wenk, C., Dawson, K.A., Newman, K.E., 2000. The effects of dietary mannaoligosaccharides on cecal parameters and the concentrations of enteric bacteria in the ceca of *Salmonella*-challenged broiler chicks. Poultry Science 79 (2), 205−211.

Swain, P., Nayak, S.K., Sasmal, A., Behera, T., Barik, S.K., Swain, S.K., Mishra, S.S., Sen, A.K., Das, J.K., Jayasankar, P., 2014. Antimicrobial activity of metal based nanoparticles against microbes associated with diseases in aquaculture. World Journal of Microbiology and Biotechnology 30 (9), 2491−2502.

Thacker, P.A., 2013. Alternatives to antibiotics as growth promoters for use in swine production: a review. Journal of Animal Science and Biotechnology 4 (1), 35.

Thiel, K., 2004. Old dogma, new tricks-21st century phage therapy. Nature Biotechnology 22 (1), 31.

Torres-Barceló, C., Arias-Sánchez, F.I., Vasse, M., Ramsayer, J., Kaltz, O., Hochberg, M.E., 2014. A window of opportunity to control the bacterial pathogen *Pseudomonas aeruginosa* combining antibiotics and phages. PLoS One 9 (9), e106628.

Twort, F.W., 1915. An investigation on the nature of ultra-microscopic viruses. The Lancet 186 (4814), 1241−1243.

Umashankari, J., Inbakandan, D., Ajithkumar, T.T., Balasubramanian, T., 2012. Mangrove plant, *Rhizophora mucronata* (Lamk, 1804) mediated one pot green synthesis of silver nanoparticles and its antibacterial activity against aquatic pathogens. Aquatic Biosystems 8 (1), 11.

Van Delden, C., Köhler, T., Brunner-Ferber, F., François, B., Carlet, J., Pechère, J.C., 2012. Azithromycin to prevent *Pseudomonas aeruginosa* ventilator-associated pneumonia by inhibition of quorum sensing: a randomized controlled trial. Intensive Care Medicine 38 (7), 1118−1125.

Vaseeharan, B., Ramasamy, P., Chen, J.C., 2010. Antibacterial activity of silver nanoparticles (AgNps) synthesized by tea leaf extracts against pathogenic *Vibrio harveyi* and its protective efficacy on juvenile *Feneropenaeus indicus*. Letters in Applied Microbiology 50 (4), 352−356.

Velmurugan, P., Iydroose, M., Lee, S.M., Cho, M., Park, J.H., Balachandar, V., Oh, B.T., 2014. Synthesis of silver and gold nanoparticles using cashew nut shell liquid and its antibacterial activity against fish pathogens. Indian Journal of Microbiology 54 (2), 196−202.

Venkatramalingam, K., Christopher, J.G., Citarasu, T., 2007. Zingiber officinalis an herbal appetizer in the tiger shrimp *Penaeus monodon* (Fabricius) larviculture. Aquaculture Nutrition 13 (6), 439−443.

Vondruskova, H., Slamova, R., Trckova, M., Zraly, Z., Pavlik, I., 2010. Alternatives to antibiotic growth promoters in prevention of diarrhoea in weaned piglets: a review. Veterinarni Medicina 55 (5), 199−224.

Walz, J.M., Avelar, R.L., Longtine, K.J., Carter, K.L., Mermel, L.A., Heard, S.O., 2010. Anti-infective external coating of central venous catheters: a randomized, noninferiority trial comparing 5-fluorouracil with chlorhexidine/silver sulfadiazine in preventing catheter colonization. Critical Care Medicine 38 (11), 2095−2102.

Wang, L., Piao, X.L., Kim, S.W., Piao, X.S., Shen, Y.B., Lee, H.S., 2008. Effects of *Forsythia suspensa* extract on growth performance, nutrient digestibility, and antioxidant activities in broiler chickens under high ambient temperature. Poultry Science 87 (7), 1287−1294.

Wang, D., Ma, W., She, R., Sun, Q., Liu, Y., Hu, Y., Liu, L., Yang, Y., Peng, K., 2009. Effects of swine gut antimicrobial peptides on the intestinal mucosal immunity in specific-pathogen-free chickens. Poultry Science 88 (5), 967−974.

Wang, K., Yan, J., Dang, W., Xie, J., Yan, B., Yan, W., Sun, M., Zhang, B., Ma, M., Zhao, Y., Jia, F., 2014. Dual antifungal properties of cationic antimicrobial peptides polybia-MPI: membrane integrity disruption and inhibition of biofilm formation. Peptides 56, 22−29.

Wen, L.F., He, J.G., 2012. Dose−response effects of an antimicrobial peptide, a cecropin hybrid, on growth performance, nutrient utilisation, bacterial counts in the digesta and intestinal morphology in broilers. British Journal of Nutrition 108 (10), 1756−1763.

Windisch, W., Kroismayr, A., 2006. The effects of phytobiotics on performance and gut function in monogastrics. In: World Nutrition Forum: The Future of Animal Nutrition, pp. 85−90.

Wright, A., Hawkins, C.H., Änggård, E.E., Harper, D.R., 2009. A controlled clinical trial of a therapeutic bacteriophage preparation in chronic otitis due to antibiotic-resistant *Pseudomonas aeruginosa*; a preliminary report of efficacy. Clinical Otolaryngology 34 (4), 349−357.

Xia, M.S., Hu, C.H., Xu, Z.R., 2004. Effects of copper-bearing montmorillonite on growth performance, digestive enzyme activities, and intestinal microflora and morphology of male broilers. Poultry Science 83 (11), 1868–1875.

Zhang, Z.F., Kim, I.H., 2014. Effects of multistrain probiotics on growth performance, apparent ileal nutrient digestibility, blood characteristics, cecal microbial shedding, and excreta odor contents in broilers. Poultry Science 93 (2), 364–370.

Zhao, P.Y., Baek, H.Y., Kim, I.H., 2012. Effects of bacteriophage supplementation on egg performance, egg quality, excreta microflora, and moisture content in laying hens. Asian-Australasian Journal of Animal Sciences 25 (7), 1015.

Zhao, X.H., He, X., Yang, X.F., Zhong, X.H., 2013. Effect of *Portulaca oleracea* extracts on growth performance and microbial populations in ceca of broilers. Poultry Science 92 (5), 1343–1347.

Zhao, L., Seth, A., Wibowo, N., Zhao, C.X., Mitter, N., Yu, C., Middelberg, A.P., 2014. Nanoparticle vaccines. Vaccine 32 (3), 327–337.

Chapter 31

Immunotherapy

Chapter outline

Immunization and use of immunotherapeutic agents will be a keystone strategy to combat antimicrobial-resistant bacteria in food animals and poultry in coming years. Active immunization with vaccines is considered among top five alternative approaches to the use of antimicrobial agents in food animals because of feasibility (Postma et al., 2015). The studies confirmed reduced antibiotic usage and associated costs of production in pigs, poultry and fishes after introduction of vaccination and improved biosecurity strategy (Morrison and Saksida, 2013; Mombarg et al., 2014; Murphy et al., 2017). Vaccination of poultry with live coccidia may also restore the environment with antibiotic sensitive populations when the same is shed by the vaccinated birds (Williams, 2002). Few studies although did not show reduction of antibiotic usage in food animals after vaccination as the vaccines could not provide protection against all the infectious diseases (Temtem et al., 2016). Passive immunization with monoclonal antibodies to bacterial proteins, lipopeptides, glycolipids or carbohydrates is an effective alternative treatment strategy if applied during the early course of the infection (Boucher et al., 2009). Improving immune status with the immunomodulators may act as a further option, although boosting immunity sometimes creates more damage associated with inflammatory response (Casadevall and Pirofski, 2009).

Cellular immunotherapy

Cellular immunotherapy is a therapeutic approach with T cell checkpoint inhibitors, engineered T cells, engineered monoclonal antibodies to tumours and immune cell antigens to boost the host immune system to combat neoplastic diseases. Immune checkpoint molecules (CTLA-4, PD-1, TIM3, Lag3) are detected on the cell surfaces (naïve and effector T cells), which can limit T cell proliferation and effector functions (Krummel and Allison, 1996). The blockade of CTLA-4/PD-1 with monoclonal antibodies can induce antitumour immunity through the generation of new T cells or reactivation of existing T cell populations (Shin et al., 2012; Dolan and Gupta, 2014). The blockers of CTLA-4 and PD-1 are approved as immunotherapeutic drugs for human patients with melanoma, renal cell carcinoma and non—small cell lung cancer. The studies are exploring distribution of PD-1 in different canine cancer cells to develop effective immunotherapy.

The engineered T cells are generated by collection of autologous T cells from the host (lymph node excision) and ex vivo modification of the cells with attachment of tumour-specific T-cell receptors or tumour antigen-specific antibodies. The engineered T cells are infused back into the host (Müller and Kontermann, 2010). Using chimeric antigen receptor technology, T cells are generated specific for CD19+ B cells and the engineered T cells after infusion showed clinical success against chronic lymphocytic leukaemia in human patients (Cruz et al., 2013). The clinical evaluation of human chimeric T cells produced success in dogs with osteosarcoma because of cross-reaction (Mata et al., 2014).

Antimicrobial Resistance in Agriculture. https://doi.org/10.1016/B978-0-12-815770-1.00031-6

Major constraint for development of cellular immunotherapy for animals included lack of availability of immune reagents and consequently human cytokines are used for in vitro propagation of animal lymphocytes.

The engineered monoclonal antibodies to tumours and immune cell antigens are major advancement in tumour immunotherapy. The monoclonal antibody developed against B-cell lymphoma of dogs (canine anti-CD20 antibody) has been approved by the United States for clinical use.

Immunomodulation

The environmental stressors such as heat, microbes, parasites, toxins (endotoxin, aflatoxin) and airborne gases (ammonia) can damage the gastrointestinal tract mucus layer of poultry and livestock. The damage can induce inflammation and immune response with loss of energy and reduced production (Arce et al., 2010). In poultry, it is indicated by reduced feed intake, loss of body weight, infiltration of heterophils in the intestine and increased pathogen load in the gut and vital organs (Quinteiro-Filho et al., 2012). Various feed additives with antiinflammatory, antimicrobial and antioxidative properties are added for protection of gut and improvement of performance in animals and birds.

An immunomodulator may be defined as any biological or synthetic substance that can stimulate or suppress either innate or adaptive or both arms of the immune system (Agarwal and Singh, 1999). Immunomodulatory property was detected in various substances such as herb/spice-based products (phytogenics), immunosaccharides, anthelmintic, stem cells, cytokines, hormones, glucocorticoids, host defence peptides, microbial products, Toll-like receptors (TLRs), vitamins and minerals.

Innate immune response in livestock and poultry is regulated by mitogen-activated protein kinases (MAPKs) and nuclear factor kappa B (NFκB) pathways through the TLRs as major pattern recognition receptors present in the surface of the immune cells. Environmental stressors including pathogens can generate proinflammatory cytokines (interleukin (IL) 1, IL-6, TNF-α), reactive oxygen species and mitogens which can activate NFκB signalling. The active NFκB can induce enhanced production of inflammatory cytokines and stunted growth in poultry (Klasing and Johnstone, 1991). The oregano, cinnamon, turmeric, purple coneflower and thyme are commonly used as phytogenics in poultry and pigs. The phytogenics can suppress TLRs, MAPKs and NFκB signalling pathways and increase the expression of antiinflammatory cytokines in animals and birds (Lubbad et al., 2009; Liang et al., 2014; Hassan and Awad, 2017). The polyphenols are major active components present in roots, leaves, flowers, fruit and seeds of the plants and it protects the plants from pests and ultraviolet irradiation (Scalbert et al., 2002). Based on the number of aromatic rings and their binding affinity, the polyphenols are classified into two varieties such as flavonoids and nonflavonoids. The flavonoids can inhibit the enzymes lipoxygenase (5-LOX) and cyclooxygenase (COX), which are associated with synthesis of prostaglandins and leukotrienes, required for inflammatory response (D Archivio et al., 2007). As a consequence, less energy is spent for innate immune response in animals and birds, and the surplus energy can be converted into growth and production. Various studies detected higher antibody titres against sheep red blood cells or Newcastle disease, higher lymphocyte count with better growth and reduced feed conversion ratio in broilers and pigs after addition of phytogenics in diet (Landy et al., 2011; Rahimi et al., 2011; Ariza-Nieto et al., 2011). Direct administration of flavonoids such as genistein, hesperidin, fermented *Ginkgo biloba* leaves, soy isoflavones in the diets of poultry and pigs improve the immune status and reduce occurrence of diarrhoea and endotoxin concentration in blood (Zhang et al., 2013; Zhu et al., 2015). In spite of all these benefits, very less numbers of polyphenols are detected, which are readily absorbed through the intestine of animals and birds (Surai, 2014).

Immunosaccharides (fructooligosaccharide (FOS), mannan oligosaccharide (MOS), polysaccharide) are functional carbohydrates that can stimulate the innate immune system directly through the pattern recognition receptors (β-glucan receptors, dectin-1) expressed by the immune cells. The FOS is present in different cereals, vegetables and fruits such as barley, wheat, rye, garlic, onion, banana and honey. It can activate immune cells through interaction with TLR2 expressed by macrophages, polymorphonuclear leukocytes and dendritic cells (Vogt et al., 2013). Similarly MOS is recognized by endocytic receptor present on the surface of macrophages and endothelial cells (Ringø et al., 2010). The interaction can induce the proinflammatory cytokines which subsequently enhances innate immunity and vaccine efficacy with increased antibody titre, phagocytic activity, growth rate and reduced pathogen load in fishes, broilers and sheep (Benites et al., 2008; Klebaniuk et al., 2008; Torrecillas et al., 2014). The alginate, chitosan and inulin are examples of polysaccharides having immunomodulatory effects in fishes (Mouriño et al., 2012).

Levamisole is an anthelmintic which can enhance the immune system through upregulation and expression of TLR 7, 8 and MyD99 and downregulation of suppression signalling pathway (JAK/STAT). Increased function of monocytes, neutrophils, dendritic cells, T cells and antibody titre were reported in dogs when levamisole was administered as adjuvant

(Zhang et al., 2009). Antibody titre and immune cell numbers were more in the levamisole and Peste des petits ruminants (PPR) vaccine treated goats than only vaccinated animals (Das et al., 2016).

Mesenchymal stem cells (MSC, mesenchymal stromal cells) are multipotent stem cells that can differentiate into various cellular lineages originated from mesoderm (Caplan, 1991). The ideal MSCs can express CD105, CD73 and CD90 and adhere to the plastic surface. In the United States, bone marrow and adipose tissue MSCs are used as therapy in animals (Cyranoski, 2013).The immunomodulatory effects of MSC are increased inflammatory cell infiltration, acinar cell necrosis, decreased pro-inflammatory cytokines and activation of T_{reg} in dogs and horses (Carrade Holt et al., 2014; Kim et al., 2016).

Various cytokines such as recombinant bovine IL-1β and IL-2, interferon-omega and liposome-IL-2 DNA complex can be used as immunomodulators in mastitis cattle and in dogs and cats to treat viral infections (Daley et al., 1991; Kuwabara et al., 2006; Veir et al., 2006). Lymphocyte T-cell immune modulator is used in dogs which can increase haematopoiesis, CD41 lymphocytes and IL-2 production required to control viral infections (Gingerich, 2008). *Staphylococcus aureus* phage lysate can enhance the phagocytic activity of macrophages against staphylococci and it is used to treat canine pyoderma (DeBoer et al., 1990).

Vaccination

Affordable, pure, safe, easy to administer in large scale and reliable vaccines can reduce the usage of antibiotics in livestock, poultry and fishes. Majority of licenced veterinary vaccines belonged to four categories such as live attenuated, killed or inactivated, toxoids and cell membrane compounds (McVey and Shi, 2010). Live attenuated vaccines are more potent as it can induce both cellular and humoural immunity. Live vaccines have a probability of reversal to the virulence phenotype and consequently are less safe. It requires low temperature to maintain the potency during storage. In comparison, killed vaccines are safer but potency is low as they cannot provide protection for long term and against emerging strains of the pathogens. Production of toxoid-based vaccines requires complex culture medium with high level of biosafety. These conventional vaccines are expensive to produce and it requires multiple boosters to generate optimum immune response (Delany et al., 2014).

Advanced vaccine technologies include whole genome sequencing of the pathogens to identify better antigens (Kremer et al., 2016). The antigens are selected through structure-based design, epitope focussing and genome-based screening (Correia et al., 2014). Comparative genome analysis software is used to detect the sequence similarity between the predicted coding sequences and known genes present in public databases (Bagnoli et al., 2011). Reverse vaccinology thus can generate 'third-generation vaccines' depending on advancement of genomics and other 'omics'. This technology cannot be used to predict carbohydrate and lipid antigens, which also act as vaccine candidates. After identification of candidate antigen, the gene for interest is cloned to generate recombinant construct. The recombinant construct is used to produce DNA vaccines, recombinant subunit vaccines and vectored vaccines. The risk for pathogenicity and toxicity is low but the recombinant antigens often have low immunogenicity because of a lack of exogenous immune activating components. Thus the adjuvants are required to be administered.

The recombinant subunit vaccines consist of short antigenic but noninfectious proteins. *Escherichia coli, Pichia pastoris* (yeast), insect cell culture (Sf9), mammalian cell lines (CHO, HEK293) and plants (alfalfa, potato, corn, peanut, strawberry) are used as platforms to produce recombinant subunit proteins. The inserted protein folding is improper in prokaryotic expression system. The proteins are inserted in native form with appropriate folding in eukaryotic platforms. Multivalent vaccine can be produced by this technique as more than one protein (of different strains/serotypes) can be inserted (Dellagostin et al., 2011). The technique generates moderate immune response which is primarily of humoural type and the adjuvants are required to be administered along with the vaccine. Several successful trials in target animals with recombinant subunit vaccines generated in different platforms were conducted. The examples included *E. coli*—made bivalent chimeric toxoid for *Clostridium botulinum* in cattle (Cunha et al., 2014), *P. pastoris*—made E2 for classical swine fever in pigs (Lin et al., 2012), Sf9-made chimeric virus-like particles (VLPs) for rabies in dogs (Qi et al., 2015), CHO cell—made tE2 for bovine viral diarrhoea in cattle (Pecora et al., 2012), potato-made spike protein for infectious bronchitis in chicken (Zhou et al., 2004), etc. Commercially available recombinant subunit vaccines include avian influenza, porcine circovirus, feline leukaemia, *E. coli* bacterin-toxoid, etc.

The vectored vaccines use an immunogenic vector to deliver antigens to the host immune system. It has two types, i.e., live vector vaccines and naked DNA vaccines. In live vector vaccines, attenuated viruses (poxvirus) or bacteria (BCG) are used as carrier of immunogenic proteins. In addition to the generation of immunity against the attenuated viruses/bacteria, the recombinant ones produce immunity against the inserted antigens. Canarypox virus—vectored vaccines are developed against rabies, canine distemper, feline leukaemia and equine influenza. Commercially available vectored vaccines include rabies vaccine for cats, canine distemper for dogs and ferrets, avian influenza/Marek's disease/Newcastle disease for poultry, etc. The naked DNA vaccines are plasmids containing viral, bacterial or parasite antigenic genes along with a strong eukaryotic promoter, a polyadenylation signal sequence and a bacterial origin of replication. The recombinant plasmids are transfected into host cells, and after translation of the antigens inserted, it can generate both cellular and humoural immunities. The commercially available naked DNA vaccines include West Nile virus for horses and infectious haematopoietic necrosis for fishes.

Vaccines used in aquaculture include bacterins and live attenuated vaccines (Toranzo et al., 2009). The bacterins used in fishes are either aqueous or oil adjuvinated. Live attenuated vaccine against *Edwardsiella ictaluri* is approved in the United States to prevent enteric septicaemia in catfish. Experimental DNA vaccine in channel catfish offered protection against herpesvirus (Nusbaum et al., 2002). Injection and immersion in a diluted vaccine solution (short or long bath) is the primary route of fish immunization in commercial aquaculture (Evensen, 2009).

Failure of vaccination is a major concern in livestock, poultry and fisheries. There are several factors detected for vaccination failure such as lack of 'match' between vaccine strains and field strains (*Streptococcus suis*, swine influenza virus, *Eimeria*), rapid mutation and emergence of new viral strains (influenza, infectious bronchitis), requirement of frequent booster (*Clostridium perfringens*), functioning immune system of the host, requirement of a lag period to generate immunity, interference with maternal antibody, incapability to control shedding of the pathogens (*Mycoplasma hyopneumoniae*), requirement of a large antigen dose (fishes), human error in vaccination route, dose and frequency of vaccination, proper vaccine handling and storage (FMD, Newcastle disease, *Theileria*) and moreover unavailability of vaccines against all important diseases. Few vaccines have undesirable side effects such as reversal to virulence causing abortions, impairment of growth, loss of productions and death (live attenuated vaccines against bovine respiratory syncytial virus, blue tongue, contagious bovine pleuropneumoniae, African horse sickness, lumpy skin disease, coccidia, etc.), horizontal transfer of the pathogen used in live vaccine to the susceptible animal population (orf) and vaccine-induced stress in fishes. Owing to high production cost and high risk of failures, the industries show lack of interest in development of veterinary or fishery vaccines. The World Organization for Animal Health (OIE) created an ad hoc group of relevant experts to make a list of diseases on priority basis to direct the policy-makers and industry for development or improvement of vaccines for livestock, poultry and fishes. The list of prioritized infections includes *E. coli*, *Eimeria*, infectious bursal disease, infectious bronchitis for broilers and layers; *Pasteurella multocida*, *Actinobacillus pleuropneumoniae*, *Lawsonia intracellularis*, porcine reproductive and respiratory syndrome virus, swine influenza virus for pigs and *Aeromonas hydrophila*, *Pseudomonas*, *Yersinia rukeri*, *Flavobacterium*, *Vibrio anguillarum*, *Piscirickettsia salmonis* and *Edwardsiella tarda* for fishes (World Organization for Animal Health, 2015).

Other approaches

Passive immunization

Application of infection-specific antibodies produces immediate but temporary protection. Administration of anti-ETEC antibodies in feed reduced the occurrence of postweaning diarrhoea in piglets (Virdi et al., 2013). The ETEC antibodies are generated from diverse sources such as immunized animal plasma, immunized hen egg powder and plants.

Plantibodies

The plants were started to be utilized as a heterologous expression system for genetically engineered antibodies during 1900 and the word 'plantibody' was coined (Wycoff, 2005). The endomembrane and secretory systems of plants are used as bioreactor to generate chimeric proteins which are later purified from the plant tissues. There are several advantages of using plants as bioreactors such as short maturation time of plants that reduces the production cost, reduced capital investment in infrastructure and easy scale-up at the commercial level (Sharma and Sharma, 2009). The plants are naturally not infected with bacteria, viruses, mycoplasma, prions and other pathogens of human and animals and thus the screening cost is low. The plants are unable to generate immune response during production of chimeric antibodies, which is a common problem in mammalian expression system (Fischer et al., 2003). High yield of quality proteins can be achieved by adaptation of a transient expression step in binary or viral vectors (Salazar-Gonzalez et al., 2015), chloroplast transformation (Jin and Daniell, 2015), subcellular targeting and the use of suppressors for gene silencing (Alvarez et al., 2010). Several successful attempts have been conducted in plants to produce recombinant antigens of livestock and poultry-associated pathogens such as *Nicotiana benthamiana* plant generated bluetongue VLPs for ruminants (Thuenemann et al., 2013), *Arabidopsis*-made VP2 for infectious bursal disease in chicken (Wu et al., 2004), strawberry-made IFN-α for gingivitis in dogs (Stoger et al., 2014), banana leaf—made GP5 for porcine reproductive and respiratory syndrome virus in pigs (Chan et al., 2013), etc. The vaccine against Newcastle disease based on the antigen prepared from cultured tobacco cells and IFN-α produced in strawberries are approved for commercial use in the United States and Japan, respectively.

However, the plantibodies are metabolized rapidly after introduction into the host body system without giving sufficient time to generate the desired immunity. Multiple doses of plantibiotics are required to be administered to generate the optimum immune responses. Other drawbacks include insufficient expression of certain antigens in plants and allergic reactions to plant glycoproteins (Stoger et al., 2002).

Hyperimmune egg yolk antibodies

Hyperimmune egg yolk antibodies are produced by repeated administration of antigens into the hens and collection of antibodies (IgY) from the egg yolks (Gadde et al., 2015). Feeding of egg yolk powder containing antibodies against neuropeptide Y improved feed efficiency and body weight of broilers when fed up to 3 weeks of age (Cook, 2004). Secretion of IL-1 during inflammation causes anorexia and muscle wasting through the production of neuropeptide Y in gut of animals and birds.

CpG oligodeoxynucleotides

The CpG oligodeoxynucleotides (CpG ODN) are motifs present in bacterial or viral genome and are recognized as 'foreign' by TLR-9 pattern recognition receptor in mammals to induce innate and Th1 type of cellular immune responses. The motifs are methylated in mammalian genome and therefore are considered as foreign when administered. Enhanced synthesis of IgG and IgA was detected in mice following the administration of CpG motif (McCluskie and Davis, 1998; Weeratna et al., 2000). The generated immunity offers protection against infectious diseases (*Listeria monocytogenes*, *Francisella tularensis*, *E. coli, Salmonella* and mycobacteria), allergy and cancer in laboratory animals, livestock and poultry (Portnoy, 1992; Gomis et al., 2003).

Antiimmunosuppressive factor

The progress of chronic infection and cancer is dependent on certain immunosuppressive factors (programmed death 1, PD-1) expressed by the effector cells. The interaction with the appropriate ligands can induce immune exhaustion of the effector cells with reduced cell proliferation and cytokine production (Day et al., 2006). Application of anti-immunosuppressive factor antibodies can reactivate the immune cells and is considered as a therapeutic strategy for chronic infections or tumour diseases in human or as an approach to enhance the efficacy of vaccines (Velu et al., 2009). The strategy can be *implemented* in future to combat the animal diseases such as Johne's disease, bovine leukaemia virus infection, etc.

Pegylation

The pegylation is the process of protein modification with covalent binding to the polymers such as polyethylene glycol. It can increase the stability of the protein by preventing proteolytic degradation and renal clearance (Molineux, 2003). The recombinant bovine granulocyte colony-stimulating factor covalently bound to polyethylene glycol was administered to periparturient dairy cows and heifers, which reduced the occurrence of clinical mastitis (Hassfurther et al., 2015).

References

Agarwal, S.S., Singh, V.K., 1999. Immunomodulators: a review of studies on Indian medicinal plants and synthetic peptides Part II: synthetic peptides. Proceedings Indian National Science Academy part B 65 (6), 377—392.

Alvarez, M.L., Topal, E., Martin, F., Cardineau, G.A., 2010. Higher accumulation of F1-V fusion recombinant protein in plants after induction of protein body formation. Plant Molecular Biology 72 (1—2), 75—89.

Arce, C., Ramirez-Boo, M., Lucena, C., Garrido, J.J., 2010. Innate immune activation of swine intestinal epithelial cell lines (IPEC-J2 and IPI-2I) in response to LPS from *Salmonella typhimurium*. Comparative Immunology, Microbiology and Infectious Diseases 33 (2), 161—174.

Ariza-Nieto, C., Bandrick, M., Baidoo, S.K., Anil, L., Molitor, T.W., Hathaway, M.R., 2011. Effect of dietary supplementation of oregano essential oils to sows on colostrum and milk composition, growth pattern and immune status of suckling pigs. Journal of Animal Science 89 (4), 1079—1089.

Bagnoli, F., Baudner, B., Mishra, R.P., Bartolini, E., Fiaschi, L., Mariotti, P., Nardi-Dei, V., Boucher, P., Rappuoli, R., 2011. Designing the next generation of vaccines for global public health. OMICS: A Journal of Integrative Biology 15 (9), 545—566.

Benites, V., Gilharry, R., Gernat, A.G., Murillo, J.G., 2008. Effect of dietary mannan oligosaccharide from Bio-Mos or SAF-Mannan on live performance of broiler chickens. The Journal of Applied Poultry Research 17 (4), 471–475.

Boucher, H.W., Talbot, G.H., Bradley, J.S., Edwards, J.E., Gilbert, D., Rice, L.B., Scheld, M., Spellberg, B., Bartlett, J., 2009. Bad bugs, no drugs: no ESKAPE! an update from the infectious diseases society of America. Clinical Infectious Diseases 48 (1), 1–12.

Caplan, A.I., 1991. Mesenchymal stem cells. Journal of Orthopaedic Research 9 (5), 641–650.

Carrade Holt, D.D., Wood, J.A., Granick, J.L., Walker, N.J., Clark, K.C., Borjesson, D.L., 2014. Equine mesenchymal stem cells inhibit T cell proliferation through different mechanisms depending on tissue source. Stem Cells and Development 23 (11), 1258–1265.

Casadevall, A., Pirofski, L.A., 2009. Virulence factors and their mechanisms of action: the view from a damage–response framework. Journal of Water and Health 7 (S1), S2–S18.

Chan, H.T., Chia, M.Y., Pang, V.F., Jeng, C.R., Do, Y.Y., Huang, P.L., 2013. Oral immunogenicity of porcine reproductive and respiratory syndrome virus antigen expressed in transgenic banana. Plant Biotechnology Journal 11 (3), 315–324.

Cook, M.E., 2004. Antibodies: alternatives to antibiotics in improving growth and feed efficiency. The Journal of Applied Poultry Research 13 (1), 106–119.

Correia, B.E., Bates, J.T., Loomis, R.J., Baneyx, G., Carrico, C., Jardine, J.G., Rupert, P., Correnti, C., Kalyuzhniy, O., Vittal, V., Connell, M.J., 2014. Proof of principle for epitope-focused vaccine design. Nature 507 (7491), 201.

Cruz, C.R.Y., Micklethwaite, K.P., Savoldo, B., Ramos, C.A., Lam, S., Ku, S., Diouf, O., Liu, E., Barrett, A.J., Ito, S., Shpall, E.J., 2013. Infusion of donor-derived CD19-redirected virus-specific T cells for B-cell malignancies relapsed after allogeneic stem cell transplant: a phase 1 study. Blood 122 (17), 2965–2973.

Cunha, C.E., Moreira, G.M., Salvarani, F.M., Neves, M.S., Lobato, F.C., Dellagostin, O.A., Conceição, F.R., 2014. Vaccination of cattle with a recombinant bivalent toxoid against botulism serotypes C and D. Vaccine 32 (2), 214–216.

Cyranoski, D., 2013. Stem cells boom in vet clinics. Nature News 496 (7444), 148.

D Archivio, M., Filesi, C., Di Benedetto, R., Gargiulo, R., Giovannini, C., Masella, R., 2007. Polyphenols, dietary sources and bioavailability. Annali-Istituto Superiore di Sanita 43 (4), 348.

Daley, M.J., Coyle, P.A., Williams, T.J., Furda, G., Dougherty, R., Hayes, P.W., 1991. Staphylococcus aureus mastitis: pathogenesis and treatment with bovine interleukin-1β and interleukin-2. Journal of Dairy Science 74 (12), 4413–4424.

Das, M., Isore, D.P., Joardar, S.N., Samanta, I., Mukhopadhayay, S.K., 2016. Immunomodulatory effect of levamisole on PPR vaccine in goats and change in haematological profile. Indian Journal of Animal Research 50 (3), 411–414.

Day, C.L., Kaufmann, D.E., Kiepiela, P., Brown, J.A., Moodley, E.S., Reddy, S., Mackey, E.W., Miller, J.D., Leslie, A.J., DePierres, C., Mncube, Z., 2006. PD-1 expression on HIV-specific T cells is associated with T-cell exhaustion and disease progression. Nature 443 (7109), 350.

DeBoer, D.J., Moriello, K.A., Thomas, C.B., Schultz, K.T., 1990. Evaluation of a commercial staphylococcal bacterin for management of idiopathic recurrent superficial pyoderma in dogs. American Journal of Veterinary Research 51 (4), 636–639.

Delany, I., Rappuoli, R., De Gregorio, E., 2014. Vaccines for the 21st century. EMBO Molecular Medicine 6 (6), 708–720.

Dellagostin, O.A., Grassmann, A.A., Hartwig, D.D., Felix, S.R., da Silva, E.F., McBride, A.J., 2011. Recombinant vaccines against leptospirosis. Human Vaccines 7 (11), 1215–1224.

Dolan, D.E., Gupta, S., 2014. PD-1 pathway inhibitors: changing the landscape of cancer immunotherapy. Cancer Control 21 (3), 231–237.

Evensen, O., 2009. Development in fish vaccinology with focus on delivery methodologies, adjuvants and formulations. Options Mediterraneennes 86, 177–186.

Fischer, R., Twyman, R.M., Schillberg, S., 2003. Production of antibodies in plants and their use for global health. Vaccine 21 (7–8), 820–825.

Gadde, U., Rathinam, T., Lillehoj, H.S., 2015. Passive immunization with hyperimmune egg-yolk IgY as prophylaxis and therapy for poultry diseases—a review. Animal Health Research Reviews 16 (2), 163–176.

Gingerich, D.A., 2008. Lymphocyte T-cell immunomodulator (LTCI): review of the immunopharmacology of a new veterinary biologic. The International Journal of Applied Research in Veterinary Medicine 6 (2), 61–68.

Gomis, S., Babiuk, L., Godson, D.L., Allan, B., Thrush, T., Townsend, H., Willson, P., Waters, E., Hecker, R., Potter, A., 2003. Protection of chickens against Escherichia coli infections by DNA containing CpG motifs. Infection and Immunity 71 (2), 857–863.

Hassan, F.A., Awad, A., 2017. Impact of thyme powder (Thymus vulgaris L.) supplementation on gene expression profiles of cytokines and economic efficiency of broiler diets. Environmental Science and Pollution Research 24 (18), 15816–15826.

Hassfurther, R.L., TerHune, T.N., Canning, P.C., 2015. Efficacy of polyethylene glycol—conjugated bovine granulocyte colony-stimulating factor for reducing the incidence of naturally occurring clinical mastitis in periparturient dairy cows and heifers. American Journal of Veterinary Research 76 (3), 231–238.

Jin, S., Daniell, H., 2015. The engineered chloroplast genome just got smarter. Trends in Plant Science 20 (10), 622–640.

Kim, H.W., Song, W.J., Li, Q., Han, S.M., Jeon, K.O., Park, S.C., Ryu, M.O., Chae, H.K., Kyeong, K., Youn, H.Y., 2016. Canine adipose tissue-derived mesenchymal stem cells ameliorate severe acute pancreatitis by regulating T cells in rats. Journal of Veterinary Science 17 (4), 539–548.

Klasing, K.C., Johnstone, B.J., 1991. Monokines in growth and development. Poultry Science 70 (8), 1781–1789.

Klebaniuk, R., Matras, J., Patkowski, K., Picta, M., 2008. Effectiveness of Bio-MOS in sheep nutrition. Annals of Animal Science 8 (4), 369–380.

Kremer, F.S., Eslabão, M.R., Jorge, S., Oliveira, N.R., Labonde, J., Santos, M.N., Monte, L.G., Grassmann, A.A., Cunha, C.E., Forster, K.M., Moreno, L.Z., 2016. Draft genome of the Leptospira interrogans strains, Acegua, RCA, Prea, and Capivara, obtained from wildlife maintenance hosts and infected domestic animals. Memórias do Instituto Oswaldo Cruz 111 (4), 280–283.

Krummel, M.F., Allison, J.P., 1996. CTLA-4 engagement inhibits IL-2 accumulation and cell cycle progression upon activation of resting T cells. Journal of Experimental Medicine 183 (6), 2533–2540.

Kuwabara, M., Nariai, Y., Horiuchi, Y., Nakajima, Y., Yamaguchi, Y., Horioka, E., Kawanabe, M., Kubo, T., Yukawa, M., Sakai, T., 2006. Immunological effects of recombinant feline interferon-ω (KT-80) administration in the dog. Microbiology and Immunology 50 (8), 637–641.

Landy, N., Ghalamkari, G.H., Toghyani, M., Moattar, F., 2011. The effects of *Echinacea purpurea* L.(purple coneflower) as an antibiotic growth promoter substitution on performance, carcass characteristics and humoral immune response in broiler chickens. Journal of Medicinal Plants Research 5 (5), 2332–2338.

Liang, D., Li, F., Fu, Y., Cao, Y., Song, X., Wang, T., Wang, W., Guo, M., Zhou, E., Li, D., Yang, Z., 2014. Thymol inhibits LPS-stimulated inflammatory response via down-regulation of NF-κB and MAPK signaling pathways in mouse mammary epithelial cells. Inflammation 37 (1), 214–222.

Lin, G.J., Deng, M.C., Chen, Z.W., Liu, T.Y., Wu, C.W., Cheng, C.Y., Chien, M.S., Huang, C., 2012. Yeast expressed classical swine fever E2 subunit vaccine candidate provides complete protection against lethal challenge infection and prevents horizontal virus transmission. Vaccine 30 (13), 2336–2341.

Lubbad, A., Oriowo, M.A., Khan, I., 2009. Curcumin attenuates inflammation through inhibition of TLR-4 receptor in experimental colitis. Molecular and Cellular Biochemistry 322 (1–2), 127–135.

Mata, M., Vera, J., Gerken, C., Rooney, C.M., Miller, T., Pfent, C., Wang, L.L., Wilson-Robles, H.M., Gottschalk, S., 2014. Towards immunotherapy with redirected T cells in a large animal model: *Ex vivo* activation, expansion, and genetic modification of canine T cells. Journal of Immunotherapy 37 (8), 407. Hagerstown, Md.: 1997.

McCluskie, M.J., Davis, H.L., 1998. Cutting edge: CpG DNA is a potent enhancer of systemic and mucosal immune responses against hepatitis B surface antigen with intranasal administration to mice. The Journal of Immunology 161 (9), 4463–4466.

McVey, S., Shi, J., 2010. Vaccines in veterinary medicine: a brief review of history and technology. Veterinary Clinics of North America: Small Animal Practice 40 (3), 381–392.

Molineux, G., 2003. Pegylation: engineering improved biopharmaceuticals for oncology. Pharmacotherapy: The Journal of Human Pharmacology and Drug Therapy 23 (8P2), 3S–8S.

Mombarg, M., Bouzoubaa, K., Andrews, S., Vanimisetti, H.B., Rodenberg, J., Karaca, K., 2014. Safety and efficacy of an *aroA*-deleted live vaccine against avian colibacillosis in a multicentre field trial in broilers in Morocco. Avian Pathology 43 (3), 276–281.

Morrison, D.B., Saksida, S., 2013. Trends in antimicrobial use in marine harvest Canada farmed salmon production in British Columbia (2003–2011). The Canadian Veterinary Journal 54 (12), 1160.

Mouriño, J.L.P., Do Nascimento Vieira, F., Jatoba, A.B., Da Silva, B.C., Jesus, G.F.A., Seiffert, W.Q., Martins, M.L., 2012. Effect of dietary supplementation of inulin and *W. cibaria* on haemato-immunological parameters of hybrid surubim (*Pseudoplatystoma* sp). Aquaculture Nutrition 18 (1), 73–80.

Müller, D., Kontermann, R.E., 2010. Bispecific antibodies for cancer immunotherapy. BioDrugs 24 (2), 89–98.

Murphy, D., Ricci, A., Auce, Z., Beechinor, J.G., Bergendahl, H., Breathnach, R., Bureš, J., Da Silva, D., Pedro, J., Hederová, J., Hekman, P., 2017. EMA and EFSA joint scientific opinion on measures to reduce the need to use antimicrobial agents in animal husbandry in the European union, and the resulting impacts on food safety (RONAFA). EFSA Journal 15 (1).

Nusbaum, K.E., Smith, B.F., DeInnocentes, P., Bird, R.C., 2002. Protective immunity induced by DNA vaccination of channel catfish with early and late transcripts of the channel catfish herpesvirus (IHV-1). Veterinary Immunology and Immunopathology 84 (3–4), 151–168.

Pecora, A., Aguirreburualde, M.S.P., Aguirreburualde, A., Leunda, M.R., Odeon, A., Chiavenna, S., Bochoeyer, D., Spitteler, M., Filippi, J.L., Santos, M.J.D., Levy, S.M., 2012. Safety and efficacy of an E2 glycoprotein subunit vaccine produced in mammalian cells to prevent experimental infection with bovine viral diarrhoea virus in cattle. Veterinary Research Communications 36 (3), 157–164.

Portnoy, D.A., 1992. Innate immunity to a facultative intracellular bacterial pathogen. Current Opinion in Immunology 4 (1), 20–24.

Postma, M., Stärk, K.D., Sjölund, M., Backhans, A., Beilage, E.G., Lösken, S., Belloc, C., Collineau, L., Iten, D., Visschers, V., Nielsen, E.O., 2015. Alternatives to the use of antimicrobial agents in pig production: a multi-country expert-ranking of perceived effectiveness, feasibility and return on investment. Preventive Veterinary Medicine 118 (4), 457–466.

Qi, Y., Kang, H., Zheng, X., Wang, H., Gao, Y., Yang, S., Xia, X., 2015. Incorporation of membrane-anchored flagellin or *Escherichia coli* heat-labile enterotoxin B subunit enhances the immunogenicity of rabies virus-like particles in mice and dogs. Frontiers in Microbiology 6, 169.

Quinteiro-Filho, W.M., Gomes, A.V.S., Pinheiro, M.L., Ribeiro, A., Ferraz-de-Paula, V., Astolfi-Ferreira, C.S., Ferreira, A.J.P., Palermo-Neto, J., 2012. Heat stress impairs performance and induces intestinal inflammation in broiler chickens infected with *Salmonella* Enteritidis. Avian Pathology 41 (5), 421–427.

Rahimi, S., Teymouri, Z.Z., Karimi, T.M., Omidbaigi, R., Rokni, H., 2011. Effect of the three herbal extracts on growth performance, immune system, blood factors and intestinal selected bacterial population in broiler chickens. Journal of Agriculture, Science and Technology 13, 527–539.

Ringø, E., Olsen, R.E., Gifstad, T.Ø., Dalmo, R.A., Amlund, H., Hemre, G.I., Bakke, A.M., 2010. Prebiotics in aquaculture: a review. Aquaculture Nutrition 16 (2), 117–136.

Salazar-González, J.A., Bañuelos-Hernández, B., Rosales-Mendoza, S., 2015. Current status of viral expression systems in plants and perspectives for oral vaccines development. Plant Molecular Biology 87 (3), 203–217.

Scalbert, A., Morand, C., Manach, C., Rémésy, C., 2002. Absorption and metabolism of polyphenols in the gut and impact on health. Biomedicine & Pharmacotherapy 56 (6), 276–282.

Sharma, A.K., Sharma, M.K., 2009. Plants as bioreactors: recent developments and emerging opportunities. Biotechnology Advances 27 (6), 811—832.

Shin, J.H., Park, H.B., Oh, Y.M., Lim, D.P., Lee, J.E., Seo, H.H., Lee, S.J., Eom, H.S., Kim, I.H., Lee, S.H., Choi, K., 2012. Positive conversion of negative signaling of CTLA4 potentiates antitumor efficacy of adoptive T-cell therapy in murine tumor models. Blood 119 (24), 5678—5687.

Stoger, E., Fischer, R., Moloney, M., Ma, J.K.C., 2014. Plant molecular pharming for the treatment of chronic and infectious diseases. Annual Review of Plant Biology 65, 743—768.

Stoger, E., Sack, M., Fischer, R., Christou, P., 2002. Plantibodies: applications, advantages and bottlenecks. Current Opinion in Biotechnology 13 (2), 161—166.

Surai, P.F., 2014. Polyphenol compounds in the chicken/animal diet: from the past to the future. Journal of Animal Physiology and Animal Nutrition 98 (1), 19—31.

Temtem, C., Kruse, A.B., Nielsen, L.R., Pedersen, K.S., Alban, L., 2016. Comparison of the antimicrobial consumption in weaning pigs in Danish sow herds with different vaccine purchase patterns during 2013. Porcine Health Management 2 (1), 23.

Thuenemann, E.C., Meyers, A.E., Verwey, J., Rybicki, E.P., Lomonossoff, G.P., 2013. A method for rapid production of heteromultimeric protein complexes in plants: assembly of protective bluetongue virus-like particles. Plant Biotechnology Journal 11 (7), 839—846.

Toranzo, A.E., Romalde, J.L., Magariños, B., Barja, J.L., 2009. Present and future of aquaculture vaccines against fish bacterial diseases. Options Mediterraneennes 86, 155—176.

Torrecillas, S., Montero, D., Izquierdo, M., 2014. Improved health and growth of fish fed mannan oligosaccharides: potential mode of action. Fish & Shellfish Immunology 36 (2), 525—544.

Veir, J.K., Lappin, M.R., Dow, S.W., 2006. Evaluation of a novel immunotherapy for treatment of chronic rhinitis in cats. Journal of Feline Medicine and Surgery 8 (6), 400—411.

Velu, V., Titanji, K., Zhu, B., Husain, S., Pladevega, A., Lai, L., Vanderford, T.H., Chennareddi, L., Silvestri, G., Freeman, G.J., Ahmed, R., 2009. Enhancing SIV-specific immunity in vivo by PD-1 blockade. Nature 458 (7235), 206.

Virdi, V., Coddens, A., De Buck, S., Millet, S., Goddeeris, B.M., Cox, E., De Greve, H., Depicker, A., 2013. Orally fed seeds producing designer IgAs protect weaned piglets against enterotoxigenic *Escherichia coli* infection. Proceedings of the National Academy of Sciences 110 (29), 11809—11814.

Vogt, L., Ramasamy, U., Meyer, D., Pullens, G., Venema, K., Faas, M.M., Schols, H.A., de Vos, P., 2013. Immune modulation by different types of β2→1-fructans is toll-like receptor dependent. PLoS One 8 (7), e68367.

Weeratna, R.D., McCluskie, M.J., Xu, Y., Davis, H.L., 2000. CpG DNA induces stronger immune responses with less toxicity than other adjuvants. Vaccine 18 (17), 1755—1762.

Williams, R.B., 2002. Anticoccidial vaccines for broiler chickens: pathways to success. Avian Pathology 31 (4), 317—353.

World Organization for Animal Health (OIE), 2015. http://www.oie.int/standard-setting/specialists-commissions-working-ad-hoc-groups/ad-hoc-groups-reports/.

Wu, H., Singh, N.K., Locy, R.D., Scissum-Gunn, K., Giambrone, J.J., 2004. Immunization of chickens with VP2 protein of infectious bursal disease virus expressed in *Arabidopsis thaliana*. Avian Diseases 48 (3), 663—668.

Wycoff, K.L., 2005. Secretory IgA antibodies from plants. Current Pharmaceutical Design 11 (19), 2429—2437.

Zhang, W., Du, X., Zhao, G., Jin, H., Kang, Y., Xiao, C., Liu, M., Wang, B., 2009. Levamisole is a potential facilitator for the activation of Th1 responses of the subunit HBV vaccination. Vaccine 27 (36), 4938—4946.

Zhang, X., Zhao, L., Cao, F., Ahmad, H., Wang, G., Wang, T., 2013. Effects of feeding fermented *Ginkgo biloba* leaves on small intestinal morphology, absorption, and immunomodulation of early lipopolysaccharide-challenged chicks. Poultry Science 92 (1), 119—130.

Zhou, J.Y., Cheng, L.Q., Zheng, X.J., Wu, J.X., Shang, S.B., Wang, J.Y., Chen, J.G., 2004. Generation of the transgenic potato expressing full-length spike protein of infectious bronchitis virus. Journal of Biotechnology 111 (2), 121—130.

Zhu, C., Wu, Y., Jiang, Z., Zheng, C., Wang, L., Yang, X., Ma, X., Gao, K., Hu, Y., 2015. Dietary soy isoflavone attenuated growth performance and intestinal barrier functions in weaned piglets challenged with lipopolysaccharide. International Immunopharmacology 28 (1), 288—294.

Chapter 32

Antimicrobial resistance: one health approach

Chapter outline

Definition of one health concept

One health concept is based on worldwide collaborative efforts of multiple stakeholders to achieve optimal and sustainable well-beings of human beings, livestock, poultry, wildlife and environment. The interdisciplinary communications should work on tier basis such as locally, nationally and globally. The approach is utmost necessary because it can reduce the chances of infectious diseases and can mitigate the effects of adversity at human—animal—environment interface. Precisely it is a collaborative venture between medical and veterinary professions with the help of wildlife specialists, environmentalists, anthropologists, economists and sociologists to ensure proper diagnosis, clinical care, surveillance of cross-species infections, vaccination, education and research on zoonotic pathogens and impact analysis of environmental changes (global warming, climate changes, etc.) on both the animal and human populations (Gibbs, 2014).

History of one health concept development

The Society for Tropical Veterinary Medicine (STVM) was established in 1978 and currently it consists of veterinarians, scientists and research scholars from 40 countries who are interested in tropical veterinary medicine. In 1999, the STVM organized a series of conferences with the theme 'working together to promote global health'. In 2001, in the second series of the conferences organized at Pilanesberg (South Africa), the pertinent issues such as control of emerging diseases, conservation and sustainable food production at the interface of domestic animals and wildlife were discussed (Gibbs and Bokma, 2002). The resolutions taken in the conferences ('Pilanesberg resolution') are considered as the keystone for the development of one health concept (Lee and Brumme, 2012). In 2004, Wildlife Conservation Society (WCS) organized a symposium on importance of wildlife diseases and ecology in The Rockefeller University (USA) and introduced the term 'One world, one health'. The resolutions, 12 in numbers and known as 'Manhattan principles', are considered as the framework of one health concept. American Veterinary Medical Association (AVMA) established a one health task force in 2006.

In global level, a joint strategy was developed in 2008 by the World Health Organization (WHO), Food and Agricultural Organization (FAO), World Organization for Animal Health (OIE) in collaboration with United Nations International Children's Emergency Fund (UNICEF) and World Bank to reduce the transmission risk of emerging diseases. One health office was established in 2009 in Centers for Disease Control and Prevention (CDC), United States. International Ministerial Conference on Animal and Pandemic Influenza (IMCAPI) in Hanoi in April 2010 recommended broad implementation of one health ('Hanoi declaration'). The tripartite concept note was also developed in 2010 by joint efforts of FAO—WHO—OIE. The World Bank and United Nations adopted the one health recommendation in 2010,

Antimicrobial Resistance in Agriculture. https://doi.org/10.1016/B978-0-12-815770-1.00032-8

which was also approved by the European Union with a commitment to work under the one health umbrella. First international one health congress was held in Australia in 2011.

Antimicrobial resistance as a one health issue

Other than combating emerging diseases and zoonoses, one health approach encompasses several 'mega-concerns' such as tackling antimicrobial resistance and climate change and ensuring food safety and wildlife conservation. One health concept has three functional domains such as animals, human and environment, and antimicrobial resistance is related with all the three domains. The resistance genes generated in the commensal or pathogens in animals or human can be transferred between them during the exchange of microbial pool (zoonosis). The resistant bugs become untreatable as antimicrobials used in animals or human are mostly the same molecule and thus the resistance generated in one can affect the others. Tackling antimicrobial resistance issue with one health approach thus increases the therapeutic lifespan of the antibiotics.

Sometimes excess antibiotics are released in the environment through different excretory systems present in the animals and human. Other than livestock and poultry manure, antibiotic residues from pharmaceutical industry, human hospitals and agricultural fields are the major sources of environmental contamination (Reinthaler et al., 2003; Larsson et al., 2007; Diwan et al., 2010). The conglomerated antibiotics contribute to the resistance gene pool ('resistome') present in the environmental bacteria. Antimicrobial resistance is thus also considered as an ecological problem (Radhouani et al., 2014). The pollution with antibiotics is more pronounced in low- and middle-income countries because of lack of rigorous enforcement of the environmental protection laws. Our studies also highlighted the role of environment in transmission of resistant bacteria (β-lactamase—producing *Enterobacteriaceae*) in pigs and ducks which were reared without antibiotics (Samanta et al., 2015, 2018; Banerjee et al., 2019).

Frequent movement of livestock, agriculture and food products and moreover the human beings throughout the world because of globalization and urbanization help in spreading and intermixing of the resistance genes. The plasmid-mediated resistance gene (*mcr-1*) to colistin was originated in human and animals in China and spread to Europe, United States and Canada (Liu et al., 2016; McGann et al., 2016). Thus antimicrobial resistance has also become a 'one world' issue.

Integrated antimicrobial intake and antimicrobial resistance surveillance

Antimicrobial usage and associated selection pressure are the major drivers for generation of antimicrobial resistance (Shallcross and Davies, 2014). It is necessary to develop a linkage between the data of antimicrobial consumption and the resistance pattern. The integrated surveillance approach for antibiotic usage and resistance can also assess the impact of antimicrobial stewardship program taken to reduce the consumption (Aryee and Price, 2015). The surveillance encompasses human behaviour, mindset and the drivers influencing the attitudes during prescription for both human and animal patients. In livestock and companion animals, the decision of prescribing antibiotics is a crucial balance between the restoring animal productivity, affordability of the owners, influence of pharmaceutical companies and the generation of resistant bugs (Rushton, 2015). The environmental factors if included in a system-based approach for surveillance will better identify the critical control points.

Fig. 32.1 shows the integrated approach of surveillance for antimicrobial consumption and resistance in animals, birds, human, food items and the environment. Two major stakeholders of the consumption pattern analysis are human and

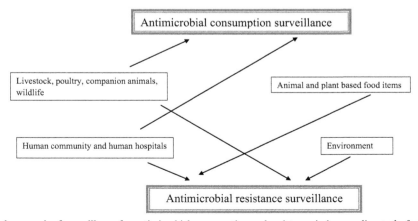

FIGURE 32.1 Integrated approach of surveillance for antimicrobial consumption and resistance in human, livestock, food items and environment.

animals. The human studies are conducted both in hospitals and community. The animal studies are conducted with the livestock, poultry, companion animals and wildlife separately. The resistance pattern analysis is performed with the commensal and pathogens isolated from human patients or healthy human in hospitals and community, respectively. Similarly the animal/environment component comprises resistance pattern analysis of the commensal and pathogens isolated from livestock (healthy and infected), poultry (healthy and infected), wildlife (healthy and infected), food items (livestock and poultry meat/eggs, meat/egg-based products, vegetables, fruits, cereals, etc.) and the environment (soil, water, plants, etc.). The collected data should be analysed in a proper way and the interpretation of analysis requires multisectoral experts from different disciplines such as human medicine, veterinary, epidemiology, statistics, environment study, food science and social science. A tiered approach with a centralized authority following the standard international guidelines for collection, processing of samples and interpretation of data is required for a successful surveillance program. The primary data generated should be available globally so that the resistant bacteria can be tracked across the international borders (Freeman et al., 2013). On the basis of prior alert, necessary steps can be taken to save the patients and to increase the therapeutic lifespan of a group of antimicrobials.

The surveillance programs at the global and national levels in different countries are enlisted in Table 32.1.

TABLE 32.1 Integrated antimicrobial resistance or antimicrobial intake surveillance program (global and national level).

Surveillance program	Nodal agency	Objectives/activities	Website with details
Advisory Group on Integrated Surveillance of Antimicrobial Resistance (AGISAR, 2008)	WHO	(a) To develop standardized sampling techniques and methodology for isolation of bacteria and detection of antibiotic resistance (b) To provide expert advice (c) To promote information sharing and supporting capacity-building for AMR surveillance and antimicrobial usage in member states	https://www.who.int
Global Antimicrobial Resistance Surveillance System (GLASS, 2015)	WHO	To support global surveillance and research to strengthen the evidence base on antimicrobial resistance (AMR)	https://www.who.int/glass/en/
Global Foodborne Infections Network (GFN)	WHO	(a) Integrated AMR surveillance (b) Intersectoral collaboration among human health, veterinary and food-related disciplines through training courses and activities	https://www.who.int/gfn/en/
WHONET	WHO	To provide free software and training to the laboratories for facilitating standardized data collection and analysis	http://www.whonet.org/
CODEX Alimentarius	FAO and WHO	AMR surveillance in humans, food animals, crops and food	http://www.fao.org/fao-who-codexalimentarius/en/

Continued

TABLE 32.1 Integrated antimicrobial resistance or antimicrobial intake surveillance program (global and national level).—cont'd

Surveillance program	Nodal agency	Objectives/activities	Website with details
Transatlantic Taskforce on Antimicrobial Resistance (TATFAR, 2009)	CDC (USA) and European Union	**(a)** To promote appropriate use of antimicrobials in human and veterinary medicine **(b)** To prevent resistant infections in hospital and communities **(c)** To improve development of new antimicrobials	https://www.cdc.gov
Joint Programming Initiative on Antimicrobial Resistance (JPIAMR, 2011)	European Commission	To support transnational research and activities in the selected areas such as therapeutics, diagnostics, surveillance, transmission, environment and interventions	https://www.jpiamr.eu/about/
European Antimicrobial Resistance Surveillance Network (EARS-Net)	European Centre for Disease Prevention and Control (ECDC)	Data collection from public health laboratories in European Union countries, data management, analysis and validation	https://ecdc.europa.eu
Central Asian and Eastern European Surveillance of Antimicrobial Resistance (CAESAR)	WHO	Network of national AMR surveillance systems and it includes all countries of the WHO European Region that are not part of the EARS-Net	http://www.euro.who.int/en/health-topics/disease-prevention/antimicrobial-resistance/about-amr/central-asian-and-eastern-european-surveillance-of-antimicrobial-resistance-caesar
Latin American Network for Antimicrobial Resistance Surveillance (ReLAVRA)	Pan American Health Organization	Surveillance of resistance in the pathogens isolated from community and hospitals	http://www.paho.org/ReLAVRA
Asian Network for Surveillance of Resistant Pathogens (ANSORP, 1996)	Asia Pacific Foundation for Infectious Diseases	Surveillance of resistance in human hospital-associated pathogens (pneumococcus) in Asia	http://www.ansorp.org/
European Surveillance of Antimicrobial Consumption Network (ESAC-Net)	ECDC	Collection of data on systemic use of antibiotics, antifungals and antivirals in hospital and community in European Union countries	https://ecdc.europa.eu
The Healthcare Associated Infection Network (HAI-Net)	ECDC	Surveillance of AMR and antimicrobial use in acute and long-term care facilities	https://ecdc.europa.eu
The European Centre for the Study of Animal Health (CEESA)	ECDC	Surveillance of AMR in healthy animals at slaughter, clinically sick food and companion animals	https://ecdc.europa.eu
European Surveillance of Veterinary Antimicrobial Consumption (ESVAC)	ECDC	Collection of harmonized data on the sales of veterinary antimicrobials (wholesalers, veterinarians and pharmacies)	https://ecdc.europa.eu

TABLE 32.1 Integrated antimicrobial resistance or antimicrobial intake surveillance program (global and national level).—cont'd

Surveillance program	Nodal agency	Objectives/activities	Website with details
The European Committee on Antimicrobial Susceptibility Testing (EUCAST, 1997)	ECDC, European Society of Clinical Microbiology and Infectious Diseases (ESCMID)	To provide technical aspects of phenotypic in vitro antimicrobial susceptibility testing	http://www.eucast.org
Danish Integrated Antimicrobial Resistance Monitoring and Research Program (DANMAP, 1995)	Ministry of Health and the Ministry of Food, Agriculture and Fisheries, Denmark	(a) AMR surveillance in human and animal clinical cases, healthy animals, locally produced and imported meat products at wholesale and retail outlets (b) Antibiotic consumption surveillance in human and animal hospitals, primary health care centres and pharmacies	https://www.danmap.org/
Swedish Strategic Programme Against Antibiotic Resistance (STRAMA, 1995)	Sweden	AMR and antibiotic consumption surveillance in human	—
Swedish Veterinary Antimicrobial Resistance Monitoring Programme (SVARM, 2000)	Sweden	AMR and antibiotic consumption surveillance in animals	https://www.sva.se/
NethMap	The Netherlands	AMR and antibiotic consumption surveillance in human	https://www.rivm.nl/isis-ar/overzichten-van-gegevens/nethmap
MARAN	The Netherlands	AMR and antibiotic consumption surveillance in animals, crops, fruits, vegetables and herbs	https://www.wur.nl/en/Research-Results/Research-Institutes/Bioveterinary-Research/Animal-health/Antibiotic-resistance-2/MARAN-reports.htm
Canadian Integrated Program for Antimicrobial Resistance Surveillance (CIPARS)	Canada	AMR and antibiotic consumption surveillance in human, food animals and food items	https://www.canada.ca/en/public-health/services/surveillance/canadian-integrated-program-antimicrobial-resistance-surveillance-cipars.html
FINRES-Vet	Finland	AMR and antibiotic consumption surveillance in food animals	—
GermVet	Germany	AMR and antibiotic consumption surveillance in food animals	—
Italian Veterinary Antimicrobial Resistance Monitoring (ITAVARM)	Italy	AMR and antibiotic consumption surveillance in food animals	—
Japanese Veterinary Antimicrobial Resistance Monitoring System (JVARM, 1999)	Japan	AMR and antibiotic consumption surveillance in food animals	http://www.maff.go.jp/nval/tyosa_kenkyu/taiseiki/monitor/e_index.html

Continued

TABLE 32.1 Integrated antimicrobial resistance or antimicrobial intake surveillance program (global and national level).—cont'd

Surveillance program	Nodal agency	Objectives/activities	Website with details
National Observatory of the Epidemiology of Bacterial Resistance to Antibiotics (ONERBA)	France	AMR and antibiotic consumption surveillance in human, food animals and food	http://onerba.org/
National Antimicrobial Resistance Monitoring System (NARMS)	USA	Monitoring antimicrobial resistance in enteric bacteria from human, retail meat and food animals	https://www.fda.gov/animal-veterinary/national-antimicrobial-resistance-monitoring-system/about-narms
Viet Nam resistance project (VINARES)	Vietnam	Monitoring antimicrobial resistance in enteric bacteria from human	—
Indian Network for Surveillance of Antimicrobial Resistance (INSAR, 2012)	India	Monitoring antimicrobial resistance in human	—
Antimicrobial Resistance Surveillance and Research Network (AMRSN, 2013)	India (ICMR)	Effective development of a stewardship program	http://iamrsn.icmr.org.in/index.php/amrsn/amrsn-network
Indian Network for Fishery and Animals Antimicrobial Resistance (INFAAR)	India (ICAR)	Monitoring antimicrobial resistance in livestock, poultry and fishery	—

Challenges of one health approach

(a) No fully standardized surveillance system for antimicrobial resistance and consumption in human, animals and environment using consensus methodology exists in several countries (WHO, 2014).

(b) No quality data is generated from the existing surveillance system because of lack of standardization and harmonization. Only 30% of the surveillance program coordinated by WHO has nationally co-ordinated body (WHO, 2012). In the European countries, only 64% of the participating laboratories follow the standard guidelines of EUCAST (ECDC-EFSA-EMA, 2015).

(c) Data are still insufficient to compare the antimicrobial resistance in different stakeholders such as human, livestock, poultry, fishery, agriculture and the environment.

(d) Substantial amount of funds are required to meet up the costs of training the staffs required for interdisciplinary work, costs of expert consultants, costs of collating the data, joint analysis and communication/sharing of results, costs for extending the coverage of surveillance program across human/animal health and the environmental sectors (Queenan et al., 2016).

(e) In low- and middle-income countries, the infrastructure should be developed for improvement of transport facility (for quick sending of biological samples into the laboratory), laboratory setup at the local level to generate primary data, training and recruitment of staffs, development of centre for excellence, enhanced collaboration between medical colleges/institutes and veterinary university/colleges/institutes to make the whole program functional.

(f) Ethical approval for interdisciplinary one health research work is a challenge, as it involves multiple institutes from different countries with variable ethical parameters (Mfutso-Bengu and Taylor, 2002).

(g) Other challenges in implementation of one health program include poor governance, corruption, lack of active citizen forum, lack of trust and respect for human rights, absence of or rapid changes in government policies, low salary with poor living standards causing brain drain of qualified staffs, etc.

References

Anti-microbial Resistance Surveillance and Research Network (AMRSN), 2013. Available at: http://iamrsn.icmr.org.in/index.php/amrsn/amrsn-network. Accessed on 05/06/2019.

Asian Network for Surveillance of Resistant Pathogens (ANSORP), 1996. Available at: http://www.ansorp.org/. Accessed on 05/06/2019.

Aryee, A., Price, N., 2015. Antimicrobial stewardship—can we afford to do without it? British Journal of Clinical Pharmacology 79 (2), 173—181.

Banerjee, A., Bardhan, R., Chowdhury, M., Joardar, S.N., Isore, D.P., Batabyal, K., Dey, S., Sar, T.K., Bandyopadhyay, S., Dutta, T.K., Samanta, I., 2019. Characterization of beta-lactamase and biofilm producing Enterobacteriaceae isolated from organized and backyard farm ducks. Letters in Applied Microbiology. https://doi.org/10.1111/lam.13170.

Danish Integrated Antimicrobial Resistance Monitoring and Research Program (DANMAP), 1995. Available at: https://www.danmap.org/. Accessed on 05/06/2019.

Diwan, V., Tamhankar, A.J., Khandal, R.K., Sen, S., Aggarwal, M., Marothi, Y., Iyer, R.V., Sundblad-Tonderski, K., Stålsby-Lundborg, C., 2010. Antibiotics and antibiotic-resistant bacteria in waters associated with a hospital in Ujjain, India. BMC Public Health 10 (1), 414.

European Centre for Disease Prevention and Control, European Food Safety Authority and European Medicines Agency, 2015. ECDC/EFSA/EMA first joint report on the integrated analysis of the consumption of antimicrobial agents and occurrence of antimicrobial resistance in bacteria from humans and food-producing animals. EFSA Journal 13 (1), 4006.

Freeman, R., Charlett, A., Hopkins, S., O'Connell, A.M., Andrews, N., Freed, J., Holmes, A., Catchpole, M., 2013. Evaluation of a national microbiological surveillance system to inform automated outbreak detection. Journal of Infection 67 (5), 378—384.

Gibbs, E.P.J., Bokma, B.H., 2002. The domestic animal/wildlife interface: issues for disease control, conservation, sustainable food production, and emerging diseases. In: Conference and Workshop Organised by the Society for Tropical Veterinary Medicine and the Wildlife Diseases Association. Wildlife and Livestock, Disease and Sustainability: What Makes Sense? Pilanesberg National Park, South Africa, 22—27 July, 2001. New York Academy of Sciences.

Gibbs, E.P.J., 2014. The evolution of One Health: a decade of progress and challenges for the future. The Veterinary Record 174 (4), 85—91.

Global Antimicrobial Resistance Surveillance System (GLASS), 2015 available at: https://www.who.int/glass/en/. Accessed on 05/06/2019.

Indian Network for Surveillance of Antimicrobial Resistance (INSAR), 2012. Available at: http://www.searo.who.int/india/topics/antimicrobial_resistance/nap_amr.pdf. Accessed on 05/06/2019.

Japanese Veterinary Antimicrobial Resistance Monitoring System (JVARM), 1999. Available at: http://www.maff.go.jp/nval/tyosa_kenkyu/taiseiki/monitor/e_index.html. Accessed on 05/06/2019.

Joint Programming Initiative on Antimicrobial Resistance (JPIAMR), 2011 available at: https://www.jpiamr.eu/about/. Accessed on 05/06/2019.

Larsson, D.J., de Pedro, C., Paxeus, N., 2007. Effluent from drug manufactures contains extremely high levels of pharmaceuticals. Journal of Hazardous Materials 148 (3), 751—755.

Lee, K., Brumme, Z.L., 2012. Operationalizing the One Health approach: the global governance challenges. Health Policy and Planning 28 (7), 778—785.

Liu, Y.Y., Wang, Y., Walsh, T.R., Yi, L.X., Zhang, R., Spencer, J., Doi, Y., Tian, G., Dong, B., Huang, X., Yu, L.F., 2016. Emergence of plasmid-mediated colistin resistance mechanism MCR-1 in animals and human beings in China: a microbiological and molecular biological study. The Lancet Infectious Diseases 16 (2), 161—168.

McGann, P., Snesrud, E., Maybank, R., Corey, B., Ong, A.C., Clifford, R., Hinkle, M., Whitman, T., Lesho, E., Schaecher, K.E., 2016. *Escherichia coli* harboring mcr-1 and blaCTX-M on a novel IncF plasmid: first report of mcr-1 in the United States. Antimicrobial Agents and Chemotherapy 60 (7), 4420—4421.

Mfutso-Bengu, J.M., Taylor, T.E., 2002. Ethical jurisdictions in biomedical research. Trends in Parasitology 18 (5), 231—234.

Queenan, K., Häsler, B., Rushton, J., 2016. A One Health approach to antimicrobial resistance surveillance: is there a business case for it? International Journal of Antimicrobial Agents 48 (4), 422—427.

Radhouani, H., Silva, N., Poeta, P., Torres, C., Correia, S., Igrejas, G., 2014. Potential impact of antimicrobial resistance in wildlife, environment and human health. Frontiers in Microbiology 5, 23.

Reinthaler, F.F., Posch, J., Feierl, G., Wüst, G., Haas, D., Ruckenbauer, G., Mascher, F., Marth, E., 2003. Antibiotic resistance of E. coli in sewage and sludge. Water Research 37 (8), 1685—1690.

Rushton, J., 2015. Anti-microbial use in animals: how to assess the trade-offs. Zoonoses and Public Health 62, 10—21.

Samanta, A., Mahanti, A., Chatterjee, S., Joardar, S.N., Bandyopadhyay, S., Sar, T.K., Mandal, G.P., Dutta, T.K., Samanta, I., 2018. Pig farm environment as a source of beta-lactamase or AmpC-producing *Klebsiella pneumoniae* and *Escherichia coli*. Annals of Microbiology 68 (11), 781—791.

Samanta, I., Joardar, S.N., Mahanti, A., Bandyopadhyay, S., Sar, T.K., Dutta, T.K., 2015. Approaches to characterize extended spectrum beta-lactamase/beta-lactamase producing *Escherichia coli* in healthy organized vis-a-vis backyard farmed pigs in India. Infection, Genetics and Evolution 36, 224—230.

Shallcross, L.J., Davies, S.C., 2014. Antibiotic overuse: a key driver of antimicrobial resistance. British Journal of General Practice 64, 604—605.

Swedish Veterinary Antimicrobial Resistance Monitoring Programme (SVARM), 2000. Available at: https://www.sva.se/. Accessed on 05/06/2019.

Swedish Strategic Programme Against Antibiotic Resistance (STRAMA), 1995. Available at: http://strama.se/about-strama?lang=en. Accessed on 05/06/2019.

The European Committee on Antimicrobial Susceptibility Testing (EUCAST), 1997. Available at: http://www.eucast.org. Accessed on 05/06/2019.

Transatlantic Taskforce on Antimicrobial Resistance (TATFAR), 2009. Available at: https://www.cdc.gov/drugresistance/tatfar/index.html. Accessed on 05/06/2019.

WHO Advisory Group on Integrated Surveillance of Antimicrobial Resistance (AGISAR), 2008. Available at: https://www.who.int/foodsafety/areas_work/antimicrobial-resistance/agisar/en/. Accessed on 05/06/2019.

WHO, 2012. Technical Consultation: Strategies for Global Surveillance of Antimicrobial Resistance. https://www.who.int/iris/bitstream/10665/90975/1/WHO_HSE_PED_2013.10358_eng.pdf.

WHO, 2014. Antimicrobial Resistance: Global Report on Surveillance. Available at: https://apps.who.int/iris/bitstream/handle/10665/112642/9789241564748_eng.pdf.

Index

Note: 'Page numbers followed by "f" indicate figures, "t" indicates tables'.

Printed in the United States
By Bookmasters